V&Runipress

Pflegewissenschaft und Pflegebildung

Band 7

Herausgegeben von
Prof. Dr. Hartmut Remmers

Thomas Foth

Caring and Killing

Nursing and Psychiatric Practice in Germany, 1931 – 1943

With 41 figures

V&R unipress

Universitätsverlag Osnabrück

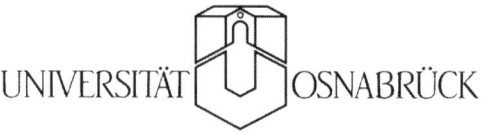

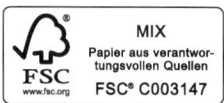

Bibliografische Information der Deutschen Nationalbibliothek

Die Deutsche Nationalbibliothek verzeichnet diese Publikation in der Deutschen Nationalbibliografie; detaillierte bibliografische Daten sind im Internet über http://dnb.d-nb.de abrufbar.

ISBN 978-3-8471-0062-1
ISBN 978-3-8470-0062-4 (E-Book)

**Veröffentlichungen des Universitätsverlags Osnabrück
erscheinen im Verlag V& R unipress GmbH.**

© 2013, V&R unipress in Göttingen / www.vr-unipress.de
Alle Rechte vorbehalten. Das Werk und seine Teile sind urheberrechtlich geschützt. Jede Verwertung in anderen als den gesetzlich zugelassenen Fällen bedarf der vorherigen schriftlichen Einwilligung des Verlages. Hinweis zu § 52a UrhG: Weder das Werk noch seine Teile dürfen ohne vorherige schriftliche Einwilligung des Verlages öffentlich zugänglich gemacht werden. Dies gilt auch bei einer entsprechenden Nutzung für Lehr-und Unterrichtszwecke.
Printed in Germany.
Titelbild: Admission Photograph of Anna Maria Buller (1931) made by the psychiatrists, with the year specification, medical record 28338.
Druck und Bindung: CPI Buch Bücher.de GmbH, Birkach

Gedruckt auf alterungsbeständigem Papier.

Inhalt

Preface 9

Foreword 13

Abstract 15

List of tables 17

List of figures 19

Acknowledgements 21

Chapter 1: Introduction 23

Chapter 2: Historical Background of the Killing of Sick Persons 29
    The Killings during the Nazi Regime 29
    Deaths in Psychiatric Hospitals before and after National Socialism .. 32
    Explanatory Approaches 34
        "Euthanasia" as "final solution of the social question" 35
        "Euthanasia" and a "Developmental Biopolitical Dictatorship" 37
    Nursing Historiography 44
        Nursing: A Powerless Occupation? 46
        Mother House Concept 48
            The Inner Organization of the Motherhouses 50
            Pastoral Power 51
        The Diversification of Nursing 53
        Governing Through Nursing 55
        The Impact of Nursing under the Nazi Regime 57

Chapter 3: The History of the Langenhorn Asylum from 1893 to 1945 . . 61
   Langenhorn before the First World War 61
      The modification of the right to complain 64
      Entry form to annual statistics at Langenhorn 70
   The First Wave: Killing Sick Persons through Starvation 78
   Langenhorn Between the Wars and During the Nazi Regime 83
   Langenhorn During the Second World War 91
   The Role of Nurses in Selecting Patients for Transfer 94

Chapter 4: Anna Maria Buller's First Admission in 1931: Analysis of the Record 97
   The Content of the Record 101
   The admission ritual and the nurses' reports 106
   The Interplay between Nurses' and Psychiatrists' Notes 136
      The text – reader conversation 138
      The conversation between Nurses' and Psychiatrists' Notes 140

Chapter 5: Transfer to House 16 (March 1931) 147
   The Medical Record in House 16 147
   The nurses' notes and the nurses' strategic position within psychiatric practice 154
   Anna Maria Buller Becomes Dangerous and the War Against the Madness Continues 159
   Enforcing the asylum's reality 176
   The Record, the Script, the Dispositif, and the Subject 179
      Fixing the subject function onto Anna Maria Buller 184
      Psychiatry interpellates Buller as subject 189
      The moralizing dimension 194

Chapter 6: The Intensification of the War against the Madness: Buller's Subsequent Admissions (1932–1943) 197
   The psychiatric dispositif 197
   Buller's First Admission to the Asylum of Langenhorn 209
   Bare Life 214
      Bare Life and the Camp 216
      Critical Remarks 217
      The Psychiatric Asylum as a Camp 221
   Buller's forced sterilization or the psychiatrist becomes a judge 223
   Admission 1936 229
   Admission 1940 233

    Shock Treatments and Psychiatric Practice 236
    Last Transfer to Langenhorn 246
    Anna Maria Buller's way into death 249
    Horrorism 251

Chapter 7: Conclusion 255

Appendix 263
    Appendix 1 – Drawings 263
    Appendix 2 – Admission Photographies of Anna Maria Buller 264

Bibliography 265
    Primary Sources 265
    Secondary Sources 266

Preface

One of the main concerns of the book series is to assist critically and to promote a theoretical- foundational discourse in nursing science and nursing education – a discourse that has been established in Germany for approximately two decades. Thus, the series should accommodate the ramifications of a discipline and a young science – not least because an action science is caught in the tension between the actual and the normative due to the logic of science. All of the books published so far are more or less oriented towards questions of normativity, which have evolved from within the course of ethical reflections on, for example, the context of global problems regarding the equitable allocation of scarce resources (staff, money) in the health care system. Nevertheless these kinds of questions can also be derived from more complex contexts and perspectives, as for example the creation of conditions which allow humans unlimited participation in the cultural achievements of life that have arisen from living and working conditions in modern societies.

Questions of normativity can also be answered from within the context of structural preconditions relating human beings to the nature of themselves and to the nature that surrounds them. It is from within this perspective that empirical-analytical aspects coalesce with those that are normative. Contemporary moral philosophy has criticized this perspective as an unduly mixing of normative and empirical claims. Nevertheless, from a critical analytical perspective it is exactly this constellation that allows for a better understanding in how far empirically backed assumptions are conditioned ex ante by implicit normative designations. This is to say that, on the one hand, scientific facts are constituted in relation to specific standards of discovery and that it should be considered that decisions for or against specific scientific research tools and observational standpoints come with prerequisites. On the other hand, our considerations aim to emphasize the fact that the structure of disciplinary knowledge – for the most part hierarchically structured knowledge is ordered, presented, and passed on – is based on implicit and tacit settings. Not only is scientific knowledge ordered according to selective relevance systems of the society, these relevance systems rather produce and codify knowledge.

These considerations are part of the well-known classical critique of ideology. According to this critique, knowledge systems cannot be perceived as free of societal interests – as a kind of removed episteme. This consideration applies not only to questions regarding the context of their application but also to questions regarding the context of discovery. After all, the historical-critical sociology of science has shown that the "triumphant success" of a knowledge paradigm was very often embedded in specific power constellations and associated with societal contexts of application.

How specific epistemological models lend structure to professional action is impressively demonstrated by Thomas Foth in the text at hand. This book evolved from a dissertation that was recently accepted by the Faculty of Health Sciences at the University of Ottawa in Canada. Psychiatric nursing care during the national socialist regime in Germany serves as his example and his empirical basis is derived from psychiatrists' and nurses' reports that are analyzed through discourse analytic and ethnographic methods. The concepts of "biopower" and "biopolitics," developed by Michel Foucault, supply the theoretical embedding for his results.

While this text focuses on the documentary practices of psychiatric nursing in Nazi Germany from a historical perspective it analytically goes far beyond a mere historiographical account. Using the example of an era that is only slowly gaining unreserved recognition by academic historians of medicine, this book uses a microscopic analysis to illuminate the hidden and therefore even more effective structural linkages between concrete action of nurses and psychiatrists and their documentation, in the form of clinical reports. Foth demonstrates that the normative discursive systems of orientation for psychiatric practice are generated through the discursive pattern of its guiding discipline, thereby generating specific modes of institutional practices and recording.

Against the backdrop of this trenchant analytical explanatory approach, most of the common patterns of interpretation regarding the active participation of nurses in the Nazi crimes appear inadequate. For example, it is not enough to ascribe certain normalization strategies to psychiatric practice in the 1930s and 1940s that led to the evaluation of a group of humans as chronic cases who were non-responsive to therapy and therefore labeled as permanently unproductive. This perspective would narrow down explanatory approaches to economic considerations, which cannot grasp the mechanisms of psychiatric identity construction. Furthermore one cannot interpret nursing participation in the killing of patients as merely the result of socio-cultural deterioration of humanitarian fundamentals. Foth rather highlights that nursing was not committed to ideological indoctrination – it was not powerless but instead played a crucial role in the construction of psychiatry.

The merit of the study at hand lies in its microscopic analysis of how vocational nursing practices were embedded within a system of scientific, social, and political exclusions under the condition of an authoritarian state. The implication that the biopolitical practices of the Nazi era were in no way unique to that regime but rather had both, historical precedents and successors after the lawsuits against physicians after 1945, is shattering.

We are happy to integrate this study in our series – a study that is rich in empirical insights – and we wish it to receive broad international attention.

Osnabrück, November 2012   Hartmut Remmers

Foreword

This book is about caring and also about killing. More precisely it is about the use of trained healthcare professionals, namely nurses and psychiatrists, to fulfill a State's objectives. Although this book focuses on psychiatric practice(s) during the Nazi regime, a time when psychiatric nurses and psychiatrists were involved in the killings of thousands of mentally ill patients, one has to bear in mind that these types of atrocities were conducted, at the time, under the rhetoric of science and ethics. Yet they share similarities with contemporary practices such as eugenics, capital punishment, and torture. The idea that some individuals had "lives not worth living", or that they committed crimes for which death was (and still is) the only retribution, had been discussed in legal and medical literature long before the Nazis' rise to power. This book clearly demonstrates to what extent. As Foth's courageous academic work clearly shows, the Nazi regime constitutes a patent example of "power over life" or what Foucault called *biopower*.

During the Nazi regime and well beyond and before it, the well-calculated killing of chronic, mentally ill patients was part of a diffuse but well-articulated biopolitical program that had a sophisticated "scientific" eugenic agenda that formed part of a politico-medical apparatus. Nurses constituted a vital part of this program through everyday nursing practice. The readers of Foth's ground breaking work, which uses a Foucauldian lens, need to understand that the analysis conducted in this book can also help us understand current unethical nursing/medical practices that are deployed in many industrialized and so-called "civilized" countries. The recent involvement of health professionals at Camp Delta in Guantanamo (Cuba) and the longstanding contribution of (para)medical personnel to the capital punishment process (especially with regards the use of lethal injection) in the United States are just some examples of health professionals involved in the dirty business of the State.

Michel Foucault's description of 'governmentality' helps us to understand how the State governs beyond its official structures, through multiple apparatuses (*dispositifs*). Foucault never neglected the State, but stressed that other apparatuses or institutions can 'conduct the conducts' of citizens. The concept of governmentality encompasses tactics, strategies, techniques, programmes, dreams and aspirations of all states that can shape the beliefs of populations. Governing today requires an active process in which the political rationalities bind themselves to technologies of government. According to Rose and Miller (1992), the articulation of these two elements is ensured by a specific form of knowledge (scientific) and the presence of an expert (professional) who serves as a mediator between political objectives and the object of intervention (citizen). The relationship between the State, its agents and agencies, and non-state actors is interactive. Today (much like it did throughout WW2), power functions well beyond the figure of the State as a unified institution. As Hall writes, the state is a 'network of institutions, deeply embedded within a constellation of ancillary institutions associated with society and the economic system' (Hall 1986, 17). Agents and agencies at a local and cellular level make sure that the broad objectives of the State are fulfilled.

What is uncovered in Foth's argument is that nursing's humanist self-identity is seriously challenged by nursing work that has nothing to do with the orgiastic caring rhetoric, deeply cherished by many influential figures in nursing. If Foth's historical research regarding psychiatric nursing under the Nazi regime accounts for an extreme case of "uncaring" practice, his powerful and bold analysis can shed light on several contemporary nursing practices in extreme contexts such as correctional and military settings. The problem of healthcare professionals serving the State's objectives is not merely an ethical one: it is also a question of the State's use of power in achieving pre-determined ends. Unfortunately, nurses are often the cogwheels of State sponsored programs and therefore complicit of ideologies that they adopted uncritically.

Professor Dave Holmes, RN
Director, School of Nursing
Associate Dean, Faculty of Health Sciences
University of Ottawa
Ottawa, Canada

December 20 2012

Abstract

Under the Nazi regime in Germany (1933 – 1945) a calculated killing of chronic "mentally ill" patients took place that was part of a large biopolitical program using well-established, contemporary scientific standards on the understanding of eugenics. Nearly 300,000 patients were assassinated during this period. Nurses executed this program through their everyday practice. However, suspicions have been raised that psychiatric patients were already assassinated before and after the Nazi regime, suggesting that the motives for these killings must be investigated within psychiatric practice itself. My research aims to highlight the mechanisms and scientific discourses in place that allowed nurses to perceive patients as unworthy of life, and thus able to be killed.

Using Foucauldian concepts of "biopower" and "State racism," this discourse analysis is carried out on several levels. First, it analyzes nursing notes in one specific patient record and interprets them in relation to the kinds of scientific discourses that are identified, for example, in nursing journals between 1900 and 1945. Second, it argues that records are not static but rather produce certain effects; they are "performative" because they are active agents. Psychiatry, with its need to make patients completely visible and its desire to maintain its dominance in the psychiatric field, requires the utilization of writing in order to register everything that happens to individuals, everything they do and everything they talk about. Furthermore, writing enables nurses to pass along information from the "bottom-up," and written documents allow all information to be accessible at any time. It is a method of centralizing information and of coordinating different levels within disciplinary systems. By following this approach it is possible to demonstrate that the production of meaning within nurses' notes is not based on the intentionality of the writer but rather depends on discursive patterns constructed by contemporary scientific discourses. Using a form of "institutional ethnography," the study analyzes documents as "inscriptions" that actively interven in interactions in institutions and that create a specific reality on their own accord. The question is not whether the reality represented within the documents is true, but rather how documents worked in institutions and what their effects were. Third, the study demonstrates how nurses were actively involved in the construction of patients' identities and how these "documentary identities" led to the death of thousands of humans whose lives were considered to be "unworthy lives."

Documents are able to constitute the identities of psychiatric patients and, conversely, are able to deconstruct them. The result of de-subjectification was that "zones for the unliving" existed in psychiatric hospitals long before the Nazi regime and within these zones, patients were exposed to an increased risk of death. An analysis of the nursing notes highlights that nurses played a decisive role in constructing these "zones" and had an important strategic function in them. Psychiatric hospitals became spaces where patients were reduced to a "bare life;" these spaces were comparable with the concentration camps of the Holocaust.

This analysis enables the integration of nursing practices under National Socialism into the history of modernity. Nursing under Nazism was not simply a relapse into barbarism; Nazi exclusionary practices were extreme variants of scientific, social, and political exclusionary practices that were already in place. Different types of power are identifiable in the Nazi regime, even those that Foucault called "technologies of the self" were demonstrated, for example, by the denunciation of "disabled persons" by nurses. Nurses themselves were able to employ techniques of power in the Nazi regime.

List of tables

Table 1: Translated diagnostic table with specified frequency for the year 1893. 72
Table 2: Statistical calculation of admissions, discharges, and cases of death, 1932. 89
Table 3: Deportation from Langenhorn 1 September 1939 to May 1945. 92
Table 4: Mortality rates in Langenhorn between 1939 and 1945. 93
Table 5: Number of treated patients and number of patients who died in Eilbektal. 246

List of figures

Figure 1: Original diagnostic table with specified frequency for the year 1893. 71
Figure 2: Original printed form with handwritten modifications. 77
Figure 3: Aerial photography of Langenhorn around 1925. 79
Figure 4: General plan of the asylum of Langenhorn, c.1925. 80
Figure 5 and 6: The folder and the front page of Anna Maria Buller's medical record in Friedrichsberg. 103
Figure 7: Psychiatrist's case history. 104
Figure 8: Nurse's reports. 105
Figure 9: Handwriting Sample of Buller. 113
Figure 10: Drawing with birthday greetings for Nurse Maria, 1931. 123
Figure 11: Fever chart for the first days of admission in 1931. 125
Figure 12 and 13: Requisition slips for laboratory analyses. 128
Figure 14: Nutrition plan and weight table. 130
Figure 15: General Plan of Friedrichsberg Asylum, 1931. 145
Figure 16: Detail of the fever chart from house 16. 148
Figure 17: Sewing room in Friedrichsberg, c. 1928. 175
Figure 18, 19 and 20: Drawings and travel diary of Buller's virtual travels to India. 187
Figure 21, 22 and 23: Some of Buller's drawings from 1931. 188
Figure 24: Self-portrait (no date). 189
Figure 25: View on the secure House 8, c. 1928. 201
Figure 26: Anna Maria Buller's perspective from House 8. 201
Figure 27: One of the halls for continuous baths in Friedrichsberg, c. 1928. 210
Figure 28: Nursing reports from Langenhorn. 213
Figure 29: Anna Maria Buller's original "diary." 231
Figure 30: Medication plan from April to September 1936. 232
Figure 31: Anna Maria Buller's drawing of House 8. 233
Figure 32 and 33: Insulin injection plan and Cardiazol injections April – June 1940. 236
Figure 34 and 35: Medication plan June 1940 – February 1941. 237
Figure 36: Anna Maria Buller's completed report sheet 1 (Meldebogen 1). 250
Figure 37, 38, 39 and 40: Some of Anna Maria Buller's drawings. 265
Figure 41: Photographies of Anna Maria Buller made by the psychiatrists. 266

Acknowledgements

Although I alone am responsible for the writing of this book, it could not have been completed without the help of many people.

I would like to thank Carmen and Katrin for the support and humour that enabled me to complete this project. I am grateful for the inspiring discussions with Katrin and I want to thank Carmen for travelling with me on this journey, not only to Canada but also spiritually. I want to further thank her for the support during the time I cared for my mother in the first years of my thesis. The deep relationship I developed with my mother at this time unwittingly supported me as well; her dementia enabled me to understand that the human condition exists beyond "normality." She taught me what it means to be vulnerable and depending on the protection and support of others.

I am particularly grateful to four persons, who, without their support and assistance, I could not have completed this thesis. Ruth Becker translated all the records from the old German script *Sütterlin* into contemporary German. Without this help it would not have been possible for me to analyse the records in the first place. Over the course of this study Ruth became a friend of mine and she gave me some precious insight in her understanding of the records.

I am overwhelmed by the support of Jayne Elliott. She helped me with the editing of my book, challenging me by questioning a lot of my taken-for-granted assumptions and forcing me to formulate my thoughts very precisely. Her comments especially on "jargon" helped me to be more precise. I am impressed by her ability to think her way into theories, and I thank her for her gracious support of my work. Without her support this book would not have been possible.

Without the assistance of Dave Holmes, Meryn Stuart, and Annette Leibing the whole project would not have been possible. I am deeply grateful for their help over these past years. I am particularly grateful for the countless intellectually stimulating discussions and also for their very practical support.

I want to thank Heiner Friesacher who introduced me to the German critical theory and the philosophy of science. I had countless discussions with Heiner about nursing science and nursing ethics and he deeply influenced my way of thinking. I want to mention Hartmut Remmers who allowed me to participate in his doctoral seminar and who enabled the publication of my book in his series. Ingo Harms supported my work through his expertise and I had many discussions with him about the killing of patients before, during, and after the Nazi regime.

Finally, I want to thank all my friends who cannot be mentioned because of limited space.

The research and writing was made possible by a grant from the Robert Bosch Foundation in Germany, the Associated Medical Services Nursing History Research Unit, and an admission scholarship from the University of Ottawa. I am indeed thankful for these sources of funding.

This book is dedicated to all the victims of the Nazi regime and all the victims of psychiatric practice.

Chapter 1: Introduction

In an early speech before the National Socialist Physicians' League, Adolf Hitler argued that he could, if need be, do without lawyers, engineers, and builders, but that "you, you National Socialist doctors, I cannot do without you for a single day, not a single hour. If not you, if you fail me, then all is lost. For what good are our struggles, if the health of our people is in danger?"[1] In 1934, Bavarian Minister Hans Schemm declared that Nazism was nothing but "applied biology."[2] These quotes highlight the important part that biology and medicine played in Nazi Germany. They also emphasize the decisive role of physicians to Nazism. What these statements do disguise is the fact that the National Socialists' health policy depended highly on nurses and their work. Generally speaking, nurses are often neglected because many historians of medicine and others seem to believe that their impact on health policy is negligible. This book is an attempt to rectify this systematic neglect and to simultaneously dispute the conception of nursing as both a powerless and benign vocation.

This book focuses specifically on psychiatric practice during the time of the Nazi regime. During this period, psychiatrists and psychiatric nurses actively participated in the killings of hundreds of thousands of their patients. Their roles in these killings can only properly be understood if their actions are seen in a broader context that includes the time before and after the Nazi regime. The idea that people had "lives not worth living" had been discussed in legal and medical literature long before the Nazis' rise to power, and, as this book will demonstrate, had already been put into practice in World War One.

When I began to work on this book, my interest was focused on the killings of nearly 300,000 psychiatric patients during the Nazi regime and more precisely, the killings that took place in the final years of the Second World War. The aim of

---

1 See Fritz Bartels, "Der Arzt als Gesundheitsfuehrer des deutschen Volkes," supplement to Deutsches Aerzteblatt, no. 68 (1938): 4–9 as cited in Robert N. Proctor, *Racial Hygiene: Medicine under the Nazis* (Cambridge, Massachusetts: Harvard University Press, 1988), 64.
2 Robert N. Proctor, *Racial Hygiene: Medicine under the Nazis* (Cambridge, Massachusetts: Harvard University Press, 1988), 64.

my research was, at that time, to highlight the mechanisms that allowed nurses to come to view some patients as living "unliveable" lives and thus able to be killed; these killings were defined by the perpetrators as "euthanasia" killings.

The earlier quotes by Adolf Hitler and Hans Schemm highlight the strong relationship between Nazi politics and biological science. The first phase of the killings, especially from 1939 to 1941, in which over 70,000 patients from more than 100 German hospitals were killed, demonstrates the close connection between scientific discourses, political rationalities, economic calculations of the killings, and nursing. The Nazi regime was a blatant example of what Foucault called "biopower."[3] The well-calculated killing of chronic, "mentally ill" patients was part of a huge biopolitical program that had a well-established "scientific" rationale to a recognized eugenic agenda. Nurses were a vital part of this program, supporting it in their everyday practice through the deliberate execution of patients. My analysis was to be based on nurses' notes in patient records obtained from one specific psychiatric hospital in Hamburg, Germany. It was meant to decipher how, based on these documents, patients were identified as having "unworthy lives," a particular construction of their identities that led to the deaths of thousands of people.

However, in the process of the analysis it became evident that certain patients were exposed to an increased risk of death much earlier than during the time of fascism. In addition, no differences could be found over time in how the notes were taken, nor were any differences identified in the content of the documentation on individual patients or in what treatment/therapies they received before, during, and after the Nazi regime. As a result, and supported by the work of some historians, my suspicions were raised that psychiatric patients were being assassinated before and after the time of the Nazi regime, implying, according to my hypothesis, that the motivation for these killings had to be investigated within psychiatric practice itself. My book is therefore a plea to expand the focus of the research of "euthanasia" killings to a broader analysis of the "murder of sick persons."

I thus shifted the focus of my analysis. Some of the records found in the archives of Hamburg were so voluminous and contained such a large number of nurses' notes that I began to question the meaning of these endless reports. It became apparent that if I wanted to understand in detail all the mechanisms at work and if I wanted to grasp the interplay between the different actors, I had to concentrate on one particular record, and for this reason, this research became a kind of case study. Nevertheless, this record was cross-read with other records

---

3 Foucault used the terms biopolitics and biopower interchangeably in order to describe the particular power constellation of biopolitics. I therefore do not delineate between biopower and biopolitics in this study.

obtained from the same asylum and with records obtained from other asylums in order to ensure that the findings in this one record were not random.

In the struggle to understand how nurses, who are usually more closely connected with the characteristics of nurturing and healing, were able to kill some of their patients, several different perspectives have emerged in the literature. Some authors have blamed the crimes committed by nurses on a combination of different factors: on their working conditions, on the political conditions of the fascist system, on the powerlessness of nurses, and on the nurses' moral fallibility (due to the lack of ethical guidelines in nursing).[4] In contrast, my research aims to highlight the mechanisms that allowed nurses to perceive patients as having lives not worth living and thus able to be killed. My analysis will center primarily on one rich medical record retrieved from the Langenhorn and Friedrichsberg asylums in Hamburg. The patient, Anna Marie Buller, was first admitted in 1931 and after multiple re-admissions over the following years, died in the asylum in Hadamar in 1943. Her medical file is particularly useful because it spans the years before and during the Nazi regime. The analysis will focus not only on the content of the nurses' notes but will also pay attention to the psychiatrists' notes in attempting to highlight the significance of the medical record in constructing patients and their identities in particular, often deadly, ways. In examining the period before the Nazi regime through this one medical file, this book is a first attempt to come to a new understanding of the mechanisms around the killings of sick persons. Evidence also exists, however, that these killings continued past the Nazi regime although more detailed research on this phase is still needed.

My analysis here tries to answer four interrelated questions: What role does the patient record play in psychiatric practice? What was the role and impact of the nurses' notes themselves? What discursive mechanisms in and around the patient record enabled nurses to contemplate the killing of "mentally ill" patients? How were the identities of patients constructed?

This book also became very personal for two reasons. First of all, as a child born in Germany in the 1960s, I grew up, like many others of my generation, with the anxiety of not knowing how involved my parents were in the Nazi regime and in the Second World War. My parents were born in the 1920s, and although

---

4 To name just a few: Hilde Steppe, "Nursing in Nazi Germany," *Western Journal of Nursing Research* 14, no. 6 (1992): 744; Steppe, "Nursing in the Third Reich," *History of Nursing Society Journal* 3, no. 4 (1991): 21–37; Ulrike Gaida, *Zwischen Pflegen und Töten. Krankenschwestern im Nationalsozialismus. Einführung und Quellen für Unterricht und Selbststudium* (Frankfurt a.M.: Mabuse, 2006); Bronwyn Rebekah McFarland-Icke, *Nurses in Nazi Germany: Moral Choice in History* (Princeton, N.J.: Princeton University Press, 1999); Susan Benedict and Jochen Kuhla, "Nurses' Participation in the Euthanasia Programs of Nazi Germany," *Western Journal of Nursing Research* 21, no. 2 (April, 1999): 246–263.

young, they were more or less active in different Nazi organizations and finished their studies in medicine shortly after the end of the war. However, my questions about their involvement with fascism and about what they knew about the Holocaust were never answered in a satisfactory manner. How they handled these questions was comparable to others of their generation, including nurses and others who had been publicly accused of crimes against humanity. Most denied any knowledge about the crimes that had been committed and above all, denied any complicity in them. Any minor deeds that they did admit to were justified by the need to obey the party.

Thus, a rift has opened between generations; large parts of family history remain blank and parents have been mute about significant aspects of their lives. Simultaneously, the younger generation developed a guilty conscience for the unknown deeds of its parents, giving rise to the urgent claim to account for their actions during the Nazi regime – a claim that is still unsatisfactorily answered. It is perhaps because of my own personal background that I never felt contented with the explanations given by the older generation nurses for their involvement in the killings, simply because their reasons sounded too familiar and their reasoning, I believed, was too comfortable.

Second, I worked for more than eight years as a nurse in psychiatry, more precisely in a center for youth detoxification. During this time I became aware of the power that nurses had in their everyday interactions with patients and how uncritically their reports on patients were made. I remember countless discussions with colleagues during shift changes over what information should be documented and how certain kinds of information might influence our perception of patients. Most colleagues were amazed at my emphasis on charting because most of them considered nurses' notes redundant and not worth talking about. Apart from any theoretical considerations, all of these personal experiences helped shape my perspective in this book and led me to focus particularly on nursing reports and the impact that they had on both psychiatric practice and patient treatment.

The dimensions of the killing of sick persons are covered in chapter 2 with a short historiography of the "euthanasia" killings and the involvement of nurses in these killings. This historiography demonstrates that the killing of sick persons was very complex and interwoven with the destruction of Jews, homosexuals, communists, Romas, Slavs, and prisoners of war. The existing historical evidence also points out that patients were already being killed before the advent of the "euthanasia" killings in 1939. A discussion of different explanatory approaches follows, where I will outline how my theoretical approach differs from mainstream history of the "euthanasia" killings. According to my perspective, Nazism must be integrated into the history of modern societies and cannot be considered simply a relapse into barbarism. The Nazi regime used modern methods in order to regulate the health of its population, and the killings of sick persons must be analyzed against the backdrop of the biopolitical agenda of the National Socialist health policy. The chapter continues with a short description of the time periods when the mortality rates in psychiatric asylums escalated. If one considers rising mortality rates within psychiatric asylums as a measure of the intentional neglect of patients with potentially deadly effects, then one has to conclude that psychiatric patients were intermittently killed during the whole first half of the twentieth century in Germany. The chapter ends by questioning the assumption that nursing was merely a powerless vocation and highlights the paradoxical situation of nurses in Germany at that time.

Chapter 3 outlines the development of the Langenhorn asylum, the focus of the empirical analysis, from its beginnings as an agricultural colony for the insane at the end of the nineteenth century. A discussion of the psychiatric system found in the city of Hamburg from 1899 to 1945 highlights the struggle of psychiatrists and medical directors to gain absolute control. The medical director's claim for power rested in his position as head of the asylum. Psychiatrists, however, began very early on to connect mental illness to genetic defects and to use these apparently "dangerous" links to set themselves up as official agents for societal protection. The annual frequency tables of the asylum in particular show how the construction of statistical tables enabled the relating of patient data to potential hereditary risks to the population. These tables also demonstrate that patients were categorized in this manner from the beginning of the century on. Under the Nazi regime these categories were used for the systematic killings of sick persons.

The subsequent three chapters focus on the file of one particular patient record.[5] Chapters 4 and 5 analyze in detail the year 1931, the year of Anna Maria

---

5 Staatsarchiv Hansestadt Hamburg 352 – 8-7, Staatskrankenanstalt Langenhorn, Abl.1 – 1995, Krankenakte 28338. This designation will be used throughout to identify Anna Maria Buller's patient record; other patient files mentioned in the text will be identified by their unique file number. The theoretical considerations and the chosen perspective for this study as described above shaped the collection of data and the method of analysis. Of the 4,907 patients who were transferred to other facilities from Langenhorn, of whom more than two-thirds were killed, 2676 records are still kept in the Archives of the City of Hamburg [Staatsarchiv der Freien und Hansestadt Hamburg]. The Langenhorn asylum was chosen because its records have already been extensively explored by historians who concentrated on a statistical analysis of the patient data in the records, aiming to explain the criteria used by psychiatrists to select patients for killing. (Klaus Böhme and Uwe Lohalm, eds., *Wege in den Tod. Hamburgs Anstalt Langenhorn und die Euthanasie in der Zeit des Nationalsozialismus* (Cloppenburg: Ergebnisse Verlag, 1993); Klaus Böhme, ed., *1893 – 1993 100 Jahre Allgemeines Krankenhaus Ochsenzoll* (Hamburg: Sozialtherapiezentrum des AK Ochsenzoll, 1993); Michael Wunder, Euthanasie in den letzten Kriegsjahren. Die Jahre 1944 und 1945 in der Heil- und Pflegeanstalt Hamburg Langenhorn, eds. Rolf Winau and Heinz Müller-Dietz, Abhandlungen zur Geschichte der Medizin und der Naturwissenschaften ed., Vol. 65 (Husum: Matthiesen, 1992),

Buller's first admission to a psychiatric asylum. These chapters concentrate closely on the record and its impact on psychiatric practice, suggesting all that ways in which she became subjectified as a schizophrenic person. This process of subjectification would be reversed in the following years – and this reversal is the focus of chapter 6. Interrupted only by short stays in her parental home, Buller spent the rest of her life in psychiatric hospitals. During this time she gradually disappeared from the record – hardly any trace of her could be found after 1941. In 1943, Buller was killed in Hadamar, which is where the book ends as well. A short conclusion follows.

36; Renate Otto, "Die Heil- und Pflegeanstalt Langenhorn in Hamburg und ihre Rolle bei den Abtransporten psychisch Kranker im Jahre 1943," unpublished Doctorate, Fakultät für klinische Medizin der Ruprecht-Karls-Universität, Heidelberg, 1992.) My qualitative analysis would therefore benefit from the results of this earlier research. The record of Anna Maria Buller was chosen because she was first admitted to hospital before the Nazi regime era and was admitted several times thereafter until 1943. Her record, which was nearly complete (at 500 pages), and covered nearly the whole period of Nazi fascism, did not differ in its construction from any of the other records found in the State archive. Furthermore, I obtained 25 records from patients who were admitted to Langenhorn in 1934 and who survived the Nazi regime. This last sample was intended to analyze any changes in the nurses' and psychiatrists' notes that might have taken place after the end of the Second World War. In the archive of the asylum at Hadamar (the facility in which Anna Maria Buller was eventually killed) I found another 30 records from patients transferred from Langenhorn.

I used the software program MAXQDA10 in my analysis to systematically evaluate and interpret the documents. The code- or category system (Code-system) that evolved over the course of the analysis was then linked to the scientific discourses found in psychiatrists' textbooks, nursing textbooks, and articles in scientific journals. This procedure permitted tracing the sources of the categories and descriptions employed by nurses and psychiatrists to describe Anna Maria Buller's behaviour. This proceeding enabled me to demonstrate that the descriptive categories employed by nurses and psychiatrists were derived from scientific discourses and to highlight the role of these notes and of the record as a whole.

Chapter 2: Historical Background of the Killing of Sick Persons

The Killings during the Nazi Regime

As a growing number of studies demonstrate, events around the killings of patients are complex and interwoven with other events that at first glance seem to be independent of them. The killings of patients during the Nazi regime must be divided into several phases. The first systematic mass destruction in National Socialism was named *Aktion T4*, after the street address of the central government agency in the Berlin *Tiergartenstraße 4*. *Aktion T4* was a centrally coordinated mass murder of patients in asylums and of residents in nursing homes for disabled people (*Heilerziehungsanstalten*). The extermination action was carried out under Hitler's orders and in cooperation with the Ministry of the Interior. Between January 1940 and August 1941, a system of selections, transports, and killing facilities assassinated more than 70,000 patients in gas chambers.[1]

During and after this "gas-killing action," an extensive but silent dying took place in psychiatric hospitals, asylums, and nursing homes for handicapped people and individuals with mental illness. Hidden, decentralized patient murders were carried out through starvation, medication, and neglect, the scope of which has proven to be so extensive that research into them cannot begin to capture every detail. Since the beginning of this newer research in the field of "euthanasia," which began in the 1990s, the number of victims has continuously escalated, with most recent attempts at quantification adding 150,000 to 200,000 people murdered under decentralized actions to the 70,200 victims of the centralized *Aktion T4*.[2]

---

1 Heinz Faulstich, *Hungersterben in der Psychiatrie 1914–1949. Mit einer Topographie der NS-Psychiatrie* (Freiburg im Breisgau: Lambertus, 1998).
2 Ingo Harms, Krankenmord in der Heil- und Pflegeanstalt Wehnen – Forschungsprobleme, in *Berichte des Arbeitskreises zur Erforschung der nationalsozialistischen "Euthanasie" und Zwangssterilisation, Tagungsband Wehnen, Herbst 2009*, ed. Arbeitskreis zur Erforschung der

In his detailed study of the Wehnen asylum, Ingo Harms illustrated how patients were killed by starvation and neglect through the subsequent *Aktion Brandt*.[3] *Aktion Brandt* evolved from 1941 onwards. Officially known as disaster medicine, it polarized the scientific community around the question of whether or not nurses and physicians had intentionally assassinated patients in hospitals. Suspicions were raised that they were killing psychiatric patients in order to obtain hospital beds for physically injured war victims. From the summer of 1942 on, the escalating air war and the disaster management needed to care for war victims, which was initially the responsibility of regional offices, became reasons for the deportation and subsequent murder of patients. The progression of the war and the increasing threats to cities as targets of severe air raids influenced central planning, at least from 1943 on.[4] In the course of this operation, asylums in the particularly endangered regions – the metropolitan areas of Berlin and Hamburg as well as the strategically important industrial zones of the Rhineland and Westphalia – were evacuated in order to make room for contingency hospitals for injured patients from these affected regions.

On 7 July 1943 the so-called barrack decree (*Barackenerlass*) allowed the construction of wooden barracks on the grounds of psychiatric asylums in order to obtain more space for psychiatric patients. Two months later the "double bed decree" (*Doppelbetterlass*) was enacted with the aim of doubling the space again by putting beds on top of existing patient beds. However, both decrees did not have the expected effects because of war conditions and the deficiency of construction materials.[5] Furthermore, the influx of deported patients to the interim asylums continued and led to the overcrowding of these outlying asylums. The "solution" in this situation was to continue with the murder of patients and most of them were killed through starvation and neglect.

Historian Peter von Rönn described conditions in the asylums to which patients from the Langenhorn asylum in Hamburg, the focus of this analysis, were deported. The asylum of Lübeck-Strecknitz, for example, was assigned as a makeshift hospital for mentally ill patients from Hamburg, necessitating the removal of the mentally ill who had been hospitalized in Lübeck to create space for the patients arriving from Hamburg. At the end of September 1941 more than 600 patients were deported from Lübeck, nearly 400 of who had earlier been

---

nationalsozialistischen "Euthanasie" und Zwangssterilisation (Münster: Klemm und Oelschläger, 2011, in print).

3 Ingo Harms, "'Wat mööt wi hier smachten...' Hungertod und "Euthanasie" in der Heil- und Pflegeanstalt Wehnen im "Dritten Reich"" (Oldenburg: Druck & Verlagscooperative GmbH, 1996).

4 Faulstich, *Hungersterben in der Psychiatrie 1914–1949*, 435–436.

5 Ibid., 308–314; Wolfgang Rose, "Der dezentrale Krankenmord. 'Euthanasie' durch Medikamente und Nahrungsentzug," in *Tödliche Medizin. Rassenwahn im Nationalsozialismus*, ed. Stiftung Jüdisches Museum (Berlin: Wallstein Verlag, 2009), 105.

transferred from the asylum at Langenhorn. Even the top officials in Hamburg's health administration – Kurt Struve, for example – had no idea where the Lübeck patients had gone. Some were transported to the asylums at Eichberg and Weilmünster; some were also transferred to Hadamar. All of these asylums were also used by Langenhorn to directly deport its patients. About four-fifths of the patients from Hamburg perished in these asylums under miserable conditions.[6] In the asylum at Eichberg chaotic conditions prevailed; barely any physicians were on staff and those that were were likely to be addicted to morphine. There were only a few nurses, leaving most of the wards understaffed or "nurse-free," and with the shortage of beds, many mattresses were placed on the floor. The patients had been abandoned.

Beyond the killing plans already described, other centrally ordered actions took place. Historians date the onset of the killing of children under the scope of the order, *Reichsausschuss zur Erfassung erb- und anlagebedingter schwerer Leiden,* to the summer of 1939, before the start of the adult "euthanasia" killings. From the summer of 1939 until the end of the war, about 5,000 children and juveniles were killed. Simultaneously, psychiatrist Paul Nitsche of Saxony developed his *Luminalscheme* that killed psychiatric patients by narcotic injection. In 1939 Nitsche, head of the Saxon asylums, ordered the psychiatrists under him to use more narcotics in order to "guard the surroundings from outrages of sick persons."[7] Nitsche's scheme was combined with the concept of "systematic weakening" (*Niederführung*) of the patients, which meant enfeebling patients by starvation in order to use smaller amounts of Luminal to kill them. Both killing methods were practiced during *Aktion T4* and during the war and characterized a regionally initiated systematic extermination of patients that took place outside the zones designated for the centralized killing action. According to historian Heinz Faulstich, the Saxony asylum's mortality rate "outside of Aktion T4" was higher than in all other regions in Germany.[8]

This Saxon killing method, known as the "Saxon special path" in the "euthanasia" historiography, was copied by psychiatric hospitals in various parts of Germany and in countless numbers of other asylums in such places as Meseritz, Hadamar, Eichberg, Uchtspringe, and the Steinhof in Vienna. However, most of the hospitals preferred to kill their patients through starvation and drew on their experiences in the 1930s. Historian Hans-Walter Schmuhl observed that in 1938, patients were already being killed through starvation.[9] Historian Ernst Klee

---

6 Peter v. Rönn, "Auf der Suche nach einem anderen Paradigma. Überlegungen zum Verlauf der NS-'Euthanasie' am Beispiel der Anstalt Langenhorn," *Recht und Psychiatrie*, no. 9 (1991): 52.
7 Faulstich, *Hungersterben in der Psychiatrie 1914–1949,* 291.
8 Ibid., 60.
9 Hans-Walter Schmuhl, *Rassenhygiene, Nationalsozialismus, Euthanasie-Von der Verhütung*

contended that the starvation method as a war measure had also already been discussed in the Ministry of the Interior in 1937.[10] Faulstich wrote that a decentralized form of starvation was already a general phenomenon in the asylums between 1933 and 1937.[11]

Other centralized plans were also carried out. The killing of 1,000 to 2,000 Jewish patients was centrally organized under a "special action" (*Spezialaktion*) in 1940.[12] In another, called "special treatment 14f13" (*Spezialbehandlung 14f13*), which was continued even after the stop of *Aktion T4*, around 20,000 concentration camp inmates were killed in the facilities used by *Aktion T4*.[13] Ultimately another 1,000 people who were classified as "criminal mentally ill persons" and who were interned in psychiatric asylums according to paragraph 42 of the criminal code, became victims of the "extermination through working" program in different concentration camps. Even in European countries raided by Germany, mentally ill persons were killed. After its annexation, Poland, for example, became an experimental field for murders that paralleled the preparations of *Aktion T4*, and at least 20,000 Polish psychiatric patients were shot, gassed, or starved to death. Together with their patients, many Polish psychiatrists and nurses were killed as well. Faulstich calculated that 80,000 people died in Polish, Soviet, and French asylums.[14] Unemployed personnel of the disbanded *Aktion T4* had found further work in the extermination camps in Eastern Europe.

Deaths in Psychiatric Hospitals before and after National Socialism

If rising mortality rates within psychiatric hospitals are seen as a measure of intentional neglect of patients with potentially deadly effects, then in 1936 and 1937, respectively, the increase in deaths that occurred in most psychiatric hospitals within the Deutsche Reich cannot be detached from the "euthanasia

   zur Vernichtung 'lebensunwerten Lebens' 1890–1945, Kritische Studien zur Geschichtswissenschaft 75 ed. (Göttingen: Vandenhoeck und Ruprecht, 1987).
10 Ernst Klee, *"Euthanasie" im NS-Staat. Die "Vernichtung lebensunwerten Lebens"* (Frankfurt a.M.: Fischer, 2009), 62.
11 Faulstich, *Hungersterben in der Psychiatrie 1914–1949*, 318.
12 Rose, "Der dezentrale Krankenmord. 'Euthanasie' durch Medikamente und Nahrungsentzug," 100.
13 Gerrit Hohendorf, "Ideengeschichte und Realgeschichte der nationalsozialistischen "Euthanasie" im Überblick," in *"Das Vergessen der Vernichtung ist Teil der Vernichtung selbst" Lebensgeschichten von Opfern der nationalsozialistischen "Euthanasie,"* eds. Petra Fuchs and others (Göttingen: Wallstein Verlag, 2008), 40–41.
14 Heinz Faulstich, "Die Zahl der "Euthanasie"-Opfer," in *"Euthanasie" und die aktuelle Sterbehilfe-Debatte. Die historischen Hintergründe medizinischer Ethik*, eds. Andreas Frewer and Clemens Eickhoff (Frankfurt, New York: Campus, 2000), 226.

action," as Faulstich indeed concluded.[15] The discovery of high mortality rates within psychiatric hospitals, asylums, and nursing homes before and after the time of fascism is a fact that has yet to attract significant historical attention. Historian Heinz Faulstich, who published a detailed study on the killings of sick persons, shed light on killings before and after the Nazi regime. He assumed that the comparative neglect of this situation by historians is due to the attempt to come to terms with the atrocious crimes of the program of "euthanasia." I believe, however, that the reasons for this neglect must be searched for in the models developed to explain the "euthanasia" killings. All of these models focus on the Nazi system of power and relate the killings to the specific circumstances that occurred under the Nazis. These models cannot explain though why the killings began before the Nazi regime and continued after the Nazis lost power, and this, I believe, is the reason why these killings have been ignored so far by historians.

It is an undisputed fact that during the First World War, starvation prevailed within psychiatric hospitals. The controversial question remains, however, whether or not this starvation was intended or was simply a consequence of war and the general famine in Germany due to the continental blockade. Historian Heinz Faulstich, who dedicated a large part of his book to this problem, assumed that the high mortality rates were apparently accepted due to the patriotic consideration that a lot of German soldiers lost their lives in the war.[16] High mortality rates in the asylums are often linked to the so-called *Rübenwinter* [turnip winter – a synonym for the winter of 1916/17 when nothing other than turnips was available as food] as well as to the influenza pandemic of 1918. As will be discussed, mortality rates in the Langenhorn asylum nearly doubled in 1916 and nearly quintupled one year later, and prolonged starvation was identified as the reason why Langenhorn had more than 1800 patients at the beginning of the war but only 1300 remaining at its end. Historian Ingo Harms also demonstrated that for the Wehnen asylum, the 1918 influenza pandemic did not play as dominant a role in the mortality rate as is generally thought.[17]

According to Klaus Dörner, reasons for the high mortality rates in asylums during the First World War could well have been due to an intentionally provoked shortage of food. The purposeful undernourishment of patients led to the death of 70,000 inmates in the asylums through starvation, and during the Second World War, this method of reducing the asylum population was simply repeated.[18] This hypothesis, however, supposed a top-down, state-organized

---

15 Faulstich, *Hungersterben in der Psychiatrie 1914–1949*, 609–620.
16 Ibid., 68. See also Harms, Krankenmord in der Heil- und Pflegeanstalt Wehnen – Forschungsprobleme.
17 Harms, 'Wat mööt wi hier smachten', 73–77.
18 Klaus Dörner, "Tödliches Mitleid," *Süddeutsche Zeitung*, 12 August 2006.

action that led to the killing of as many victims as did *Aktion T4* during the Nazi regime. Even though the intentional nature of these killings cannot be proven, the fact that mortality in nursing homes and psychiatric asylums exceeded that in the general population cannot be denied.[19]

The increase in mortality during the period of hyperinflation in 1923 was merely the peak of a famine that did not end with the First World War ceasefire but rather lasted late into the 1920s. Patients in psychiatric hospitals were hit especially hard. According to Faulstich, a general consensus now perceives psychiatric patients as victims. The economic misery that continued after the end of the war suspended their right to live.[20]

Faulstich's 1998 study leaves no doubt that in the postwar period, deaths within psychiatric hospitals in all four zones of occupation did not come to an end, leaving the high mortality rates in need of explanation. Although the author relates these deaths once again to an avoidable lack of food, he rejects the idea that any occupying power was intentionally withholding food. He emphasized that food distribution was organized by and under the responsibility of German authorities.

Explanatory Approaches

Most historians working in the fields of the history of medicine and of nursing focus on the killings (or what they refer to as "euthanasia") under the Nazi regime, neglecting the fact that these events were taking place both before and after this time. Historian Hans-Walter Schmuhl, for example, asserted that "after nearly three decades of intensive research we are far from a generally accepted interpretative model of the genesis of the "euthanasia" program of the National Socialists.[21] Historian Uwe Kaminsky stated too that it would be an almost impossible endeavour to provide an overview of the development of the research in the field of National Socialist "euthanasia" and to give an account of the present state of research.[22]

---

19 Faulstich, Hungersterben in der Psychiatrie 1914–1949, 63.
20 Ibid., 82.
21 Hans-Walter Schmuhl, "Die Genesis der "Euthanasie." Interpretationsansätze," in *Die nationalsozialistische "Euthanasie"-Aktion "T4" und ihre Opfer*, eds Maike Rotzoll and others (Paderborn: Ferdinand Schöning, 2010), 66.
22 Ibid., 15. An overview of the literature to the beginning of the 1990s can be found in Michael Burleigh, "Surveys of Developments in the Social History of Medicine: III. 'Euthanasia' in the Third Reich: Some Recent Literature," *Social History of Medicine* 4, no. 2 (1991): 317–328; Michael Burleigh, ed., *Confronting the Nazi Past: New Debates on Modern German History* (New York: St. Martin's Press, 1996). A synopsis of the research can be found as well in Faulstich, *Hungersterben in der Psychiatrie 1914–1949*. A widespread bibliography can be

"Euthanasia" as "final solution of the social question"

Two main explanatory models exert considerable influence on the debate about the origins of the "euthanasia" programs. One approach, which incidentally could also be used for explaining the genesis of the Holocaust, can be found in the groundwork provided by Götz Aly and his collaborators. According to them, the "euthanasia" actions were planned and carried out mainly by a more or less homogeneous "expertocracy" legitimized under Hitler's authority (*Führerermächtigungen*). These experts pursued a purportedly rational, economic, and demographic political program. The aim of the "final solution of the social question" was to select and exterminate the "useless."[23] In Aly's hypothesis, the rationale of the killings was based on the above-mentioned plans of psychiatric experts to reorganize and "modernize" the German psychiatric system under a divided plan, which would provide "active" therapy for the treatable, and concurrently, would exterminate the non-treatable, unproductive, and chronically ill patients.

The explanation of "euthanasia" as the final consequence of a health and social policy in a capitalistic industrial society was most clearly developed by scholar Klaus Dörner. The National Socialists, along with members of the traditional bureaucracy and human sciences, saw using Germany as their "historic mission" to prove to "the rest of world once and for all that a society, once freed from its whole social burden by taking the painful risks of finally solving the social question – even if it meant losing a third of its whole population – would be able to set free the total potential of industrialization and become economically, militarily, scientifically, and certainly culturally, invincible."[24] According to Dörner's hypothesis, industrialization in the nineteenth century was only realizable when a population was released from its obligation to care for family members. Hence a modern system of institutionalization and professionaliza-

---

found in Christoph Beck, *Sozialdarwinismus, Rassenhygiene, Zwangssterilisation und Vernichtung 'lebensunwerten' Lebens – Eine Bibliographie zum Umgang mit behinderten Menschen im 'Dritten Reich' und heute* (Bonn: Psychiatrie Verlag, 1995).

23 Götz Aly, *'Endlösung'- Völkerverschiebung und der Mord an europäischen Juden* (Frankfurt a.M.: Fischer, 1995), 50–55; Aly, Götz. Medicine Against the Useless. In *Cleansing the Fatherland. Nazi Medicine and Racial Hygiene*, edited by Götz Aly, Peter Chroust and Christian Pross (Baltimore and London: Johns Hopkins University), 22–99. Press, 1994.; Götz Aly, Medizin gegen Unbrauchbare, in *Aussonderung und Tod. Die klinische Hinrichtung der Unbrauchbaren*, edited by Götz Aly, Angelika Ebbinghaus, Matthias Hamann, Friedemann Pfäfflin, Gerd Preissler, Beiträge zur nationalsozialistischen Gesundheits- und Sozialpolitik: 1 ed. (Berlin: Rotbuch Verlag, 9–74; Götz Aly, ed., Aktion T4 1939–1945-Die 'Euthanasie'-Zentrale in der Tiergartenstrasse 4 (Berlin: Hentrich, 1989); Aly, "Erwiderung auf Dan Diner," *Vierteljahreshefte für Zeitgeschichte* 41 (1993): 621–635.

24 Klaus Dörner, Tödliches Mitleid. Zur Frage der Unerträglichkeit des Lebens (Gütersloh: Paranus, 2002), 60.

tion of care took place. "The onset of modernity around 1800 is not only characterized by the marketization of the economy and the industrialization of work but also by the elimination of caring for family members unable to work."[25] The decoupling of economy and science from a religious and philosophical idea of what it means to be human enabled the perception that "up to a third of society was a drain on society and thus what to do with these people was seen as a question of financial costs."[26]

Dörner's position was close to that of sociologist Zygmunt Bauman, who argued that the Holocaust was a symptom of this kind of rational modernity.[27] Dörner's model was sharply criticized by historian Dirk Blasius, who focused on its teleological tendencies.[28] In the end, Dörner's explanation is based on a Marxist analysis of capitalism, and Schmuhl pointed out that in Marxist analyses the social question of the nineteenth century was synonymous with the "labour question" of the proletariat. Dörner's model adopted the social question to the *Lumpenproletariat*, which in Marxist theory is the lowest, most degraded stratum of the proletariat, and described those members of the proletariat, especially criminals, vagrants, and the unemployed, who lack class consciousness.[29] However, even if one concedes that regarding everything – even human beings – as objects of use is inherent in capitalism, nothing at all is explained. This is the Marxist idea of reification as developed by Georg Lukacs. Emphasizing the primacy of socio-economic factors in this kind of historical analysis always produces the same results. Distinguishing between structures and the "rest" constructs the historical subject as a rational being and does not allow for "irrationality" or "free will." This approach thus cannot explain why many assassinations were carried out in a more or less unorganized manner and independently from orders issued under the centralized planning actions.

---

25 Klaus Dörner, "Die soziale Frage und der Diskurs um 'Euthanasie'," in *Die nationalsozialistische 'Euthanasie'-Aktion 'T4' und ihre Opfer. Geschichte und ethische Konsequenzen für die Gegenwart*, eds. Maike Rotzoll et al (Paderborn: Ferdinand Schöning, 2010), 44; Dörner, *Bürger und Irre. Zur Sozialgeschichte und Wissenschaftssoziologie der Psychiatrie* (Frankfurt a.M.: Europäische Verlagsanstalt, 1984).
26 Klaus Dörner, "Anstaltsalltag in der Psychiatrie und NS-Euthanasie," *Deutsches Ärzteblatt* 86, no. 11 (1989): B-534-B-538.
27 Zygmunt Bauman, *Modernité et Holocauste* (Paris: Complexe, 2008).
28 Dirk Blasius, "Das Ende der Humanität. Psychiatrie und Krankenmord in der NS-Zeit," in *Der historische Ort des Nationalsozialismus. Annäherungen*, ed. Walter H. Pehle (Frankfurt a.M.: Fischer, 1990), 47–70.
29 Schmuhl, "Die Genesis der 'Euthanasie'. Interpretationsansätze," 67.

"Euthanasia" and a "Developmental Biopolitical Dictatorship"

For a long time research assumed that there was a close interrelationship between eugenics and "euthanasia." Schmuhl explained "euthanasia" as the endpoint in the radicalization of Nazi health policy on race and genetics and related it to the general political conditions under the "Third Reich." The pre-history of the Nazi program of "euthanasia" can be found in the discussions on racial hygiene in the 1890s, in its apparent triumphal procession in science, society, and state during the time of the Weimar Republic, and finally, in its elevation to state doctrine in 1933. The interconnections between government and party institutions enabled extraordinary, confidential, and even extra-legal interventions that were justified by an apparently increasing threat of racial impurity.[30] The succession of forced sterilizations, the abortions performed due to eugenic indications, and the "euthanasia" of children seemed to manifest this radicalization of eugenic ideas. This position was criticized by historians like Michael Schwartz and others, who emphasized that the concept of eugenics was politically polyvalent and adopted by different political parties and systems, implying that a categorical difference existed between eugenics and euthanasia.[31] An international comparison underlines this aspect: eugenic movements existed in democracies – the USA, Canada, Great Britain, Scandinavia, Switzerland, etc. – and in authoritative states or dictatorships such as those found in National Socialist Germany or Stalinist Soviet Union.[32]

Schmuhl later refined his thesis, underlining the interrelationship of eugenics

---

30 Schmuhl, Rassenhygiene, Nationalsozialismus, Euthanasie-Von der Verhütung zur Vernichtung 'lebensunwerten Lebens' 1890–1945, 129–145.
31 Michael Schwartz, "Rassenhygiene, Nationalsozialismus, Euthanasie? Kritische Anfragen an eine These Hans-Walter Schmuhls," *Westfälische Forschungen* 46 (1996): 604–622.
32 See, for example, Mark B. Adams, ed., *The Wellborn Science: Eugenics in Germany, France, Brazil, and Russia* (Oxford: Oxford University Press, 1990); Stefan Kühl, *Die Internationale der Rassisten. Aufstieg und Niedergang der internationalen Bewegung für Eugenik und Rassenhygiene im 20. Jahrhundert* (Frankfurt a.M.: Campus, 1997); Kühl, *The Nazi Connection: Eugenics, American Racism, and German National Socialism* (Oxford: Oxford University Press, 1994); Volker Roelcke, "The Establishment of Psychiatric Genetics in Germany, Great Britain and the USA, circa 1910–1960: To the Inseparable History of Eugenics and Human Genetics," *Acta Historica Leopoldina* (48), no. 48 (2007): 173–190; Volker Roelcke, "Mentalities and Sterilization Laws in Europe during the 1930s: Eugenics, Genetics, and Politics in a Historic Context," *Der Nervenarzt* 73, no. 11 (Nov, 2002): 1019–1030; Roelcke and Gerrit Hohendorf, "Akten der "Euthanasie"-Aktion T4 gefunden," *Vierteljahreshefte für Zeitgeschichte* 41, no. 3 (1993): 479–481; Peter Weingart, "Eugenics–Medical Or Social Science?" *Science in Context* 8, no. 1 (Spring, 1995): 197–207; Peter Weingart, Kurt Bayertz and Jürgen Kroll, eds., *Rasse, Blut und Gene. Geschichte der Eugenik und Rassenhygiene in Deutschland* (Frankfurt a.M.: Suhrkamp, 1992).

and euthanasia on the same discursive level.[33] He defined discourse as a "'ruling mode of speaking' that determines what can be talked about and in which language – and what supposedly should remain silent."[34] According to Schmuhl, it was apparent that since 1890, discussions about eugenics and the "extermination of life unworthy of life" were based on the same premises: "the categorization of humans and groups of humans according to their worth, the move to biologize the social, the absoluteness of the supra-individual community of origin, the abolishment of the idea of human rights anchored in natural rights, the exclusion of illness, disability, feebleness, old age, pain, and suffering from the *conditio humana*."[35] Despite appearing to coincide with the theoretical perspective of this book, Schmuhl's definition of discourse in my view is imprecise and rough. Schmuhl is right in defining discourses as historically delineable possibilities of thematic speech, which define the borders of meaningful speech and coherent social acting. He nevertheless neglects the fact that language does not function merely as a mirror of reality but rather it works in the construction of social reality and in the perception of what is perceived as "natural," a second dimension because language is a medium that dictates its conditions on speech. Foucault argued that regimes carry (and disseminate throughout the space they occupy and the subjects they organize) their own truth, and that indeed, a regime of truth is a precondition of power.[36] It appears to me as if Schmuhl used the concept of discourse more in order to "prove" his original assumption that "euthanasia" was a radicalized form of eugenics. In the end, he remained within the more traditional framework of the history of ideas and insisted that socio-economic conditions and the specific circumstances of the Second World War were decisive moments generating the mass assassinations of patients. At this point, Schmuhl is no longer arguing from a discourse theory perspective.

Schmuhl defined the "Third Reich" as a "developmental biopolitical dictatorship" aimed at controlling "birth and death, sexuality and reproduction, body and genetic dispositions."[37] The point of reference for this political entity was the collective subject of "people," defined as a bio-organic body. The developmental

---

33 Hans-Walter Schmuhl, "Eugenik und "Euthanasie"-Zwei Paar Schuhe? Eine Antwort an Michael Schwartz," *Westfälische Forschungen* 47 (1997): 757–762.
34 Schmuhl, "Die Genesis der 'Euthanasie.' Interpretationsansätz," 69.
35 Ibid.
36 Wendy Brown, *Regulating Aversion. Tolerance in the Age of Identity and Empire*. (Princeton: Princeton University Press, 2008); Michel Foucault, *L'ordre du discours*. (France: Gallimard, 2007); Foucault, *Les mots et les choses. Une archéologie des sciences humaines*. (France: Gallimard, 2007).
37 Hans-Walter Schmuhl, "Das "Dritte Reich" als biopolitische Entwicklungsdiktatur. Zur inneren Logik der nationalsozialistischen Genozidpolitik," in *Tödliche Medizin. Rassenwahn im Nationalsozialismus* (Göttingen: Wallstein Verlag, 2009), 8–21.

biopolitical dictatorship was based on two pillars – one on health and heredity and the other on race. According to Schmuhl, these related streams were under scientific leadership that aimed to establish a stratified society. At its top would emerge a social egalitarian, biological homogeneous *Volksgemeinschaft* (or folk community) in which class disparities would be resolved. The relevance of the biosciences within the National Socialist state thus cannot be overestimated. As Schmuhl stated, the "scientists from these disciplines envisioned – even before 1933 – a technocratic model of policy counseling through which 'scientific expertise' would dissolve politics into multiple factual constraints, political decision processes would become 'rational' solutions, with the consequence that science and technology would take the place of politics." Schmuhl described this process as "reciprocal instrumentalization of science and politics."[38]

I also use the term biopolitic in this book, but I am taking a more Foucauldian perspective than Schmuhl. I argue that Schmuhl loses some critical potential in his understanding of the concept. The role of racism, for example, has a specific strategic function in Foucault's conception of biopower, which I feel becomes somewhat blurred in Schmuhl's approach. Whereas biopower from a Foucauldian perspective is a particular mode of governing that is bound to multi-level technologies of power, Schmuhl's conception of the term tended to reduce biopolitics to a biologized social. He reduced biopolitics to a kind of "social engineering" through eugenics. He and other historians have perceived the ideas behind eugenics and the actions of carrying out "euthanasia" killings as imposed by a coercive dictatorship and its technocratic elite. But as historian Michael Burleigh has emphasized, the procedures of sterilization and "euthanasia" were not always imposed top-down by a coercive state apparatus.[39] And as this analysis demonstrates as well, many German doctors and nurses made their decisions based on their own understanding of eugenics. In the context of a widespread campaign of propaganda and public education, even parents often requested eugenic measures for their own children.[40] Canadian historian Robert Gellately takes this aspect as the focus of his book, *Backing Hitler*. In it, he highlighted the broad participation of Germans in Nazism and emphasized that the explanatory model of the Nazi regime as a brutal police state, which forced its citizens into cooperation with the state, cannot capture its effectiveness.[41] Based on an analysis of documents from the archives of the former Nazi Secret State Police (*Geheime Staatspolizei, GeStaPo*) Gallately argued that the police system

---

38 Ibid., 9.
39 Michael Burleigh, *Death and Deliverance: "Euthanasia" in Germany 1900–1945* (Cambridge: Cambridge University Press, 1994).
40 Burleigh, *Death and Deliverance*; Robert Gellately, *Backing Hitler: Consent and Coercion in Nazi Germany* (New York: Oxford University Press, 2009).
41 Ibid.

could only have functioned so effectively because of the voluntary cooperation of Germans. It was not the case that secret police agents were everywhere; on the contrary, a low level of staff coverage made it impossible to control the population as a whole. Many police arrests were enabled only because many Germans voluntarily informed on their neighbours or acquaintances to the police.[42] Gellately further contended that the Germans would have known everything about the crimes committed by the Nazi regime and concluded that most Germans agreed with these crimes.[43] In discussing the "euthanasia" killings, Gellately emphasized that most relatives of patients who were killed did not want to know too much about the killings and

> numerous German families were prepared to accept the murder of their closest relatives without protest, even with approval. By so doing, they created the psychological conditions for the genocidal policies carried out in the years to come. If people did not protest even when their relatives were murdered, they could hardly be expected to object to the murder of Jews, Gypsies, Russians, and Poles.[44]

Biopolitics under the Nazi regime cannot be reduced to a simple killing of the unfit. As historian Robert Proctor highlighted in his book, the Nazi's attempt to defeat cancer was the most decisive and vigorous attack on the disease then known to humankind; German cancer research was the most advanced in the world by the time Hitler assumed power in 1933, and the anticancer measures likely caused the disease to decline among the post-1945 German population.[45]

Throughout the world over the course of the twentieth century, there was not a clear distinction between preventive medicine and eugenics, between the pursuit of health and the elimination of unfitness, between consent and compulsion. Sociologist Nikolas Rose emphasized that even "under National Socialism ... a coincidence between generalized biopower and dictatorship [developed] that was at once absolute and retransmitted throughout the entire social body ... [which was] a complex mix of the politics of life and the politics of death."[46] Proctor's book has shown especially that biopolitics under the Nazi regime entailed

---

42 Robert Gellately, "Denunciation as a Subject of Historical Research," in *Denunciation in the 20th Century*, ed. Inge Marszolek (Kölln: Quantum, 2001), 16–29.
43 Silke Schneider, "Diskurse in der Diktatur? Überlegungen zu einer Analyse des Nationalsozialismus mit Foucault," in *Foucault: Diskursanalyse der Politik. Eine Einführung*, eds. Brigitte Kerchner and Silke Schneider (Wiesbaden: VS Verlag, 2006), 123–144.
44 Gellately, *Backing Hitler*, 107.
45 Robert Proctor, *The Nazi War on Cancer* (Princeton: Princeton University Press, 1999).
46 Nikolas Rose, *The Politics of Life Itself: Biomedicine, Power, and Subjectivity in the Twenty-First Century* (New Jersey: Princeton University Press, 2007), 58.

not merely the exercise of state power but strategies for governing life developed by many other authorities. Nazi doctors and health activists, not acting solely under the direction of a sovereign state, waged war on tobacco, sought to curb exposure to asbestos, worried about the overuse of medication and X-rays, stressed the importance of a diet free from petrochemical dyes and preservatives, campaigned for whole-grain bread and foods high in vitamins and fiber, and supported vegetarianism.[47]

My book demonstrates that the decisions doctors and nurses made in regard to the killings of patients were not forced by the state or by a technocratic elite but rather were deliberately made by the psychiatrists and nurses themselves in the Langenhorn asylum based on scientific categorizations and internalized normative conceptions. This is an impressive example of what Foucault called "self-techniques" and "self-regulation."[48] Understanding biopolitics as being composed of different power technologies and carried out by a multiplicity of authorities and experts independently from "state apparatuses" forces one to analyze the connecting lines between eugenics, "euthanasia," and biopower in psychiatric practice as such. Furthermore, this perspective enables one to understand why the killings of patients were carried out independently of central planning, as I demonstrated above, and why sick persons were being killed both before the National Socialists came to power and continued after the end of the Second World War.

Society under the Nazi regime must be analysed as a society of regulation and the decisive element in such a society is the norm. The norm operates, on the one hand, towards a body that power tries to discipline and, on the other hand, towards a population that power tries to regulate. A normalizing society is, according to Foucault, a society

> in which the norm of discipline and the norm of regulation intersect along an orthogonal articulation. To say that power took possession of life in the nineteenth century, or to say that power at least takes life under its care in the nineteenth century, is to say that it has, thanks to the play of technologies of discipline on the one hand and technologies of regulation on the other, succeeded in covering the whole surface that lies between the organic and the biological, between body and population.[49]

Biopolitics discovered population as a scientific and political problem, as a biologic problem of power engaged with collective phenomena that influence economy. These phenomena are random and unpredictable in detail, but they establish constants on a collective level, which can be detected at the level of

---

47 Ibid., 58; Proctor, *The Nazi War on Cancer*.
48 Michel Foucault et al., *Technologien des Selbst*, trans. Michael Bischoff (Frankfurt a.M.: Fischer, 1993).
49 Michel Foucault, *Society must be Defended: Lectures at the Collège De France 1975–1976*, eds. Mauro Bertani, Alessandro Fontana and François Ewald, trans. David Macey (New York: Picador, 2003), 253.

populations. Biopolitics use mechanisms that are very different to those used by the disciplines. First of all, it uses statistical surveys and global measurements, intervening on a global level by installing a regulatory mechanism and trying to establish a kind of homeostasis.

If the Nazi regime is analysed from this perspective, it becomes a blatant example of modern population policy that was from the beginning connected to multiple detailed statistical surveys. During the Nazi regime, most of the data were evaluated with the newest technologies. The administration systematically used punch cards to enable the analysis of large amounts of data. Even the Holocaust was organized by using these technologies (and could not have been realized without this technological support) and the company IBM gained notoriety because it delivered the infrastructure enabling these data collections and analyses.[50] The same is true for the organization of the killings of sick persons and the capturing of so-called hereditary risks. The former president of the German statistical society (*Deutsche Statistische Gesellschaft*), Friedrich Zahn, noted in 1940 that "statistics is closely related to the National Socialist movement." As he continued,

> the demographic policy enjoys the particular interest of the State. It is not anymore solely a quantitative population policy but rather has developed into a qualitative and psychological population policy and therefore demands from statistics increasing and deepened insights, which can be implemented using the energy of our Führer.[51]

Under the direction of the police, the health and welfare administration, and the statistical office of the German Reich, an efficient system of different registers, censuses, registration laws, and identification cards developed after 1933. All these measurements aimed to register and classify the population. In 1933 and 1939, population censuses were carried out but they were not the only actions of registration: the work book (*Arbeitsbuch*) (1939), the health family register (1936), the obligation to register (1938), the German People's Party (1939), and finally, the personal identification number (1944) were the bureaucratic preconditions for a graded system of gratification and penalty, for selection and extermination. With the raw material of the population census from 1939, a register was installed for all non-Aryan peoples within the German Reich; it contained the names, dates and places of birth, places of residence, occupation, and "grade of crossbreed." The political office for matters of race (*Rassenpolitisches Amt*) of the German National Socialist Worker Party (NSDAP) began in 1934/35 to install a "register of asocial elements" (*Assozialenkartei*), followed in

---

50 Edwin Black, *IBM und der Holocaust. Die Verstrickung des Weltkonzerns in die Verbrechen der Nazis* (München: Ullstein, 2002).
51 Götz Aly and Karl Heinz Roth, *Die restlose Erfassung. Volkszählen, Identifizieren, Aussondern im Nationalsozialismus* (Farnkfurt a.M.: Fischer, 2005), 12.

1935/36 by the special register of Jews, Gypsies, and other "foreign ethnics" (*Fremdvölkischer*). From 1934 on, "hereditary sick persons" were registered by the health administration. Especially in the latter cases, nurses played a decisive role because they were mainly the ones who reported these persons.[52] Historians Götz Aly and Karl Heinz Roth described the effectiveness of statistics for population policy as follows:

> Only through the work of statisticians with anonymous data do people become part of "problem areas" with their own so-called fertility probability, with their own probability of divorces, their own social behaviour, etc. Thus people are indexed by character profiles that can be differentiated endlessly and, even more important, can be randomly combined. Only then is it possible to further subdivide people in the process of population politic and social politic. By this means, it becomes possible to enact laws, decrees, and regulations for ever-smaller groups of people. These laws, decrees and regulations become less and less comprehensible and understandable.[53]

This perspective enables one to integrate Nazism into the history of modern societies. Nazism was not a simple relapse into barbarism but rather used modern statistical methods in order to regulate the health of its population. The other side of a biopolitical society of regulation is that certain elements are excluded from the normal range of its population and defined as biologically dangerous. Killing the other within a system of biopolitics becomes acceptable if a biological danger is targeted and if the elimination of this danger will strengthen the race; it is not a question of victory. In a normalizing society, race or racism is the precondition that makes killing acceptable. Darwin's theory of evolution developed out of this background of biopower and became the means to imagine colonial relations, the necessity of war, criminality, the phenomena of madness or mental illness. The concept of evolution became the frame through which to imagine killing and the potential of war. War did not only eliminate the opposite race, but it also regenerated one's own race through a selection of those battling for life. Seen from this perspective, psychiatry becomes one of the key sciences in biopolitics, because it is the psychiatric expert who is in charge of demarcating the border between what has to be considered as normal and what must be defined as a biological danger to populations. As we will see in the course of this book, psychiatrists in Hamburg fought from the end of the nineteenth century on to be acknowledged as the sole source of expertise able to decide which individuals might present a danger to society. Psychiatry's decisive

---

52 Ulrike Gaida, "Eugenik im Deutschen Reich und im Nationalsozialismus," in *Quellen zur Geschichte der Krankenpflege. Mit Einführungen und Kommentaren*, ed. Sylvelyn Hähner-Rombach (Frankfurt a.M.: Mabuse, 2008).
53 Aly and Roth, *Die restlose Erfassung*, 8.

position in the governing of populations enabled the killing of psychiatrist patients before and after the Nazi regime.

Nursing Historiography

Contrary to the large body of research on the "euthanasia" killings that historians in the field of social history of medicine have developed, the current state of research in the history of nursing is comparatively limited. As the brief description above highlights, medical historians have not only carried out countless regional studies but they have also entered into a theoretical debate about how eugenics, "euthanasia," and their connections should be classified and what the rationales were behind these killings. Over the course of this lengthy process, which began with the Nuremberg trial and has encompassed more than 50 years of research, the complexity of the "euthanasia" killings becomes apparent as well as the fact that these killings cannot be detached from the Holocaust.

However, nurses seem to be irrelevant and are strangely absent in these studies, which is astonishing if one considers that without nurses, the whole "extermination program" could not have been possible. If nurses are mentioned at all, conclusions historians have reached have followed similar patterns. Henry Friedlander, for example, assumed that psychiatric nurses were always dependent on their physician bosses and became willing helpers in the machinery of sterilization and "mercy killings."[54] Michael Burleigh explained that there was "no great psychological mystery about why these 'carers' became killers." Nurses were complicit because they were tired, frustrated, and were already desensitized to the suffering of others. Many had internalized common pejorative attitudes about the mentally ill and saw nothing in the patients in front of them to change their minds.

In March 1984 a group of German nurses tried to critically assess the role of nurses during the Nazi regime. The authors understood their work as an attempt to write nursing history from below, as an engagement of nurses with their own history. Their book, *Nursing during National Socialism*, was edited by nurse Hilde Steppe and by 2001, nine editions had appeared.[55] This book seems to have set the research parameters because subsequent nursing history studies have not gone beyond this book's framework. To my knowledge, regional studies about the involvement of nurses in the killings of sick persons in specific asylums have

---

54 Henry Friedlander, *The Origins of Nazi Genocide: From Euthanasia to the Final Solution* (Chapel Hill: University of North Carolina Press, 1995); Burleigh, *Death and Deliverance*.
55 Hilde Steppe, *Krankenpflege im Nationalsozialismus* (Frankfurt a.M.: Mabuse, 2001).

not been published, implying that little is known about the nature of nursing work.

Most of the nursing history studies carried out so far have tried to draw an all-embracing picture of nurses' roles in the killings of patients. For this reason Steppe's political appraisal of the "euthanasia" killings was never contradicted and seemed to establish consensus in the scientific community.[56] For Steppe, "race hygiene ideologies and capitalism's interest in profit must be considered as the main reasons for the deadly logic of the National Socialist extermination politics."[57] This approach resonates with Dörner's view of "euthanasia" as the final solution of the social question. According to Steppe, the main criteria for killing patients centered on their inability to work because psychiatric patients were only of interest to the system if they could be used as cheap labour. Another consensus persists in the question of the relation between eugenics and "euthanasia." Similar to Schmuhl and his early work, most nursing historians seem to be convinced that "euthanasia" was the culmination of a process of radicalization of Nazi policies on race and health genetics.[58] Furthermore, Steppe's study was based on the assumption that killings were centrally planned and systematically carried out, an assumption that is refuted by newer research in the field of "euthanasia" and especially contradicts the perspective of this book. For Steppe and others with similar perspectives, nurses can only be perceived as helping to actualize the program. Steppe also clearly distinguished between killings in asylums and the killing that took place during the Holocaust, a position most nursing historians accept without contradiction. Again, newer research in the history of medicine highlights how interwoven were these different aspects of killings. Despite these insights, research in nursing history can roughly be subdivided into nurses in concentration camps,[59] nurses in psychi-

---

56 Ibid., 143; Phil Barker and Gary Rolfe, "Psychiatric Nursing: Living with the Legacy of the Holocaust," *Journal of Psychiatric and Mental Health Nursing* 9 (2002): 365–375; Maria Berghs, Bernadette Dierckx de Casterlé, and Chris Gastmans, "Practices of Responsibility and Nurses during the Euthanasia Programs of Nazi Germany: A Discussion Paper," *International Journal of Nursing Studies* 44, no. 5 (Jul, 2007): 845–854; Warren T. Reich, "The Care-Based Ethic of Nazi Medicine and the Moral Importance of What We Care About," *American Journal of Bioethics* 1, no. 1 (2001): 64–74.
57 Steppe, *Krankenpflege im Nationalsozialismus*, 142.
58 Sylvia A. Hoskins, "Nurses and National Socialism – a Moral Dilemma: One Historical Example of a Route to Euthanasia," *Nursing Ethics* 12, no. 1 (Jan, 2005): 79–91; Ulrike Gaida, *Zwischen Pflegen und Töten. Krankenschwestern im Nationalsozialismus. Einführung und Quellen für Unterricht und Selbststudium* (Frankfurt a.M.: Mabuse, 2006); Ulrike Gaida, "Eugenik im Deutschen Reich und im Nationalsozialismus" 531–543.
59 See especially Susan Benedict, "The Nadir of Nursing: Nurse-Perpetrators of the Ravensbrück Concentration Camp," *Nursing History Review*, 11 (2003): 129–146; Benedict and Jane M. Georges, "Nurses and the Sterilization Experiments of Auschwitz: A Postmodernist Perspective," *Nursing Inquiry* 13, no. 4 (Dec 2006): 277–288; Barbara L. Brush, "Nursing

atric asylums, and nurses in killing facilities. Other research concentrates on the involvement of nurses in specific aspects of eugenics or "euthanasia," as in, for example, children's "euthanasia."[60]

Most of the studies mentioned above used testimonies of nurses who killed patients and analyzed them from an ethical perspective. Authors agree that the involvement of nurses in these crimes can only be understood against the backdrop of the specific situation of nursing in Germany. I want to summarize very briefly these undisputed assumptions. Most of these studies began with historical overviews of the development of nursing as a vocation in Germany, highlighting the fact that German nursing was particularly powerless due to its traditional connection to the Protestant and Catholic churches.[61] Because of this connection, German nurses were trained to obey and to understand themselves as subordinated to physicians and religious authorities. The Nazi system was thus said to have exploited this condition by indoctrinating nurses with race ideologies, reorganizing their vocational organizations, and using psychological methods in order to brainwash nurses to do their duty and follow orders even if their conduct fell outside the realm of moral acceptability. Nursing historian Susan Benedict and historian Jochen Kuhla developed an analytic framework for understanding nurses' participation that seems to have provided the basis for many other studies: ideological commitment, obedience, religion, nursing education and nursing professional organizations, putative duress, and economic factors.[62]

Nursing: A Powerless Occupation?

This book seeks to extend this analytical framework, because it does not ask why nurses voluntarily participated in the killings of patients, but rather how the

---

Care and Context in Theresienstadt." *Western Journal of Nuring Research* 26, no. 8 (Dec 2004): 860–871.

60 Susan Benedict, Linda Shields, and Alison J. O'Donnel, "Children's 'Euthanasia' in Nazi Germany," *Journal of Pediatric Nursing* 24, no. 6 (2009): 506–516.

61 Hilde Steppe, "Das Selbstverständnis der Krankenpflege in ihrer historischen Entwicklung," *Pflege* 13 (2000): 77–83; Hilde Steppe, "Nursing in Nazi Germany," *Western Journal of Nursing Research* 14, no. 6 (1992):744; Hilde Steppe, "Nursing in the Third Reich," *History of Nursing Society Journal* 3, no. 4 (1991): 21–37; Steppe, *Krankenpflege im Nationalsozialismus*; Rebekah Bronwyn McFarland-Icke, *Nurses in Nazi Germany: Moral Choice in History* (Princeton: Princeton University Press), 1999; Gerhard Fürstler and Peter Malina, "Ich tat nur meinen Dienst." Zur Geschichte der Krankenpflege in Österreich in der NS-Zeit (Wien: Facultas, 2004); Christoph Schweikhardt, "Krankenpflege im Nationalsozialismus," in *Quellen zur Geschichte der Krankenpflege. Mit Einführungen und Kommentaren*, ed. Sylvelyn Hähner-Rombach (Frankfurt a.M.: Mabuse, 2008), 554–564.

62 Susan Benedict and Jochen Kuhla, "Nurses' Participation in the Euthanasia Programs of Nazi Germany," *Western Journal of Nursing Research* 21, no. 2 (Apr 1999): 259–260.

killings were carried out in an ordinary psychiatric asylum and what role the nurses took in these killings. This kind of research tries to "explore the territory of active participation, the *own-active participation of the many*."[63]

The question of "the own-active participation of the many," however, is still not satisfactory answered for nurses' participation in the killings of their patients. This book demonstrates that nurses participated in these killings not merely because they were forced to do so but rather because scientific discourses cast certain lives as unworthy of living. In order to understand these mechanisms, I concentrate on the crucial role that nurses played in the construction of "lives unworthy of living" through the observations and reports that they documented in the medical record. The book also attempts to break new methodological ground by using a discourse theory approach to the history of nursing, as will be demonstrated in the following chapters. As a first step I will analyze in some detail the organizational forms of nursing since the nineteenth century and will focus on the question of whether nurses were simply part of a "powerless profession" or if they must rather be seen as both powerless and powerful. Such a perspective enables an analysis of the impact of nurses on health policies, not only during the Nazi regime but also in modern societies. What follows is not meant to be an in-depth analysis of nursing history since the nineteenth century. The aim is to develop a critical perspective on the assumption that nurses were always powerless and that this powerlessness was the foundation for the actions of nurses during the Nazi regime.

The following overview starts with a brief summary of how nursing developed in the nineteenth century. Special emphasis will be put on the organization and aims of motherhouses. Nurses in these motherhouses were in a somewhat paradoxical situation: they had few personal liberties and were subordinated to both the directors of the motherhouses and to physicians, but outside the motherhouse they provided a form of pastoral care and were considered competent employees in hospitals and parishes where they worked primarily autonomously. Because pastoral care allowed nurses to have a commanding influence over populations, nursing had significant theoretical and powerful importance in the governing of modern societies. At the end of the nineteenth century and at the beginning of the twentieth, so-called free sisterhoods emerged that tried to act as a counterbalance to the strict hierarchy of the motherhouse system. Nevertheless, the working and living conditions of the free sisters were

---

63 Alf Lüdtke, "Alltagsgeschichte: Stand der Diskussion und Perspektiven," in Alltag in der Pflege – Wie machten sich Pflegende bemerkbar? Beiträge des 8. Internationalen Kongress zur Geschichte der Pflege 2008, eds. Andrea Thiekötter and others (Frankfurt a.M.: Mabuse, 2009), 20.

shaped by the same concept of "religious calling" that influenced the lives of those in the traditional system.

The last part of this summary outlines the emphasis the National Socialist government put on the importance of nursing to their health policies. An analysis of pastoral power reveals why Nazi politicians depended on the work of nurses to implement these policies. Racial biology was an integral part of nursing discourse long before the Nazis came to power. Nurses openly supported the Nazi regime and were an important pillar of its racist policies and thus the apparent powerlessness of a professional nurses' organization cannot account for the special significance that nursing gained under the Nazi regime.

Mother House Concept

According to historian Susanne Kreutzer, it was taken for granted that a "good" nurse would consider her occupation more of a vocation than a job until well into the 1950s in West Germany.[64] For nurses, nursing was not labor but service. The large motherhouse sisterhoods of Caritas, the Inner Mission, and the German Red Cross dominated nursing in Germany before, during, and after the Nazi regime. Joining a sisterhood meant that women vowed to subordinate their "lives completely to the service of the community and to the service of the sick and needy."[65] In return, the motherhouse provided training, lifelong support, and a minimal amount of pocket money.

It was during the nineteenth century that the motherhouse system developed into the dominant form of nursing organization in the German Reich, and it remained relatively unchanged well into the second half of the twentieth century. From the nineteenth century on, nurses claimed particular requirements for the education of nursing trainees and the Protestant and Catholic Churches had a crucial impact on the development of "modern nursing care."[66] The Protestant Church, for example, reinstalled the formerly well-known office of the Dea-

---

64 Susanne Kreutzer, "Die Einheit von Leibes- und Seelenpflege als Kern des tradierten christlichen Pflegeverständnisses," in *Transformationen pflegerischen Handelns. Institutionelle Kontexte und soziale Praxis vom 19. bis 21. Jahrhundert*, ed. Susanne Kreutzer (Göttingen: V&R unipress, Universität Osnabrück, 2010), 109–130; Kreutzer, "'Before, We Were Always There-Now, Everything is Separate': On Nursing Reforms in Western Germany," *Nursing History Review*, 21, (2008): 180–200.
65 Ibid., 180.
66 Norbert Friedrich, "Christentum und Krankenpflege – Einige historische Anmerkungen," in *Quellen zur Geschichte der Krankenpflege*, ed. Sylvelin Hähner-Rombach (Frankfurt am Main: Mabuse-Verlag, 2008), 52; Anna Sticker, *Die Entstehung der neuzeitlichen Krankenpflege. Deutsche Quellenstücke aus der ersten Hälfte des 19. Jahrhunderts* (Stuttgart: Kohlhammer, 1960).

coness that had been most popular in Protestant parishes in the Netherlands. Theodor Fliedner especially, supported by his two spouses Fredericke (1800–1842) and Caroline (1808–1892), shaped a religious ideal of community-integrated service that was realized through practical charity.[67] Although the focus of the motherhouse was on sending nurses out to work in communities, this model was not meant to be limited to the parish nurse (comparable to what we call public health nurses nowadays) but was used for nurses working in hospitals as well. The motherhouses considered themselves communities for life: places of service and faith for unmarried women. Deaconesses should be "servants of Lord Jesus, servants of the sick for Jesus' sake, and servants among one another."[68] Work should be regarded as "charity service" based on Christian faith and not as a profession or means of livelihood.[69] The parish deaconess was regarded as the "crown of the Female Diaconate,"[70] and her work was based on strict boundaries. "Every Deaconess who wants to fulfill the duties of her office to please the Lord and to the contentment of the direction [of the motherhouse] in order to serve the one who suffers must be governed by the love of Christ, which becomes her inner law. Then she is less in need of external laws to guide her behavior."[71] Fliedner described the nurse as a woman "who is always ready to serve [and therefore] will never elevate herself or try to dominate. She will do good quietly and unassumingly and will always strive to deny her own desires."[72] At the center of the Deaconess' work stood the devotion of the missionary and the companionship of the neighbor – her curing role was not her primary function. "The noble sacred office of nursing care emerges in its whole solemnity as well as in its fullest significance at the bedside of the dying. Here, where the assistance of the physician has already found its limit, the love of the nurse is still relentlessly active to assist her sick person with caring hands and mild mind in the hour of fight and dissolution, in order to provide him with relief and comfort."[73]

---

67 Anna Sticker, *Friederike Fliedner und die Anfänge der Frauendiakonie. Ein Quellenbuch* (Neukirchen/Vluyn: Neukirchener Verlag, 1961).
68 House rules and service regulation for Deaconesses in the Deaconess-establishment in Kaiserswerth as cited in Friedrich, *Christentum und Krankenpflege-Einige historische Anmerkungen*, 53.
69 Kreutzer, "Before, We Were Always There-Now, Everything is Separate," 180.
70 Susanne Kreutzer, "Nursing Body and Soul in the Parish: Lutheran Deaconess Motherhouses in Germany and the United States," *Nursing History Review* 18 (2010): 137.
71 Friederike Fliedner as cited in Sticker, *Friederike Fliedner und die Anfänge der Frauendiakonie. Ein Quellenbuch*, 359.
72 Sticker, *Die Entstehung der Neuzeitlichen Krankenpflege. Deutsche Quellenstücke aus der ersten Hälfte des 19. Jahrhunderts*, 271.
73 Ibid., 278.

The Inner Organization of the Motherhouses

The motherhouses were disciplinary institutions and organized, according to American sociologist Erving Goffmann (1961), along the lines of "total institutions." A primary characteristic of the total institution is the isolation of the inhabitants from the wider community; they live within an enclosed, formally administered life and are excluded from decisions concerning their fate.[74] Foucault used an abstract model of the panopticon, developed by Bentham, to analyze the functional operation of disciplinary power.[75] The panopticon is a circular building with a watch tower in its center. Around the center is a circle of cells arranged so that every individual is accommodated alone. This individual is visible from the tower at all times but in contrast, the tower windows have blinds so inmates cannot see when they are observed and when they are not. Individuals gradually perceive that their behaviour is under permanent visibility and observation, and eventually learn to observe themselves through the eyes of their observers and to control themselves according to imposed norms.[76] During the eighteenth century a number of disciplinary institutions emerged that functioned according to the principles of the panopticon. One such example was the monastery, which was based on the organizational principle of making the single individual visible and controllable. Disciplinary power functioned by measuring and, either explicitly or implicitly, evaluating the behavior of individuals according to a norm, and an aberration from this norm could be either registered or sanctioned.

The motherhouse in Kaiserswerth adopted elements of the monastic organizational principle from the Catholic sisterhood of the "Sisters of Mercy."[77] In the motherhouse, the barracks-like accommodation enabled an all-embracing surveillance of the deaconesses that included their behavior inside and outside of work. Fliedner conceived of a strict regulation; not only was the worker's performance controlled but also her daily routine. "They were furthermore urged to regularly perform "self-inspections" by means of a questionnaire. With this technique nurses should learn to self-monitor themselves regarding their compliance with the rules and norms."[78] This explanation described Fliedner's

---

74 Erving Goffman, *Asylums: Essays on the Social Situation of Mental Patients and Other Inmates* (New York: Doubleday and Co., 1961).
75 Michel Foucault, *Discipline & Punish: The Birth of the Prison*, trans. Alan Sheridan (New York: Vintage Books, 1995).
76 Foucault, "Panopticism," in *Discipline & Punish*, 195–228.
77 Jutta Schmidt, *Beruf Schwester: Mutterhausdiakonie im 19. Jahrhundert* (Frankfurt a. M.: Campus, 1998); Sticker, *Friederike Fliedner und die Anfänge der Frauendiakonie. Ein Quellenbuch*.
78 Doris Arnold, "Pflege und Macht. Der Beitrag Foucaults," in *Pflege-Räume, Macht und Alltag*, ed. Sabine Braunschweig (Zürich: Chronos, 2006), 158.

definition of the "the inner law" of the nurse. It also highlights that power has a productive effect; the disciplinary system in the motherhouse profoundly shaped the nurses not only because they acquired technical knowledge but, most importantly, they learned to develop personal attributes such as obedience and self-denial, which were considered to be the basis for nursing care understood as charitable activity.

Nevertheless the motherhouses were one of the few institutions in nineteenth-century Germany that provided women with sound training and a lifelong occupation, offering them a socially approved way of living and working outside marriage. Motherhouses ran their own charitable hospitals and, in addition, entered into contract with other institutions. Kreutzer emphasizes that in this way "the influence of motherhouses extended far beyond their immediate locality."[79]

Pastoral Power

The deaconess was considered a "Christian mother of the parish" and charged with a wide spectrum of tasks "including nursing, social service work and pastoral care or "care of the soul," to distinguish it from the work of parish pastors. At the center of the Christian understanding of nursing was the idea of nursing body and soul together."[80] Apart from providing nursing care in the strictest sense, nurses were also to perform pastoral functions and provide patients with religious strength. Part of a Christian nurse's obligation was to listen to the sick person, to pray with him or her, and to strengthen his or her faith.[81] The motherhouses trained nurses to work in parishes and hospitals since they maintained their own confessional hospitals and as well contracted with secular hospitals to send their nurses to work there.

The Christian interpretation of sickness assured nurses an independent, religious-based role within the German health care system. The medical fraternity in the confessional institutions had to struggle to implement its biomedical understanding of health and sickness that was based purely on scientific concepts.[82] As Kreutzer pointed out, "The great importance of nursing is docu-

---

79 Kreutzer, "Before, We Were Always There-Now, Everything is Separate," 182.
80 Hans-Walther Schmuhl, "Ärzte in Konfessionellen Kranken- und Pflegeanstalten 1908–1957," in *Beruf und Religion im 19. und 20. Jahrhundert*, eds. Frank-Michael Kuhlemann and Hans-Walther Schmuhl (Stuttgart: Kohlhammer, 2003), 176–194.
81 Kreutzer, "Die Einheit von Leibes- und Seelenpflege als Kern des tradierten christlichen Pflegeverständnisses," 109–130; Karen Nolte, "Pflege von Sterbenden im 19. Jahrhundert," in *Transformationen pflegerischen Handelns. Institutionelle Kontexte und soziale Praxis vom 19. Bis 21. Jahrhunderts*, ed. Susanne Kreutzer (Göttingen: V&R unipress, Univerität Osnabrück, 2010), 87–107.
82 Hans-Walther Schmuhl, "Ärzte in Konfessionellen Kranken- und Pflegeanstalten 1908–

mented, for example, in the by-laws of the *Henriettenstiftung* [one of the big German motherhouses] in which nursing care was defined as the main task of the motherhouse. Medicine, according to the self-definition of the foundation, was seen as only part of nursing care."[83] The strong hierarchical position of nurses was also demonstrated by the fact that physicians were not represented in the administration of the hospital until the end of the 1970s. The traditional administrative structure of the confessional hospitals was controlled by the theological head as represented by the Mother Superior.[84] The portrayal of nursing as subordinate to medicine cannot be maintained for the confessional hospitals. Rather, physicians and nurses were considered complementary occupational groups with distinct roles in curing patients.

Fliedner's idea for the motherhouse was to train nurses to send out as "country missionaries" to combat illness, poverty, and faithlessness, particularly in poor communities. This "inner mission" was based on the underlying assumption that material and spiritual impoverishment were closely related. "It was hoped that deaconesses, because their training was [considered] non-academic, would have more immediate contact with the poor than pastors."[85] Fliedner's concept was anything but apolitical. Nurses were deemed able to influence the behavior of the people they cared for due to their ability to get to know patients in their personal family settings and to the intimate knowledge that they gathered, available to no other professional group. Furthermore, the parish nurse was often the first contact in cases of illness and other emergencies, because the next doctor was usually far away.[86] Nurses therefore had to have trusting relationships with their patients and their families. "When they succeeded in fulfilling their various tasks and integrating themselves into parish life, they acquired a prominent position in their communities – a high social standing that was also based on their specific expertise."[87] From this perspective, nurses in both parishes and hospitals were indispensable to the governing of modern societies, and, as will be demonstrated in the course of this chapter, Nazi politicians especially appreciated this aspect of these nurses.

1957," in *Beruf und Religion im 19. und 20. Jahrhundert*, eds. Frank-Michael Kuhlemann and Hans-Walther Schmuhl (Stuttgart: Kohlhammer, 2003), 176–194.
83 Susanne Kreutzer, "Fragmentierung der Pflege. Umbrüche pflegerischen Handelns in den 1960er Jahren," in *Transformationen pflegerischen Handelns*, ed. Susanne Kreutzer (Göttingen: V&R unipress, Universität Osnabrück, 2010), 172.
84 Ibid., 112.
85 Kreutzer, "Nursing Body and Soul in the Parish," 137; Karen Nolte, "Telling the Painful Truth: Nurses and Physicians in the Nineteenth Century," *Nursing History Review*, no. 16 (2008): 115–134.
86 Kreutzer, "Nursing Body and Soul in the Parish," 138.
87 Ibid., 141.

The Diversification of Nursing

In the last third of the nineteenth century the Kaiserswerth motherhouse system and confessional nursing care at large came under increasing scrutiny. Industrialization, urbanization, and the differentiation within societies led to new approaches in nursing. Furthermore, motherhouse nurses were numerically no longer able to meet the need for nurses and they were becoming less welcomed because of their allegiance to the motherhouse rather than to physicians. New organizational forms emerged, like the Protestant Deaconess Association, for example, which was founded in 1894 by pastor Friedrich Zimmer and which consciously tried to distinguish itself from the motherhouse system by its structure as a cooperative.[88]

At the beginning of the twentieth century, so-called free sisterhoods were founded as an alternative to the motherhouse system. Their members did not establish a permanent bond with their sisterhood and they received a salary for their work, although they were at the bottom of the salary scale. The working and living conditions of the free sisters were shaped, however, by the same concept of "religious calling" that influenced the lives of their religious counterparts. Like the motherhouse sisters, they lived in hospital residences and often worked 70 to 80 hours per week. It was understood that they would be single.[89]

Against this backdrop nursing developed into an ideal occupation for "middle class" women. The professional ethical frame was constructed around the principles of Christianity, unpaid (which actually meant priceless) nursing care, and the main ideas of pastoral care became paramount for these sisterhoods too. These principles were nearly identical with middle-class feminine morality. The cornerstone of "good secular nursing care" became obedience, altruism, self-denial, and humility. The development of German nursing in this way, in which it was understood as pastoral care and invaluable, explains why it was consequently so difficult to organize around waged labour. If "self-denial is a vocational element (this is to say, it is a precondition for nursing care) it is nearly impossible to ask for something or to formulate demands in the interests of employees. Attempts of this kind were consequently outlawed as "socialist turnovers."[90]

Nurses sympathetic to the middle-class feminist movement (above all Agnes

---

88 Friedrich, *Christentum und Krankenpflege-Einige historische Anmerkungen*, 55.
89 Kreutzer, "Before, We Were Always There-Now, Everything is Separate,"181; Marianne Schmidbauer, *Vom Lazaruskreuz zur Pflege aktuell: Professionalisierungsdiskurse in der deutschen Krankenpflege 1903–2000* (Königstein/Taunus: Ulrike Helmer Verlag, 2002).
90 Steppe, *Krankenpflege im Nationalsozialismus*, 35.

Karll, 1868–1927[91]) who complained that the motherhouse hierarchy was too rigid, founded the *"Berufsorganisation der Krankenpflegerinnen Deutschlands (B.O.K.D.)"* [German Nursing Association] in 1903. For these women, obtaining personal, individual "liberty" was a priority, and for them, "free nursing," in opposition to motherhouse nursing, was an emancipatory step.[92] Jewish nurses, too, organized into an association in 1893 in Frankfurt am Main, and even though this association oriented itself to existing models (e. g. motherhouses), it developed an independent nursing tradition that was very important for Jewish parishes.[93]

But the price these different sisterhoods had to pay was high: they still had to deny themselves and obey physicians. This paradoxical situation was reflected in the journals of that time, where side-by-side articles described the exploitative aspects of every-day nursing at the same as they waxed eloquent about the self-fulfillment a woman could realize only in nursing.[94] Nursing as a German occupation was a paradigmatic example of the gender-specific division of labour.

Nursing in Germany was paradoxical. On the one hand, the strong emphasis on obedience as a valued nursing trait and the internalization of patriarchal civil morality provided assurance that nurses would not question the structures that made them subordinate and required their unquestioning obedience. On the other hand, nurses assumed a very powerful position vis-à-vis their patients and within the health care system because they mobilized a large repertoire of techniques to influence the conduct of their patients, they had acquired a distinct body of knowledge, and they possessed an independent sphere of action with respect to physicians. A historical analysis of the role nurses played in the killing of thousands of their most vulnerable patients must consider this paradoxical position of nurses in Germany. Such an analysis must also consider the significance of nursing for the government of modern societies, because it was this aspect of nursing that made it so valuable to the Nazi regime.

---

91 Anna Sticker, *Agnes Karll, Die Reformerin der deutschen Krankenpflege. Ein Wegweiser für Heute zu ihrem 50. Todestag* (Stuttgart: Aussaat, 1984).
92 Steppe, Das Selbstverständnis der Krankenpflege in ihrer historischen Entwicklung, 77–83.
93 Friedrich, *Christentum und Krankenpflege-Einige historische Anmerkungen*; Hilde Steppe, *'…dem Kranken zum Troste und dem Judenthum zur Ehre…'* (Frankfurt a. M.: Mabuse, 2006).
94 Steppe, *Krankenpflege im Nationalsozialismus*, 36.

Governing Through Nursing

"Government," is understood here in a "nominalistic" manner.[95] It is neither a concept nor a theory but rather a perspective that emphasizes the heterogeneity of authorities, who tried to govern the behavior of citizens, as well as the heterogeneity of strategies and means deployed by these authorities.[96] Governmentality describes a new characteristic of governing that developed in sixteenth-century Europe. It was intertwined with the invention, operationalization, and institutionalization of specific forms of knowledge, disciplines, tactics, and technologies, which were all related to the governing of health, self, children, and state. This new rationality of governing was related to the emergence of the large territorial and administrative states and the colonial empires, as well as to the challenges to religious leadership by the reformation and counter-reformation. The appearance of diverse discourses around the government of the family, the self, and the state constituted a revolutionary break with the Machiavellian conception of power, which had assumed that the power of the prince had to be guaranteed through sovereign power.[97] Henceforward, government must be more than the "right disposition of things" because it must be concerned about the "common welfare and salvation for all."[98] This new rationality of government[99] comprised several crucial features that political scientist Wendy Brown has described:

> First, governing involves the harnessing and organizing of energies in any body – individual, mass, international – that might otherwise be anarchic, self-destructive, or simply unproductive. And not only energies but needs, capacities, and desires are harnessed, ordered, managed, and directed by governmentality. Governing thus concerns what Foucault calls 'the conduct of conduct' – it orchestrates the conduct of the body individual, the body social, and the body politic. Second, as the conduct of conduct, governmentality has multiple points of operation and application, from individuals to mass populations, and from particular parts of the body and psyche to appetites and ethics, work and citizenship practices. Third, far from being restricted to rule, law, or other visible and accountable power, governmentality works through a range of invisible and nonaccountable social powers, of which Foucault's best example is pastoral power. And fourth, governmentality both employs *and* infiltrates a number

---

95 Nikolas Rose, *Powers of Freedom. Reframing Political Thought* (Cambridge: Cambridge University Press, 2005).
96 Ibid., 22.
97 Michel Foucault, *Sécurité, Territoire, Population. Cours au Collège de France. 1977–1978* (France: Gallimard Seuil, 2004).
98 Terry Johnson, "Governmentality and the Institutionalization of Expertise," in *Health Professions and the State in Europe*, eds. Terry Johnson, Gerald Larkin and Mike Saks (London: Routledge, 1995), 8.
99 Foucault, *Sécurité, Territoire, Population*, 47.

of discourses ordinarily conceived as unrelated to political power, governance, or the state. These include scientific discourses (among them medicine, criminology, pedagogy, psychology, psychiatry, and demography), religious discourses, and popular discourses. Governmentality, then, draws on without unifying, centralizing, or rendering systematic or even consistent a range of powers and knowledges dispersed across modern societies.[100]

The "art of government" paved the way for a "science of government." Population became the core object of governance and political economy became its core scientific knowledge.[101] This new form of governing required an ensemble of institutions, processes, analyses, calculations, reflections, and tactics, which all together constitute governmentality, "a very specific albeit complex form of power."[102] From the eighteenth century onward, expertise became a crucial part in the process of governing. Like the formalistic, bureaucratic, and administrative machinery, expertise became the foundation of political power. By now, one could only govern rightly under the condition that the liberty, or a certain form of liberty, was really respected.[103] Furthermore, expertise had an epistemological character, because it comprised specific conceptions of how, for example, spaces, persons, problems, and objects should be governed, and it comprised specific forms of languages. Hence, all government projects included a certain element of rationalization. Political rationality and expertise performed by "experts of truth" were from the beginning on intertwined.[104]

It is in this context that nursing became a vital aspect in the government of populations because of its ability to influence the conduct of conduct. As the analysis of the motherhouse system emphasized, nurses were a powerful group of experts in the provision of health care. They were in direct contact with individuals, communities, groups, and populations, and due to their subordinated, nonacademic position they were able to develop and maintain a particularly trusting relationship with people. Only nurses were able to reach into the finest ramifications of society – they possessed a kind of microscopic power. Nurses were powerful because they were able to influence and to form individuals through their interventions, and moreover, they possessed a scientific "savoir" that was broadly accepted as true.[105] Nurses operated within a network of power relations that was determined on the one hand by society, and, on the other hand, constituted by nurses themselves.

---

100 Brown, *Regulating Aversion*, 80 (original italics).
101 Foucault, *Sécurité, Territoire, Population*.
102 Johnson, *Governmentality and the Institutionalization of Expertise*, 8.
103 Foucault, *Sécurité, Territoire, Population*, 47.
104 Rose, *Powers of Freedom. Reframing Political Thought*, 30.
105 Dave Holmes and Denise Gastaldo, "Nursing as Means of Governmentality," *Journal of Advanced Nursing* 38, no. 6 (2002): 557–565.

Nursing interventions were regulated through disciplinary and pastoral power, which distinguishes nursing from other health care professions. Pastoral power developed from the relation between a pastor (as a leader) and an individual or congregation. The pastor is thought of as a shepherd of his flock, who, while knowing every single sheep, is also concerned for the well-being of the flock. In the western world pastoral power developed into an individualizing form of power, which knows its subjects in great detail and is linked to expert knowledge. Holmes describes pastoral power as a power technique "which penetrates souls, decodes hearts, and reveals the most intimate secrets. It seeks disclosure of unconsciousness; it penetrates the soul and acts upon it to ultimately direct it."[106]

The most important tool to generate this kind of power is the confession and the key element is confidence; the aim is to discover the inmost secrets of patients. Pastoral power produces a complete knowledge about the individual, an important element in enabling the governing of the individual. Confession is the encouragement to speak and it is carefully stimulated by the nurse. Fliedner's idea of the nurses' "inner mission" integrated the pastoral use of confession, introspection, and self-examination into the day-to-day work of nurses and made all these characteristics an integral part of nursing care. Although at the end of the nineteenth century and the beginning of the twentieth century new forms of nursing organizations emerged, the conception of nurses as the ones responsible for the care of the soul survived, as did the idea that nursing care should be regarded more as "charity service" than as a profession or means of livelihood.

The Impact of Nursing under the Nazi Regime

For nurses, racial biology was an integral part of nursing discourses long before the Nazis came to power, as can be demonstrated in contemporary nursing journals. For example, in February 1930, a certain Dr. T. Fürst asked the rhetorical question: "Is the woman able to practically support the program of racial-hygiene?" in the nursing journal *Unter dem Lazaruskreuz*, and answered the question with "yes" all around.[107] This journal was the official organ of the

---

106 Dave Holmes, "Police and Pastoral Power: Governmentality and Correctional Forensic Psychiatric Nursing," *Nursing Inquiry* 9, no. 2 (2002): 86; Holmes and Gastaldo, *Nursing as Means of Governmentality*, 557–565.
107 Dr. T. Fürst, "Kann die Frau im Dienste der praktischen Rassenhygiene mitarbeiten?" in *Unterm Lazaruskreuz*, 1930, 13–15 as cited in Gaida, *Zwischen Pflegen und Töten. Krankenschwestern im Nationalsozialismus. Einführung und Quellen für Unterricht und Selbststudium*, 30.

German Nursing Association (*B.O.K.D.*) and was by no means a right-wing journal. Fürst meant by "woman" the public health nurse whom he described as "the soul of welfare" and whose task should be the clarification of the causal relation between the "social need for help and congenital predisposition."[108]

It was not only physicians like Dr. Fürst who made an argument for the impact of nurses in the politics of eugenics but nurses themselves also campaigned for eugenics to be considered an urgent task for nursing. Historian Ulrike Gaida discusses an article written by nurse Minna Bahnson in 1930 in *Unterm Lazaruskreuz*, entitled "Three requirements for population policy."[109] Bahnson noted that physician Bonne calculated the financial charges evolving from accommodation and care of "inferiors" (people with disabilities), concluding that the state had to pay more than two milliards [billions] Marks [approximately US$ 476.190 476 in 1938] per year for these "sick persons" and that this money was lost because these humans were "worthless, if not even harmful" to the entire nation. For example, Bahnson noted, "in the case of the completely moronic children in Bethel [a protestant institution for the accommodation of people with disabilities and a psychiatric asylum] one can no longer speak of 'human beings' at all, which means it would be better if they were erased from time." Bahnson openly supported the assassination of people with disabilities in this article, providing her theoretical basis for the killings. It must be emphasized that these articles appeared three years before the Nazis came to power and nine years before the official start of the "euthanasia" killings. Nurses openly supported the Nazi regime and were an important pillar of its racist policies. As Gaida emphasized, the number of cases of people with purported potential hereditary defects reported to the health authorities by nurses far exceeded the number of cases reported by physicians.[110] Nurses did so in the clear consciousness that their reports might lead to severe consequences for those they reported on.

The quotes from Adolf Hilter and Hans Schemm in the introduction highlight the important part that biology and medicine played in Nazi Germany. They also emphasize the important role of physicians to Nazism, and in a talk just after the National Socialists came to power in January 1933, the Deputy Leader of the Reich's medical profession provided a blueprint of the future of nursing under the Nazis:

---

108 Ibid.
109 Minna Bahnson, "Drei Forderungen zur Bevölkerungspolitik," in *Unterm Lazaruskreuz*, 1930, 58–59 as cited in Gaida, *Zwischen Pflegen und Töten. Krankenschwestern im Nationalsozialismus. Einführung und Quellen für Unterricht und Selbststudium*, 30.
110 Ibid., 139.

> The requirements which German nurses in social and medical service have to meet in the new state are completely different from the previous period in many respects. The new state does not only want to look after the sick and weak; it also wants to secure a healthy development of all national comrades, and also to improve their health, if their inherited biological predisposition allows for it. Above all, the new state wants to secure and promote a genetically sound, valuable race and, in contrast to the past, not to expend an exaggerated effort on the care of genetically or racially inferior people. Of course, such people must be looked after, but no longer be supported and promoted at the cost of the more valuable people.[111]

Nurses under the Nazi regime had a biopolitical task that was openly acknowledged and propagated by Nazi politicians. Seen from this perspective, nursing became a state-supporting vocation, which obviously enhanced the status of nurses in Nazi society. This might be one reason why nurses supported the Nazi health policy so broadly and uncritically. Nevertheless, it must be emphasized that the two recognized confessional associations differed in their attitude to the "Law for the Prevention of Hereditary Diseased Offspring" [*Gesetz zur Verhütung erbkranken Nachwuchses*] that regulated the forced sterilization of so-called mentally ill patients and criminals. On the Protestant side, the central committee of the "Inner Mission" welcomed the legislation whereas the Caritas Association of the Catholic Church dismissed it.[112] Cases are documented in which the Catholic nurses refused to assist in these surgeries.[113] However, all confessional nursing organizations supported the aims of Nazi health policy. As Nazi politics on nursing stated, nurses were to lead and educate patients in questions of health. The Nazi regime well acknowledged the specific capacity of nurses to influence people's behavior in questions of sickness and well-being, but as the above suggests, this capacity was understood to be a task supporting the state. In order to carry out the will of the state, nurses had to clearly understand their work as political activity based on political consciousness. The chief physician of the Rudolf-Heß-Krankenhaus in Dresden, Dr. Hermann Jensen, wrote in 1934:

> ...with us every national comrade [*Volksgenosse*] must be a political soldier. I use the word "political" here very consciously even though I know that the connection between nurse and politics will be rejected in many places. ... Because for us politics means:

---

111 Dr. Friedrich Bartels as cited in Suzanne Hahn, "Nursing Issues During the Third Reich," in *Medicine, Ethics, and the Third Reich: Historical and Contemporary Issues*, ed. John M. Michalczyk (Kansas City: Sheed and Ward, 1994), 143–144.
112 Jochen-Christoph Kaiser, "Konfessionelle Wohlfahrtspflege im Nationalsozialismus. Caritas und Innere Mission," in *Caritas und Diakonie in der NS-Zeit. Beispiele aus Niedersachsen*, ed. Hans Otte (Hildesheim: Olms, 2001), 56.
113 Christoph Schweikhardt, ""Der Stosstrupp 1937/38 rückt in Würzburg ein!" Eine Fallstudie zur Ausbildung einer NS-Krankenschwester am dortigen Luitpoldkrankenhaus," *Historica Hospitalium* 22 (200/2001): 111.

active participation in the life of our people's community and active pursuit in the service of the nation. That is what is called politics! And that is what the nurse has to do with politics. Especially today she cannot deprive herself of these obligations to this end. She occupies too important a position in the frame of our people's community.[114]

The Nazi regime tried to harmonize the different German nursing sisterhoods and organizations, attempting to enforce political conformity in nursing by implementing a bundle of organizationally and bureaucratically regulatory actions. Historian Christoph Schweikhardt concluded, however, that it was much easier for the regime to bring the non-confessional nursing associations under its control than it was for the Nazi regime to get access to the confessional sisterhoods. As has been shown, these sisterhoods had been under the protection of the churches and their educational institutions had been established as non-governmental institutions with a high degree of autonomy during the empire.

For example, the NS nursing sisterhood, founded under the Nazi regime and aimed to organize nurses in one association, remained smaller than the larger faction of nurses who were still organized in traditional nursing associations. Until 1939 the NS sisterhood contained 10,000 nurses, but in contrast 21,599 nurses were in the Imperial Association of Free Nurses, 14, 595 in the German Red Cross, 46,500 in the Protestant Diaconia Fellowship, and around 50,000 in the Catholic Caritas Sisterhood.[115] These numbers of nurses outside the NS Sisterhood support the argument that nurses were not coerced by an omnipotent Nazi organisation and clearly indicate the enormous influence of confessional nursing organizations on nursing in Germany. There was actually no need to push for the unification of nursing, because most of the nursing organizations, both non-confessional and confessional nursing associations, did not resist Nazi politics and even openly supported fascist health policies. The influence of confessional nursing continued even after the end of Second World War and into the late 1960s.[116]

---

114 Dr Hermann Jensen, "Sinn, Zweck und Ziel der NS-Schwesternschaft," in *Zeitschrift der Reichsfachschaft Deutscher Schwestern und Pflegerinnen*, 1934, 137–140 as cited in Gaida, *Zwischen Pflegen und Töten. Krankenschwestern im Nationalsozialismus. Einführung und Quellen für Unterricht und Selbststudium*, 112.
115 Schweikhardt, *Krankenpflege im Nationalsozialismus*, 558; Birgit Breiding, *Die Braunen Schwestern. Ideologie, Struktur, Funktion einer nationalsozialistischen Elite* (Stuttgart: Franz Steiner Verlag), 176
116 Kreutzer, Die Einheit Von Leibes- und Seelenpflege als Kern des tradierten christlichen Pflegeverständnisses, 109

Chapter 3: The History of the Langenhorn Asylum from 1893 to 1945

Langenhorn before the First World War

In 1888, the medical director of Hamburg's academic psychiatric asylum at Friedrichsberg, Dr. Wilhelm Reye, first proposed the foundation of an agricultural institution to the city's hospital council (*Krankenhauskollegium*), the executive committee of the Senate of Hamburg for Hamburg's hospitals. At this time, Friedrichsberg was the central asylum for the city of Hamburg, and he believed that a new institution would free up space in the overcrowded established asylum. According to his perspective, the rapid rise of industrialization and the consequent growth of Hamburg's population had increased the number of mentally ill persons needing hospital care. At the start of the industrializing period, Friedrichsberg had held 1200 beds but now that capacity had to be increased.[1] Based on a report mandated by health authorities, it was determined that the proposed "colony for the insane" should be reserved for mentally ill persons who were supported by welfare and whose insanity was likely long-term but who could work. The report determined that in order to address this need for more space, a manor should be purchased and several houses, constructed along the lines of the pavilions in Friedrichsberg, should be built to house about 200 patients. Central administrative buildings and coverage areas should be added to provide support for the increased number of patients.

Based on this report of May 1888, the health authorities mandated public health officer Dr. C. Reinhard to analyze possible solutions, and he proposed to develop a new agricultural colony, for which he had a precise vision.

> It is important that the whole must appear, as far as possible, as a wealthy village, because then the sick persons will feel more comfortable. That is why the residential houses must avoid being all the same size and constructed in the same style, since an awkward monotony would be created that unintentionally evokes the idea of modern

---

1 Klaus Böhme, ed., *1893–1993 100 Jahre Allgemeines Krankenhaus Ochsenzoll* (Hamburg: Sozialtherapiezentrum des AK Ochsenzoll, 1993), 8.

proletarian quarters near the factories. It would be best to construct houses for forty, thirty, and twenty mentally ill persons and to further sub-divide the former two into two sections.[2]

The health authority decided to purchase an area of 185 acres called "fir tree pasture" (*Tannenkoppel*) situated far outside of Hamburg, in Langenhorn. The organizational plan designated Friedrichsberg as the exclusive referring institution for the new colony. Reinhard recommended that the direction of the institution should be assigned to a psychiatrist under whom all employees would be subordinated, while he himself would answer to the medical director of Friedrichsberg.[3] It was also determined that male patients would work on the farm and in the workshops, with female patients in the kitchen, the sewing centre, or in the garden. After completion of the first four 50-bed houses to care for the patients (male patients in houses one and two, and female patients in houses 21 and 22), the agricultural colony for the insane (*Landwirtschaftliche Kolonie für Geisteskranke*) was officially inaugurated on 1 April 1893. As of that date, the colony accommodated 119 patients, where 99 % of the male patients and 88 % of the female patients were working.

The first annual report defined the agricultural asylum as an institution designed for the "admission of quiet and chronically ill patients with the ability to work."[4] This report also emphasized the health benefits of the colony's location, as it resided within a forest and thus in an area without traffic. Furthermore, the report highlighted the "open-door-system" (*Offene-Türen-System*) that it claimed produced a village-like atmosphere at the colony. However, this ideal was apparently never quite realized. By 25 April 1895, the public health officer, Dr. Deneke, described the quality of the accommodations in a letter to the Medical Council (*Medizinalkollegium*). "Hitherto the existence of a colony in Langenhorn cannot be perceived; the asylum with its checkered buildings distributed in a confined space has nothing in common with a rural settlement." According to Deneke, Langenhorn seemed to be a "military complex of buildings like those one would find on a firing range."[5]

Nevertheless, the "open-door-system" was understood as a continuation of the "no-restraint-principle," which had been introduced in 1861 by Ludwig Meyer with the intent to abolish coercive treatment in Friedrichsberg. The precondition for this system was the "selection of suitable sick persons," as noted by

---

2 Ibid., 10.
3 Michael Wunder, *Euthanasie in den letzten Kriegsjahren. Die Jahre 1944 und 1945 in der Heil- und Pflegeanstalt Hamburg Langenhorn*, eds. Rolf Winau and Heinz Müller-Dietz, Abhandlungen zur Geschichte der Medizin und der Naturwissenschaften ed., Vol. 65 (Husum: Matthiesen, 1992), 36.
4 Ibid.
5 Böhme, *1893–1993 100 Jahre Allgemeines Krankenhaus Ochsenzoll*, 15.

the annual report. At the end of 1894, the asylum housed 150 male and 49 female patients, with the nursing auxiliary force made up of 11 male guards and 4 female guards.[6]

In 1894, plans were developed to enlarge Langenhorn again. Dr. Theodor Neuberger, a senior psychiatrist at Friedrichsberg and Langenhorn's medical director from 1898 on, supported the idea of transferring patients unfit for work from Friedrichsberg to Langenhorn, because the number of patients able to work was limited and Friedrichsberg needed a certain number of working patients in order to maintain its own infrastructure. The patient population (*Krankenbestand*) in Friedrichsberg had changed significantly, according to Neuberger, because through the transfer or discharge of "orderly, quiet patients that are able to work, many beds had become free and were now taken up by partly unreliable, unsocial, or even physically sick persons." He claimed that "pavilions must be constructed in Langenhorn for patients who were not constantly able to work and for restless mentally ill patients" in order to create normal conditions in Friedrichsberg.[7] On 5 April 1897, the health authority approved Neuberger's concept and began the construction of new houses at Langenhorn.[8] Surveillance houses were constructed to accommodate "anti-social" and patients perceived as dangerous to public safety. Observation houses for semi-quiet patients were also built, as well as rural houses to accommodate quiet sick persons who were relatively free to circulate. From this point on, Langenhorn treated many different categories of mentally ill persons and consequently, the open-door system was practically abandoned. Accordingly, the name was changed on 20 March 1899 to "Lunatic Asylum Langenhorn" (*Irrenanstalt Langenhorn*), and altogether now accommodated 500 patients.

From 1896 to1899, Langehorn experienced on average an increase of 72 patients per year. Responding to this steady growth, Neuberger prepared a position paper (*Denkschrift*) demanding a second enlargement of 860 beds, with a view to a subsequent increase of 1400 beds.[9] He justified his claims of expanding the institution on the basis that the nearby major city of Hamburg was producing larger numbers of mentally ill persons and mentally ill criminals, and that the city was not providing any relief for its lunatic asylums through "family care." Neuberger's report was accepted but it must be emphasized that the Provincial state government of Hamburg counted the construction of a specifically secured house (House #9) for the accommodation of mentally ill criminals a high priority

---

6 Ibid., 16.
7 Theodor Dr Neuberger, "Die Irrenanstalt Langenhorn," in *Deutsche Heil- und Pflegeanstalten für psychisch Kranke in Wort und Bild*, ed. Johannes Bresler (Halle: Marhold, 1910), 311.
8 Ibid., 313.
9 Böhme, *1893–1993 100 Jahre Allgemeines Krankenhaus Ochsenzoll*, 19; Wunder, *Euthanasie in den letzten Kriegsjahren*,37.

and approved its construction in 1902, while the general enlargement of Langenhorn did not take place until 1904–1906. From 1904 onward, Langenhorn admitted patients directly without them first being admitted to Friedrichsberg, and took in remand prisoners from the penitentiary of Fuhlsbüttel to observe their mental state, as well as people who came into conflict with the law due to a mental illness. From this moment on, Langenhorn had a vital position in the penitentiary system of Hamburg.

During these years, three events regarding patient treatment are noteworthy. The first two aspects are related to a planned modification of the "Ordinance concerning the Regulation of the Service for the Insane" (*Verordnung betreffend das Irrenwesen*) which had been in force since 1899 and was modified due to organizational changes in the asylums in Hamburg. The first issue concerned the patients' right to complain, while the second centered on the question of who had legal responsibility for the decision to discharge patients from the asylum. The third event highlights modifications in the upkeep of the statistical annual register. All three aspects are discussed here in some depth because they caused disputes between psychiatrists on the one side, and the administration, police, and medical officers on the other, highlighting how resolutely the psychiatrists fought for their right to gain absolute control over the asylums in Hamburg and the patients.

The modification of the right to complain

As mentioned above, the provincial government of Hamburg designated Langenhorn as a facility able to admit convicted offenders and remand prisoners. As a result, a debate took place within the Medical Council regarding patients' right to complain about both their treatment and the conditions in Hamburg's asylums. The critique of the asylum medical directors (especially director Neuberger at Langenhorn) illustrates the self-understanding of psychiatrists in Hamburg at that time, and underlines the degree to which these psychiatrists cared about ensuring their own reach of power outside any kind of control. The fight for this uncontrolled power rose to the surface in 1906, and again in the 1920s and 1930s when the question arose as to whether or not patient incapacitation had to be a pre-condition for compulsory hospitalization.

The right to complain was regulated by paragraph six of the "Medical Ordinance" (*Medizinalordnung*) that was instituted in December 1899 and modified in 1904. According to the later modification, residents and their relatives had the right to complain to the Commission of the Medical Council for the Regulation of the Service for the Insane (*Kommission des Medizinalkollegiums für das Irrenwesen*). The management of the asylum had to provide complainants with the necessary writing utensils to submit their complaint and had to forward complaints to the commission, which was composed of representatives from the Senate of Hamburg and psychiatrists from Hamburg asylums.[10] This modification became the focus of a long-lasting conflict between the health authorities and the medical directors of Hamburg's asylums. At the end of 1906, Dr. Neuberger argued in his defence that the number of complaints had increased since the secured house for "deranged criminals and lunatics dangerous to public safety" had been inaugurated in November 1905.

> From December 1905 to 20 October 1906 the management of the asylum had to forward 40 complaints to the commission of the medical council. Of these 40 submissions, 39 derived from a stock of only 50 sick persons, all of them accommodated in the secured house. Of the rest of the sick houses that are occupied by around 600 residents, only one complaint was admitted since December 1905. The sick persons appealing from the secured house (20) were all, except for one, previously convicted criminals. In looking over their records one can find particular sick persons with 28, 22, 20, 16, 12, 9, 8, 7, 5, 4, 3 etc. reported previous convictions, among them 14 people who will always need care (*Pfleglinge*)[11] from the hard labor penal facilities (*Zuchthaus*).[12]

Furthermore, Neuberger argued that in Friedrichsberg between 1900 and 1906, only 61 complaints were submitted by "sick persons who had no previous convictions and who were not criminals," because they want to be discharged earlier and "this wish finds enough attention by the medical directors of the asylums." Although he described the "ordinary Lunatic" as "less harmful" as compared to those considered "criminal," he assumed that all mentally ill persons were dangerous and only differed in danger by degree. Criminal lunatics, however, were "pathologically uncritical and inclined to hold the physician responsible for their incarceration in the asylum, even though the physicians would be happy if they could discharge these lunatics." Neuberger believed that these patients used their right to complain to take revenge on psychiatrists, hindering patient treatment and perhaps more importantly, weakening the

---

10 *Amtsblatt*, Public Law 152, (1904): 915.
11 The German term "Pflegling" is difficult to translate into English. It is a term that is no longer in use in Germany. The term could approximately be translated as a "care dependent sick person" but the German term implies a normative dimension because it reduces the recipient of care to someone who will have to depend on care provided by others for his or her whole life. This term was used only in administrative records and in publications and thereby automatically connected to economic considerations, because someone who depends on care is an economic burden. In this study the translation 'care dependent sick person' is used as translation.
12 Staatsarchiv HH 352–8-7 Staatskrankenanstalt Langenhorn 147 (hereafter StArch, Langenhorn Administrational Record LAR 147). Neuberger, 1906, position paper to Senate of Health [n.d., n.p.].

position of the psychiatrist. Neuberger summarized his arguments by stating that

> through the right to complain the correct treatment for the individual sick person is hindered. Rather, frequent excitements and impairments are caused that could have been averted, and the position of the physician towards the sick person becomes more difficult because the position of the physician will be decreased, which disturbs the work of the physician.[13]

Neuberger supported his arguments by using a former decision of the Higher Regional Court of Hamburg (*Hanseatisches Oberlandesgericht*) from 1888. According to this legal decision, the medical director of the asylum decided on all matters concerning the sick person based on what was determined to be best for his or her healing process. Only the medical director of the asylum could determine how far patients' rights extended, a conclusion that was based on the sick person's condition or the reasons for his or her incarnation. Neuberger argued that, in the city of Hamburg, the patient's right to complain superseded the medical director's control over the patient and hence, contradicted the older judicial order. He contended further that sick persons were granted the right to complain because of the "lay public's" impression that "mentally healthy persons could be taken to the asylum and be detained there." He claimed that this fear was completely unfounded because "it could be scientifically demonstrated that a truly healthy person…was not kept in an asylum, but rather, the asylums kept only those persons who were proven to be mentally ill."[14] The paper ended with the request to withdraw the right to complain from inmates of public asylums.

Neuberger could not get his ideas entirely accepted, but his argument highlighted several important aspects. Although his paper began by rejecting the right of criminal inmates to complain, it became obvious that its true aim was to reject this right for all asylum inmates. Neuberger's justification for rejecting these claims revealed his fear over reducing the power of the asylum's medical director. If inmates of the asylum had the right to complain, then the absolute will of the medical director was jeopardized because mentally ill persons could not assess the damages that they might cause to themselves or their surroundings. Furthermore, someone lacking psychiatric knowledge could neither make informed decisions about inmates' complaints nor understand their pathological background. The scientific knowledge that psychiatrists possessed precluded them assigning patients to an asylum if they were not mad, implying that only psychiatrists were able to assess the need for asylum care. As well,

---

13 Ibid.
14 Ibid.

throughout the course of his paper, Neuberger distinguished between different classes of inmates.

Along with arguing against patients' right to complain, Neuberger also protested against a planned modification of the "Ordinance concerning the Regulation of Service for the Insane" (*Verordnung betreffend das Irrenwesen*) regarding the legal authority over patient admissions and discharges. Questions regarding this issue would flare up many times during the next 25 years, and the germ of Neuberger's arguments would resurface again and again.

Paragraph 13 of this draft regulated the discharge of patients from the asylum, with section 4 introducing a kind of rubber stamping of decisions to discharge patients who were considered incapacitated but whose reasons for admission had been judicially abolished. In these cases, according to the draft, these patients should be immediately discharged.[15]

> Regarding Paragraph 13: section 4 has to be omitted.
> Discharging patients because their perceived incapacitation has been legally revoked or abolished raises several objections. Revoking the incapacitation of sick persons does not prove that they are mentally stable or that treatment in an asylum is not necessary, but only serves to inhibit the threat of legal recourse by them. Not every form or every degree of mental disturbance qualifies for the label of incapacitation, a designation which should only be issued if the sick person is unable to take care of legal concerns. The need for treatment or incarceration in an asylum cannot be determined by a court order or a refusal to consider patients incompetent.[16]

In order to highlight the danger that might arise if decisions on admission and discharge were delegated to the legal system, Neuberger narrated a fictitious story about a "psychically disordered man" whose admission was revoked and who became a major danger to public safety outside the asylum. Note the type of mentally ill person Neuberger had in mind:

> I am especially concerned about the degenerative feeble-minded who are observed to have less obvious symptoms of mental disorder in the asylum but whose pathological incapability comes to the fore once they are left to their own resources. Then they demonstrate that *they are not able to conduct a moral life* due to the pathological organisation of their brains.[17]

This last sentence highlights what Neuberger seemed to acknowledge as the real purpose of psychiatry – the appraisal of a "moral conduct of life," which could only be estimated by an expert who possessed the scientific knowledge of psy-

---

15 Staatsarchiv HH 352 – 3 Medizinalkollegium II L 1d Bd 1, p. 80 – 94 (hereafter StArch, Medical Council MC II L 1d Bd 1). Neuberger, position paper regarding the planned modification of the "Ordinance concerning the Regulation of Service for the Insane."
16 Ibid., 97.
17 Ibid., 97 – 98. [emphasis mine]

chiatry. The inability to "conduct a moral life" was suggested 20 years later by Neuberger's colleague, Dr. Kankeleit, a psychiatrist from Langenhorn who in 1925 published an article "What do the inferiors cost the state?" (*Was kosten die Minderwertigen den Staat?*). The article dealt primarily with the social Darwinist theory of devolution, which would take place through uncontrolled reproduction of "inferiors," and he claimed that Germany needed sterilization laws modeled on those in the United States. As evidence, he cited the example of one particular family.

> An examination of 709 out of the 834 direct offspring of Ida Jukes, born in 1740, revealed that 106 were illegitimate, 181 were prostitutes, 142 were beggars and vagabonds, 64 were accommodated in poorhouses, and 76 were criminals (among them 7 murderers). All in all they had served 116 years of prison, received 784 years public welfare and had cost the state 5 million Marks for 75 of those years in prison, welfare, and direct damages. In the fifth generation all the women were prostitutes and all the men criminals.[18]

Neuberger, however, had explicitly mentioned the "degenerative feeble minded" whose prominent characteristic centered on the difficulty of determining the pathological disorder from which they suffered. Although they might have seemed "normal" at some periods of time, over time psychiatric experts could unmask their "abnormality." The degenerate thus represented a state of abnormality rather than one of illness. Neuberger's linking of the "moral conduct of life" and the theory of degeneration was no coincidence but rather described the self-concept of psychiatry at that time. In his examination of the development of modern psychiatry, Michel Foucault emphasized that the most important part of the theory of degeneration was the perception that the "degenerated" person was abnormal. According to him, the theory of degeneration provided psychiatry the opportunity to fold any kind of deviance, discrepancy, or "retardation" into a diagnosis of degeneration, allowing for a wide-ranging interference in human behaviour. Even more importantly, directly relating deviant behaviour with theory allowed psychiatry to extend its power beyond its traditional focus on curing. The idea of incurability had formerly represented a kind of psychiatric horizon, since it defined the effective limits of treatment for diseases that had been perceived as essentially curable. Nevertheless, from this moment on, psychiatry appeared to be more the technology of the abnormal, and when the status of abnormality was fixed by heredity onto the individual, the project of curing no longer made any sense.[19] Kankeleit made this correlation

---

18 Dr Kankeleit, "Was kosten die Minderwertigen den Staat?" Hamburger Anzeiger, 21, no12 (1925): 10.
19 Michel Foucault, *Les Anormaux. Cours au Collège de France. 1974– 1975*, eds. François Ewald and others (Paris: Seuil/Gallimard, 1999).

visible when he argued that, although it would be easier and less expensive to "re-integrate the inferiors as viable members into society," the power of psychiatry was insufficient to achieve this goal. As he asserted in the case of children, "however successful the care, it can only reform but it can never transform inferiors into normal humans."[20]

Foucault also argued that as the pathological content of the psychiatric domain disappeared, so too did the therapeutic dimension of psychiatry.

> Psychiatry no longer seeks to cure, or in its essence no longer seeks to cure. It can offer merely to protect society from being the victim of definitive dangers represented by people in abnormal condition (and this actually occurs at this time). With the medicalization of the abnormal and by dispensing with the ill and the therapeutic, psychiatry can claim for itself the simple function of protection and order.[21]

The notion of heredity allowed psychiatry to take on a generalized social defense role and at the same time, provided it with the grounds to interfere into the sexuality of the family. Psychiatry set itself up as the scientific protector of society, and as it became the science of the biological protection of the species, it reached the zenith of its power. This contention of social authority helps explain the intense struggle with the legal system during the first 30 years of the twentieth century over defining who was considered a danger to society and the need for asylum custody. It was on the basis of claims that psychiatry's role as the general defender of a society was being eroded from within that psychiatrists claimed the right to substitute for the judiciary.

At this point, this psychiatric reasoning introduced the kind of racism that Foucault defined as scientific racism of biopolitics (see page 43) and which explains why German psychiatry functioned so smoothly under Nazism. This racism, which was based on the linkages between notions of degeneration and heredity, was racism against the abnormal – "against individuals who, as carriers of a condition, a stigma, or any defect whatsoever, may more or less randomly transmit to their heirs the unpredictable consequences of the evil, or rather of the non-normal, that they carry within them."[22] As already emphasized in the last chapter, this kind of racism does not function as prevention or as defence of one group against another, but rather its aim is to detect inside a group the elements that may constitute a danger.

> Certainly, there were very quickly a series of interactions between this racism and traditional Western, essentially anti-Semitic racism, without, however, the two forms ever being coherently or effectively organized prior to Nazism. We should not be

---

20 Kankeleit, Was kosten die Minderwertigen den Staat?, 10.
21 Michel Foucault, *Abnormal. Lectures at the Collège De France 1974–1975*, eds. Arnold I. Davidson and others, trans. Graham Burchell (USA: Picador, 2003), 316.
22 Ibid., 316–317.

surprised that German psychiatry functioned so spontaneously within Nazism. The new racism specific to the twentieth century, this neoracism as the internal means of defense of a society against its abnormal individuals, is the child of psychiatry, and Nazism did no more than graft this racism onto the ethnic racism that was endemic in the nineteenth century.[23]

The self-conception of psychiatry in Hamburg was based on the basic approach that it was responsible for the detection of dangerous elements within society and that only the psychiatric expert could carry out this important task. Psychiatric discourse enabled relating every aspect of abnormal behavior to ideas of heredity and degeneration, as the development of record keeping in Langenhorn demonstrates.

Entry form to annual statistics at Langenhorn

An analysis of Langenhorn's annual statistics reveals that they became part of the broader context, described above, that influenced which aspects of inmates were highlighted in the annual report and accordingly, what was noteworthy about them. Among the existing sources from Hamburg's public record office (*Staatsarchiv Hamburg*) is a folder that contains handwritten and typewritten duplications of Langenhorn's annual statistics from 1893 to 1924.

These statistics were part of the asylum's annual reports for the health authority and became part of the foundation of yearly statistics collected by the government of the German Empire. From the year of its inauguration in 1893 and in the years following, Langenhorn's annual report contained a completed data entry form. This printed form was originally just a single page subdivided into three parts, and directions indicated that the form had to be completed each year by all asylums and was to include the asylum's name and the province wherein it resided. It is noteworthy that this form from the beginning designated Langenhorn as a "lunatic asylum," even though until 1899 it was considered a "colony for the insane." Evidently, the government administration did not differentiate between the status of an asylum and a colony before that date, suggesting that apparent differences between asylum and colony were artificial from the beginning. In reality, no real difference existed between the two. Furthermore, these entry forms were signed by the medical director or his representative, indicating that they were well aware of the name. In fact, the form did not even permit any other designation, implying that from the beginning, Langenhorn was officially counted as an asylum. The second part of the form requested general information about admitted patients, including gender and

---

23 Ibid., 317.

the number of inpatient days. The third part of the form, entitled "specified frequency," was designed as a table. (See Figure 1 and Table 1)

The specified frequency table classified Langenhorn's patients into four categories that were not, in fact, very selective. Though there seemed to be little purposeful difference between the categories, it is interesting to observe that already by 1893, heredity was a decisive criterion to sort inmates. How heredity was "proven" is evident by analyzing the admission forms, which posed questions about the patient's family history. (See the chapter on the analysis of the records.) A proven hereditary defect meant nothing more than a perceived "abnormality" in the inmate's family history; this could include a remote relative who drank or who had drawn attention because of a criminal offense or other wrongdoing.

The basic structure of the annual statistics persisted over the years, although the table details were modified somewhat. For example, in 1900, additional institutions were obliged to keep annual statistics and this requirement was expanded to include any "institution for mentally ill persons, epileptics, idiots, feeble-minded persons, and persons with neurological disorders." This expansion added additional categories by which to classify patients. In 1902, the table listed 11 different categories of mental illnesses including hysteria, chorea, tabes, and "other illnesses of the nervous system." Furthermore, alcoholism and "morphinism and other narcotic intoxications" were further subdivided into two distinct categories. Langenhorn, however, used only the first four categories over the years (those from the 1893 form) to classify inmates.

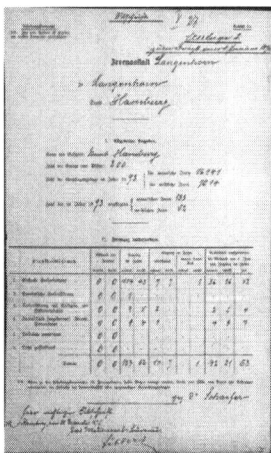

Figure 1: Original diagnostic table with specified frequency for the year 1893.[24]

---

24 Staatsarchiv HH 352–8-7 Staatskrankenanstalt Langenhorn 139. Annual Reports (hereafter StArch LAR 139).

Table 1: Translated diagnostic table with specified frequency for the year 1893.

Kind of illness	Stock on January 1		Admissions during year		Reduction over the year				Heredity proven in "the stock" at January 1 and admissions during the year		
	M	F	M	F	General		through death		M	F	Total
					M	F	M	F.			
1. Simple mental disorder	0	0	114	43	7	7	-	1	36	16	52
2. Paralytic mental disorder	0	0	1	-	-	-	-	-	-	-	-
3. Mental disorder with epilepsy, with hysterioepilepsya	0	0	9	5	2	-	-	-	2	2	4
4. Imbecility (congenital), idiocy, cretinism	0	0	9	4	1	-	-	-	4	3	7
5. Delirium potatorum	0	0	-	-	-	-	-	-	-	-	-
6. Not mentally ill	0	0	-	-	-	-	-	-	-	-	-
Amount	0	0	133	52	10	7	-	1	42	21	63

Nevertheless, the table imposed a relationship between heredity and other factors. In 1902, it listed not only "proven heredity" but also the category "proven alcohol abuse," suggesting a connection between mental illness, heredity, and alcoholism that did not exist in 1893. Furthermore, the construction of the table itself made it obvious that the two variables of "heredity" and "alcoholism" were thought to intersect with one another. Not only were the two columns drawn side by side, but the figures were also often entered congruently, giving the impression that alcoholism automatically increased the hereditary risk for the inmate's offspring to become mentally ill. Inversely, "abnormal events" in the inmate's family history were considered threats to the inherited traits of inmates, automatically increasing their risk of alcoholism. Clearly, the way in which the table was constructed affected the relationship between different categories, and consequently how they were perceived. It imposed a range of assumptions on the reader who, without any knowledge or understanding of psychiatric scientific discourse of the time, could understand that mentally ill persons could be classified into four distinct categories of mental illnesses that were all inheritable (even though their inheritance might not yet be "proven" in every case) and were connected to alcohol consumption in so far as alcoholism might have been the cause for the mental illness, or at least involved in its development. Furthermore, the table suggested a relationship between hereditary risk, alcoholism, and mental illness through its construction, making something visible that was invisible prior to its existence. This ability of annual statistics – to make certain aspects visible whilst others are rendered invisible – is used extensively in the years to come.

Further substantiation of this observation can be found in the drafts of these annual statistics. These handwritten drafts were also designed as tables but they contained more extensive and detailed information than was found in the annual statistics. Each year, a few tables were constructed for the male and female wards respectively, where each sick person was listed by first and last name, his or her date of birth, and date of admission. Adjacent to each other, the next three columns were entitled "statistical diagnosis," "psychiatric diagnosis," and "hereditary burden, alcohol abuse." The column under statistical diagnoses was further subdivided into numerous psychiatric diagnoses. "Simple mental disorder," for example, was broken down in 1903 into the following diagnoses: dementia praecox, catatonia, paranoia, dementia senile, degenerative mental disorder, etc. The next column contained information about alcohol abuse and hereditary burden, and ignoring the mutual exclusivity of these factors by combining them into one column strengthened the impression that an interrelation existed between them. At the end of the table, the cases were counted according to their statistical categories and were then analyzed in relation to hereditary and alcohol abuse. For example, the draft from 1903 counted 20 new (male) admissions with the statistical diagnosis of "simple mental disorder." According to the table, four of these admissions had a proven hereditary defect and were diagnosed with alcohol abuse. Furthermore, that same year, of the four people who were admitted with the statistical diagnosis of "paralytic mental disorder," one had a proven hereditary fault and was coincidentally abusing alcohol. The drafts highlight how interrelations between different diagnoses were actively constructed through the manner in which specific information was combined. They also pointed out that an enormous amount of work was required to create the annual statistical report, since the published tables condensed and displayed complex information in such a manner that it could be grasped at a glance.

This simplified table required several translation steps. First, the information from the admission record had to be inserted into the draft's hand-drawn table. In this first "simplification" stage, the patient's history was reduced to his or her name, place of birth, and psychological diagnosis. Any abnormal events noted were translated into a hereditary burden. Alcohol consumption became the potential for "alcohol abuse." Through this translation process, the individual disappeared and became merely one number in the statistical table. Consequently, the huge amount of work necessary to create these short tables disappeared; the necessary effort can only be guessed at by the size of the drafts, which contained many hand-drawn tables and handwritten information. For 1903, for example, the draft comprised more than 20 pages – practically a small booklet.

The next part of the draft, concerned with the "reduction in stock" over the year, was divided into two distinct tables. The first table addressed the discharged sick persons and was designed in exactly the same manner as the admission table. Even here the variables of hereditary factors and alcohol abuse were explicitly listed. Nonetheless, the last table in the draft, on the deceased inmates of the asylum, is the most interesting, although as the number of deaths rose, this table was abandoned. This table is laid out in exactly the same manner as the others except for the last column on the patient's cause of death, which was accompanied by a particular diagnosis. Neither the causes for discharge or death were published in the annual statistics; however; in a manner similar to the handling of the admission forms, the discharge tables followed the same translation process in reducing information to single figures.

In 1908, the drafts were more formalised, as the former hand-drawn tables became printed forms with formally titled columns. The titles remained the same as those from previous years, except for the column entitled "hereditary burden, alcohol," which was subsequently modified to either "able to work or bedridden." To indicate that a patient was hereditarily tainted or abused alcohol, the capital letters "H" (for *hereditas*) or "A" (for alcoholism) were used. The table was further enlarged through two additional hand-drawn columns, one for "committed by the police, transferred from *Fuhlsbüttel* (the jail house of Hamburg) for observation," and the other for "with criminal record of imprisonment or forced labour penalty." These alterations corresponded to the previously noted change in 1904 that allowed Langenhorn to directly admit prisoners from Hamburg's penitentiary. The increased complexity of the table allowed for more correlation of diverse factors. In the case of Anna Magdalena (all names are pseudonyms) for example, the statistical diagnosis of "simple mental disorder" was transformed into the psychiatric diagnosis of "dementia praecox." According to the table, she was hereditarily tainted because her "father was a drunkard;" as a result, she was not able to work but she was not bedridden. Friedrich Wilhelm had a statistical diagnosis of "simple mental disorder," but his psychiatric diagnosis marked him with "degenerative feeblemindedness," and the insertion of an A and H demonstrated that he was considered both an alcoholic and hereditarily tainted. Unlike Anna, he was able to work and was committed by the police (or came through the jail of *Fuhlsbüttel*).[25] This information had a huge impact on the narrative of patients' situations and prognoses, because it enabled editing and summarizing particular aspects of a person

---

25 Annual Report from 1908, StArch LAR 139.

without knowing any details about them, demonstrating once again how a table constructed specific correlations and functioned as a statement. Even more importantly, the categories used in this 1908 table were similar to those used 31 years later under the Nazi regime as "report sheets" (*Meldebogen T4*) for the systematic recording of mentally ill persons. The tables regarding the discharged patients and those deceased did not undergo any modifications during these years; the cause of death was still noted and the deceased's names were listed.

A further, albeit short-lived modification to these tables illustrated the ongoing efforts to compress and codify patient information. In 1909, the column entitled "able to work or bedridden" became a distinct category. The two columns introduced earlier regarding the patients' criminal records were abandoned, and in their place the category "able to work" was differentiated into the four discrete columns of "able to work," "able to work at all," "bedridden," and "can occasionally be occupied." Coded with small letters from "a" to "d," the state of the patient could thus be represented by a combination of letters and figures. For example, Albert Reinhard Gustav was coded as H2 A2c, which is to say that he was diagnosed as "paralytic" (represented by the figure 2, because "paralysis" was the second diagnosis in the list of diagnoses in the annual statistics), hereditarily tainted (represented by the capital letter H), alcohol addicted (represented by the capital letter A), and bedridden (represented by the small letter c).[26] This combination of letters and figures presented complex information about a patient in a succinct manner, and even though this system of compressed information did not outlast the year 1909, it nevertheless highlighted enduring efforts to compress information into the smallest units possible. (See Figure 2). This year was also the first year that the patient's cause of death was no longer differentiated. Only the names and the statistical diagnoses of the deceased were listed thereafter. These considerations highlight the fact that discursive statements are not solely linguistic but can contain any kind of linguistic structure. Important forms of statements are figures, statistics, and maps.[27] Accounting, for example, forms a body of knowledge that often competes with the knowledge of other experts, but calculative devices allow it to direct actions within organizations and within society.

Figures are an indispensable part of complex technologies used by governments. Only through using figures does it become possible to intervene in specific areas and to demarcate the delineations and inner characteristics of populations, economies, and societies.[28] From 1900 on, the Langenhorn ad-

---

26 Annual Report from 1909. StArch LAR 139.
27 Nikolas Rose, "Numbers," in Nikolas Rose, *Powers of Freedom. Reframing Political Thought* (Cambridge: Cambridge University Press, 2005), 197–232.
28 Ibid.; Peter Miller, "Accounting as Social and Institutional Practice: An Introduction," in

ministration through asylum statistics was anxious to summarize different aspects of patients' diagnoses and biographies into a single combination of figures and letters. In doing so, relations between the different aspects of the person were implicitly established by statistics; annual statistics became statements of their own about the relationship between, for example, alcoholism and degeneration. These statistics demonstrate that language is a medium that dictates its conditions on speech and installs "regimes of truth."[29] Subjects do not pre-exist discourses but are constructed through "regimes of truth." The latter is also the objective of this book: to reconstruct empirically how patients became subjects in the medical record.

This is what happened in the construction of these tables. Sociologist of science and philosopher Ian Hacking who understands his work as supporting Foucault's theoretical concept of biopower refers to the open and subversive effects of statistical operations.[30] Hacking demonstrated that any category has its own history, which is influenced by two vectors. The first vector, according to Hacking, is the "labelling from above" emanating from a community of experts, which creates a reality. Distinguishable from this first vector is the vector "autonomous behaviour" of the persons labelled in such a manner. This second vector generates a pressure from the bottom up, which creates a reality that any expert has to consider. Hacking calls this "dynamic nominalism," which remains an intriguing doctrine, arguing that numerous kinds of human beings and human acts come into being hand in hand with our invention of the categories labelling them.

> It is for me the only intelligible species of nominalism, the only one that can even gesture at an account of how common names and the named could tidily fit together ... [O]ur spheres of possibility, and hence ourselves, are to some extent made up of our naming and what that entails.[31]

The analysis thus far has suggested that important patient information was compressed into a format that retained the most data in a minimal amount of space. After 1914, however, a further modification left deceased patients unnamed and anonymous. This change occurred at precisely the moment when the number of deaths began to rise dramatically, due more or less to the intentional starvation of sick persons in German asylums during the First World War. Even

---

Accounting as Social and Institutional Practice, eds. Anthony G. Hopwood and Peter Miller (Cambridge: Cambridge University Press, 1994), 1–39.
29 Michel Foucault. *L'archéologie du savoir.* (France: Gallimard, 2008).
30 Ian Hacking, "Making Up People," in *Reconstructing Individualism: Autonomy, Individuality, and Self in Western Thought*, eds. Thomas C. Heller, Morton Sosna and David E. Wellbery (Stanford: Stanford University Press, 1986), 222–237; Ian Hacking, "Biopower and the Avalanche of Printed Numbers," *Humanaties in Society* Band 5 (1982): 279–295.
31 Hacking, Making Up People, 227.

though a direct correlation between this change in bookeeping and the murder of sick persons cannot be explicitly proven, it is noteworthy that all records concerning the increase in mortality rate in Langenhorn from 1913–1917 were oddly incomplete. Furthermore, by omitting the individual names of victims, the patients lost their identity and could not be grieved for. It is as if they were reduced to a single figure; the dead lost their status as individualised dead.

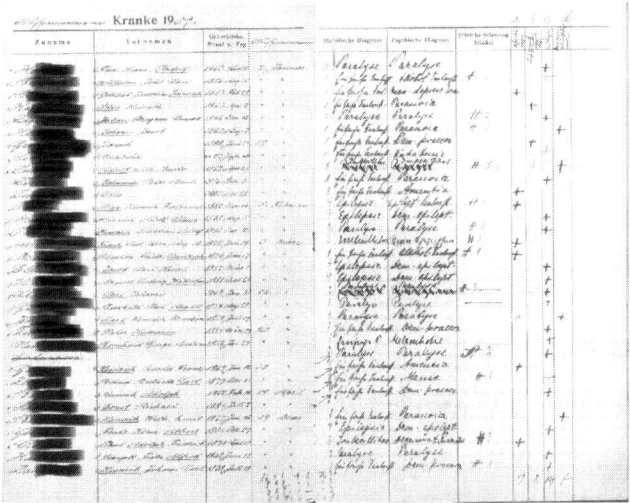

Figure 2: Original printed form with handwritten modifications.[32]

Although the statistical table was resumed in its initial form in the 1920s, it never became as detailed as in the years between 1893 and 1908. The patients were individually listed with their names, but neither their ability to work nor a differentiation between statistical and psychological diagnoses was resumed. Even the causes of death were never again listed after the war.

---

32 StArch LAR 139.

The First Wave: Killing Sick Persons through Starvation

From 1910 to 1914, a third enlargement of Langenhorn took place with the bed capacity increased to 2000. This enlargement was again justified due to overcrowding at Friedrichsberg and to the steady increase in the number of mentally ill persons needing admission, which was again blamed on the facility's proximity to the city.[33] At that time, the idea evolved that a third asylum should be built near Langenhorn. In a letter from 10 February 1910 to Dr. Schröder, the mayor of Hamburg, Neuberger cautioned against building "open houses." He warned that the type of sick people who must be "supervised more or less intensely or that are not fit for less-secured housing accommodations" were estimated to make up the majority of the future patient population.[34] Neuberger further claimed that the planned new asylum should contain at least four pavilions, each one with 30 to 35 beds for class III patients who were mostly clerks and civil servants (*Büroangestellte*). These four pavilions, he wrote, should be divided into

> two for males and two for females. On each side, one pavilion would be assigned to secure care-dependent sick persons ("*Pfleglinge*"), those who required continuous care and were in need of monitoring, whereas each side of the II. hospital [Langenhorn] would accommodate the more harmless and sick persons eligible for a freer therapy.[35]

As Neuberger's letter suggested, the grounds of Langenhorn were subdivided by a road with each side segregated by sex. Asylum construction was a technology of individualization and physical control, with the focus on the patient as an object of control rather than on having a disease amenable to therapy. One suspects that debates over restraint were not so much arguments between promoters of restraint and non-restraint but were more concerned with the mechanism (mechanical or architectural) best suited to the psychiatric practice of rationality. Debates in Hamburg over this issue were no different from other European countries.[36] The desire for control and segregation was a central mechanism behind asylum construction; Langenhorn was a disciplinary space. However, architectural organization also expressed a distinct division of labour, since space within the asylum was distributed in accordance with a hierarchy of labour; volume and status overlapped to ensure that those who inhabited the

---

33 Wunder, *Euthanasie in den letzten Kriegsjahren*, 37.
34 Staatsarchiv HH 352–8-7 Staatskrankenanstalt Langenhorn 8 (hereafter StArch LAR 8). Letter from Dr. Neuberger to Dr. Schröder, 10 February 1910 [n.p.].
35 Ibid.
36 Lindsay Prior, "The Architecture of the Hospital: A Study of Spatial Organization and Medical Knowledge," *The British Journal of Sociology* 39, no. 1 (March 1988): 86–113.

higher echelons of the disciplinary apparatus obtained the largest amount of space. (See Figures 3 and 4) As sociologist Lindsay Prior has argued,

> the greatest amount of space is assigned to the supervisors, less to the keepers, yet still less to the menial functionaries. It is an architecture of social hierarchy which echoes throughout the nineteenth and twentieth centuries, and serves to underpin the strict division of tasks which define modern medical practice.[37]

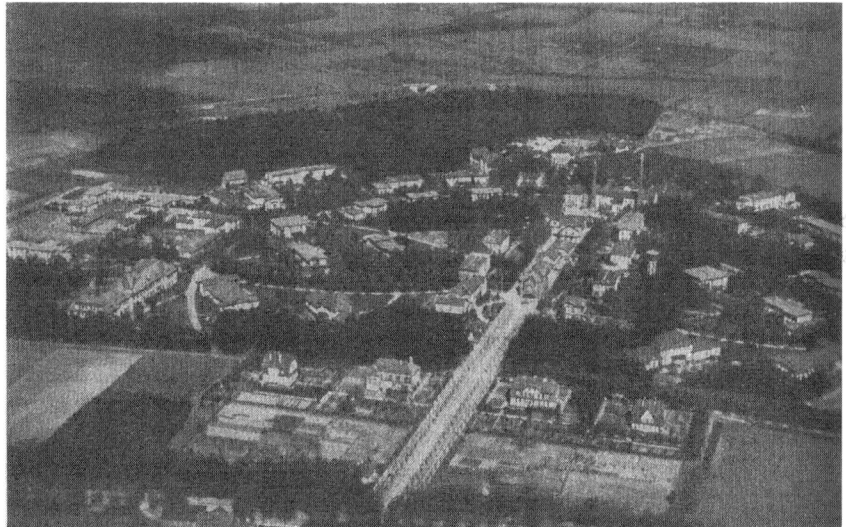

Figure 3: Aerial photography of Langenhorn around 1925.[38]

The onset of the First World War prevented any expansion at Langenhorn, nor was a third asylum ever built. A 1913 tally of all people living and working in the asylum demonstrated that 10 psychiatrists, 34 clerks, 3 nurses, 341 guards (211 males and 130 females), and 181 supervisors, workers and mechanics attended to the needs of 1809 inmates.[39] This breakdown meant that each psychiatrist supervised approximately 180 inmates and each nurse approximately 603 inmates – though supported by 344 guards – which left each guard responsible for approximately 5 inmates. According to this bed capacity, Langenhorn exceeded the size of Friedrichsberg.

---
37 Ibid., 106.
38 Dr. Gerhard Schäfer and Rudolf Birkenstock, "Staatskrankenanstalt Langenhorn," in *Hygiene und soziale Hygiene in Hamburg. Zur neunzigsten Versammlung der deutschen Naturforscher und Ärzte in Hamburg im Jahre 1928*, ed. Gesundheitsbehörde Hamburg (Hamburg: Paul Hartung Verlag, 1928), 200.
39 StArch LAR 139 [n.p.]. Tally of all people living and working in the asylum from the year 1913.

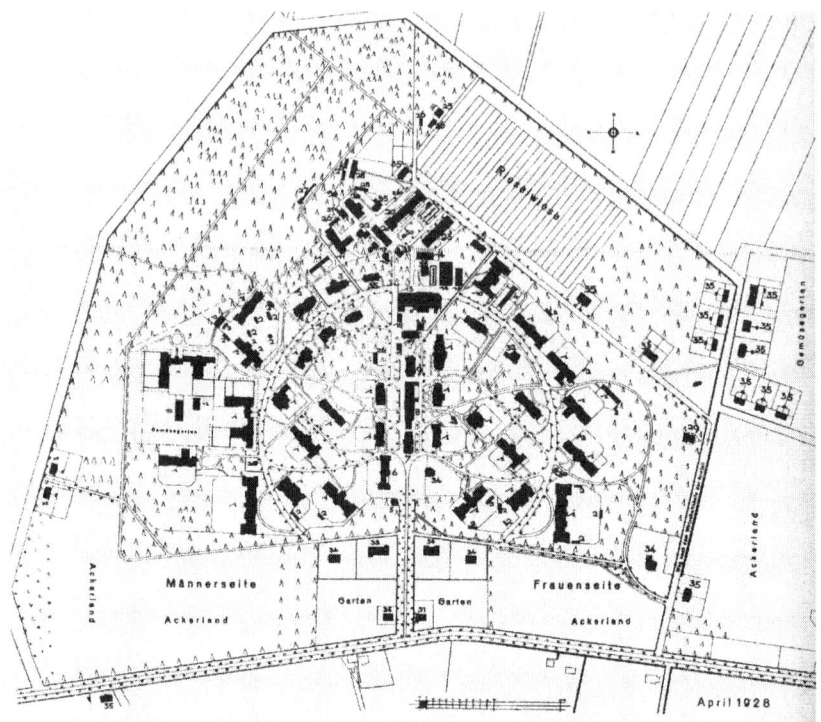

Figure 4: General plan of the asylum of Langenhorn, c.1925. Explanation: Left: men's side (*Männerseite*); Right: women's side (*Frauenseite*) 1) houses for mentally ill patients, 2) halls for tuberculosis treatment, 3) X-ray, 4) nursing school, 5) Emergency room and pharmacy, 6) administrative building, 7) house for social and religious events, 8) kitchen building, 9) warehouse, 10) laundry, 11) workshop, 12) houses for occupational therapy, 13) machine house, 14) coal storage, 15) well houses, 16) water towers, 17) bathhouse, 18) disinfection house, 19) workshop, 20) stables, 21) slaughterhouse, 22) cold storage house, 23) barn, 24) cart scale, 25) warehouse for agricultural machines, 26) warehouse, 27) bowling alley, 28) greenhouses, 29) morgue, 30) guard houses, 31) gatehouse, 32) residence of the medical director, 33) residence of the administrative director, 34) residences for senior physicians and ward physicians, 35) residences for civil servants and clerks.[40]

During the First World War, many of the male personnel were called up to war service. At the end of 1914, 8 physicians and 282 civil servants and staff, including 179 guards and chief warders, had been drafted. Two years later most of the guards had gone. At this time, since almost 2000 patients were accommodated in Langenhorn, temporary staff was engaged and tradesmen took over the duties of the guards and nurses. Regardless of temporary staff hires, the

---

40 Schäfer und Birkenstock, *Staatskrankenanstalt Langenhorn*, 208.

quarterly report from October 1917 mentioned that no guards were available to monitor the secured houses.[41]

With the beginning of the war in August 1914, all development had stopped at the Langenhorn asylum, and the proposed fourth enlargement was abandoned. At the outbreak of war, Langenhorn had more than 1800 patients but only 1300 remained at the end. Incomplete statistical records reveal the reason for this decline. Shortly before war broke out, approximately 100 patients per year died in the asylum. This number nearly doubled in 1916 and nearly quintupled one year later.[42] The increasing mortality rate was the result of a catastrophic lack of supplies during wartime, which plagued Langenhorn as well as other asylums in the German Reich where hospitalized mentally ill patients became victims of a prolonged starvation.[43] In his function as the medical director of Langenhorn, Neuberger wrote a striking letter to Mayor Schröder on 5 June 1917 in which he pointed out that

> we imposed such severe restrictions on the nutrition of sick persons and personnel that now we have achieved a limit beyond which we cannot go without considerable damage to the inmates of the asylum. The body weight of the patients has continuously and exceedingly diminished.[44]

Neuberger wrote his letter more than four years after the mass mortality began, and thus this protest seems comparatively gentle given the extent of the starvation in Langenhorn. Furthermore, quarterly reports from Langenhorn to the hospital council gave the impression that the mass deaths occurring in the asylum were not as alarming as believed. Neuberger had earlier written that

> [t]he general regulations regarding the reduction in food rations for the individual sick person, especially for men, have resulted in a more or less decrease in weight that is quite remarkable, nevertheless, one could not say that this weight loss is, in general, especially considerable. It does not appear to be more than the weight loss that occurs in civilians living under the same conditions outside the asylum. We make sure that by cooking a combination of potatoes and cabbage, turnips or roots, along with the permitted amount of meat, that the sick persons at least receive a filling portion food at lunchtime ... Even though here and there some sick persons, especially those who were well known as big eaters, complain about too small portions, one has to emphasize that, in general, conditions due to the war are accounted for in an understanding manner

---

41 Staatsarchiv HH 352-8-7 Staatskrankenanstalt Langenhorn 16a (hereafter StArch LAR 16a). Quarterly Report from Oct. 1917 [n.p.].
42 StArch LAR 16a [n.p.]. Annual Reports of the years 1916 and 1917.
43 Böhme, *1893-1993 100 Jahre Allgemeines Krankenhaus Ochsenzoll*.
44 Neuberger as cited in Klaus Böhme and Uwe Lohalm, eds., *Wege in den Tod. Hamburgs Anstalt Langenhorn und die Euthanasie in der Zeit des Nationalsozialismus*, Forum Zeitgeschichte ed., Vol. 2 (Cloppenburg: Ergebnisse Verlag, 1993), 28.

and that even though the food rations are significantly reduced during war time, many patients are content.⁴⁵

Considering that in the first quarter of 1917 the death toll of patients who died from starvation exceeded that of the entire year of 1913, this letter makes a mockery of the conditions that they had to endure. Not wanting to alert the health authorities to this shocking phenomenon, Neuberger manipulated his statistics. Although he mentioned the increasing number of asylum deaths in the quarterly report of 14 April 1917, he compared the body count only from the first three months of the years spanning 1914 to 1917: 32 in 1914, 27 in 1915; 40 in 1916, and 99 in 1917. These flawed reference points – especially since the mortality rate had already begun to increase in 1914 – played down the extent of starvation in Langenhorn. Even though the patient death rate was accelerating in 1917, in his 12 July quarterly report of that year Neuberger wrote that

> recently the health status of the sick persons has become better. In an annual medical report that I received from the *Provinzial-Heil-und Pflegeanstalt Kreuzburg O.-S.* [another German asylum] I found a notice stating that the number of deaths in 1916 had doubled over 1915, due to the reduced food conditions. In Langenhorn, we counted 158 deaths and in 1916, we had [only] 208.⁴⁶

The increasing deaths of Langenhorn patients were further trivialized by comparing them to another asylum, which had nothing to do with Langenhorn. By referencing the degree of severity in this other asylum, the mass starvation of sick persons in Langenhorn appeared more moderate. In this situation as well, Neuberger used the years 1915 and 1916 as a comparison, withholding the fact that the number of deaths increased fivefold compared to 1913.

As previously highlighted, the manner in which the annual statistics were handled during wartime suggests that the reasons for the mass mortality rate were covered up. Recorded causes of death only add to this evidence. To a large extent, those who died of starvation were officially classified as dying from cardiac insufficiency. The striking increase in numbers of dead persons from this diagnosis occasioned the health authority (*Medizinalamt*) to ask officials at Langenhorn if this phenomenon could be explained by undernourishment. As they answered, "in such similar cases that can be conceived as due to undernourishment, we specified the cause of death as due to cardiac insufficiency."⁴⁷

It is important to note that these strategies in dealing with the more or less intended assassinations of sick persons are exactly the same methods employed

---

45 StArch LAR 16a [n.p.]. Letter from Neuberger to the health authority, 24 January 1917.
46 Ibid.
47 Staatsarchiv HH 352 – 8-7 Staatskrankenanstalt Langenhorn 110 (hereafter: StArch LAR 110) [n.p.].Letter from the administration of Langenhorn to the health authority, no signature, 1916.

in a systematic manner during the Nazi regime. The asylums in Hamburg were inspected every year by the Commission for the Regulation of the Service for the Insane (*Kommission für das Irrenwesen*), which provided an annual report about the situation in Langenhorn. Each year the Commission had no complaints; the increasing number of deaths received no mention.[48] Furthermore, psychiatrists of the Weimar Republic appeared to agree on the results of starvation in German asylums from 1914 to 1918: "situations exist, in which the weal and woe of the stronger may override the right to live of the feeble," was their response.[49] That these events had a decisive impact later is highlighted by the fact that the "Euthanasia planner" of the Nazi regime 20 years later referred to these incidents. Dr. Rautenberg, head of Hamburg's main health authority (*Hauptgesundheitsamt*) under the Nazis, referred to these events during the legal proceedings against him regarding his involvement in euthanasia actions.

> The first time I heard about euthanasia endeavours was at the end of the First World War, when the food situation became disastrous after the serious years of war while the asylums were full of mentally ill persons. At that time the question was raised – an unworthy life is an unnecessary eater.[50]

From 1914 to 1919 the number of inmates decreased in Langenhorn and Friederichsberg by approximately 40 % and 35 %, respectively. Since only 1305 patients remained in Langenhorn,[51] the decrease in numbers enabled the first large conversion of psychiatric beds into space for the treatment of physical illnesses. The freed-up beds were used for the treatment of tuberculosis, and at this point, the asylum was renamed the Public Hospital Langenhorn (*Staatskrankenanstalt*). Using the asylum as a pulmonary sanatorium, however, lasted only 12 1/2 years.

Langenhorn Between the Wars and During the Nazi Regime

Not until the years 1927/28 did the occupancy rate regain the scale of the pre-war years with a total of 1846 psychiatric patients. Once again, talk developed in Hamburg about the overcrowding of public asylums. By 1925, two position papers from Langenhorn and Friedrichsberg had alerted the health authority

---

48 Staatsarchiv HH 352–8-7 Staatskrankenanstalt Langenhorn 17 (hereafter: StArch LAR 17) Annual reports of the Commission for the Regulation of the Service for the Insane, n.p.
49 Wunder, *Euthanasie in den letzten Kriegsjahren. Die Jahre 1944 und 1945 in der Heil- und Pflegeanstalt Hamburg Langenhorn*, 38.
50 Böhme, Klaus and Uwe Lohalm, eds. *Wege in den Tod. Hamburgs Anstalt Langenhorn und die Euthanasie in der Zeit des Nationalsozialismus* (Cloppenburg: Ergebnisse Verlag, 1993).
51 Böhme, *1893–1993 100 Jahre Allgemeines Krankenhaus Ochsenzoll*, 24.

that the situation in both hospitals had become unsustainable. Both of the medical directors at Langenhorn and Friedrichsberg argued that the number of patients forced not only quantitative changes in the asylums, but also qualitative changes due to an increase in the severity of mental illnesses observed. The number of surveillance rooms in Friedrichsberg exceeded the number of those offered in any other German asylum. According to the authors, the number of chronically ill patients had increased and developing therapeutic treatments, especially so-called fever therapies, necessitated a more intensive observation of the patients. Underlying these complaints was the implicit suggestion that asylum space should be alleviated by transferring chronically ill patients to other facilities.[52] On 20 October 1926, Dr. Gerhard Schäfer, medical director of Langenhorn, proposed a modification of the penal code to allow for specific facilities that were half way between psychiatric asylums and prisons in order to accommodate especially those inmates deemed to have diminished capabilities. He named these institutions "inter-institutions" (*Zwischenanstalten*)

> [which did not necessarily need] to be accommodated in new construction. A portion of mentally inferiors ... resides in psychiatric asylums [but] a much larger segment can be found in prisons. I suggest designating and installing specific small prisons or independent parts of bigger prisons to be used exclusively as "inter-institutions."[53]

Schäfer's petition demonstrated that Hamburg's psychiatrists had begun very early on to differentiate between cases that should be kept in facilities with a more "prison like" character as opposed to those more like hospitals. This distinction enabled psychiatrists to transfer patients according to such criteria as their potential danger to society, their ability to work, and the chronic nature of their illness.

The health authorities adopted parts of this proposed strategy, but instead of constructing a third asylum in Hamburg, they decided to discharge patients deemed chronically ill from Langenhorn to a network of other asylums outside the city. The Lippische Heilanstalt Lindenhaus, for example, agreed to accommodate 60–65 patients, and the city of Lübeck received budgetary funds to build houses in Heilanstalt Strecknitz, which would accommodate 400 psychiatric patients from Hamburg.[54]

---

52 Staatsarchiv HH 352-8-7, Staatskrankenanstalt Langenhorn 9 (hereafter StArch LAR 9), Copies of the position papers, one entitled "Memorandum regarding the Development of Care for lunatics in Hamburg," Langenhorn, 12 January 1925 and the other, "Memorandum regarding the Development of the Provision of Care for Lunatics in Hamburg," Friedrichsberg, 24 August 1925, [n.p.].
53 Staatsarchiv HH 352-8-7, Staatskrankenanstalt Langenhorn 12 (hereafter: StArch LAR 12), Position paper of Dr. Schäfer regarding the "Intended Reorganization of Hospital Order Treatment (Penal Code)," 20 October 1926, [n.p.].
54 Peter Delius, *Das Ende von Strecknitz: die Lübecker Heilanstalt und ihre Auflösung 1941: ein*

Psychiatrists determined clear criteria that dictated the kind of patients to be transferred to these external facilities. Langenhorn's medical director highlighted the reasoning behind the transfers in a letter initiated by a father's complaint to the health authority of Hamburg over his daughter's transfer to Strecknitz and his subsequent request to relocate her back to Langenhorn. To explain his actions, the medical director wrote that

> [t]he pat.[patient] was treated here [in Langenhorn] for schizophrenia from 2.8.1930 to 26.8.1937 and then transferred to Strecknitz/Lübeck. With short interruptions, this sick person has demonstrated throughout the years a completely catatonic disorder often accompanied by severe agitation, which was the reason why she had to be kept in an isolation room most of the time. The mother of the sick person was treated here for a long time for the same condition and was then discharged as reformed. Because we have had numerous referrals from Friedrichsberg, room had to be made and therefore even patients with good family support have to be transferred. Sick persons who rarely receive visits or no visits at all were already transferred long ago.[55]

This short excerpt demonstrates that the criteria for the transfers to Strecknitz were the same as those employed by the Nazi administration during "*Aktion T4.*" One criterion for transfer depended on the chronic nature of the illness, with the assumption that patients were incurable and needed extended care. This distinction between "hopeless" and curable cases was an integral part of psychiatric practice, including that at Langenhorn. In 1931, a specific department with 400 beds was established there to accommodate "care-dependent" sick persons. This department required lower hospital and nursing charges and alleviated other overcrowded welfare institutions in Hamburg by admitting their patients as well. Another criterion was the frequency of visits to a patient. The fact that sick persons who did not receive any visits were already transferred long ago illuminates a routine procedure that had existed for years, and therefore was not invented by the Nazis.

During this period, many facilities for the mentally ill were involved in transferring hundreds of patients to other facilities. The manner in which these transports were organized foreshadows the way transfers took place during the Nazi regime. For example, Langenhorn received a group of displaced patients from Farmsen, a welfare institution. When the medical director complained about the condition in which some of these patients arrived, Farmsen's director replied that

---

Beitrag zur Sozialgeschichte der Psychiatrie im Nationalsozialismus (Kiel: Malik-Verlag, 1988).

55 Staatsarchiv HH 352–3, Medizinalkollegium II L1d Bd.2 (hereafter: StArch MC II L1d Bd 2), 52, Letter from Langenhorn to the health authority of Hamburg regarding a complaint of a husband of a former patient of Langenhorn, 24 November 1937.

[d]uring the quick transfer of 230 inmates from Farmsen to Langenhorn, Farmsen was in a difficult situation. The inmates wanted to stay in their familiar environment and expressed their aversion by protest actions, states of excitation, and attempts to escape. Therefore, it was necessary to smoothly evacuate the number of inmates requested by Langenhorn ... Even in the male group, a certain number were informed at the last minute about their transfer and therefore could not accordingly be treated ... In order to relieve their anxiety, inmates suffering from a disease that drove them to collect things were allowed to collect and keep their so-called property.[56]

I suggest that this evidence conflicts with earlier research that assumed large patient transfers took place only after the closure of Friedrichsberg in 1934.[57] Furthermore, it clearly highlights the fact that these transfers, a strategy adopted by the Nazi administration, were more or less hidden from patients and their families as early as 1932. Long before the Nazis came to power a sophisticated selection system was already in place in Hamburg. From early on, a hierarchical system of institutions had enabled the dispersion of psychiatric patients according to their perceived prospects for cure, their tendency to become dangerous, and their ability to work, etc. – an organizational structure that was further developed and refined in the years to come. Since only Friedrichsberg undertook any therapeutic treatment, only patients believed curable remained there. Patients considered incurable were sent to Langenhorn, and if considered a hopeless case, were kept in the care-dependent department or further transferred to external facilities.

However, the transfer process initiated great controversy around who held responsibility for deciding which patients were to be admitted to asylums. In order to reduce the numbers of admissions in general, a welfare administration attempted to enforce a stricter admission procedure under the guidance of a medical officer in the years 1931 and 1932. This procedure was called "combing out," (*Auskämmen*),[58] a method decisively rejected by the then medical director of Friedrichsberg, Prof. Dr. Wilhelm Weygandt. He especially protested against the idea that medical officers and the police should decide whether or not patients were a proven danger to public safety, a precondition for compulsory admission. According to Weygandt, only the psychiatrist in the asylum was able to detect the patient's delirium and it was only within the asylum that the mentally ill person would display all of the symptoms to help determine his or

---

56 Staatsarchiv HH 352–8-7, Staatskrankenanstalt Langenhorn 15 (hereafter StArch LAR 15) Memo in order to prepare for a meeting of the medical and administrative directors of Hamburg's asylums and nursing homes with the Senator of Health, 16 March 1932, n.p., no signature.
57 Michael Wunder, "Die Auflösung von Friedrichsberg – Hintergründe und Folgen," *Hamburger Ärzteblatt* 44 (1990): 128–131.
58 StArch AR 15, Minute of the meeting of the medical and administrative directors of Hamburg's asylums and nursing homes with the Senator of Health, 29 April 1932, n.p.

her level of danger to public safety. He argued that the current approach to proving the danger of patients prior to their admission had resulted in serious consequences and casualties: "One lunatic whose admission was delayed because his danger to the public had yet to be proven, indeed proved his danger by assassinating his family."[59]

Although he believed that all mentally ill persons were potentially dangerous, Weygandt nevertheless maintained that only the psychiatrist was able to make this determination. He also rejected the idea that asylum administrators should encourage families of mentally ill persons to support their "harmless" maniac members as long as possible in order to reduce the stress on the asylums, stating that next of kin, as "inferiors," were unable to estimate the real magnitude of the illness.

> The idea of influencing the next of kin to keep the harmless sick person in the family means to act in a medically irresponsible manner. Most of the family members are wrongly convinced of the harmlessness of their patient family member and one has to continuously convince them not to take them carelessly out of the asylum.[60]

The medical director of Friedrichsberg advocated for the central position of the psychiatrist within the welfare system. In 1923, he had already complained in a letter to the health authority about "sweetheart reports" issued by general practitioners who wanted to preserve the right to admit to the asylum, and affirmed that these medical officers did not have the appropriate knowledge to make these kinds of decisions.[61] However, the regulations of the "Ordinance concerning the Regulation of the Service for the Insane" from 1900 remained in effect. Mentally ill persons who became disruptive could be admitted directly to an asylum by the police and the police then had to initiate a subsequent examination by a medical officer to approve the admission.

The controversy about the legal responsibility for admission to an asylum and the duration of hospitalization was once again taken up in 1934 because of a specific case about a compulsory admission to Friedrichsberg. The debate centred on whether or not patients needed a legal designation of incapacitation before being admitted to the asylum, with the implication that they could be automatically discharged and thus bypassing the need for the decision of a medical expert if this judgment was overruled. As described earlier, this same controversy had taken place around the year 1906, and, as had been feared before, the medical director perceived that this legal requirement would infringe

---

59 StArch AR 15, Position paper to the health authority, 2 April 1932, n.p.
60 Ibid.
61 Staatsarchiv HH 352–3, Medizinalkollegium II L5 Bd.3 (hereafter StArch MC II L5 Bd.3), Letter from Weygandt to the health authority, only specification of the year 1923, n.p.

on the right of psychiatrists to decide what was best for their patients irrespective of their legal status.

> The question of whether a sick person can be discharged from the asylum is in many cases a question of subjective estimation – a so-called relative indication...Only the expert physician is able to decide; he can demand that the necessary confidence is given to him.[62]

However, psychiatric claim to authority over admissions and discharges was finally legalized on 21 February 1934, when the Nazi administration modified the previous ordinance by eliminating the commitment that every admission had to be reviewed by a medical officer. In the end, the psychiatrists had achieved their goal.

Historian and philosopher Robert Castel has analysed this long-lasting dispute, ostensibly about the development of psychiatry as a "political science," for France. He argued that this kind of power

> constituted an assault upon the principle of the separation of powers. There was no longer, on one side, the administration, the transmission belt of the executive power and guardian of public order, and on the other, the magistracy, the guarantor of liberties because it possessed a monopoly of the decisions that could suspend that guarantee. A third power, the medical one, was legitimized and ensured a new balance between the two others. The sacredness of the principles of law gave way before the practical rationality that was presented by expertise.[63]

Nonetheless, at a meeting of 29 April 1932 attended by all medical and administrative directors of Hamburg's psychiatric asylums, Hamburg's medical officer, and the senator of the health authority, administrative director Kressin, emphasized that admissions to Hamburg's asylums had diminished continuously. In 1929, 2653 people had been admitted to the asylums while 2543 had been discharged or died in the same period, giving in absolute numbers an increase of only 110 persons. Over the next two years, the total number of admissions declined over each previous year's admissions by 232 in 1930 and by 513 in 1931. Furthermore, in 1931, the *discharges and deaths outnumbered the admissions by approximately 65 persons.*[64]

---

62 Staatsarchiv HH 352 – 3, Medizinalkollegium II L1d Bd.2 (hereafter StArch MC II L 1d Bd.2), 42 – 43. Position paper of the medical director Prof. Dr. Rittershaus to the president of the health administration regarding the complaints of a former patient, 26 September 1934.
63 Robert Castel, *The Regulation of Madness: The Origins of Incarceration in France* (Great Britain: University of California Press, 1988), 189.
64 StArch LAR 15 [emphasis mine], Minute of a meeting of 29 April 1932 attended by all medical and administrative directors of Hamburg's psychiatric asylums, Hamburg's medical officer, and the senator of the health authority.

Table 2: Statistical calculation of admissions, discharges, and cases of death presented by administrational director Kressin, April 1932.[65]

Years	Discharges (absolute numbers)	Percent (discharges compared to admissions)	Cases of death (absolute numbers)	Percent (cases of death compared to admissions)
1929	2229	84 %	314	11.9 %
1930	2155	89 %	320	13.3 %
1931	1702	90 %	254	13.4 %

These percentages are suggestive, especially when viewed against the backdrop of the events during and after the First World War. As the number of admissions had decreased, the percentage rate of discharges had increased, and more importantly, the percentage of deaths was also rising in the same time period. Nevertheless, in the same meeting, medical officer Dr. Holm suggested that it might be possible, by further "combing out" less serious cases, to shut down one asylum. This idea was realized a few years later. It was also emphasized that Langenhorn had generated a financial surplus of 5 % in 1931.

The years after the takeover of the Nazi regime were characterized by a dramatic increase in the number of psychiatric beds crammed into the same asylum space. Two events aggravated the situation for Langenhorn: the closure of Friedrichsberg and the revision of the Greater Hamburg Act (*Groß-Hamburg-Gesetz*).

In 1934/35, the psychiatric asylum of Friedrichsberg was closed down, a decision based on economic grounds. Patients were to be distributed among Langenhorn, Strecknitz, and a new asylum to be built, the Clinic for Psychiatric and Nervous Diseases at Eppendorf (*Psychiatrische und Nervenklinik Eppendorf*). In Langenhorn, a hutment [a kind of barracks] was to be erected to accommodate the transferred patients from Friedrichsberg. Most historians have emphasized the economic dimension of the so-called Friedrichsberg-Langenhorn Plan,[66] but there is another interesting aspect to this restructuring of Hamburg's asylums. On 7 October 1934, the Provincial State Government of Hamburg had declared that

> curable sick persons shall be provided with the utmost medical care. Incurable sick persons shall be kept in custody and their medical support should be reduced to a justifiable minimum. Physicians will not engage with this group inside the framework

---

65 Ibid.
66 Wunder, *Die Auflösung von Friedrichsberg – Hintergründe und Folgen*; Angelika Ebbinghaus, Heidrun Kaupen-Haas and Karl Heinz Roth, *Heilen und Vernichten im Mustergau Hamburg. Bevölkerungspolitik im Dritten Reich* (Hamburg: Konkret Literatur Verlag, 1984).

of the proposed university hospital, nor should these patients be used for scientific research since that will increase the cost of their care.[67]

At this time, the Nazi administration officially legalized the already established practice of selectively sorting patients into different categories. Fourteen days later, the Provincial State Government decided to reduce the number of patients in Langenhorn in order to economize on the planned barracks. The result of this restructuring was that Langenhorn was described even by the Senator of Health, Martin Ofterdinger, as a "madhouse," since the most severe cases were transferred there.[68]

Simultaneously, through the revision of the Greater Hamburg Act (*Gross-Hamburg-Gesetz*), densely populated town areas became part of the administrative district of Hamburg and thus Langenhorn came within the district's catchment area. Two other asylums in cities near Hamburg, Lüneburg and Neustadt, also became part of the district. All three institutions played an important role as intermediate asylums during the time of the "euthanasia" action under the Nazi regime. Langenhorn was renamed a Treatment and Nursing facility (*Heil-und Pflegeanstalt*) in 1938, belying its future use.

The politics of the medical fraternity board of Hamburg can be assessed by referring briefly to its position on the sterilization of mentally ill persons. On 8 March 1933 the Nazi Senate in Hamburg was legally established, a change of power that had significant consequences for Hamburg's health policy and especially for the inmates in the asylums. As already mentioned, the "Ordinance concerning the Regulation of the Service for the Insane" was modified in 1934. A year before this event, the Federal Government in Berlin had adopted two fundamental laws: the "Law for the Prevention of Genetically Diseased Offspring" (*Gesetz zur Verhütung erbkranken Nachwuchses*) or the "Sterilization Law" (14 July 1933) and the "Law against Dangerous Habitual Criminals and their Restriction Order" (*Gesetz gegen gefährliche Gewohnheitsverbrecher und über Maßregeln der Sicherung und Besserung*) (24 November 1933). The former became effective at the beginning of January 1934; the latter had been in place since November 1933. Both laws were connected through their concern with genetics and the certain assumption that criminality was genetically determined.

Hamburg's medical fraternity broadly supported the sterilization law of July 1933.[69] Even ten years prior to the Nazi takeover of power and the enactment of this law, Hamburg's health authority had distributed a questionnaire to all

---

67 Staatsarchiv HH Hochschulwesen II, Gb 11, Bd. 1, p. 4, Declaration of the Provincial State Government of Hamburg, 7 October 1934.
68 Staatsarchiv HH Hochschulwesen II, Gb 11, Bd. 1, p. 12, Position paper by senator of health Ofterdinger, December 1934 [no exact date].
69 Böhme and Lohalm, *Wege in den Tod*, 41.

asylums, nursing homes, and schools for mentally or physically handicapped children in the city. The goal of the questionnaire was to assess the thinking about sterilizing specific residents in these institutions. Among other things, it asked if sterilization based on eugenic considerations was already taking place and tried to elicit public opinion on this issue. Friedrichsberg denied that people were already sterilized in Hamburg but, at the same time, gave a differentiated list of those people whom the medical directors considered cases that should be sterilized: "15 epileptics, 30 feeble minded, 5 idiots."[70] After the law was passed, Schäfer, Langenhorn's medical director, provided detailed instructions on how to overcome resistance against sterilization from both mentally ill people and their family members.[71]

Langenhorn During the Second World War

From 1939 on, Langenhorn became the interim "storage facility" for all Jewish patients in Schleswig-Holstein and Hamburg and the starting point of their deportation elsewhere. Although a so-called children's special ward (*Kinderfachabteilung*) was established during these years, the asylum otherwise functioned as an admission, interim, and distribution institution from which inmates were transported to various other asylums. Although the number of beds in Langenhorn was reduced by half in these years, the number of treatments was reduced only by approximately a third, meaning that more patients were cycling through the same number of beds.[72] The number of admissions and discharges for the year 1944 resembled those from 1931; at this time, when Langenhorn had 1220 beds available, 1321 patients were admitted, with 1147 being discharged or transferred and 497 dying. Despite the high number of admissions, the occupancy rate decreased.[73] Nor were the nurses outnumbered: an estimated nurse to patient ration in the years 1944/45 is 1 to 3.7.[74] According to the statistical analysis of medical historian Michael Wunder, transports of patients were put together during the war years and sent off; the table below (Table 3) compares

---

70 StArch MC II L5 Bd.3, questionnaire mailed to all asylums, schools, education institutions, nursing homes, etc. by the health administration of Hamburg, 1924.
71 Dr. Gerhard Schäfer, "Über einige Aufgaben des Arztes bei der Durchführung des Gesetzes zur Verhütung erbkranken Nachwuchses," *Ärzteblatt für Hamburg und Schleswig Holstein* 1, no. 15 (1934): 136–137.
72 Wunder, *Euthanasie in den letzten Kriegsjahren. Die Jahre 1944 und 1945 in der Heil- und Pflegeanstalt Hamburg Langenhorn*. The idea of "treatments" is being used in much the same way that we would use the number of hospital days.
73 Ibid., 45.
74 Ibid., 46.

the absolute number of transports in relation to the number of treatments to derive the deportation rate.

Table 3: Deportation from Langenhorn 1 September 1939* to May 1945**[75]

Year	Deported patients
1939*	04.72 %
1940	05.50 %
1941	33.39 %
1942	11.75 %
1943	33.55 %
1944	12.67 %
1945**	01.97 %

The heyday years of deportation were 1941 and 1943. Under *Aktion T4*, in 1941 the central medical commission required a report sheet on "euthanasia" (*Meldebogen-Euthanasie*) from every asylum within the German Reich. That deportations were taking place before the required use of the report sheet strengthens the evidence that selections and transports were already part of the practice at Langenhorn before the Nazi regime. For example, all of the Jewish patients were deported and killed in 1940. As could be expected, the evacuation rate declined in 1942 because at this time the central office in Berlin was reorganized and the *Aktion T4* was terminated. However, because the year 1943 in Hamburg was characterized not only by nights of bombings but also by the process of changing the largest number of psychiatric beds into acute care treatment beds in Langenhorn, the deportations continued and even intensified. As Wunder has demonstrated in his research, selections and transfers of patients were integrated into Langenhorn's everyday routine.

The total number of patients transferred from Hamburg during these years amounted to 4600. Only two transports took place in the city without the involvement of Langenhorn, and thus, the total number of transferred patients from Langenhorn was 3848. However, even though a large number of patients were transferred elsewhere, the death rate in Langenhorn alone remained astonishingly high. If the number of treatments is related to the absolute number of deaths, the following mortality rates evolve.[76]

---

75 Ibid., 47.
76 Ibid.

Table 4: Mortality rates in Langenhorn between 1939 and 1945.[77]

Year	Deaths
1939	05.73 %
1940	05.79 %
1941	07.56 %
1942	12.49 %
1943	10.36 %
1944	17.74 %
1945	20.53 %

At the 1960s' war crimes tribunal in Hamburg, the Polish court-appointed expert Jozef Radzicki issued a report for the prosecution in which he assumed that an annual mortality rate of 4 % in the asylums during the pre-war years was considered normal. An increase of mortality to 8 % could be perceived as average to normal during wartime itself. Any mortality rate beyond this limit must be evaluated as intentionally caused and precipitated.[78] Based on the above calculations, the annual mortality rates from 1942 onward were above 10 % and as such, could be considered abnormal. However, if the mortality rate was already elevated in the interwar years, as I have suggested, then the scope of these crimes seems even larger, because the calculation base of Radzicki's report was already biased. This suspicion is also supported by the research of historians Ingo Harms and Heinz Faulstich.[79]

Evidence also exists to support the contention that the killing of sick persons continued in Langenhorn after the end of the Second World War, even though no exact number of treatments exists from 1946 on. Asylum statistics reveal that 553 patients died in 1946 and 371 in 1947, indicating that many deaths continued after the end of the war.[80]

---

77 Ibid., 48.
78 Staatsanwaltschaft HH Az. 147 Js 58/67, Bl. 3315–3419.
79 Harms, Krankenmord in der Heil- und Pflegeanstalt Wehnen – Forschungsprobleme; Ingo Harms, 'Wat mööt wi hier smachten...' Hungertod und 'Euthanasie' in der Heil- und Pflegeanstalt Wehnen im 'Dritten Reich' (Oldenburg: Druck & Verlagscooperative GmbH, 1996); Heinz Faulstich, Die Zahl der "Euthanasie"-Opfer, in "Euthanasie" und die aktuelle Sterbehilfe-Debatte. Die historischen Hintergründe medizinischer Ethik, eds. Andreas Frewer and Clemens Eickhoff (Frankfurt/New York: Campus, 2000), 218–234; Faulstich, Hungersterben in der Psychiatrie 1914–1949. Mit einer Topographie der NS-Psychiatrie (Freiburg im Breisgau: Lambertus, 1998).
80 Arthur Kreßin, Das allgemeine Krankenhaus Langenhorn in Hamburg: 1950 (Hamburg: Wöll, 1950).

The Role of Nurses in Selecting Patients for Transfer

Nurses, especially head nurses (*Oberpfleger*), played an important role in selecting patients for transfer. They compiled the proposed lists that were then countersigned by the psychiatrists, a procedure verified by the comments given after the war by surviving patient "W." He also believed that nurses chose patients that "they wanted to get rid of."[81] Dr. Saupe, senior physician in Langenhorn during the Nazi regime, described the selection process in his testimony at the tribunal as follows:

> It is not that the most severe cases were transferred outward. On the contrary, only those patients who were physically healthy enough to withstand the transports, and patients whose next of kin did not live in the immediate proximity, were selected; bedridden patients were not at all transferred outward.[82]

Nurse Heinrich Roßburg also testified in 1946 that nurses had their own criteria for selecting patients for different places. "The selection of the patients was done by the head nurses and the physicians examined the cases. The head nurses naturally attached great weight to the fact that the so-called good worker, whom we could use here, preferably stayed here." This procedure was further confirmed by the testimony of Dr. Knigge, medical director of Langenhorn during the Second World War, in his 1946 defence. If a transport was planned, the "hospital administration compiled a list of patients hand in hand with the head nurses and the superintendents."[83]

Because financial reasons often dictated that asylum personnel carry out the transportation of patients themselves, numerous nurses therefore came in contact with "euthanasia" facilities. This is especially true for the transfers to the killing facility at Meseritz-Obrawalde. As one nurse reported, "we drove our sick persons in a car to the Meseritz asylum. There, they went into a house and were distributed to different wards. We delivered the medical and administrative records to the administration as well as the patients' valuables and other belongings. Afterwards, we drove back."[84] Another nurse reported that "I participated two or three times in transports of mentally ill patients to Meseritz ...Indeed, we never stayed long in Meseritz, but rather drove back again shortly after. Nevertheless, here and there I occasionally spoke to former patients."[85] Likewise, nurse Sch. reported that she saw "in Meseritz a few familiar faces that

---

81 Böhme and Lohalm, *Wege in den Tod*, 116.
82 Staatsanwaltschaft HH 147 Js 58/67, Bd, 1 u, 2, Bl. 17.
83 Staatsanwaltschaft HH 147 Js 58/67, Bd, 1 u, 2, Bl. 45.
84 Ibid., 116.
85 Ibid.

were with us for a long time in House 9 and who were criminal patients. They were on the loose there."[86]

In their testimonies, all of the nurses denied that they knew patients were murdered at Meseritz, although the patients themselves knew very early on what really happened there. Letters written by family members before or after the death of their sons or daughters suggest that their loved ones knew what was going on. During his admission to the academic medical centre at Eppendorf, Fritz Niemand, a patient who survived Meseritz, reported that he had already heard from other patients what the transfer to Langenhorn and the selections made there signified. In Langenhorn the patients lived in continuous fear of being transferred. Numerous testimonies of patients during the trials after 1945 proved that the events in asylums like Meseritz were understood by all inmates and visitors, and this knowledge could not be suppressed.

I want to stop the listing here because the aim of this book is not so much to demonstrate that the nurses were conscious of what they were doing, even though they probably were. As repeatedly stressed throughout the previous chapters, this book is more interested in considering the mechanisms that made the assassination of sick persons possible. The next two chapters attempt empirically to trace the complex interplay among the technologies, the nurses, psychiatrists, and administrators, which enabled these bureaucratically administered killings. As already mentioned in the last chapter, the book therefore concentrates on one patient record and traces the suffering of Anna Maria Buller.

---

86 Ibid., 117.

Chapter 4: Anna Maria Buller's First Admission in 1931: Analysis of the Record

Anna Maria Buller was first admitted to the psychiatric hospital (Friedrichsberg) in 1931 when she was 18 years old. She had originally been admitted to the general hospital, Barmbek, on a suspected diagnosis of influenza, but was transferred to Friedrichsberg within the first week of her illness because her behaviour was classified as "abnormal." From then on, she spent the rest of her life confined to either Friedrichsberg or the Langenhorn asylum, a period of 12 years interrupted only by more or less short stays in her parental home. Her diagnoses included schizophrenia, dementia, dementia praecox, and feeble mindedness. In 1935, she was sterilized against the will of both herself and her family. She endured any number of treatments, including shock therapy with the drugs Cardiazol, Insulin, Eugenozym (an unlicensed medication) in combination with Digitalis, Morphium-Scopolamine, or Paraldehyde, as well as continuous baths, isolation, and forced bed rest, to name a few. In addition, her problematic refusal to eat upon being first admitted resulted in the use of a feeding tube. She was eventually killed in Hadamar on 6 July 1943 after being diagnosed with tuberculosis of the bone, likely her final "death sentence."

The ability to summarize the "institutional biography" of this woman 69 years after her assassination demonstrates the capacity of records. The record preserves a documentary biography and a documentary reality of its own, which is activated at the moment it is read. Patient records in psychiatric asylums and other hospitals have gained in importance in German historiography in recent years and are of importance in research on "euthanasia" killings. In this kind of research the record has often been considered a medium for the mere storage of information, and researchers have used it primarily to confirm whether or not these records represented events accurately.

In contrast, in this book I will argue that the records must also be analyzed independently from their content. In order to grasp how the record functioned in psychiatric practice it is necessary to focus on the production of representations within the records and how these representations were used.[1] Documents and letters, even if they were written by the patients or their relatives themselves, were always written in the consciousness that they would become part of the record. This awareness is thus one reason why they cannot be considered the authentic voice of the patient.[2] This book is taking the theoretical perspective that the record must be perceived as a technology operating within a network in which it assumes the functions of translation and coordination. Patient records highlight the fact that "discourses themselves must be understood as 'technologies' that do not impact institutions and technical apparatuses from the outside, but rather constitute, penetrate, and regulate them."[3] Only through the interplay of semiotic-discursive and technical-material structure can the effects of power and truth be understood.

This kind of analysis of technologies enables us to grasp how knowledge is inscribed onto the practical exertion of power, authority, and dominance. Using a metaphor of heterogeneous networks allows us to perceive power to be the result of a more-or-less-successful coordination or alignment of different actors. Here the Foucauldian analysis of power meets up with the "sociology of translation" of Actor Network Theory (ANT), according to which every interaction with other humans is mediated by objects of various kinds. Technological objects define and distribute roles to human and non-human actors and are linked to various inscription devices. Technologies of psychiatric practice are not static, but rather become "[sites] of struggle, a relational effect that recursively generates and reproduces itself." As sociologist John Law contended, power effects evolve "in a relational and distributed manner, and nothing is ever sewn up."[4] Networks are oriented to establish and maintain a specific order but they continuously attempt to resist and limit other possibilities of ordering. The analysis of such "ordering struggles" is at the core of ANT. According to Law, "[t]he object is to explore and describe local processes of patterning, social orchestration, ordering and resistance. In short, it is to explore the process that is often called translation, which generates ordering effects such as devices, agents, institutions, or organisations."[5]

This definition resembles Foucault's perspective on power, which also as-

---

1 Marc Berg, "Practices of Reading and Writing: The Constitutive Role of the Patient Record in Medical Work," *Sociology of Health and Illness* 18, no. 4 (1996): 499–524; Lindsay Prior, *Using Documents in Social Research* (London: Sage, 2008), 3–5.
2 Dorothy E. Smith, *Institutional Ethnograph: A Sociology for People* (Oxford: Alta Mira Press, 2005).
3 Hannelore Bublitz, *Diskurs*, Einsichten – Vielsichten ed. (Bielefeld: transcript, 2003), 58–9.
4 John Law, "Notes on the Theory of the Actor Network: Ordering, Strategy and Heterogeneity," Centre for Science Studies, Lancaster University, http://www.lancs.ac.uk/fass/sociology/papers/law-notes-on-ant.pdf (accessed 24/01/2012).
5 Ibid.

sumes that power is not a static entity that can be owned but one that develops and changes in relationship to other objects or actors.[6] To analyze how power functions means to analyze power microscopically and to follow it in all its ramifications of capillary activities. Only from this perspective can the functioning of power be fully grasped, and this will be the approach taken in the following analysis of one particular medical record.

Along with an analysis of the patient record, I will also illuminate the significant roles that nurses played within these "ordering struggles." Law demonstrated that social actors can never be reduced to their mere physical corporeality but must be thought of as parts of a structured network of heterogeneous interrelations, or to put it another way, as social actors who emerge through networks. Human actors are therefore "generated in networks that pass through and ramify both within and beyond the body. Hence the term, actor-network – an actor is also, always, a network."[7] The patient record, too, is the result of a manifold interplay of different processes, instruments, reports, and measuring data. In the words of Bruno Latour, they are the result of different "inscription devices," which can be defined as apparatuses or specific configurations of objects that are able to translate "substance" into written documentation.[8] Latour and Steve Woolgar demonstrated in their laboratory studies how laboratory rats and the chemicals used on them were transformed into paper. Inscriptions appear as a direct image of the original substance and they are relevant because, on the one hand, any inscription can be combined with any other and, on the other hand, paper is a medium that guarantees the conservation of these inscriptions beyond time and space. Latour used the term "immutable mobiles" to characterize this ability of documents.[9] From the moment of their creation, these diagrams and images become the object of scientific disputes and function as evidence for the substances that they represent, even though these substances themselves can only be "seen" in the form of these inscriptions. In other words, the successful alignment of different inscriptions evolves into a "hard fact," and as more inscriptions are gathered together in order to prove the existence of a fact, it becomes difficult to deny this fact. In the

---

6 Michel Foucault, *Il faut défendre la société. Cours au College de France. 1976* (France: Gallimard Seuil, 1997); Michel Foucault, "Governmentality," in *Power. Essentials Works of Foucault 1954–1984*, ed. James D. Faubion (London: Penguin Books, 1994), 201–222; Foucault, "The Subject and Power," in *Michel Foucault: Beyond Structuralism and Hermeneutics*, eds. Hubert L. Dreyfus and Paul Rabinow (Chicago: University of Chicago Press, 1983), 208–226.
7 Law, "Notes on the Theory of the Actor Network," 4.
8 Bruno Latour and Steve Woolgar, *Laboratory Life. The Construction of Scientific Facts* (Princeton, New Jersey: Princeton University Press, 1986); Latour, *Science in Action* (Cambridge: Harvard University Press, 2003).
9 Bruno Latour, "Visualisation and Cognition: Thinking with Eyes and Hands," *Knowledge and Society*, no. 6 (1986): 7.

case of the psychiatric patient records, the body of the patient, for example, which is translated into fever charts, medication tables, laboratory results, weight tables, etc., is first and foremost constituted. Everyday institutional life and the psychic parameters of patients are translated respectively into psychiatrists' and nurses' notes. The patient record thus acts as a "mediator" because it mediates the interrelations that function and act through the record.[10] The material activities and production stages that were necessary to construct the network of the patient record are invisible. The patient record appears as nothing more than a resource of information but it actually intervenes into the interactions of psychiatric practice; the record, as linguist John Austin stated for speech acts, is also *"performativ."*[11] This simplifying effect Law described as "punctualisation," which occurs each time networks are perceived as "network packages – routines – that can, if precariously, be more or less taken for granted in the process of heterogeneous engineering."[12] Punctualisation makes it difficult for actors to recognize the active part that these simplified networks play in interactions because they work silently "behind their backs," strengthening their effectiveness. Latour used the term "black boxing" to highlight the fact that these simplified networks appear to the actors as black boxes whose complexities only emerge if the network encounters a kind of problem, because only in these moments does it become necessary to open them in order to find the fault that led to the problem. In these moments the complexity of the internal structure of the black box becomes apparent. The aim of the following analysis is to open the "black box" and to make visible the functioning of the patient record as mediator.

The above explanations highlight why I decided to analyze primarily one record in depth. Opening the "black box" of this patient record reveals such a complex network that it was not possible to analyze all the details in a completely organized fashion. The record is the product of a multitude of interactions between both human and non-human actors.

The following overview summarizes the terms used in this analysis to describe the different parts of the record. The records from Langenhorn are unusual in one aspect, because strictly speaking, they consist of two case histories – one from Langenhorn and one from Friedrichsberg. As research on records from

---

10 Bruno Latour, *Reassembling the Social. An Introduction to Actor-Network-Theory* (New York: Oxford University Press, 2005); Latour, "Pragmatogonies. A Mythical Account of how Humans and Nonhumans Swap Properties," *American Behavioral Scientist* 37, no. 6 (1994): 791–808.
11 John L. Austin, *Zur Theorie der Sprechakte (How to do things with words)*, trans. Eike von Savigny (Stuttgart: Reclam, 2002); Judith Butler, *Excitable Speech. A Politics of the Performative* (London: Routledge, 1997).
12 Law, "Notes on the Theory of the Actor Network," 5.

other hospitals has revealed, the record normally remained in the admitting asylum and was not given to patients who were transferred to take with them or, if it was sent, the record was returned to the admitting asylum.[13] That this situation was different in Hamburg highlights once again how close Friedrichsberg and Langenhorn were interconnected, and the fact that both records were available enables analysis of the interplay between these two asylums. However, the administrative record (*Personalakte*) remained in Friedrichsberg, which is to say that only the administrative records from Langenhorn were available for this analysis. The medical record or patient record in Langenhorn is a collection of all patient documents consisting of administrative record and case history/medical history:

- Administrative record: Administrative processes of all kind, court decisions, correspondence, index of clothes, letters from relatives to the medical director, report sheet "*Aktion T4.*" The administrative record identification number is the connection between the inside world of the asylum and the outside world.
- Case history/medical history: Psychiatrists' and nurses' notes, collections of evidence on the patient's madness (the record often contains drawings from the patients, patients' letters, and other materials), reports of extraordinary events.

The Content of the Record

Patients and their histories are actively produced through the written case history record that, like other forms of histories, follow a chronological time frame. As will be seen in this book's patient records, only psychiatrists were allowed to write a patient's history. Nurses merely produced "reports," and their writings were therefore called "nursing reports." Psychiatrists constructed the history; nurses delivered the constitutive parts.

A patient's raw medical record was a kind of booklet of empty, unlined pages, each with the printed heading "case history" and a column to the left side of the page for the date. The first page of this booklet, entitled *Staatskrankenanstalt Friedrichsberg Hamburg*, was the only pre-printed form in the booklet. At the top of this page was a space to enter a file number and the name of the admitting psychiatrist. Allocating patients a number brought them into being as a case. Other spaces on the form asked for patients' names, their date of birth and address, their occupation, and their date of admission to the asylum. Space was

---

13 Ulrich Müller, "Metamorphosen: Krankenakten als Quellen für Lebensgeschichten," in *"Das Vergessen der Vernichtung ist Teil der Vernichtung selbst." Lebengeschichten von Opfern der nationalsozialistischen "Euthanasie,"* eds. Petra Fuchs and others (Göttingen: Wallstein, 2007), 80–96.

also reserved for information on how the patient arrived in the asylum (on foot or "*m. San. Kol.*," meaning through sanitary unit) and from where. All of these blanks were filled in by hand by an admitting clerk – an informed assumption because the handwriting is very exact and suits the formal obligations of administrative handwriting of that time.

Once the standard demographic information was completed, two additional spaces were required to be filled in – one for the definition of the illness and the other for the admittance-attestation. The fact that the handwriting conveying this information was less legible and less exact implies that it was supplied by the psychiatrist (an observation strengthened by examining physicians' handwriting throughout the record). The formal spaces on the form are thus divided between personnel, with most of the non-medical information being completed before the psychiatrist transcribed the patient's medical information. The layout of the front page, with its specific arrangement of printed key terms and empty spaces, was structured to create a narrative. The front page prescribed the linearity of the patients' story because the administrator could enter only the information requested by the form. The story formed the introduction to the entire medical record.

Following is the front page information from the Friedrichsberg asylum for patient Anna Maria Buller, with the handwritten parts marked in italics.

Name: *Anna Maria Dorothea Buller*
Place of birth: *Hamburg*
Date of birth: *28.1.13*
Occupation: *Advertisement Designer*
admitted the *18.II.1931*
illness: *Schizophrenia*
comes m. San. Kol. *v. d. A. K. Barm*bek [from the General Hospital Barmbek]
Last residence: *Wagnerstr. 47 hptr* [ground floor], *Bullerd.* [at the] *parents*.
Admittance-Attestation: *Schizophrenia, catatonic clinical picture. Negativism (refuses any food consumption, completely withdrawn). Temporary states of agitation with hallucinations.*
signed *Dr. Reuter*.[14] (See Figure 5 and 6)

---

14 Staatsarchiv Hansestadt Hamburg 352 – 8-7, Staatskrankenanstalt Langenhorn, Abl.1 – 1995, Krankenakte 28338 (hereafter Patient Record (PR), Friedrichsberg Medical Records Section (hereafter FMR), psychiatric notes (hereafter PN). This designation will be used throughout to identify Anna Maria Buller's patient record; other patient files mentioned in the text will be identified by their unique file number.

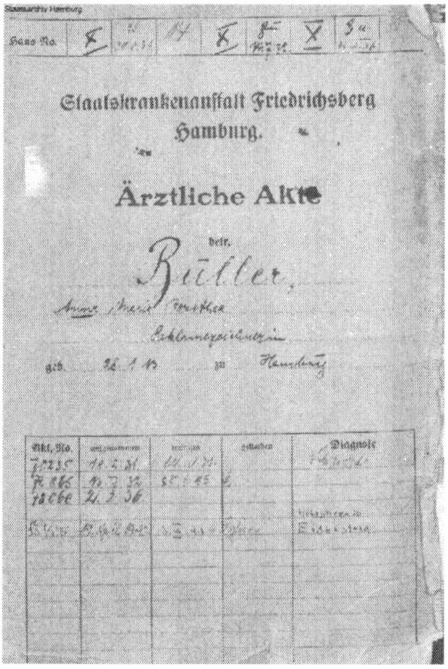

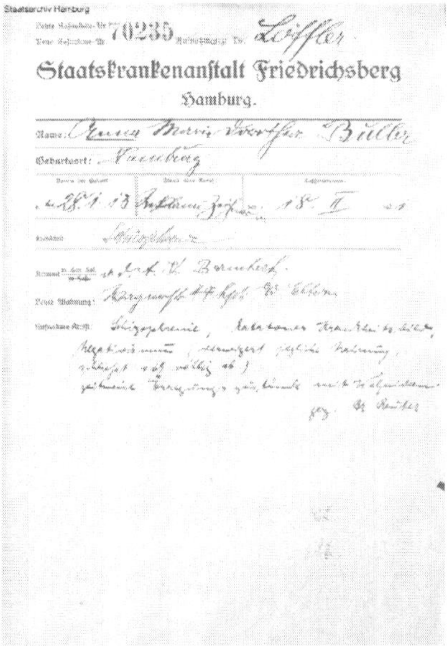

Figure 5 and 6: The folder and the front page of Anna Maria Buller's medical record 28338 in Friedrichsberg.[15]

The abbreviations used made the front page comprehensible only to those working in this specific organizational context. From Buller's form, we can discern her diagnosis, the definition of her illness, that she did not arrive voluntarily (she was brought by sanitary unit) and that she was already hospitalized elsewhere before she arrived in the asylum. The form also revealed that she lived with her parents, and that the physician who diagnosed her was not the same psychiatrist who admitted her to Friedrichsberg (we know this because the name of the admitting psychiatrist on the top of the form was different from the "Dr. Reuter" who signed the diagnosis, who was probably the medical officer.) How the diagnosis was obtained or why Buller had been admitted to the general hospital of Barmbek is not perceivable to the reader. Furthermore, reading the first few pages of the record reveals that a lot of work was necessary to obtain the information assembled on the front page, work that was obviously invisible if one went no further than the first page. The front page formed a frame for other psychiatric observations that had a significant impact on how patients like Buller would be described in the notes, and how the record as a whole would be constructed.

The booklet, which made up the core of the record, contained psychiatrists' notes, laboratory results, and other official medical documents. All of the papers

---

15 PR, FMR, PN.

in the booklet used by psychiatrists were officially designed and printed forms, providing a kind of status that helped to legitimize their work. Except for the booklet, all other kinds of documents in the record, including the nurses' notes, are found at the end (or are part of the administrative record), making them more difficult to find. As such, what counts as legitimate information is already defined by the material appearance of the record.

The notes written by psychiatrists and nurses differed more than in the content they contained. First, the psychiatrists wrote their remarks in ink (or sometimes their secretaries used a typewriter) on printed, unlined forms in which they were prompted to note only the date of their writing. Psychiatrists thus were at liberty to decide how much to write and in what way. As described above, the pages of the patient's record are fastened together into a kind of booklet, and are not numbered consecutively. In Buller's case, her name was not even marked on the top of every page. In other words, psychiatrists had available an unregulated space in which to write their case histories, a space that was entirely controlled by them and whose writing was often very difficult to decipher. (See Figure 7)

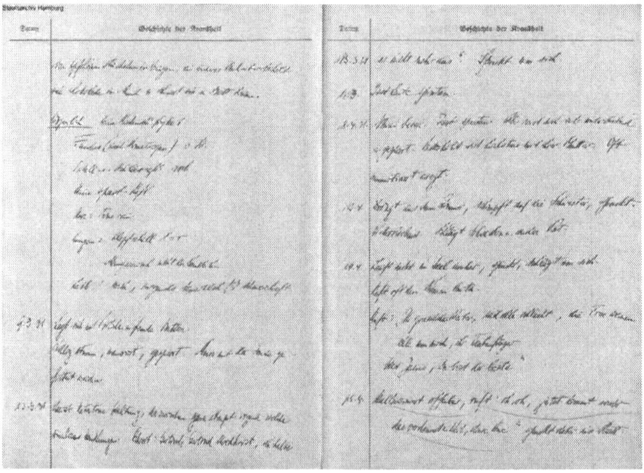

Figure 7: Psychiatrist's case history, medical record 28338.

In contrast to the forms provided to physicians, the ones supplied to the nurses in Friedrichsberg were very specific. Nursing reports were written on lined sheets of paper with headings in bold print. The overall construction of the form resembled the construction of a copybook used to practice handwriting in elementary school. (See Figure 8) The left edge was to remain empty to facilitate binding. Nurses were forced to organize their reports: they needed to number each page consecutively and to add the patient's name and file number (in this case, those of Buller) as well as the date in specific spaces on the form. The nurses' notes were thus highly regulated by the material construction of the form.

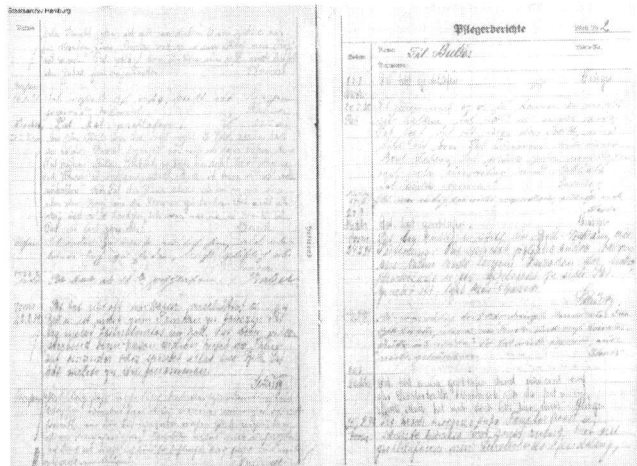

Figure 8: Nurse's reports, medical record 28338.

Most of the nursing notes at Friedrichsberg contained initials and some underlining from psychiatrists who controlled the nurses' entries and used them in their own notes to make clear that they had observed what the nurses described. The notes are also much more legible than those written by the psychiatrists, even though the nurses wrote in pencil (only the head nurse occasionally wrote in ink). The fact that they were written in pencil and thus relatively faint, however, gives the impression of the writing being more childlike, and thus the writer as more subordinate. This is to say that the material construction of the forms enforced a certain way of entering information and represented, in a concrete manner, the entire organization of psychiatric practice – a strategic interplay of different parts arranged around the absolute power of the psychiatrist.

Although they represented the largest part of the patient record, I argue that the formal appearance of these notes, which directed and controlled the observations of nurses, the nature of their being written in pencil, and their position at the back of the medical file, suggests that nurses and their work were considered subordinate within the hierarchical organization of psychiatric treatment at Friedrichsberg.

I argue further, however, that these same elements have continued to influence historical research, in that historians themselves have tended to ignore nursing notes. Until recently, a vast number of nursing reports have continued to be destroyed simply because they have been considered uninformative and thus unimportant. Yet, as I contend in the case of Friedrichsberg, the material from these nursing documents contained critical information and useful observations on which psychiatrists themselves based their medical decisions. Without the nurses' notes, the psychiatrists' notes could not have existed. This is what is meant by the term "strategic" power distribution: nurses' information could only be useful if it was written in a standardized, easily readable manner and in an efficient style that enabled the psychiatrist to read through the notes in the shortest amount of time possible. Dr. Enge, medical director of the asylum of Strecknitz-Lübeck in the 1930s, emphasized the significance of clearly written nursing reports that suggested a style significantly different from that of physicians.

> In order to allow the physician to inform himself rapidly and comprehensively about the condition of a sick person and to be informed about all incidents some demands must be fulfilled, demands that concern more the formal nature: articulate writing! Well-arranged ordering![16]

The admission ritual and the nurses' reports

Following the chronology of Anna Maria Buller's medical file enables demonstrating the record's ability to initiate or influence a chain of action within psychiatric practice, and the role that it played in constructing the identity of patients. The introductory narrative at the front highlights the fact that Buller was first admitted to the general hospital at Barmbek before she was transferred to Friedrichsberg. The following pages, which contain an excerpt from her file at Barmbek, are written in the same handwriting as that on the front page, inferring that an office clerk at Friedrichsberg copied the case history from Barmbek. Buller was originally admitted to Barmbek on 12 February 1931 with a diagnosis of "Morbus Internes (possibly the flu)."

> Patient's history: Information provided by mother: <u>No nervous diseases in the family.</u>
> Family's health history: nothing to mention.
> Pat. [patient] has never been seriously ill. She is an apprentice of an advertisement designer. The parents did not notice anything specific, except for her demeanour which has been somewhat staring and empty lately. Since yesterday, [Buller] has been very restless and strange in her behaviour. She apparently said that all people were against her and she did not know why. The doctor diagnosed her with the flu and admitted her to hospital. On Sunday (8.2.) she was tobogganing; the mother did not know anything about it. She had not slept for 3 nights and did not feel good during the days. She

---

16 Dr Enge, "Beobachtungsberichte des Pflegepersonals," *Geisteskrankenpflege. Monatsschrift für Geisteskranken- und Krankenpflege* 37, no. 1 (1933): 113–115.

constantly talked about dying. She was to die; the mother should not worry about it, everybody had to die. The mother should cut open the artery on the wrist so that the soul could be released. Yesterday 38 °C temperature. Before Sunday, the parents did not notice anything....[17]

This part of the physician's report from the Barmbek hospital summarized the mother's testament as to why her daughter should be admitted. She had not noticed anything unusual in her daughter's behaviour "before Sunday" and she and the general practitioner considered the changes in Buller's behaviour to be the result of a potential flu. The manner in which the note was written demonstrates that the physician had directed the interview and that he was concentrating primarily on the patient's somatic symptoms. He described her as a "tiny pat. [whose] every movement seems weak, limp and without energy," lying "in bed with her eyes closed and [reacting] to all stimulation in a sluggish and slow manner."[18] Even more unusual behaviour still elicited no comments that Buller might be mentally ill. "(15.2) Completely withdrawn. Doesn't answer, doesn't eat. Most of the time, she lies in bed uncovered, hair untidy in her face. Lifted her arms up straight in the air for a long time, without moving."[19] Not until three days later was she finally transferred to Friedrichsberg.

The public health officer who examined her at Barmbek in order to refer her to Friedrichsberg translated the observations from Barmbek into the psychiatric diagnosis that would later become the admittance attestation to the new institution. Unlike the previous physician, he did not focus solely on somatic aspects of her illness alone but rather interpreted the symptoms provided by the mother's interview and the Barmbek physician's notes as a mental illness. "Schizophrenia, catatonic clinical picture. Negativism (refuses any food consumption, completely withdrawn). Temporary states of agitation with hallucinations."[20]

Obtaining the psychiatric diagnosis from the copied case history from Barmbek nevertheless took a great deal of work, as it rearranged and transformed observations to fit into a specific diagnostic frame. For example, the reported observation from Barmbek "arms up straight in the air for a long time, without moving" was translated into a "catatonic clinical picture." "Hardly accepts any food, lies in bed apathetically" became "negativism (refuses any food consumption, completely withdrawn)." Agitation and continual muttering about being poisoned by food was explained by her experiencing "temporary

---

17 PR, FMR, PN.
18 Ibid.
19 Ibid.
20 Ibid.

states of agitation with hallucinations."²¹ Nonetheless, while the Barmbek physician did not acknowledge that Buller's symptoms might suggest she was mentally ill, she was receiving Luminal, a commonly prescribed psychiatric sedative at this time.²² It was not until she reached Friedrichsberg, however, when a psychiatrist there noted that she had developed a "Luminal exanthema,"²³ that we discover she was receiving this drug on a regular basis.

From the moment that Buller received her psychiatric diagnosis, her record began to follow what seemed to be a predetermined course that was guided by her diagnosis. The terms used in the diagnosis would accompany her throughout her multiple stays in the psychiatric hospital. The diagnosis became the hidden pattern of psychiatrists' observations, functioning even retroactively to sustain a certain direction and coherence in these observations not possessed prior to the diagnosis. Simultaneously, the diagnosis linked Buller's Barmbek history with that obtained in the Friedrichsberg asylum, corresponding to published guidelines on examination techniques. Author Wilhelm Weygandt, who had been become medical director of Friedrichsberg in 1908, contended that the history of the patient should be written in a chronological sequence and psychiatrists should "describe the past [of the patient] as far as possible in an objective manner."²⁴ Following these guidelines, Buller's clinical history was actually rewritten during her first examination in Friedrichsberg.

Nevertheless, the admission examination had an alternate motive. It followed a particular scheme that was more or less the same for every admission to Friedrichsberg, one that could be described as a kind of ceremony or ritual. Furthermore, it was also the first demonstration of the medical power that ruled the asylum, conveying to the patient that he/she had entered into a specific space where the distribution of power had nothing in common with the "ordinary world." As stated by Eugen Bleuler, influential Swiss psychiatrist who introduced the concept of schizophrenia,

> during the admission no lies and no false promises are to be applied (…) In cases of emergency it is preferable to use violence or narcotics, because the sick person is most likely to forgive them afterwards. Nevertheless, violence is often unnecessary if one acts with caution. Most sick persons can be persuaded, without being ruffled, of the ne-

---

21 Ibid.
22 Patrick Kwan and Martin J. Brodie, "Phenobarbital for the Treatment of Epilepsy in the 21st Century: A Critical Review," *Epilepsia*, 2004, Wiley Online Library, http://onlinelibrary.wiley.com.proxy.biBulleruottawa.ca/doi/10.1111/j.0013–9580.2004.12704.x/full (accessed 1/24/ 2011).
23 Hannes Weber Dr., "Luminal und Luminal-Exanthem," *Klinische Wochenzeitschrift* 20, no. 1 (1922): 998–999.
24 Wilhelm Weygandt, *Forensische Psychiatrie. II. Teil. Sachverständigentätigkeit*, ed. Vereinigung wissenschaftlicher Verleger, Sammlung Göschen ed. (Berlin, Leipzig: de Gruyter & Co, 1922), 22.

cessity of the decision [to be admitted to the asylum] – but in such an authoritative way that they feel that any discussion is useless and enough people are around who are capable of enforcing the will in case of resistance. One cannot forget that it is very rare to persuade the sick person to back down through logic itself, but rather through the appearance of the one who applies the logic....[25]

According to Bleuler, the physical appearance of the psychiatrist alone should be sufficient to convince the patient that any resistance was futile. As such, the "logic" of the asylum was physically imposed on the patient, hinting at the rationale behind psychiatric practice.

The admission ritual was also characterized by a power imbalance that implied neither reciprocity nor equal exchange; Bleuler even characterized the admission of mentally ill persons as an "internment."[26] The admission "exploration" (as Friedrichsberg psychiatrists called it) appeared as a threefold usurpation of the patient's body. First, communication during the exploration did not exist as a free, equal linguistic exchange but rather was marked by the power of the psychiatrist. The patient was not encouraged to freely recount his or her experiences; instead, the psychiatrist posed questions that patients were compelled to answer in order to "convict" the madness. According to Weygandt, the "assessment of the mental condition" was the most important part of the examination and he developed a long list of questions and "special methods" in order to establish the psychic status and the mental performance of the patient.[27] Nevertheless, this could only be a preliminary assessment because the patient's status had to be regularly verified, and if necessary, rectified through observations and by repeating the interview.

Even though psychiatrists did not appear to personally address Buller during the admission ritual in 1931, a power imbalance can be observed during her stay in the asylum and on the occasions of her subsequent admissions to Friedrichsberg in the years to come. The questions psychiatrists asked revealed that they possessed information that was not obtained directly from the patient but was derived from other sources, including documents and interview transcripts. Weygandt had also emphasized that the examination was to begin with research for records and other documents

> that should underlie the expert report. Particularly, one should reclaim school reports especially in cases when the disorders reach back to adolescence. Furthermore, depending on the circumstances, one should reclaim reports of the time in the armed forces. In addition, any medical histories from earlier stays in hospitals or asylums

---

25 Eugen Bleuler, *Lehrbuch der Psychiatrie* (Berlin: Springer, 1923), 163; Eugen Bleuler, *Lehrbuch der Psychiatrie*, eds. Manfred Bleuler and Josef Berze (Berlin: Springer-Verlag, 1943).
26 Bleuler, *Lehrbuch der Psychiatrie*, 162.
27 Weygandt, *Forensische Psychiatrie. II. Teil. Sachverständigentätigkeit*, 27.

come into consideration even though some parts of the content of the patient's history, as far as they concern the history obtained from the patient himself or from his next of kin, must be critically considered.[28]

Information on Buller was derived from her record at Barmbek and the detailed information provided by her mother. However, the psychiatrist apparently did not entirely trust her mother's statements, or even Buller herself, as her later admissions demonstrate. Dr. Enge, medical director of the asylum of Strecknitz-Lübeck, too, had written that the next of kin "are sometimes abnormal themselves and therefore suppress facts," or they mix "popular conceptions, unclear associations into their statements."[29]

Psychiatrists asked patients questions unrelated to their personal situation that appeared to follow a specific formula. Other records revealed that these kinds of questions were standardized and were used to check "mental capacities." Weygandt described the course of this examination procedure, which could be characterized more as an interrogation. Against the backdrop of information obtained from school records, medical histories from other hospitals, military reports, and testimonies obtained from family members, etc., he believed that the psychiatrist was to question the patient for basic demographic information and then probe five areas of concern: heredity, birth and infanthood, childhood and adolescence, maturity, and illness. Every detail seemed to be important in the context of the mental illness. Questions about heredity, for example, were meant to uncover not only mental or nervous illnesses of blood relations but also instances of possible alcoholism, criminality, instability, wastefulness, or any other striking characteristic, which more than anything else demonstrated psychiatric concerns for moral behaviour. Other questions, for example, could focus on the course of the mother's pregnancy and aspects of infant nutrition, or delve into such wide-ranging areas as whether or not the patient was lively or quiet, had wet the bed, had tried to run away from home, coped well with school or military service, performed well at work, or masturbated.[30] Finally, the psychiatrist was encouraged to ask about the illness itself.

> What are the causes of the actual illness? Supposed psychic influences, sorrow, excitements, fear. Febrile illnesses, metabolism, lues, poisons like alcohol, morphine, cocaine, nicotine, plumb, sleeping pills. Regarding women, menstruation, pregnancy, birth, confinement, breastfeeding, climacteric period. Exhaustive circumstances.
> In what manner did the condition change? Suddenly or gradually? Changes in character? Weakness of memory? Excesses? Wastefulness? Changes in speech and script.

---

28 Ibid., 19.
29 Enge, "Die Vorgeschichte (Anamnese) und ihre Bedeutung für die Krankheitsfeststellung (Diagnose)," *Geisteskrankenpflege. Monatsschrift für Geisteskranken- und Krankenpflege* 37, no. 6 (1933): 89.
30 Weygandt, *Forensische Psychiatrie. II. Teil. Sachverständigentätigkeit*, 22–23.

> Resentments, world-weariness, aptitude to self-murder? Obsessive ideas. Bodily functions; sleep disorder, digestion, headache, dizziness, faints, cramps? Confusion, misperceptions, delusional ideas, excitements, memory, striking behaviour, bizarre gestures, unresponsiveness, dysfunctional reactions?[31]

From this list it becomes very clear that nearly any aspect of a patient's behaviour could become a symptom related to the diagnosis of a mental illness. However, only the psychiatrist could assess the interrelationships between the different dispositions and symptoms. Although diagnostic indications could be deduced from hereditary elements, they were warned that it would be a fault to overestimate the hereditary burden.[32]

Bleuler (1943) emphasized not only the significance of the questions but also the way in which they should be asked.

> Of utmost importance is the manner of questioning. First of all, one has not to antagonize the patient, if possible at all; awkward aspects are set aside till the end. If possible one tries to gain confidence – of course without pretending anything. An examination under false pretences must be declined. If a patient does not talk one does not try to go further, but rather examines the body and occasionally poses a question that can be easily answered: Does this hurt, or the like, to make the patient talk. One observes certain things on mentally and bodily dimensions without patients noticing...[33]

This advice also highlighted the fact that the admission ritual was a strategic procedure used to provoke certain answers from the patient in order to "trap" the madness and convict the patient of his or her illness. Weygandt's own catalogue of questions was so extensive that the patient could only be "cornered" and forced to surrender.[34] Even so, he wrote, depending on the case, parts of the examination could be deepened. "In the case of a person with delusive ideas one has to go into detail about his pathological perceptions and the possible development of a system of delerium."[35] If these "experimental-psychological examination methods" were not sufficient to trap the madness, one could apply even "more complicated experiments like, for example, [asking patients to] consecutively add up figures."[36] And if this acceleration in the interrogation technique was still insufficient to provoke the decisive symptoms, Weygandt advised psychiatrists to resort to chemicals to settle the case.

---

31 Ibid.
32 Ibid., 24.
33 Bleuler, *Lehrbuch der Psychiatrie*, 107.
34 Weygandt, *Forensische Psychiatrie. II. Teil. Sachverständigentätigkeit*, 28–32.
35 Ibid., 32.
36 Ibid.

So they administered cocaine (0.05 subcutaneous) in order to test for epilepsy and with a congruent disposition it was occasionally, but rather rarely, possible to cause a kind of epileptic seizure. I think it is more efficient not only in the case of suspected epilepsy, but also in the case of different types of degeneration to conduct an alcohol experiment. This means letting the person concerned quickly intake a bottle of wine, normally a sweet wine [Süßwein] with approximately 100 gr alcohol. Sometimes a kind of epileptic seizure, even with fixed pupils, is initiated [but]more often more slight disorders occur such as vertigo, headache, excitability.[37]

By now, it is clear that the function of the admission ritual was to expose the patient's central symptoms through specific layered techniques of questioning, and if necessary, through the application of chemicals, an aspect of the admission ritual that is analyzed in more detail below.

Also of interest to Bleuler was not only what the patient said, but the manner in which he or she spoke. "For the sick persons talking, their inflection can be abnormal, too loud, too low, too fast, too slow, through the fistula, grumbling, grunting, staccato, precipitous and so on....Speech manners often express a certain complex."[38]

Madness was apparently traceable even in a patient's writing, made visible by a kind of "unconscious" confession that was manifested through the act of writing. According to Bleuler, the "written statements correspond[ed] to oral statements. Abnormalities in style [were] frequent."[39] Buller refused to provide a writing sample when she was asked to do so one day prior to her interrogation by the psychiatrist in Friedrichsberg. A nurse conducted the writing exercise, and the fact that Buller was not seen by a psychiatrist until the next day implies nurses, as representatives of the psychiatrist, supplemented the admission procedure by rituals of their own. This will be further analyzed below. With each predetermined sentence, Buller was either forced to acknowledge the power of the nurse as the representative of the psychiatrist's power (like a teacher who dictates a text) or reveal her madness through her inability to write, if for instance she was not able to compose a grammatically correct sentence. In both cases, the act of writing was literally a demonstration of power by the psychiatrist and his representatives. (See Figure 9)

---

37 Ibid., 33.
38 Bleuler, *Lehrbuch der Psychiatrie*, 305.
39 Ibid., 308.

Figure 9: Handwriting Sample of Buller. The nurse noted: "Patient does not write".
Medical record 28338.

In some records, patients were asked to write their own biography. Enge called this exercise the "autoanamnesis" (*Autoanamnese*), meaning that the case history was based on the information obtained from the sick person. This autoanamnesis, which included a questionnaire and an unstructured written biography, was "of utmost importance. The manner in which a sick person is able to express himself, his capability to depict and to summarize something he experienced, his hand writing, his mistakes in language and spelling, give important reference points for the assessment." The written biography was synonymous with patients' "confession…of the history of [their] madness."[40] The inability or unwillingness of Buller to provide a writing sample became a demonstration of uncooperative behaviour and offered further evidence for her diagnosis.

Attempts to capture the mental state of the patient through the interrogation procedure were supplemented by a physical examination, which followed a thoroughly detailed and systematic process at Friedrichsberg that Weygandt had laid down.[41] This kind of examination was meant to help the psychiatrist link the psychic and the physical state of the patient.

Bodily symptoms found through the physical examination served to provide evidence for a particular mental illness diagnosis. When counterposed against the "catatonic clinic picture" that had described Buller's state on admission to Friedrichsberg, the slack muscle tone found at her physical exam only made her

---

40 Enge, "Die Vorgeschichte (Anamnese) und ihre Bedeutung für die Krankheitsfestellung (Diagnose)," 87–88.
41 Weygandt, *Forensische Psychiatrie. II. Teil. Sachverständigentätigkeit*, 22–23

mental illness more visible. The examining psychiatrist's failed attempt to provoke a reaction through "rough needle pricks" only underlined how "withdrawn" she was. The "narcoleptic" state of the patient could not be altered by speaking to her, nor did it change during a lumbar puncture. Even the "much greater resistance to blood work" was perceived as a sign of instability.[42]

In conjunction with the diagnosis, the description of these physical findings acted to introduce other observations. At the same time, however, her pre-determined diagnosis installed a kind of frame that made some aspects visible and others invisible. For example, no one mentioned that Buller had been heavily sedated, not only by the Luminal she had received in Barmbek but also by an injection of another heavy sedative, Morphine-Scopolamine, that she received in Friedrichsberg prior to her admission procedure and which had been marked only on the "fever chart."[43] These drugs may well have been implicated in the creation of Buller's catatonic state. Demonstrating the "power" of the record, she may well have received this last injection as a preventative measure because of the physical aggression recorded in the notes of both the psychiatrists and the nurses.

Physical examinations were attempts to map mental illness on the body. As Bleuler wrote, "due to an aberration of the brain, which is the cause for most of the brain illnesses, very often the bodily development gets off track. A huge number of sick people endure many more malformations than healthy people do."[44] Of the six areas of bodily symptoms connected to mental illnesses that he listed, the fourth was especially noteworthy.

> Bodily symptoms are the expression of an abnormal constitution that includes the whole personality and pre-disposes to psychic disorders: including first and foremost the "signs of degeneration" (…) subnormal size, cranial deformations…irregular tooth position, underdeveloped teeth…deformations of the genitals…Regarding the schizophrenic, those forms that are related to dumbing down on average have more signs of degeneration than those that are less severe.[45]

However, Weygandt "caution[ed] against overestimating the signs of possible devolution" (*Entartungszeichen*) or characteristics of degeneration or *stigmata hereditatis*.

> Only in cases of a large occurrence [of degenerative signs] the conclusion by analogy is allowed: If the miscellaneous organism, particularly in the range of the ectoderm, tends to deviate in serious extent from normal development then the assumption is obvious

---

42 PR, FMR, PN.
43 Ullrich Hinrichs, "Über Dauerschlafbehandlung mit Scopolamin-Paraldehyd bei Geisteskranken," *Zeitschrift für die gesamte Neurologie und Psychiatrie* 105, no. 1 (1926): 626.
44 Bleuler, *Lehrbuch der Psychiatrie*, 120.
45 Ibid.

that the central nervous system and the cerebral cortex too, as carriers of the psychic functions, seen from their disposition have a certain tendency to deviations from the normal development.[46]

Three constitutive aspects of psychiatric rationale appear in this short paragraph. First of all, the degeneration of the body was somehow related to mental degeneration. Second, it was not possible to draw direct conclusions from the existence of bodily signs of degeneration to probable mental degeneration. Owing to their medical expertise, only psychiatrists were able to draw the right conclusions regarding the impact of bodily signs on the mental state. Third, Weygandt's statement regarding deviations from "the normal arrangement and the normal development" highlighted the fact that psychiatrists dealt with distinctions between "normal and "abnormal," although he considered it difficult to clearly differentiate the two. The predominant number of "cases of mental disturbance do not show their deformity at first sight," he wrote, but rather a scientific diagnostic was necessary "even more for bodily disturbances in which the sick persons sense the illness themselves."[47] Lay persons, according to Weygandt, could only imagine a kind of "prototype" of lunacy which in reality equated only to a few of the most severe cases. They could not recognize the "average" mentally ill person, because his or her illness was not visible at first sight and waited to be discovered by the psychiatric expert. As this thinking suggests, psychiatric discourse at this point always related mental illness with a somatic component of degeneration and searched for the cause of the illness in the corporeal constitution or in the biography of the mentally ill person. Assuming that a degenerative constitution was a foundation for madness meant that the patient could not be cured because of the unchangeable nature of the constitution.

Since all of Buller's laboratory results were negative, the body disappeared in the psychiatrist's notes. As Bleuler had noted, it was often impossible to find an anatomical essence of schizophrenia "despite numerous efforts."[48] Only the nurses attempted to control specific bodily functions of the patient though the use of fever charts or handwritten forms that they themselves had designed. As Buller's file evolved, a clear distinction was drawn between the bodily life of the patient, which was represented on these forms, and the psychic life, which was represented in the nurses' and psychiatrists' notes. The body appeared to be mysteriously absent. It was no longer a question of which behaviour or which manner of speech belonged to which damaged bodily function, it became more a

---

46 Weygandt, *Forensische Psychiatrie. II. Teil. Sachverständigentätigkeit*, 26.
47 Ibid., 46–47.
48 Bleuler, *Lehrbuch der Psychiatrie*, 122.

matter of whether or not a certain conduct, such as hearing voices, etc. should be classified as madness or not. As Bleuler stated:

> The whole difficulty lies in the fact that there is no definition of "illness" and that there cannot be one. It is so easy to examine how a human is and how he reacts and then from the factual, instead from the term, to draw the consequences and to determine our action.[49]

An investigation into the genetic disposition was always part of the admission ritual, although the reason it was not given the same weight in all clinical records likely depended on the admitting psychiatrist. In Buller's file, an examination of her hereditary background was already part of the report from Barmbek and the Friedrichsberg psychiatrist had recorded "no abnormality detected."

In schizophrenia, Bleuler believed that heredity or "congenital disposition [was] of critical importance" and considered schizophrenia to be a "heredodegeneration" even though he admitted that no medical sound idea existed for the causes of schizophrenia.[50] The term heredodegeneration, a combination of "heredity" and "degeneration," implied that the cause was to be found in the patient's family history, that it was possible to locate the reason for the illness in former events that had induced a degeneration of a family member and was later passed on. The inability to find an organic cause of illness could be balanced by a kind of "virtual body," the "body of the family." Through heredity, it was possible to re-introduce a pathological "material substratum" and give the illness certain physicality.

Even though physicians could not distinguish any former event in Buller's family medical history as a cause for her pathological "disposition" during her 1931 admission, by the first draft of the medical report for the sterilization process in 1935, an alcoholic grandfather had suddenly been found. A "faulty" family history invented a new body because the illness, no matter what its nature might have been, could be passed off as a "meta-organic substrate" of madness from previous generations. The body was in reality the whole body of the family and the search for inherited traits replaced the individual body through a material correlation. As Foucault contended, psychiatrists attempted to construct a meta-individual "analogon."[51]

In Buller's case, the psychiatrist possessed information from the Barmbek record and he used his knowledge to construct a "biographic corpus" that included family, occupation, marital status, and medical observations. The admission ritual was the first step towards fixing this documentary identity onto

---

49 Ibid., 125.
50 Ibid., 328–329.
51 Michel Foucault, *Le pouvoir psychiatrique. Cours au collège de France. 1973–1974*, eds. François Ewald et al (France: Seuil/Gallimard, 2003), 272.

individuals and, consequently, forcing individuals to recognize themselves in their documentary histories and in the documented events that took place during their stay in the asylum. For this reason, the interrogations were repeated regularly, which also served to emphasize the status of the psychiatrist as a doctor in a twofold manner: either patients showed their symptoms and in showing them, demonstrated that they were really sick, or they "confessed" their madness. In both cases the result demonstrated that they were really in need of treatment by a physician.

Buller's psychiatrist noted during the admission procedure to Friedrichsberg in February 1931 that:

> 19.2.31 Mother (addition to details in B [Barmbek])
> On Feb 9th in the morning she said to mother: "Mum, what a bad person I am!" Reproaches herself because she had told a colleague that she liked the business she was working in. She did not want to get professional training although she did not want to miss school before. After school she lay down in bed, then she became frightened: "You my dear, I have to leave you now...,etc." At night often [had] anxiety attacks. "My soul wants to get out..." Next day, same timidity: that is why in hospital. In previous evening, at a 2nd doctor's, she did not speak at all. Last school Humboldtstr. At the age of 12 in the upper. At the age of 16, graduated from school. Now advertisement designer with Ortmann, Pohlstr. She did not want to be there at all, did not like the boss. Because at school she was told she was talented, she became a designer. Formerly, all in all quiet. Interests: only drawing and reading heavy, difficult books: Dostojewski, Schopenhauer, Zola. Never went out, did not dance, only went out with mother, was very attached to her. At school very hard working, punctual, conscientious. Felt very unhappy with her nose (broke back of nose when falling as child) and rejected. No interest in men. She loved nature and animals. Very economical, humble.'[52]

In detailing the reasons for admitting Buller, the psychiatrist made choices in considering which information was deemed important to develop a picture of the illness and thus what should be included in the admission report. Using quotations and reported speech as stylistic devices suggested an authentic objectivity on the part of the psychiatrist, which was further emphasized by his assertion that this additional information (to the report from Barmbek) was obtained from Buller's mother when Buller herself kept silent. However, the direction of the report from Barmbek and the one written by the psychiatrist at Friedrichsberg differed considerably. Much of the Barmbek account was structured around symptoms and behaviours that appeared to stem from the pivotal event of her developing the "flu." In comparison, the Friedrichsberg psychiatrist, who was aware of the information contained in the Barmbek record, was more concerned with detecting early signs of madness in Buller's biography.

---

52 PR, FMR, PN.

The physician at Barmbek believed that the precipitating event for Buller's illness was her flu-like illness, and this diagnosis seemed to shape his admission report. His suspicions were strengthened by the facts that she had been tobogganing on 9 February 1931, had not slept for three days afterwards, and now had a fever; all in all, she had not felt well during this time. Her parents reportedly had also not noticed anything different about her "before Sunday." Although the physician noted some "restless and strange" behaviour (and her gaze was "somewhat staring and empty"), he did not initially consider these definite signs for an underlying mental illness.

The Friedrichsberg psychiatrist also believed that 9 February was a significant date related to Buller's admission. However, he was more interested in the conversation her mother had reported from that day ("Mama what a bad person I am!"), as well as Buller's confession to a colleague that she liked her work, when in reality she did not. Connecting these sentences seems to suggest that the psychiatrist believed she felt guilty about something that was normally not worth mentioning. He ordered these and other details in such a way so as to provide an alternative framing to her illness. Although Buller had not wanted to miss school before, he emphasized that she now did not want to attend and lay down immediately after coming home, indicating that something had been wrong for longer than previously thought. He reported her "anxiety attacks" at night that left her anxious and frightened, feelings that she had shared with her mother ("my soul wants to get out"). The use of "etc." and ellipses indicated that these were only some examples of her confused thinking, and her refusal to speak suggested to the psychiatrist that her condition had rapidly worsened. Thus, the reasons for Buller's admission to Barmbek were transformed from the physical "morbus internes (flu?)" into the psychiatric diagnosis of schizophrenia.

The Friedrichsberg psychiatrist was also determined to trace the development of her illness from much further back than his Barmbek colleague. Highlighting Buller's discontent with her present job could perhaps be seen as a sign that, despite her talents, she had been pressured into this kind of work. The report hinted that her extreme attachment to her mother and her lack of interest in men, dancing, and going out was inappropriately gendered behaviour. Reading "heavy, difficult books" was suggested as somewhat abnormal despite apparent model childhood behaviour, and her unhappiness with her appearance pointed to psychic consequences from a broken nose.

With these admission notes, a new kind of "documentary temporality" was introduced.[53] A "documentary temporality" was one of Enge's declared aims of

---

53 Smith, *Institutional Ethnography. A Sociology for People*; Dorothy E. Smith, *Writing the Social. Critique, Theory, and Investigations* (Canada: University of Toronto Press, 2004);

the admission ritual, in that the prehistory of the case had to focus on the time of the outbreak and on the different mental and physical events that took place.[54] How Buller's behaviour was perceived to be mental illness lies in the manner in which the report was constructed. Labelling Buller as a schizophrenic meant that all other aspects of her history become nothing more than evidence to support the officially recognized mental illness. Sociologist Dorothy Smith called this the "authorization rules," which are part of an official account and that instruct the reader as to what criteria to use in determining the adequacy of the description and credibility of the account. The actual events are not facts per se.

> A fact is something which is already categorized, which is already worked up so that it conforms to the model of what the fact should be like. To describe something as fact or to treat something as fact implies that the events themselves – what happened – entitle or authorize the teller of the tale to treat that categorization as ineluctable. "Whether I wish it or not, it is a fact. Whether I will admit it or not, it is a fact."[55]

Buller's account was based on the testimony of her mother, someone whom we would usually feel had her daughter's best interests at heart. In these circumstances it was not even necessary that Buller had a voice, because the version was legitimized by the fact that it was given by her mother. The willingness of the psychiatrist, as the approved medical authority, to translate the mother's testimony into the official history, gives this account a privileged status. Any alternative account could only be speculative because the organization of this privileged status was constructed by people who were part of the event. However, an alternative interpretation was also made impossible by the lack of sufficient information. One feature of official accounts is that they do not contain irrelevant material, material which neither establishes the adequacy of the authorization procedures nor contributes to the conceptual organization. The construction of an alternative account that denies Buller's mental illness is not possible on the basis of the available evidence and its organization. This account became the foundation for all the events that occurred in the future: 10 years later this first admission account would continue to be consulted.

However, this account and the way it was constructed has even deeper implications. In supporting Buller's psychiatric diagnosis with evidence from her history that included her very constitution as a cause for her illness, the psy-

---

Smith, "The Social Construction of Documentary Reality," *Sociological Inquiry* 44, no. 4 (1974): 257–268; George W. Smith, "Policing the Gay Community: An Inquiry into Textually-Mediated Social Relations," *International Journal of the Sociology of Law*, no. 16 (1988): 163–183.

54 Enge, "Die Vorgeschichte (Anamnese) und ihre Bedeutung für die Krankheitsfeststellung (Diagnose)," 89.

55 Dorothy E. Smith, "'K. is Mentally Ill:' The Anatomy of a Factual Account," *Sociology*, no. 12 (1978): 35.

chiatrist constructed her from the beginning as a chronic and even an incurable case. This is to say, from the beginning he considered Buller to be a "hopeless" case; the disturbances that occurred early in her childhood indicated that something, however hidden, existed underneath and demonstrated a form of degeneration even if it was not yet possible to find the source.

The search for the individual history is, according to Foucault, the attempt to demonstrate that, on the one hand, madness already existed before it expressed itself as real illness and on the other, that these signs were not yet the madness itself but rather the conditions of possibility. These signs were not really pathological, because in that moment they were nothing more than symptoms of an illness, but rather something like implicit signs that were related in a specific way to the illness in order to be marked as signs or dispositions. The illness was thereby separated from the individual context and placed within a frame that could be characterized as "abnormal." Abnormality was simultaneously the individual condition of possibility for madness and the precondition to demonstrate that what needed treatment were effectively pathological symptoms. A web of abnormality was the precondition enabling reasons for admission to be transformed into pathological symptoms. In this part of the admission ritual something like a "horizon of abnormality" was thus established.[56] As Enge implicitly acknowledged:

> Of utmost importance is the *detection of the original disposition*. [original emphasis]. Poor mental ability (*Verstandesbegabung*), which later often becomes obvious in belated language development, points to mutagenic influences and, to a higher degree, it points to *pathological processes that were already established before or after birth* (syphilis, infectious diseases). Imbecility combined with pedantry is often found at an early state as concomitant of true epilepsy. The different forms of psychopathic disposition are mostly prefigured at an early state by a great vividness of the phantasy and pathological fiddling, by excitability, anxiousness, abjection or hilarity, saintliness, increased self-worth. Through behaviour it is possible to infer a shy, closed, stubborn constitution, an absence of will or adventurousness (*Unternehmenslustig*), lack of stability, cantankerousness, domination by one's physical desires (*Triebhaftigkeit*), criminal affinities, or different forms of psychopathy. *Nearly every acute mental illness has its precursors.*[57]

As this short extract illustrated, virtually any behaviour could be marked as a sign of mental illness, precursors that could be adequately interpreted only by psychiatrists.

The Friedrichsberg account on Buller transformed the reasons for her admission into actual psychiatric symptoms. Whereas the admission to Barmbek

---

56 Foucault, *Le pouvoir psychiatrique. Cours au collège de France. 1973–1974*, 271–275.
57 Enge, "Die Vorgeschichte (Anamnese) und ihre Bedeutung für die Krankheitsfeststellung (Diagnose)," 89. [emphasis mine]

took place due to a kind of helplessness on the part of her mother because her daughter's behaviour had changed, this behaviour became in Friedrichsberg the symptoms of schizophrenia, and at the end of the admission ritual, Buller's diagnosis had transformed into fact.

Nonetheless, as Bleuler and Weygandt previously suggested, the admission ritual had a more far-reaching objective. The purpose of the interrogation was to reduce the illness to its "main symptom," not only to make the subject acknowledge this absolute core but also to effectively actualize it during the interrogation. It could be actualized in two different ways, either by means of a patient's confession like "yes, I hear voices," because in that moment the symptoms would be fixed to the individual in the form of a first-person statement, or by provoking a crisis, for example, by triggering hallucinations, an epileptic seizure, or a bout of hysteria. This is what Weygandt attempted to obtain though his administering the "alcohol test" or cocaine. The "rough needle pricks" and "pricks in the system" that Buller experienced could be considered attempts to provoke a kind of aggressive reaction, efforts that were finally successful during the struggle to obtain her blood work.

This part of the admission ritual that aimed to provoke a situation in which patients could not avoid acknowledging their madness had a direct relevance to the development of psychiatric practice. Admitting madness meant that patients also admitted that they were actually ill, in need of a physician and of being interned, and that they were the kind of patients for whom psychiatric asylums were built. This moment Foucault called the "double enthronement" (*double intronisation*), when, on the one hand, the interned individual was "enthroned" as a sick person and on the other, when the interning individual was "enthroned" as psychiatrist and physician.[58]

Interrogations can be analyzed on three different levels. The first level concerns the dimension of the disciplinary character as analyzed above. Foucault described the aim of the second level of the interrogation as

> ...constituting a medical mimesis in psychiatric questioning, the analogon of a medical schema given by pathological anatomy: first, psychiatric questioning constitutes a body through the system of ascriptions of heredity, it gives body to an illness which did not have one; second, around this illness, and in order to pick it out as illness, it constitutes a field of abnormalities; third, it fabricates symptoms from a demand for confinement; and finally, fourth, it isolates, delimits, and defines a pathological source that it shows and actualizes in the confession or in the realization of this major and nuclear symptom.[59]

---

58 Foucault, *Le pouvoir psychiatrique. Cours au collège de France. 1973–1974*, 273.
59 Michel Foucault, *Psychiatric Power. Lectures at the Collège De France, 1973–74*, eds. Jaques Langrange et al, trans. Graham Burchell (New York: Palgrave Mac Millan, 2006), 275.

The interrogation recreates in a way exactly the elements that characterize the differential diagnosis in organic medicine in a form of a "mimesis" or "analogon." For the third level of the interrogation is the level at which,

> ...through the play of sleights of hand, exchanges, promises, gifts and counter-gifts between psychiatrist and patient there is the triple realization of conduct as madness, of madness as illness, and finally, of the mad person's guardian as doctor.[60]

The psychiatrist had two functions in the everyday life of the asylum: the interrogation and the round. A psychiatrist made rounds through all departments of his asylum every morning in order to transform discipline into therapy – to control all the small wheels of the system, to inspect all disciplinary mechanisms, and to transform those parts into a therapeutic apparatus solely through the presence of the psychiatrist. The interrogation consisted of summoning the sick person to demonstrate his or her symptoms, and through these symptoms, to transform the psychiatrist into a recognized doctor. The whole disciplinary field functioned by means of these two rites, and to preserve these functions is why this ritual had to be re-enacted from time to time.

Portions of these rites are clearly recognizable in the records under study here. As initials and underlining in the nurses' notes attest, psychiatrists maintained control over nursing information. Almost every paper that found its way into the patient record had to be signed by the medical director or his representative. Only at the moment that psychiatrists used fragments of the nurses' notes in their own notes did nursing observations become an approved official part of the record. These mechanisms will be highlighted in more detail over the course of this analysis.

Completing the case history of a patient was one objective of a stay in the asylum and this objective was an important aspect of nursing work. According to Enge, it was important that the nurses not only understood the importance of the patient's biography, in order to determine the causes for his or her mental illness, but also that they realized the process of gathering information about the patient's prehistory never ended during the patient's stay in the asylum. According to Enge, nurses must assist

> at times to complete the case history. Their constant interactions with patients allow the development of mutual trust, so that many a sick person confides in them more quickly and with less reserve than with their physicians. Therefore I feel free, if I know the exact skills, the psychological understanding and the discretion of a nurse, to give this particular nurse the order to obtain the pre-history.[61]

---

60 Ibid.
61 Enge, "Die Vorgeschichte (Anamnese) und ihre Bedeutung für die Krankheitsfeststellung (Diagnose)," 90

This short section touches on the specific relevance of nursing within psychiatric practice. As will be suggested, nurses occupied a kind of strategic position, because the "mutual trust' relationship between the patient and the nurse enabled the psychiatrist to gather information that he himself was not able to obtain. This specific relationship between nurses and patients is sometimes reflected in the record. In some records, letters were found in which patients emphasized their appraisal of particular nurses. Anna Maria Buller's record contained, for example, a drawing with birthday greetings for a nurse named Maria. (See Figure 10) Something similar was never found for psychiatrists. However, the strategic relationship between nurses and psychiatrists is illustrated in the interplay between their separate records.

The nurses were often the first hospital personnel the patient encountered when entering the institution, especially if the patient had been transferred from another hospital. Most were provisionally admitted by nurses and only over the next few days were they officially admitted by the psychiatrist. Like the admission rituals carried out by psychiatrists, admission procedures undertaken by nurses also had a ceremonial character, although with some important differences. While physician admission rituals were meant to demonstrate the power of the psychiatrist through making the patient understand their behaviour as madness, to realize that madness was illness, and to apprehend that they were under the control of the psychiatrist, nurses admission measures had a purely disciplinary aim that targeted the patients' body.

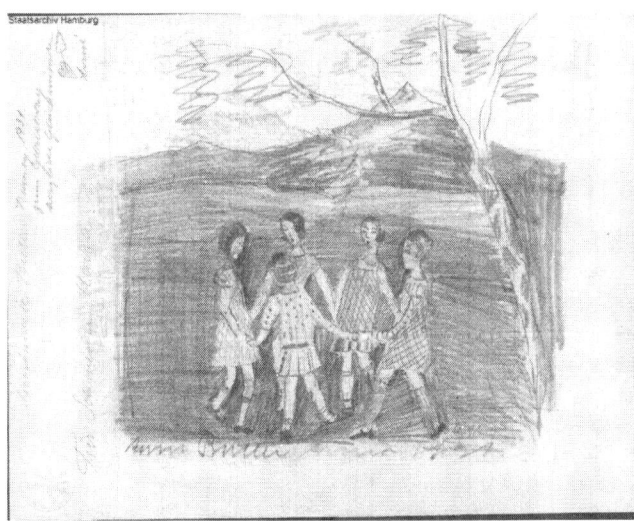

Figure 10: Drawing with birthday greetings for Nurse Maria, 1931. Patient record 23883.

This focus began the moment the patient arrived on the ward. A Langenhorn nursing school textbook described the procedure.

> Every arrival is guided to the ward and gets a bath as a start; if he resists it despite persuasion the physician must be informed. The bath functions not only to clean the sick person but also provides a means to inspect his body for something like wounds, skin rashes, vermin (hairy parts!), abdominal ruptures and others. Also the clothing is to be reviewed during the bath (valuables, arms, vermin). After the bath the sick person has to be weighed and, if not decided otherwise, to be put to bed and kept under constant surveillance.[62]

This procedure was also routinely carried out in Friedrichsberg when patients were admitted from home, but not when patients like Buller were transferred from another hospital. The meaning of the bath obviously extended beyond a simple cleansing of a patient's body; it signified the starting point for appropriating patients' bodies, because they were not only weighed and measured but every bodily function as well that was deemed beyond "normal range" became the target of specific nursing interventions.

Nurses used different forms to record their work, compiling individual fever charts, for example, from the moment patients were admitted to Friedrichsberg. Buller's fever chart was drawn up on the day of her admission, as was a weight table, the latter suggesting that the admitting nurses were already informed of her refusal to take any food. (See Figure 11) As other medical records demonstrate, the routine procedure was to weigh the patient on the day of admission, to note the weight in the fever chart, and to check the weight sporadically during a patient's hospitalization, if at all. In Buller's case, however, her weight was noted not only on the fever chart but also on a weight table. As we will later see, "facts" on the record had the ability to initiate further action, recalling sociologist Bruno Latour's concept of "chains of action."[63]

---

62 Ludwig Scholz, *Leitfaden für Irrenpfleger* (Halle a. d. Saale: Carl Marhold, 1920), 71; Ludwig Scholz, *Leitfaden für Irrenpfleger* (Halle a. d. Saale: Carl Marhold, 1904). This textbook was used throughout the period under study in the Langenhorn nursing school. It was first published in 1900 and was reprinted thereafter until WWII. The textbook can be considered the standard text on the education of nurses in the German Reich. The medical director of Langenhorn conducted an inquiry of several German asylums to decide what textbook to use for nursing education at the school, with the result that he chose Scholz's textbook. StArHH 352-8/7 Nursing staff. Education, inauguration of the school of Nursing for the lunatics (*Pflegepersonal. Ausbildung. Eröffnung der Irrenpflegeschule*). Scholz was also the main editor of the journal *Nursing for the Lunatics* (*Die Irrenpflege*), which in 1930 was renamed *Nursing for the Mentally Ill* (*Die Geisteskrankenpflege*).
63 Latour, "Reassembling the Social. An Introduction to Actor-Network-Theory," 47.

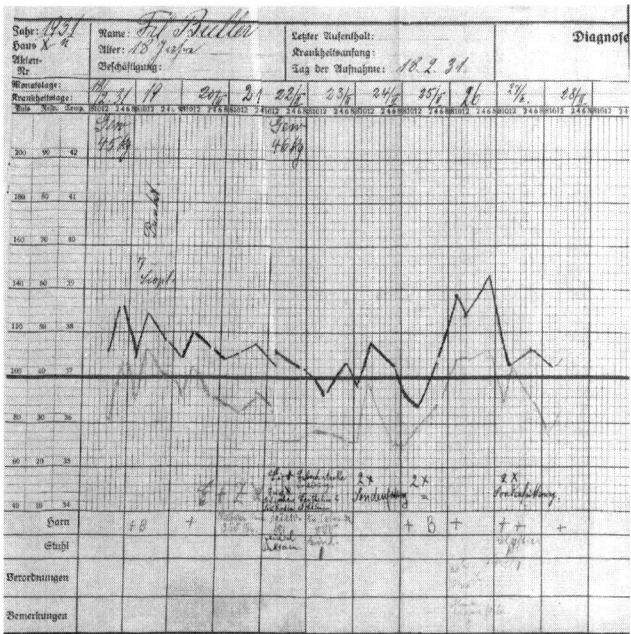

Figure 11: Fever chart for the first days of admission in 1931. Medical record 28338.

Different forms suggest that there was a perceived need for continuous observation of particular bodily functions. For example, the fever chart predetermined the need for regular monitoring of body temperature and pulse, and that these and other factors (prescriptions, urine output, etc.) should be recorded in a predefined manner that was controlled by the construction of the chart. These charts also determined who was allowed to write on the form and above all, who was allowed to enter what factors into the form. The writing of remarks, for example, was a task reserved for physicians, whereas temperature, pulse, defecation, weight, tube feeding, and medications were recorded by nurses. Occupying a pivotal position between psychiatrists and nurses, fever charts are especially interesting, because they were always compiled at least for the patient's first couple of days in the asylum and they sometimes initiated further consequences. The fever chart was thus a complex "inscription" because it graphically represented patient corporeality. As a kind of map, the fever chart integrated large amounts of different data onto one single form, relating this information in a specific way to make certain interrelationships visible. The fever chart was further connected to a wide range of "inscriptions devices," such as clinical thermometers, clocks, centrifuges, and catheters, and served both to initiate a series of organizational reactions and to facilitate the mutual co-ordination of individual nurses. The record had much more than an auxiliary role, however, because not only did it represent this co-ordination of work but it also initiated and mediated it. The record was a material form of semipublic memory; it was a *"structured distributing and collecting device,* where all the tasks concerning the patient's trajectory must begin and end."[64] Scribbling a "+B" (bacteria found in urine) onto the fever chart resulted in Buller's repeated catheterization, a detailed analysis of her catheterized urine, and the repeated verification of her body temperature, illustrating the pivotal role that these inscription devices played within the asylum. The record afforded the ability for "action at distance:" the act of writing on the nutrition chart about Buller's refusal to eat, for example, channelled a wide range of asylum resources around and through her body.[65] A forced feeding was ordered for Buller, for which it was necessary to bring her to a treatment room, find two nurses to hold her down, engage a psychiatrist to introduce the tube, prepare a specific diet, observe that she did not vomit afterwards, and so on. The patient's body was rendered transparent through further disciplining and material rewriting and through the production of comparable and combinable inscriptions that could be listed on a few sheets of paper. As sociologist Marc Berg, wrote, "the availability of such an over viewable, durable and moveable set of inscriptions allow[ed] physicians the opportunity to extend their gaze across time and space."[66] The patient's body was disciplined through different interventions and made transparent by translating bodily functions into charts and lists (inscriptions). In the end, the patient became nothing more than sheets of paper.

Divisions on the chart prescribed when the specific information had to be charted, structuring nurses' time and thus entering the sequential nature of the fever chart into the temporal organization of asylum work.[67] Each day was divided into two-hour stages. The column in the middle of each day, however, was a little broader than the others, signifying that the days were further subdivided into four two-hour columns, which resulted in eight-hour segments (According to the chart, the asylum day was only 16 hours) The chart was thus constructed in such a manner that nurses entered their information during the morning and evening shifts. The chart enforced the idea that particular kinds of recordings had to be carried out in a predefined manner but other fields in the chart could be used for purposes other than what was intended.

The chart was laid out as an x-y axis graph, with the temporal dimensions of hours, days, and weeks charted along the x-axis, and the measurements of pulse,

---

64 Berg, "Practices of Reading and Writing," 499–524. [emphasis in original]
65 Latour and Woolgar, *Laboratory Life: The Construction of Scientific Facts*, 245; Latour, *Science in Action*.
66 Berg, "Practices of Reading and Writing," 511.
67 Paul Atkinson, *The Clinical Experience: The Construction and Reconstruction of Medical Reality* (Farnborough: Gower, 1981).

respiration, and temperature placed along the y-axis. The "normal" range of the latter measurements lay on a curve highlighted in bold in the middle of the graph, making them easy to monitor, to see their relation to each other and to other entries on the chart, and to note whether or not they were outside the normal range.

Within specific limits, however, the form could be adjusted to meet organizational necessities. The complex temporal structure of the asylum could only be maintained through a material infrastructure of lists, schedules, and so forth. Moreover, while the chart format structured the nurses' time during their working day, the psychiatrist could choose on their own when to take notes or when to carry out specific tasks. The differential valuation of time between the professional groups in the asylum was built into the very structure of the record.

Nevertheless, the form did not simply determine the course of action it mediated nor did it just impose its structure on those working with it. It was not an uncomplicated intermediary between the "intentions" of those who ordered particular tasks and the activities of those who performed it. Certain fields, especially at the top of the form, were not filled in. On Buller's record, for example, no one had written anything about the origins of her illness, her diagnosis, or her occupation. As ethnologist Harold Garfinkel contended, some indices were considered simply superfluous for the performance of everyday work, a fact that he stated was a general feature of record keeping in psychiatric asylums.[68] The fields on the lower part of the fever chart were also only partially used; for example, not one single record had the space for "comments" filled in, not necessarily surprising since it was a fairly limited space in which to enter remarks for psychiatric patients. However, in many records, examinations, laboratory results, prescriptions, and interventions, etc., were entered on the fever charts even though they were not designed for this kind of detail. The fact that these forms were sometimes used in a manner other than that prescribed by their organizational structure highlights the fact that rules were constantly re-interpreted or overridden. Berg called these instances "repair work," because it suggested an ongoing elaboration of what was or needed to be written down and what had to be done. "The continuous working around and re-interpreting of the record's content allow the record to function – to distribute and collect, and thereby transform the very work of those who bring it alive."[69]

A kind of "insider knowledge" was necessary to read these charts. For example, although different colours were used to register body temperature and the pulse (red and black, respectively), most of the information entered on the

---

68 Harold Garfinkel, "Good Organizational Reasons for 'Bad' Clinic Records," in *Studies in Ethnomethodology* (Cambridge: Polity Press, 2010): 186–207.
69 Berg, "Practices of Reading and Writing," 513.

fever chart was written in a "code-like" style, necessary not only because the space on the chart was limited, enforcing the use of abbreviations, but also because the entries were part of a "special discourse."[70] (On the delineation between different discursive formations see the analysis below.) And although the red "E+Z ø" indicated that Buller's urine was free of protein and sugar, the code "+B" revealed some bacteria, and she was catheterized three consecutive times to obtain sterile samples. The "Einl." in the "feces" column meant that she had received an enema, a successful procedure that was repeated four days later with a "clyster."

The first entries on Buller's fever chart, begun on the afternoon of her admission on 18 February 1931, were her body weight (45 kg) and temperature. Because her temperature was considered elevated and her weight low, these entries initiated a cascade of interventions in the days to come. The next day, the word *Punkt* (for *Punktion* or puncture) revealed that a lumbar puncture had been carried out. This procedure in turn led to new inscriptions – new recordings – when the psychiatrist filled out more lab requisitions. (See Figure 12 and 13) He sent the specimens he obtained to the laboratory for testing, and the results of the tests came back in diagram or table form, which were then posted on the chart by the laboratory assistant. From this moment on, these inscriptions became parts of the medical record, with Buller's internal bodily functions translated into graphs and figures.

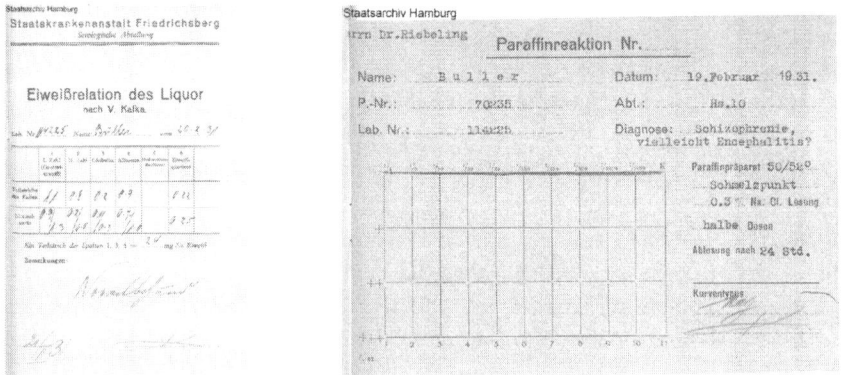

Figure 12 and 13: Requisition slips for laboratory analyses. Medical record 28338.

---

70 Jürgen Link, *Versuch über den Normalismus. Wie Normalität produziert wird* (Göttingen: Vandenhoeck und Ruprecht, 2006).

The fact that no abnormal physiological results were found supported, in a reverse manner, the diagnosis of schizophrenia. Laboratory analyses, obeying a rationality of "differential diagnosis" could only "prove" the physical symptoms of something like paralytic dementia or encephalitis because no laboratory measures enabled relating any specific mental illness to pathological processes in the brain. Buller's psychiatrist, who had written "schizophrenia, perhaps encephalitis?" implied that there were only two diagnostic possibilities. Because the results falsified the hypothesis that Buller might have been suffering from encephalitis, the actual diagnosis of schizophrenia was verified. Like the interrogation during the admission examination, the laboratory analyses recreated what Foucault had called a form of "mimesis" or "analogon" to organic medicine. Simultaneously, they served as objective evidence of Buller's schizophrenia and thereby underlined the chronic nature of her condition. If no pathological cause could be found, the cause of the disease therefore lay in what Bleuler had described as "heredogeneration"– in her constitution – implying that no hope for a cure existed. From the beginning then, the laboratory analyses constructed her condition as "hopeless."

Anna Maria Buller's weight (46 kg) was recorded again on 22 February. In combination with the fever chart, the weight table led to the construction of a nutrition plan. (See Figure 14) The nutrition plan was not a standardized form but was designed by the nurses themselves, who apparently also participated in establishing conditions that enabled surveillance of their work. Even though written in pencil, it was an official part of the medical record, and contributed to the organization of their daily work as well as to the number of interventions carried out on the patient. Most notably, however, the nurses had also inserted a column for the psychiatrist's signature, suggesting that he was expected to monitor the entries in the table.

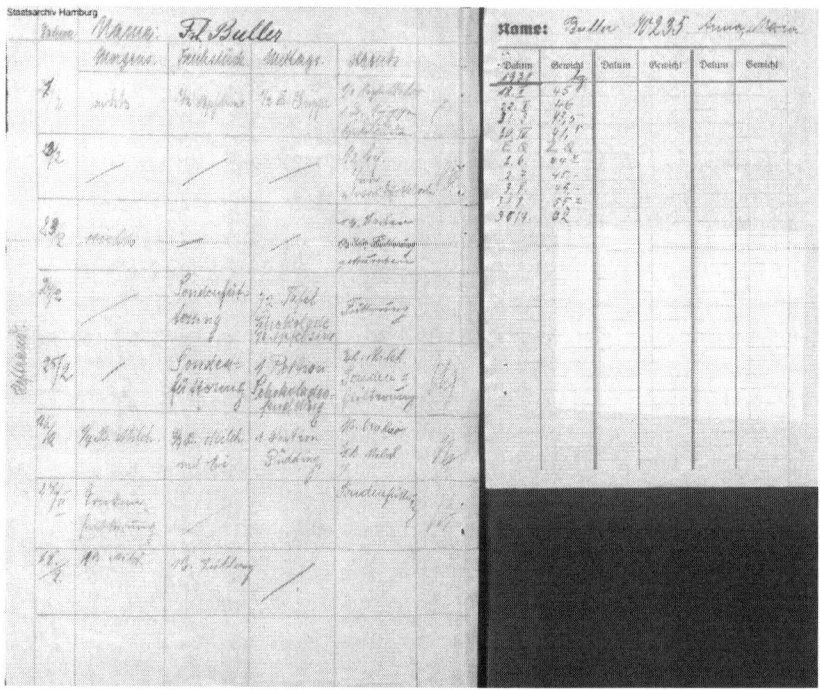

Figure 14: Nutrition plan (left) and weight table (right). Medical record 28338.

The nutrition table was a consequence of the weight table, but it also resulted from the medical record from Barmbek where it had been reported that Buller had refused to eat. From this point on, the nutrition "problem" was provable "objectively." In other words, different tables and diagrams had made Buller's refusal of food visible – neither the family members nor Buller herself had mentioned this aspect before – and it became the target of several disciplinary technical and nursing interventions. This "objective" information was supplemented by nursing reports in the medical file. Six days after Buller's admission to Friedrichsberg, both the data collection and the reports had not only led to the realization that her food intake was insufficient but also that she actually actively resisted any attempt to feed her. Buller's "aggressive-negativistic" conduct then led to the decision to feed her by force, a procedure that did not help to increase her weight. On the contrary, by 13 April 1931, she weighed just 41.5 kg.

As further analysis of the nursing notes demonstrates, the tube feeding was perceived as more a kind of educational intervention: the forced feeding was not aimed primarily at achieving a weight increase but rather to convince Buller to start eating on her own accord. However, the interplay between the different inscription devices that dealt with Buller's weight loss demonstrates that the represented and the representation are wholly interdependent. The represented did not simply predate its representation; rather, the former only existed because of the latter and vice versa. Only by reading the weight table and the nutrition plan was it perceived, and proved, that Buller had insufficient nutritional intake. The practices of reading and writing the record, then, are practices of reading and writing patients' bodies, as well as their subjectivities. As Berg noted,

> the practices of representation are indistinguishable from the activities they supposedly represent. The intertwining of this distributing and collecting device with the hospital's organizational routines is what allows physicians to travel through a patient's body from behind their desk, to cross temporal, bodily and professional boundaries....[71]

Nevertheless, that the documents directed the perceptions of the nurses becomes obvious when Buller was readmitted to Friedrichsberg in 1936 and again in 1940. Although the nurses' notes mentioned that she was not eating sufficiently at those times, no nutrition plans were laid out. Although by 1936 the patient had lost more than 12 kilograms from her first admission to Friedrichsberg, her eating disorder is merely mentioned in the notes but never systematically observed and accordingly, did not become a target of nursing intervention. In 1940, no weight chart was even instituted, and thus neither Buller's weight nor her nutritional intake was monitored. At these points her weight was not a primary concern, and because it was not the subject-matter of specific inscriptive devices in the record, Buller thus did not "have" an eating disorder.

From 24 February on, Buller was force fed twice a day. (The German translation of the word *Fütterung* refers to the feeding of animals, somewhat unusual in special medical discourse when one would expect a word like *Sondenernährung*, which would be closer to the idea of nutrition.) Such a complex fever chart enabled viewing all relevant information of the patient's bodily functions at a glance, or to use the terminology of Actor-Network Theory, all the bodily functions were translated onto the fever chart.[72] Furthermore, according to Garfinkel,

> [t]he expressions, the remarks that make up these documents [patient records] have overwhelmingly the characteristic that their sense cannot be decided by a reader without necessarily knowing or assuming something about a typical biography and typical purpose of the user of the expressions, about typical circumstances under which such remarks are written, about a typical previous course of transactions between the writers and patient, or about a typical relationship of actual or potential interaction between the writers and the reader. Thus the folder contents, much less than

---

71 Berg, "Practices of Reading and Writing," 511.
72 Latour, *Reassembling the Social,* Latour, *Science in Action*; Bruno Latour, *We have Never been Modern* (Cambridge, Massachusetts: Harvard University press, 2002); Latour and Woolgar, *Laboratory Life.*

revealing an order or interaction, presuppose an understanding of that order for a correct reading.[73]

Using abbreviations in the medical record was directed towards an economy of effort, since reports that were too long wasted the time of the writer as well as the reader, who wanted quickly to find the relevant information. However, the brevity and (seeming) incompleteness of these records worked since both reader and writer were part of the asylum medical personnel and were familiar with the language associated with those positions.[74] As this analysis has attempted to demonstrate, all bodily functions became the target of observations and interventions. Each was translated into an inscription in order to detect and correct possible "malfunctions" of, in this case, Buller's body. More importantly, by collecting physiological parameters and graphing them on, for example, the fever chart, it became possible to make visible trends that had not yet been physically manifested. As the following analysis demonstrates, this ability was an important aspect of psychiatric practice, and one that applied to nurses' notes as well. Trends and tendencies not yet materialized can be said to be in a "space of possibility," still in the process of becoming and thus in a purely virtual state. Although Buller's eating disorder, for example, was not yet fully developed, it became the target of multiple interventions in the hope of retarding any further progression. The struggle over the "virtual" behaviour of patients is the focus of the next section.

As previously mentioned, Buller was first admitted to Friedrichsberg on 18 February 1931 by the nurses.

> Afternoon, 18.2.31. New admission.
> Pat. lay in bed quietly, didn't answer questions, shouted out loud at certain times "I want to see my sister Gertrud, she is next door." Pat. only drank.
> (Ha.) [nurse's signature][75]

As was the case for the psychiatric admission ritual that followed, this first entry contained nearly all the points that would guide future observations and reports on Buller, and all of these that are mentioned in these first few sentences were also part of the admittance attestation. The "general consideration (*Betrachtung*) of the sick person" was one of the "most important means" of obtaining a correct "detection of the disease (*Krankheitsfeststellung*)."[76] For example, according to Enge, a "comparatively simple aid for the detection of a disease is the position in the bed (*Bettlage*), the attitude and posture of the sick person. It can be perceived

---

73 Garfinkel, "Good Organizational Reasons for 'Bad' Clinic Records," 201.
74 Berg, "Practices of Reading and Writing,"513.
75 PR, FMR, nurses' notes (hereafter NN).
76 Enge, "Krankheitsfeststellung durch bloße Betrachtung," *Geisteskrankenpflege. Monatsschrift für Geisteskranken- und Krankenpflege* 40, no. 9 (1936):129.

at a glance."[77] As the first clause revealed, Buller was on bed rest, a typical nursing directive for psychiatric patients during these years, and one that presupposed an understanding of the usual nursing procedures for a correct reading.[78] Unusual activities in bed, however, might typically indicate a brain disorder. The phrase "did not answer questions" was more revealing, in that

> ...from the overall conduct of some sick persons by mere observation, without using any other method of examination, one very often obtains certain proofs of a disease. If one has for example a sick person who reacts to every advance (*Annäherungsversuche*) stiffly and with hostility, does not talk, freezes in a bodily position, always repeats the same movements, grimacing etc. then the diagnosis schizophrenia is not difficult to make.[79]

From this perspective, the nurses had already confirmed the diagnosis of schizophrenia, supporting Enge's contention that it was "possible to perceive the suffering of a sick person 'at a glance.'"[80]

Although the psychiatric admission note had attempted to decipher the hidden truth of Buller's mental illness, the nursing records appeared to be less "directional;" nurses were apparently observing signs that might be connected to madness. The use of direct speech, as if the patients were speaking for themselves, was an important strategic function of nurses' notes within the medical record that will be addressed later. Thus, in this short paragraph all the aspects of her diagnosis are assembled, and they will form the core of further observations about her during her stay in Friedrichsberg over the next few months.

On 19 February:

> Night: Pat. slept. (Du.)
> 19.2. [Morning]: Pat. shouted continuously until 8[am]: "Muthorst, Gertrud, aunty Hertha, Misses Kort I am still alive, one wants to kill me. Help, help, murder, murder, you villains, you beasts want to poison me. Help, help." Pat. could not be calmed down, took off her shirt, refused food, only drank. Pat. resists everything. Beats and lash out with feet. (Ge)
> 19.2. [Afternoon]: After coffee, Pat. was very lively, again and again sat upright in bed, laid her head over the barrier board (*Steckbrett*)[81] and shouted: <u>Cut off my head quickly, very quickly.</u>" Then pat. cried: "Now I won't see any of you ever again." Then,

---

77 Enge, "Die Vorgeschichte (Anamnese) und ihre Bedeutung für die Krankheitsfeststellung (Diagnose)," 88.
78 Philipp Seibert, "Zur Pflege Geisteskranker," *Geisteskrankenpflege. Monatsschrift für Geisteskranken- und Krankenpflege* 44, no. 12 (1940): 149.
79 Enge, "Krankheitsfeststellung durch bloße Betrachtung," 138.
80 Ibid.
81 The "barrierboard" (*Steckbrett*) was a board that was inserted into the bed sideways in order to prevent the patient from getting out of the bed. As the notes in other records demonstrate, this was a routine precautionary measure, especially on surveillance wards.

> coffee time, pat. spat out everything, ate well for dinner. Food had to be given. Pat. slept well after dinner. (Schmi.) [all underlined passages here and hereafter in the original] Night: Pat. was very restless and noisy. Threw around the bedding, did not let herself be touched, lashed out. (Du.) *M*. [Initialed by psychiatrist]
>
> 20.2. [Forenoon]: Pat. slept until 11 [am] became again very agitated, threw herself around in bed, shouted: "Please hack off my head, I have done wrong I want to die. O what a bunch of people are they, animals, beasts are they. O my head, my head hurts so badly." Pat. lashed out during feeding and clenches the teeth tightly. (Ge.)[82]

For the first three days, the nurses charted regularly on Buller, although it was more frequent when events occurred that seemed noteworthy. Most entries consisted almost exclusively of quoting Buller, supplemented by the context in which she uttered her statements. One of the textbooks used at that time in the nursing schools at Langenhorn and Friedrichsberg pointed out that, since nurses spent more time than physicians with patients, their observations were of particular importance and that patients might be more willing to confide in them.[83] Apart from suggesting that psychiatric practice could not function without nurses, the text also spoke to the strategic position nurses occupied in relation to their patients. As the author emphasized, "[the nurse] must be on his [*sic*] guard against giving an account of his personal opinion, but should rather factually report what he himself has noticed, *without connecting it to any judgment*."[84] Enge, too, believed that nurses should only offer descriptions of what they observed themselves, "the conduct of the sick person, all his doings, his talk, his moods, his habits and particularities, his bodily condition."[85] The psychiatrist

> wants to form his own opinion about the condition of the sick person. In order to do so he does not need an alien judgment but rather the knowledge of what happened during his absence. At this point very often mistakes are made with best intentions. It is not correct if the nurse reports, for example, that "The sick person hears voices and believes that he or she is being persecuted." The physician wants to hear how the sick person behaves, for example, if he sits up and takes notice, if he stares into the distance, if he moves defensively or offensively: the physician wants to hear what the sick person says. The physician wants to draw the conclusions himself.[86]

Nursing students at Langenhorn and Friedrichsberg were taught which descriptive categories and conceptual structures were important,[87] and the nurses'

---

82 PR, FMR, NN.
83 Scholz, *Leitfaden für Irrenpfleger*, 71–73.
84 Ibid., 72. [original emphasis]
85 Enge, "Beobachtungsberichte des Pflegepersonals," 115.
86 Ibid., 114–115.
87 Scholz, *Leitfaden für Irrenpfleger*, 72–73.

notes from Buller's first three days in Friedrichsberg replicated these requirements. Everything the patient did became a sign of the underlying disease.

The use of direct speech implied that the nurses were reporting the exact image of events that had occurred, as if the madness was speaking for itself. It granted their notes a certain authenticity and their "objective, empiricist" language only strengthened this impression. A single quote from Buller often stood as an exemplar for all of the statements she had made during an eight-hour shift, and was thus necessarily taken out of context. However, as sociologist Dorothy E. Smith suggested, this practice constructed "an account of behaviour so that it can be recognized by any member of the relevant cultural community as mentally ill type behaviour." She called this a "cutting out" procedure, accomplished "by constructing relationships between rules and definitions of situations on the one hand" and descriptions of mentally ill behaviour "on the other such that the former do not provide for the latter."[88]

Reporting in the asylum was done within the context of background knowledge and an understanding of normal courses of action. For example, Buller was assigned complete bed rest when admitted to the asylum, a fact that was not mentioned in the nurses' notes because it was a usual asylum-wide admission procedure. Thus, her behaviour in bed (sitting upright, laying her head over the barrier board, throwing herself around) was considered noteworthy because it deviated from the expected behaviour of lying quietly when on bed rest. This "observed" behaviour was enabled, or at least facilitated, by a form of institutional organization,[89] and its effects were similar to the trends made visible when various inscription devices were combined on the fever chart. It was the organization of asylum rules and regulations that provoked observation and classification of Buller's behaviour by both nurses and psychiatrists.

However, there is another dimension to the nurses' notes, because their thinking took place at the moment of writing – it was a "thinking in action" that was intertwined with artefacts. As Berg noted, "what we consider to be 'intellectual tasks' in fact often appear to be highly embodied activities."[90] Latour termed this aspect "thinking with eyes and hands,"[91] or "thinking is craftwork."[92] It is through writing that observations transform into manageable problems for the asylum's working routine.

---

88 Smith, "K. is Mentally Ill," 50.
89 Erving Goffman, *Asylums: Essays on the Social Situation of Mental Patients and Other Inmates* (New York: Doubleday and Co., 1961).
90 Berg, "Practices of Reading and Writing," 499–524.
91 Latour, "Visualisation and Cognition: Thinking with Eyes and Hands," 1–40.
92 Latour, *Science in Action*.

The Interplay between Nurses' and Psychiatrists' Notes

In the process of writing, the nurses and the psychiatrist constructed a "clear case" on Buller
On 20 February 1931, Buller's psychiatrist wrote that

> At night restless and noisy, lashed out with her feet. Today in the morning also agitated: "Please, cut off my head. I have done wrong. I want to die..." Refuses food in an aggressive-negativistic manner. Liquor results proved negative (see attached).[93]

His report more or less summarized the first three days of Buller's admission to the asylum, consisting almost entirely of information from the nurses' notes but reordering and representing them in a specific way. As Berg contended, representation involves the active work of ordering and is involved in the very event it represents: "'Representation' is not the (social) attaching of 'meaning' through which the (natural) world achieves its existence ... 'the social,' as a pure category, is a chimera: practices always also include artefacts, architectures, paper, machines."[94] As previously mentioned, psychiatrists underlined key features in nurses' notes that they included in their own notes. In this instance, the first sentence is a combination of the nurses' notes from 19 February. "Restless and noisy" came from the night nurse, and "lashing out with the feet" was noted in the afternoon. The psychiatrist's report, however, suggested that this behaviour occurred every night because it no longer specified when these events were observed. The next sentence was taken as is from the nursing notes of 20 February but in using the term "also," the psychiatrist implied that Buller had been excited throughout the night, when in fact she had slept until 11 a.m. before becoming agitated. While the nurses may have noted that Buller had had a bad headache and wished to cut off her head, this kind of context is absent in the psychiatrist's note. His simple but terse statement on Buller's refusal to eat translated the detailed nursing descriptions into medical terms that had already been mentioned in the admittance attestation. The nurses' note implied that she was being fed against her will (again using the German verb *füttern*) which might well have explained her active resistance. In defining this problem in diagnostic-medical terms it became a medical problem and a symptom that must accordingly be treated. Moreover, the psychiatrist's note became the official version of Buller's observed behaviour, helping not only to shape and maintain the course of Buller's asylum stay but also to illuminate the hierarchical relationships between Buller and the psychiatrist and between psychiatrists and nurses.

---

93 PR, FMR, PN.
94 Berg, "Practices of Reading and Writing," 500.

The record functioned as a kind of "mediator,"[95] because it mediated the relations that acted and worked through it, transforming social interactions due to its "documentary capacity." The "documentary capacity" of documents and texts in social organization refers to their ability to crystallize and preserve words detached from their local history. Through the materiality of documents, the meaning of lived processes is transformed, made and remade, at each moment of its course. Rather than being enforced by a sovereign individual, social consciousness is externalized by documents and texts, thereby objectifying reasoning, knowledge, memory, etc.[96]

Two interrelated coordinating functions of the medical record within the asylum can be distinguished. First are the textually coordinated work processes, which construct the institutional realities that make the actual actionable. This is a form of "fashioning institutional representations." From this perspective, the record establishes an "organizational time" by transforming the sequences of local events into another time frame; organizational judgment or information thus becomes an objectified documentary rather than a subjective process. Second, as seen in the translation from the nurses' to the psychiatrists' notes, "hierarchical forms of intertextuality in which texts on one level establish frames, concepts, and so on, [are] operating on and in the production of institutional realities."[97] As Smith wrote,

> [t]he work of fitting the actualities of people's lives to institutional categories that make them actionable is done at the front line. The categories, questions, or other particulars are governed by and responsive to frames established at a more general level.[98]

The medical record is activated through practices of reading and writing: "These practices, in which the record is turned to, leafed through, read, used for jotting, communicated through, dispatched, form a crucial side in the sociotechnical organisation of medical work." Without these practices the record would be without relevance. All of these activities "allow it to have its mediating role in the organization."[99] These interrelations of people and paperwork formulate the conditions so that the psychiatrist can be a psychiatrist, the nurse can be a nurse, and the patient becomes the diagnosed mentally ill person.

---

95 Latour, *Reassembling the Social*; Latour, "Pragmatogonies," 800.
96 Smith, *Institutional Ethnography*, Dorothy E. Smith, "Textually Mediated Social Organization," *International Social Science Journal* 36, no. 1 (1984): 59–76.
97 Smith, *Institutional Ethnography*, 186.
98 Ibid.; George Smith, "Policing the Gay Community," 180–183.
99 Berg, "Practices of Reading and Writing," 501.

The text – reader conversation

The practices of reading and writing were crucial "in the production of the very possibility of *"doctoring."*[100] The process of writing demonstrated the psychiatrist's competence and his intellectual qualities. Every entry in the medical history entailed the active production of a historical piece of information with the result that every bit of information was transformed into a symptom of illness. The psychiatrist's paperwork was a crucial feature in this transformative process, allowing it to create a representation of "the patient." As Berg maintained, "its value lies in the very fact that it is a highly selective, distanced, abstracted 'representation.'"[101] Furthermore, the patient is put into the temporal or psychiatric order of a mentally ill person's life span. Through the record the patient is integrated into a kind of a biography of the mentally ill. Through the writing of the patient's medical history, he or she becomes part of a "new temporality": the temporality of the psychiatric order. The psychiatrist's notes are not simple recordings; his reading and writing cannot be disentangled from his thinking. The reordering of events as outlined in the medical history under study here demonstrate the simple but significant phenomenon that the psychiatrist's own inscriptions become part of the information resources he had available as an element of the "thought processes" themselves.[102]

This analysis suggests that texts are active, not static, and thus are crucially significant in the asylum. The direct engagement of readers with texts "activates" them, creating a connection between the local bodily being and the translocal organization of "ruling relations,"[103] which Smith described as "objectified forms of consciousness and organization, constituted externally to particular places, creating and relying on textually based realities."[104] In bringing these different levels (local/translocal) together into one dimension, the text can be viewed as actively organizing institutional relations. "Documents in action" construct particular visions of the world and structure identities of those served by the asylum in specific ways, whether they are known as patients, clients, or the criminally insane.[105] Records are therefore "enrolled" in routine activity because they direct activities or serve as props in interaction; they enable the asylum to "perform."

---

100 Ibid., 504. [emphasis in original].
101 Ibid.
102 Latour, "Visualisation and Cognition: Thinking with Eyes and Hands;" David Gooding, "Putting Agency Back into Experiment," in *Science as Practice and Culture*, ed. Andrew Pickering (Chicago: University of Chicago Press, 1992), 63–112.
103 Smith, *Institutional Ethnography*, 102.
104 Ibid., 227.
105 Ibid., 102.

Nevertheless, it is important to recognize that not only is the text active but also the reader. A kind of "conversation" between the text and the reader takes place; text and reader enter into a dialogical relationship or a "duplex action."

> Texts have this capacity for a dialogic or dual coordination, one as they enter into how the course of action in which they occur is coordinated and the other in how the text coordinates a local and particular course of action with social relations extending both temporally and spatially beyond the moment of the text's occurrence.[106]

Texts are read by a specific person in a particular local setting, but unlike conversation, they remain the same no matter how many times they are read – i.e., the written words remain on the page for others to see and to read. This does not mean that every reader understands or interprets the words in exactly the same manner (on the contrary), but rather that the text itself (i.e., the words on the page) remains unchanged in its materiality as a written text. This characteristic of written text within the record is crucial to the role that it plays in institutions. The text remains unchanged by the history of its reading and is unresponsive to the reader's engagement with the text. This characteristic of written texts is crucial for their role in institutions, because it is

> key to the effect of institutional standardization across multiple local sites of people's work. It produces for any institutional participant reading the text a standardizing vocabulary, subject-object structure, entities, subjects and their interrelations, and so forth. They are the same for all readers, and as readers talk or otherwise act to coordinate across situations in relations to the text, it regulates the discourse effective amongst them. Sure, they may use other speech genres, some of which resist the institutional, but even resistance adopts the standardizing agenda, if only as foil.[107]

To govern the asylum is a mode of action, which depends on a reality constructed through documentary processes. Writers of texts and their readers are separated in time and space, and texts can be read by different individuals, in different places, and at different times. These characteristics thus allow documents to coordinate people's activities translocally, and they play an important role in standardizing social organization in institutions. Through the text-reader conversation, readers are caught by the text's temporal order and detached from their local bodily presence. "When we read, the text contains our consciousness; it lifts us out of locally oriented awareness," and this containment of consciousness enables readers to recognize the "active" part that texts play in coordinating people's work.

The reader activates the text, and in so doing, becomes the text's agent; the reader responds to it in whatever way. The activated text is playing a crucial part

---

106 Ibid., 103.
107 Ibid., 108.

in organizing definite sequences of action. One possible way of coordinating individuals within an institution is to initiate a sequence "that is involved in coordinating more than one individual in an institutional course of action."[108] Smith used the term "processing interchange" to characterize this form of work organization. "At each processing interchange, a text enters and is processed. It may then be passed on as modified or checked, or a new text built from resources of the original is produced and passed on. The individual whose case is organized in this process has been constituted textually." The institutional schedule organizes the life of this individual. Who the individual is, how he or she is recognized, and how he or she may be required to perform "are established in the texts that make up the record of the case."[109]

The conversation between Nurses' and Psychiatrists' Notes

The mechanisms analyzed above can be detected in every note in Buller's medical record. For example, the next note written by the psychiatrist is found on 22 February 1931, two days after the previously analysed entry.

> Stuporous. Refuses food. Often asks for water but does not drink. In the afternoon she refuses food saying: "I mustn't, I am so bad." Stuporous, with closed eyes.
> Luminal exanthema: [drug] received from 10.2.–18.3. 2.0[110]

His note was based on nursing records from 20 February to 22 February:

> 20.2.31 After: Pat. is quiet, answers hesitantly questions. (Ha.) *M.* [psychiatrist's initial] Night: Pat. slept. (Du.)
>
> 21.2. Foren [forenoon]: <u>Until coffee time pat. was very agitated, said: "O father why did you do such wrong and why do I have to pay for it. Pay for your deeds, mother, Gertrud help me. Nurse give me a lot of water I am burning, fast fast I can't take it anymore." When pat. received the water she poured it all over the bed to extinguish the fire. Pat. makes herself stiff and becomes violent when one want to take care of her. Pat. eats almost nothing.</u> (Ge.)
> After: At times, pat. cries quietly but does not finish a single sentence, suddenly stops. (Ha.)
> 21/22.2. Night:Pat. fell asleep at 11 [pm]. (Str.) *M.*
>
> 22.2.31 Foren: <u>Pat. very often asked for water, spilled it in bed and cannot be made to drink. Pat. stayed in bed, mostly indifferent. Is very resistent when being fed, clenches her teeth or spits everything in the bed. Pat.consumed almost nothing.</u> (Schm.)
> After: Pat. was very <u>apathetic on various occasions,</u> asked for water of which she also

---

108 Ibid., 170.
109 Ibid., 171.
110 PR, FMR, PN.

always drank a few sips; <u>during visiting time pat. did not accept anything from her relatives</u>, spat everything out and said: <u>"I am not allowed to, I am so bad."</u> <u>Lay there her eyes closed almost all the time.</u>[111]

Since the psychiatrist reported on his patients only every two or three days, his opening assumptions that she was "stuporous" and "[refusing] food" characterized time between the notes. This was thus another effect of the notion of "documentary time" because time not mentioned in the record became time that did not exist. Buller's "local" time was detached from the "documentary time" in the record, enabling more than 72 hours of the "asylum lifetime" to be compressed into just three short words. Three days of her life were contained in 26 lines of the nursing record, but they were further compressed in the psychiatrist's note. This decisive capacity not only caused periods of "local embodied time" to vanish, it also implied that the undocumented periods were not worth documenting. Furthermore, the psychiatrist translated the underlined words "indifferent" and "apathetic" from the same day into the medical term "stuporous." Although the nurses had focused more on Buller's resistance and her indifference had been only a minor point in their eyes, in the psychiatrist's note it had become a clear symptom of her schizophrenia, and his reporting of her "closed eyes" only further emphasized this idea.

Buller's stupor and her refusal to eat became the main focus of the psychiatrist's medical reports from that point on and both, it should be noted, were already part of the admittance attestation. While the physician noted that Buller often refused to drink the water she had asked for, the nurses had stated she had taken some sips, and that she had poured out the water because she thought her bed was burning, a context missing from the psychiatrist's report. Once again, he ordered all the symptoms to fit the frame of the diagnosis. The "rule violations" that the nurses recorded (does not stick to bed rest, becomes violent if one tries to care for her, does not adequately react to her relatives, etc.) are marshalled to illuminate schizophrenic behaviour. And while nurses had at least used the word "patient" when they had written about her, Buller as an individual vanished completely in his note.

The longer Buller stayed in the asylum as well, the shorter the notes from the medical personnel became; they began to resemble a telegram more than anything else.

On 25 February 1931, three days later, the psychiatrist wrote that

Whines, at times timidly. Otherwise stuporous. Since yesterday tube feeding.[112]

---

111 PR, FMR, NN.
112 PR, FMR, PN.

The nurses' notes from 23 to 25 February recorded that

> 22.2. Night: Pat. slept. (Jü.) M.
>
> 23.2.31 Pat. moans "o, o, I cannot stand it, I cannot stand it." Pat. often leans across the bed and lets Pat. T. lift her out of bed, became very restless and lively. Did not eat anything. (Ys.)
> 23.2. After: Pat. was quiet, did not speak, slept a lot. (Sa.)
> Night: Pat. slept. (Sch.)
>
> 24.2.31 Foren [Forenoon]: Pat. lay in the bed quietly and silently. Got a feeding. Pat. spat out any other food. After a lot of convincing from her mother, the Pat. consumed some chocolate and some orange. Pat. often vomits; does not urinate. (Sch.)
> 24.2. After [Afternoon]: Pat. was quiet until 8 o'clock, [then]surged out of the bed, stood by the window and shouted: "Mama I'm dying!" Pat. did not eat or drink anything. (Sa.)
> Night: Pat. had little sleep, stood continuously on the window sill, held on to it tightly and shouted "Mommy, mommy please get me out of here." (Jü.)
>
> 25.2. Foren: Pat. crawled onto the window sill in the morning and looked out. Otherwise she was quiet, slept a lot and consumed only chocolate pudding apart from the tube feeding. Pat. does not react to questions. (Sch).
> 25.2. Night: Pat. slept a lot. (Ru.)
>
> 26.2. Aftern.:Pat. slept a lot, got a feeding.(Hu.)[113]

This sequence illustrated that, in comparison to the nurses' note, those written by the psychiatrist had become even less detailed. Again, the psychiatrist had compressed the three intervening days between notes, and again, it confirmed what had already been decided about her behaviour. This time, however, no sentences had been underlined in the nursing notes. Although the first clause in the psychiatrist's note is taken from the nurse's chart on the 23rd of the month, the word "stuporous" cannot be found, unless it was implied from the nurse's statements on the 24th. Furthermore, from the recordings on the fever chart it is perceivable that Buller had developed a high body temperature (39 °C) but to the psychiatrist, her behaviour seemed to be nothing more than an aggravation of her mental condition, and indeed, the term "whines" can be viewed as pejorative.

Nevertheless, the overall picture in the nurses' notes is one of patient resistance to asylum treatment – both to the nursing treatments (adjustment to the asylum schedule, bed rest, repeated catheterizations, clysters, etc.) and to the medical interventions (lumbar puncture, blood work, examination, interrogation, Luminal and Scopolamine injections, etc.), and from 24 February, to the forced feedings. All these interventions had taken place over this period of

---

113 PR, FMR, NN.

reporting on Buller, but were never mentioned in either the nurses' or psychiatrist's notes.

Buller's behaviour evolved in the record through the active interplay between these two sets of notes. On 26 February the psychiatrist noted

> 27.2.31 Sore throat. Stuporous, autistic. Only spontaneous comments: "I want to die, I don't want to live anymore."
>
> 28.2.31. Unchanged in stupor. Transferred to House 16.[114]

Compare his note with those of the nurses from 25 to 28 February.

> 25.2.31: Night: Pat. slept. (Si.) M.
>
> 26.2.31: Foren [Forenoon]: Pat. lay still, ate some milk and custard. (Li.)
> After: Pat. lay still in bed, sleeps a lot. Pat said once: "I want to die, I don't want to live any longer." Otherwise does not answer questions. (Ru.)
>
> 26/27.2.31: Night: Pat. slept. (Si.) M.
> 27.2.31: Foren: Pat. lies continuously with her eyes closed, lets saliva drool out of her mouth, only ingested feeding. (Fr.)
> 27.2. 31:After: <u>Pat. was absolutely apathetic, lay with her eyes closed very quietly in her bed, only after the light was switched off did Pat. sat up in bed and look at her environment.</u> (Hu.)
>
> 27/28 31:Night: Pat. slept with short interruptions. (Si.) M.
>
> 28.2.31: Foren: Pat. lays in bed quietly, does not answer questions. (Ru.)[115]

The psychiatrist's note from February 27 began with a medical diagnosis that was also written in pencil on the fever chart. This chart also noted that Buller had developed a high fever for which she had received throat compresses (*Halsprignitz*) and chest embrocation with "Transpulmin." Although these bodily symptoms may well have explained Buller's apathetic behaviour, the frame of reference in which the nurses and physicians were operating contained within it the possibility that other conditions could be ignored. The term "autistic" was also an escalation of "stuporous" because it implied a disconnect with her surroundings, an aspect that became more emphasized after Buller's transfer to another ward in March 1931. The words "only spontaneous remarks" built on this impression since Buller appeared to be giving "kneejerk" reactions to stimuli rather than being connected to real events occurring around her. And while the psychiatrist seemed to suggest that Buller's wanting to die was an example of her general state of mind over this time, the nurses' notes revealed that she had made this remark only once.

---

114 PR, FMR, PN.
115 PR, FMR, NN.

In his last two notes from February 1931 in particular, the psychiatrist seemed to be focused only on verifying Buller's admission diagnosis to support the decision to transfer her. Observing newly admitted patients closely in order to decide their future placement within the asylum was a routine procedure at both Friedrichsberg and Langenhorn, but it is clear that decisions to transfer were based more on disciplinary rather than on medical considerations. The plan to transfer Buller to House 16, one of the 11 so-called treatment houses for women in Friedrichsberg, confirmed not only her diagnosis but also the degree of trouble the asylum personnel thought she might cause. (See Figure 15) This impression is emphasized by the fact that all record keeping broke off between 28 February and 4 March, when the fever chart indicated that her "treatment" began again in House 16. Thus, for nearly one week, no detailed reports were written on Buller, another indication of what I have termed "documentary time." The fact that this one week was not worth noting automatically implies that Buller's week was so "empty" and so monotonous that nothing important enough occurred to add to what was already known about her. The record enabled the literal disposing of a patient through non-observance; if the represented (the patient) and the representation (of the patient) were wholly interdependent, then not being represented in the record signified that the formerly represented disappeared and became non-existent. Buller's "non-existence" during that last week in February is strengthened by the content of the psychiatrists' notes from House 16, which continued to emphasize her stuporous and autistic state as well as her refusal to eat; nothing had apparently changed. The "documentary time" of the record gave the impression that Buller was already, at the end of February 1931, an "empty human shell" (*leere Menschenhüllen*),[116] a concept discussed in more detail in the next section.

---

116 Karl Binding and Alfred Hoche, *Die Freigabe der Vernichtung lebensunwerten Lebens. Ihr Maß und ihre Form (1920)* (Berlin: Berliner Wissenschaftsverlag, 2006), 51.

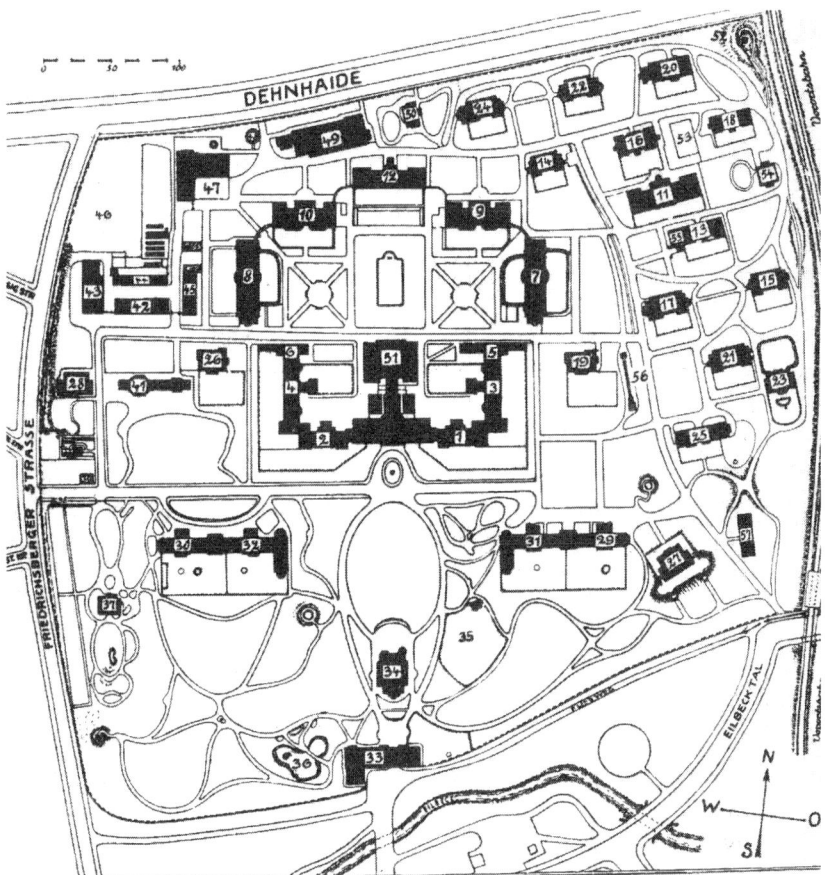

Figure 15: Friedrichsberg Asylum, 1931.[117]

Explanation: 1 and 27, open section for men; house 2, open section for women; 7, for agitated men; 8, for agitated women; 9, reception men; 10, reception women (Anna Maria Buller was admitted to this house); 5, 11, 13, 15, 17, 19, 21, 25, treatment houses for men; 4, 6, 12, 14, 16, 18, 20, 22, 24, 26, 28, treatment houses for women (Anna Maria Buller was transferred to house 16); 23, house for adolescents; 29, 31, nursing homes for men; 30, 32, nursing homes for women; 33, administration; 34, concert hall; 35,game enclosure; no. 36. Lake; 37, residence of the director; 38, gatehouse; 39, residency of work master; 41, morgue; 42, 43, 44,workshops; 45, stable; 46, nursery; 47, machine house; 48, water tower; 49,laundry; 50, residence for civil servants; 51, kitchen; 52, vantage point; 53, tennis court; 54, residence of senior physician; 55, surgery house; 56, bowling alley; 57, animal shed.

---

117 Wilhelm Weygandt, ed., *Die Staatskrankenanstalt Friedrichsberg* (Hamburg: Paul Hartung Verlag, 1928), 187.

Before continuing, it is useful to examine two other aspects of the nurses' notes that involved the frequent use of different types of statements. First was the oft-repeated phrase "did not answer questions," implying both that the patient was obligated to answer the questions posed by nurses, and that a hierarchical relationship between nurse and patient existed: it was the nurse who asked and the patient who was to answer. Although it is unclear exactly what kinds of questions were asked, it is likely that they were designed to test Buller's mental status. Not answering the questions only confirmed her mental derangement and isolation.

Second, nurses' observations included every detail of a patient's life in the asylum, a phenomenon made possible by the structure of asylum life that enabled such boundless scrutiny. For example, the nurses provided detailed descriptions of Buller's behaviour during visiting hours, sometimes "quoting" what she had said to her mother or reporting on her activities after switching off the light. The emphasis on this type of reporting suggests that nurses had a clear idea of what "normal" behaviour in the asylum should be like. Nurses' use of the word "lively," which in general has no negative connotation, became a synonym for a behaviour that lay somewhere between quiet and agitated. The term "quiet" itself usually meant that patients did not disturb ward routines, but they could also be too quiet, which then referred more to them being apathetic and non-talkative.

The bed played a central role in these perceptions – more than 480 entries alone in her medical file between 1931 and 1943 (Buller's entire hospital "career") were related to her bed. We have already seen some of these comments: "[lying] with her eyes closed very quietly in her bed," suggested that she was expected to lie in bed with her eyes open but not make a disturbance. Sleeping during the day, rather than just at night, was evidence of illness. Even the simple fact of sitting upright in the bed could become an indication of abnormal behaviour. The same thing applied to descriptions of restlessness – throwing the bedding, shouting from the bed, etc. In general, it appeared that there was a certain "code of conduct" around bed behaviour, a set of rules that could also be applied to other activities.

Nevertheless, the nurses not only observed Buller's behaviour but they also actively intervened to correct what they conceived as misbehaviour. With the transfer to house 16 not only the content of the notes changed but also Buller's treatment. This will be highlighted in the next chapter.

Chapter 5: Transfer to House 16 (March 1931)

The Medical Record in House 16

The transfer from House 10 (the admission ward) to House 16, where it was expected that she would remain in her vegetative state, confirmed Buller's diagnosis of schizophrenia. The nurses resumed their notations on the fever chart on 4 March, the psychiatrists' notes recommenced on 6 March, and the nurses' notes started again on 9 March. The only information available is that preserved on the fever chart and these entries are of particular interest, because they highlight once more the interplay between the recording of Buller's physical parameters and the production of a particular behaviour brought about through the application of miscellaneous techniques (here especially the administration of drugs) which was observed later on and described in the nurses' and psychiatrists' notes (See Figure 16).

The fever chart functioned in the same manner as described for her admission earlier in February. Bacteria were apparently found in Buller's urine, and she still received an enema every second day and a tube feeding twice a day (reduced to once a day from 12 March on). A significant difference, however, was Buller's behaviour was not only observed and registered in every detail but also active interventions took place that influenced this behaviour. These interventions were partly chemical and partly educational, changing both the character of the nurses' notes and how nurses ecorded these interventions. Buller's behaviour can only be grasped by an analysis of the interplay of different human and non-human actors. Questions arise as to what extent the behaviour observed by the nurses and recorded in their notes was a result of their own interventions. When Buller arrived at House 16, the nurses began another fever chart, somewhat surprisingly since it was usually maintained only during the first days of admission. They may have begun this new chart because of her high temperature on 26 February, and likely the diagnosis of "sore throat" had raised doubts that this was the sole cause for the fever. Another urine examination was also carried out.

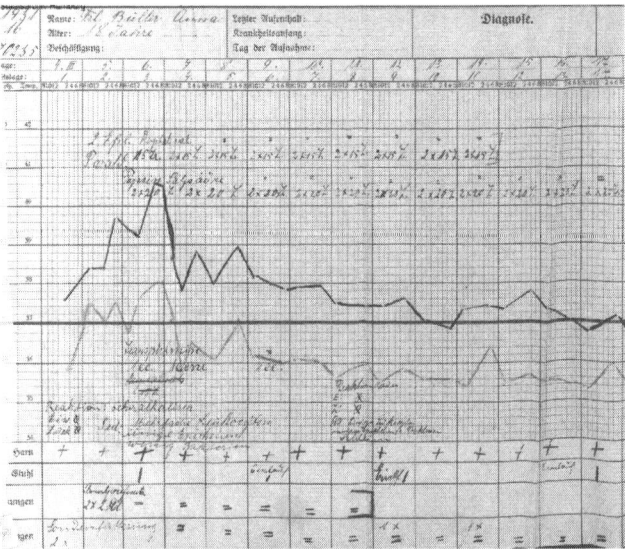

Figure 16: Detail of the fever chart from house 16 (cutout). Patient record 28338.

Against the backdrop of stuporousness and apathy that had described Buller's state at the end of February, she was prescribed a 10-day course of Digitalin (Digitalis) and Paraldehyde beginning on 4 March. Obtained from the seeds of the common foxglove, Digitalin was used not only in the treatment of cardiac arrhythmias but also appreciated as a narcotic in psychiatry, with the theory that the increased pulse rates accompanying an agitated state would drop, thereby calming the patient.[1] She was administered Digitalin even though its efficacy had already been widely questioned.[2] In Buller's case, the combination of drugs was meant to sedate her, but the fact that they were administered before a careful observation of her behaviour had been carried out highlights once more the

---

[1] In his Handbook for practical pharmacology from 1851, Lessing listed Digitalis under the category of "narcotics" and described four nervous diseases that were qualified for treatment with it (mania, asthmatic cramps, alcoholic delirium, and epilepsy). Michael B. Lessing, *Handbuch der praktischen Arzneimittellehre. Für Studierende, praktische Aerzte, Physicats-Aerzte und Apotheker*, 6. ed., Vol. 2 (Berlin: Verlag von Albert Förstner, 1851), 42–43.

[2] *Geisteskrankenpflege* had warned physicians in 1934 not to use the drug as a sedative. Nowadays we know that psychiatric problems were often manifestations of digitalis and may range from mild disorientation, lethargy, or restlessness to full blown delirium; or in other words, psychiatric problems in relation to the application of digitalis could be defined as "iatrogenic disorders." Dr. H. Witetzki, "Über die Anwendung und Verabreichung von Arzneimitteln bei Geisteskranken," *Geisteskrankenpflege. Monatsschrift für Geisteskranken- und Krankenpflege* 38, no. 3 (1934), 92–96; M. K. Shear and M. Sacks, "Digitalis Delirium: Psychiatric Considerations," *International Journal Psychiatry Medicine* 8, no. 4 (1977–1978): 371–381.

power of the record. The apparent need to administer chemical sedation was based solely on the notes from her file and the drugs seemed to be a kind of prophylactic measure. However, as the comparison with other records demonstrates, drugs were rarely documented or discussed in the actual notes. Evidence of their use appeared only on medication cards or fever charts.

It should also be emphasized that while clinical observations in the admission ward helped to verify a diagnosis, in House 16 these same activities became treatment measures – interventions in order to adjust patient conduct and physiological parameters. For example, because it had been noted in House 10 that Buller had begun to vomit after tube feedings, she was medicated with a combination of Pepsin and hydrochloric acid in House 16. The House 10 notes initiated interventions in House 16, demonstrating that the assignment of non-human actants (feeding tube) prompted the intervention of further actants (Pepsin and hydrochlorid acid).

On 6 March a kind of a medical readmission on Buller was done in House 16 although in the psychiatrist's note, the administration of the different drugs was never mentioned.

> 6.3.31 Lies in bed mostly completely apathetic with eyes closed, even soils the bed. Does not react to any call. Must be tube fed. When she is sat on a chair undressed, she doesn't change her position at all; when put to bed, she lets herself be dragged there, with her feet dragging along the floor.
> In between though, she does act spontaneously and abruptly: jumps out of bed, joins another patient in bed and hugs her, or steps on the window sill naked, and similar things. A few times, the mother managed to get her to eat some slices of an orange, another time though she kept the chocolate in her mouth and smeared it all over the bed.[3]

The first part of the psychiatrist's description concerned Buller's catatonic state, the core of her admission diagnosis. Buller's condition, however, had worsened dramatically by now; she seemed to have lost any connection to her environment and was not reacting to any stimulation, even becoming incontinent. Not eating, which in House 10 had been considered a sign of negativism, became now another characteristic of her extreme withdrawal – a withdrawal so profound that she required tube feeding.

The psychiatrist's wording could have been copied from Bleuler's Textbook of Psychiatry (*Lehrbuch der Psychiatrie*).

---

3 Staatsarchiv Hansestadt Hamburg 352-8-7, Staatskrankenanstalt Langenhorn, Abl.1-1995, Krankenakte 28338 (hereafter Patient Record (PR), Friedrichsberg Medical Records Section (hereafter FMR), psychiatric notes (hereafter PN). This designation will be used throughout to identify Anna Maria Buller's patient record; other patient files mentioned in the text will be identified with their unqiue file number.

> Sick persons do not move by themselves. If one puts them in an arbitrary, even uncomfortable position, they keep it over a long period of time...Some sick persons resist the passive movement of their limbs; in other sick persons one can model their limbs like a wax statue.[4]

The description of Buller in the psychiatrist's note resembled what psychiatrist Alfred Hoche had termed the "mentally dead." In his book that he had written with German jurist Karl Binding in 1920, Hoche argued for the legal killing of patients who were in "conditions of ultimate incurably idiocy" (*Zustände endgültigen unheilbaren Blödsinns*) and who he claimed had no value for society or for themselves. He divided this group into two large groups, those cases in which mental death was acquired late in the course of their life but who once had been mentally fully fledged, or at least had been mentally average, and those in which the brain alteration developed due to "congenital conditions" or because it had been "acquired in early childhood."[5]

According to Hoche, the first group contained those with senile dementia, paralytic dementia, arteriosclerotic alterations of the brain, and the huge group of "juvenile processes of idiocy (Dementia praecox)."[6] From this perspective Buller was considered part of the latter group since dementia praecox was another term for schizophrenia. Although he believed that equal degrees of idiocy could occur in both groups, Hoche argued that one had to consider

> a difference in the condition of the mental inventory, even though it might be comparatively the same, like between a disorderly pile of stones that was never touched by a building hand and the ruins of a collapsed building....In our consideration these two groups of mentally dead persons must be differentiated as well as the relation of them to their environment. Among those who acquired their condition very early a rapport with their environment never existed, whereas those who acquired their condition late in life might have had an abundant connection. Their environment, their relatives and friends therefore subjectively have a completely different relation to the latter; mentally dead persons of this kind might have acquired a completely different "affection value" (*Affektionswert*); they have feelings of piety, of thankfulness; numerous, perhaps strongly sentimental memories are connected to this perception, and all this happens even in the case when they do not respond to their environment.[7]

Hoche contended that it was not difficult for physicians, especially alienists and neurologists, to identify mentally dead persons, because these people had no clear imagination, no feelings, wishes, or determination. They had no possibility of developing a "world view" (*Weltbild*), no relationship to their environment,

---

4 Bleuler, *Lehrbuch der Psychiatrie* (Berlin: Springer, 1923), 116.
5 Karl Binding and Alfred Hoche, *Die Freigabe der Vernichtung lebensunwerten Lebens. Ihr Maß und ihre Form (1920)* (Berlin: Berliner Wissenschaftsverlag, 2006), 48.
6 Ibid., 49.
7 Ibid.

and most importantly, they lacked self-consciousness or the possibility of becoming conscious of their own existence. They had no subjective claim to life because they had only simple, elemental feelings such as are found in lower animals. A mentally dead person therefore was not able "to raise a subjective claim to life nor [was] he able to perform any kind of mental process."[8]

All of Hoche's criteria relating to the idea of mentally dead persons can be viewed in the short psychiatrist's note on Buller from 6 March 1931, perhaps already sealing her fate. The record as a whole can be read as the narrative of how Buller came to be viewed as a hopeless case, or as the record's folder indicated, how Buller entered a "final state" (Endzustand) (See photograph of record's folder figure 1). As in the case of the admission ritual in February 1931, the psychiatrist's note functioned as a kind of introduction as to how Buller should be described and what seemed to be noteworthy about her behaviour into the future.

In the first few weeks in House 16, the focus of the records from both the nurses and psychiatrists was on Buller's refusal to eat and on her sudden mood changes that ranged between complete withdrawal and wild, unpredictable activity. This behaviour was deemed dangerous, adding a new dimension to the perspectives of the medical personnel.

Psychiatrist's note:

9.3.31. Prefers to lie down in other patients' beds. Completely dumb, mannerism (*maniriert*), blocked (*gesperrt*). Must be tube fed.

13.3.31 Most of the time in catatonic state, in between though very abrupt senseless actions. Screams: "Gertrud, Gertrud Mordhorst, I cannot take it anymore." Spits.

14.3. Eats spontaneously today.[9]

Nurses' notes:

9.3.31: Pat. lies down in other beds, and often stands up in the bed. Pat. did not speak or eat. (Me.)
Aftern: Kept quiet all afternoon, drank a cup of coffee by herself. At times sat up in bed. (No.)
Night: Pat. slept throughout the night. (Schi.) H.

10.3.31 Morning: Pat. was out of bed a lot. Otherwise quiet. Pat. spat out everything she had in her mouth. (Me.)
Night: Pat. slept with interruptions; pat. wet the bed once. (Schi.) H.

11.3.31 Morning: Pat. got out of the bed and said: "My mother is not a scrubbing brush." To the remark that the pat. would get cold feet outside the bed, pat. answered

---
8 Ibid., 54.
9 PR, FMR, PN.

"That does not matter, at least I will be dying that way." Later pat. was quiet.
Aftern: Repeatedly said to her mother that she wanted to die and that she was so bad. Drank $\frac{1}{2}$ cup of cacao, after the feeding she immediately wet the bed. Fell asleep right away. At 9 pm drank another cup of cacao by herself. (No.) *H.*

12.3.31 Morning: Pat. ate $\frac{1}{2}$ cup of cacao and $1\frac{1}{2}$ Zwieback. Otherwise pat. was quiet. (Me.) *H.*

13.3.31: Pat. was tube fed, otherwise lay apathetically in bed. (Mü.)
Aftern: Suddenly cried out loud and jumped out of the bed screamed repeatedly: "Gertrud, Gertrud Mordhorst! I can't take it anymore" while trembling all over her body. After a short period of time she went back to bed again quietly. (No.) *H.*

14.3.31 Morning: Pat. lay still in bed, vomiting a lot. Pat. consumed $\frac{1}{2}$ cup of milk and $\frac{1}{2}$ cup of soup, solid food pat. spat out. (E.)[10]

The same mechanisms are at work in these last records as were analyzed in detail in an earlier section. Elements found in the psychiatrist's note were clearly taken from the nurses' notes with the typical generalizations, transformations, and reordering of events. For example, the psychiatrist's remark that Buller was "most of the time in a catatonic state" is contrasted with the nurses' opinion, which seemed to emphasize her active behaviour. Buller's spitting was also charted three days earlier by the nurses than what the physician reported.

Some particular aspects of this passage are significant. First, the psychiatrist had written that Buller "preferred" to lie in other patients' beds, a term that implied a degree of intentionality, and in this case, a kind of intentional wickedness, since it was against the rules of the asylum and therefore unacceptable to the staff. Second, the sentence following contained a sequence of medical terms on Buller's mental condition that were found within the diagnostic frame of schizophrenia as it was understood at the time. He used the expression "completely dumb," but according to the nurses, Buller was not speechless. The term "mannerism" helped to strengthen the impression that Buller had worsened. Mannerism had been introduced by Emil Kraepelin in his theory of "dementia praecox," from which Eugen Bleuler had developed his theory of schizophrenia. According to Kraepelin, "another prominent symptom of this stage of the disease [sc. dementia praecox] is the mannerisms in facial expression and speech. Accompanying speech is a peculiar gesticulation, winking of the eyes, senseless shaking and nodding of the head."[11] Bleuler specified that many schizophrenic people adopted particular poses.

---

10 PR, FMR, PN.
11 Emil Kraepelin, *Psychiatrie: ein Lehrbuch für Studierende und Ärzte*, Vol. 2, Klinische Psychiatrie (Leipzig: Barth, 1922), 181.

Some try over years, for example, to act like Bismarck [the former Imperial Chancellor]; others want to present themselves as something special, almost always in an overblown (*gespreizter*), made up (*gemachter*), caricatured manner. Sometimes, however, only some actions are changed or carried out in an elaborate manner: Before ingesting a bite, people will knock their food three times on the plate, they will put the food on the fork seven times and again it will be thrown down before they get it to the mouth.[12]

The word "blocked" (*gesperrt*)' inferred that Buller was unapproachable and made up part of what early psychiatrists called "autism." According to Bleuler, being blocked was one characteristic of schizophrenics because they lost "contact with reality; the less severe cases inconspicuously here and there, and the more severe ones completely."[13] When coupled with the psychiatrist's observation of Buller's catatonic state and senseless actions, these three terms summarized, re-ordered, and again condensed the nurses' notes to allow the psychiatrist to sum up her whole medical history in a succinct fashion.

This sequence also highlights another important mechanism functioning in the medical record. How "what really happened" evolved in the medical file has already been analysed. The previous examples on Buller from House 16 demonstrate, however, that information from diverse sources was constantly being compressed into short statements to determine the "truth" of "what really happened" and "what was the case." As the examples above show, the psychiatrist condensed the information gleaned from all notes written while Buller was in House 10 – the nurses' notes, her tests etc. – to create a concise statement of the relevant problems and their histories. Buller's history was thus selectively re-written. Detailed descriptions embodied in the House 10 records sink back into pages that are no longer "actual," as was shown by the notes written on 6 and 9 March that summarized all the available information in the first two sentences. These continuous re-formulations and condensations were crucial for the functioning of the record; at particular points in Buller's psychiatric career, her whole history was compressed into a few words. This ongoing re-summarizing also contributed to the "construction of narratives in which the ambiguities, the ad hoc and fluid character of the medical work [were] lost,"[14] a concept that becomes particularly clear in a comparison of the notes from the psychiatrist and the nurses at the beginning of March 1931. Whereas the nurses' notes were ambiguous and did not describe Buller's behaviour as clear-cut even though nursing observations were guided by specific charting categories, these ambiguities were eliminated in the psychiatrist's note. These reconstructions were

---

12 Bleuler, *Lehrbuch der Psychiatrie*, 311.
13 Ibid., 293.
14 Marc Berg, "Practices of Reading and Writing: The Constitutive Role of the Patient Record in Medical Work," *Sociology of Health and Illness*,18, no. 4 (1996): 519.

"needed to *produce* an account ordered enough to enable action or to communicate what [was] going on."[15] As illustrated, each and every one of the three terms employed by the psychiatrist reflected a history of repeated reconstructive work. As Berg noted, the medical record (re)constructs the present and enables an "accountable, 'adequate' rendering of the Now and its History." It is an iterative process of summarizing that aids to construct a history which seamlessly and rationally predates and underpins the current "present." A history emerges in which the nurses' notes in particular naturally "lead to certain diagnostic conclusions, which then lead to a rational, therapeutic intervention." The interactive processes that shaped Buller's trajectory were replaced "by a clear-cut, step-by-step temporal sequence (observation → diagnosis → intervention), matched by a clear-cut causality underlying this sequence, and by a circumscribed and fitting set of 'signs and symptoms.'"[16] From this perspective, what occurred after 14 March in House 16 could be described as a kind of permanent educational intervention based on the appraisal that Buller was a severe case, as proven by the psychiatrist's notes.

> The multitude of ad hoc articulations made, the wide array of elements involved, the way these elements were (re)constructed: all this is erased in this post hoc reification of a trajectory's history. Also, in this final mediation, the record ultimately deletes itself: it erases all traces of its own constitutive role in the production of medical work. It becomes no more than the simple "carrier" of information, a mere re-enactment of events-a humble object.[17]

The nurses' notes and the nurses' strategic position within psychiatric practice

As already mentioned earlier, the nurses' notes differed not only in the material appearance (written in pencil, highly regulated by the material construction of the forms, etc.) but they also differed from those written by the psychiatrist in the language that they used and the focus of their writing. The nurses were far less specific about the various psychological signs and symptoms that they noted. The psychiatrists later underlined key terms and events that seemed to fit into their diagnostic frame, translating the nurses' descriptions into medical terminology. The nurses' notes appear as a kind of empirical database and the psychiatrists' notes seemed to be nothing more than inductively generated as-

---

15 David Gooding, "Putting Agency Back into Experiment," in *Science as Practice and Culture*, ed. Andrew Pickering (Chicago: University of Chicago Press), 76. [original emphasis]
16 Berg, "Practices of Reading and Writing," 519.
17 Ibid., 520.

sumptions; this interplay gives the record its scientific character. Apart from the fact that the nurses' notes were very detailed and those written by the psychiatrists were not, the reports also emphasized different areas. The nurses were mostly concerned with rule violations (in the end the patient became conspicuous by deviating from expected behaviour) but the psychiatrists focused primarily on gathering symptoms. From the nurses' viewpoint, it appeared that any behaviour became a pathologic sign. Either the patient was too quiet (did not answer questions) or too lively (disturbed the regular course of action).

Nevertheless, even the nurses' observations appeared to be led by the diagnosis, which was especially clear in 1940 when they assessed Buller's behaviour somewhat differently from that occurring during her earlier admissions. From 1931 to 1936, Buller's behaviour had always been interpreted from within the diagnostic scheme of catatonic schizophrenia and "negativism." In 1940, however, the diagnostic frame changed when she was diagnosed with "dementia praecox," indicating that she was becoming completely stupified. This changed resulted in the nurses now considering Buller helpless. The interrelation between diagnosis and nurses' observations is also traceable in Buller's refusing to eat, since the major efforts spent in feeding her in March and April 1931 appear to have been neglected later, even though her nutritional situation was apparently still as severe. But because the concern over her nutrition never again became part of the official diagnosis, it seemed to the nurses not to be worthy of note.

However, the nurses' notes also differ in other respects. They are characterized by a kind of tension resulting from the attempt to write in a scientific, neutral manner with bad grammar and in a Hamburg dialect. On the one hand, the nurses always used the term "patient" when they wrote about Buller and they never used personal pronouns such as "I" or "me." When they reported their own impressions and observations, they often referred to themselves as "the nurse" or they even used the impersonal "one." For example, on 28 April 1931, one nurse wrote on Buller that "if one tries to put on her shirt she throws it," or again, on 31 May, "one tried to play a few games with her." The notes resembled a kind of laboratory report, with the date and time of observations written as if the reported events were observed with a distant, all-seeing gaze. On the other hand, the reports were written in the everyday spoken style used by Hamburg's proletarian class. For example, on 17 April 1931, one nurse wrote that "in the morning pat. was loud and agitated, threw her lunch on pat. Baade[18] her bed," or later that day, Buller apparently "repeatedly stood high up in bed naked or lay down in pat. Baade her bed." The turn of speech "pat. Baade her bed" was typical of Hamburg's spoken dialect. Another example occurred on 31 May 1931 when

---

18 All patients' names are anonymous.

the nurse wrote that "only as her mother left, she ran after her," a particular word-order construction particular to those from Hamburg.

The fusion of "medical discourse" with everyday language was also illustrated through the use of particular terms that were characteristic of Hamburg's dialect. For example, nurses used the adjective "nakedly" instead of "naked" (*nackend* instead of *nackt*) but the psychiatrists always used "naked." This combination of different kinds of discursive formations also led to peculiar overblown language at times as well. For example, the word "high" as in "stood high up in bed" is redundant, since someone already standing up in bed cannot get higher. Nevertheless, the nurses were attempting to show that standing high up in bed was worse than just standing up in bed. The nurses' use of the expression "did not ingest dishes" in place of "did not eat," was also somewhat pretentious. Again, on 15 April 1931, the nurse reported that the "Pat. sits nakedly in bed for the entire afternoon, tears apart her shirts, or runs around the dormitory like this; lies down in patient Kuscher her bed and holds on to her so tightly that the same can hardly be freed. For tea time, the patient demands coffee, when passed using the hand (*hinreichen*) she knocked the coffee into the nurse's face and threw the cup against the window." This passage demonstrates the nurses' efforts to write as much as possible in a neutral, objectified language. They often used the phrase "the same," as noted on 27 April 1931, "when the patient's mother came, the same tried to feed the patient." And rather than using the words "to give the coffee," they wrote "when passed using the hand."

The long sentences, arbitrarily subdivided by commas, also suggest that the nurses were not used to writing long passages. The way the nurses wrote has been termed "interdiscourses," a hybrid form of discourse that mediates between specialized discourses, in this case, medical discourse, and what Jürgen Link called elementary discourse, which is a kind of everyday discourse.[19] This perspective enables illustrating the structured character as well as the originality of "what people are saying;" the significance of establishing legitimacy and subjectification for everyday knowledge therefore can also be pointed out. The empirical findings demonstrate the relations between special knowledge and

---

19 Jürgen Link, "Dispositiv und Interdiskurs. Mit Überlegungen zum 'Dreieck' Foucault-Bourdieu-Luhmann," in *Foucault in den Kulturwissenschaften*, eds. Clemens Kammler and Rolf Parr (Heidelberg: Synchron, 2007), 219–238; Jürgen Link, "Diskursanalyse unter besonderer Berücksichtigung von Interdiskurs und Kollektivsymbolik," in *Handbuch Sozialwissenschaftliche Diskursanalyse 1: Theorien und Methoden*, eds. Reiner Keller, Andreas Hirseland and Werner Schneider, Vol. 1 (Opladen: VS Verlag, 2006), 407–430; Link, "Warum Diskurse nicht von personalen Subjekten 'ausgehandelt' werden. Von der Diskurs- zur Interdiskurstheorie," in *Die diskursive Konstruktion der Wirklichkeit. Zum Verhältnis von Wissenssoziologie und Diskursforschung*, eds. Reiner Keller and others (Konstanz: UvK, 2005), 77–99.

everyday knowledge.[20] "Interdiscources" have the ability to combine parts of specialized and elementary discourses in order to transform specialized discourses and make them become more understandable for "lay persons" and a part of unquestioned everyday knowledge. In the nurses' notes, these discursive formations of medical knowledge merge with everyday discourse.

Seen from this perspective, the journal *Irrenpflege* (from 1930 on renamed *Geisteskrankenpflege*) can be perceived as a forum for this interdiscourse, because leading psychiatrists published along with nurses and translated the special psychiatric discourse into an interdiscourse. However, different discursive formations are, according to Link, also characterized by a different power distribution; special discourses are more "powerful" than "interdiscourses" because they connect to knowledge considered "true." Nevertheless, in the case of the nurses' notes, the interdiscourse became powerful because of its material form in the record. As already highlighted, the nurses' notes initiated a cascade of ever-simplified inscriptions that allowed the production of unquestionable facts and the translation into the special discourse. They are the basis for decisions on how to proceed with Buller. For example, on 11 May 1931 the nurses reported that Buller tried to climb "over the fence, said she wanted to walk towards her mother," which one week later the psychiatrist translated into "because she tried to climb over the garden fence, she was transferred to House 14 on 12.5." The nurses' recorded observations thus implied direct consequences for patients, as further analysis will demonstrate, and they highlighted the strategic position of nurses within psychiatric practice. The notes seemed somehow less scientific than those written by psychiatrists and one could even argue that they appeared "unarmed." The nurses functioned, however, as the physician's "optical canal" through which his "scientific" or objective gaze could flow. This delegated gaze could only be performed by those who were at the bottom of the asylum hierarchy and whose discourses, observations, and relations enabled the constitution of this concentrated medical gaze. Only those at the bottom had this power, for only they were able to observe and report on "madness"as an everyday part of their job. In order to do so the nurses were below the patients they served; denials of their services must appear as pure consequences of asylum rules or the result of a psychiatrist's order.

> The nurse must keep in mind that he [sic] is not the superior but rather the servant and protector of the sick person....If the nurse must carry out an order that would likely provoke the sick person he has to draw on the fact that he must follow the request of the

---

20 Anne Waldschmidt et al., "Diskurs im Alltag-Alltag im Diskurs: Ein Beitrag zur empirisch begründeten Methodologie sozialwissenschaftlicher Diskursforschung [69 Absätze]," *Forum Qualitative Sozialforschung / Forum: Qualitative Social Research* 8, no. 2 (June 2007), accessed 02/15, 2010.

physician but avoid any criticizing (*Bekritteln*) of the request, if only with the words "I am sorry, but ,..."[21]

As nurse Georg Roos described this strategic interplay, the nurse must "report to the physician everything he [observes] about the sick person" but a decision about a change in "therapy lies outside his competency." The sick person not only needs the assistance of the nurse "but behind the nurse must stand the authority of the physician." The physician lays out the "scientific treatment plan and the nurse is the one who carries it out. Therefore the nurse is subordinated to the physician." Nevertheless, according to Roos, the "work of the nurse is not worth less. It is very difficult work and not everybody, not even the physician, is able to cope with it."[22]

These remarks suggest that juxtaposing the idea of "the powerful physician" versus "the powerless nurses" does not grasp the essence of psychiatric practice. According to Foucault, power is not something that one group owns but rather develops within relationships; power becomes effective through relays and specific disseminations, reciprocal endorsements and different potentials. The power of psychiatrists only becomes effective through the interplay of physicians with other groups within the psychiatric system. This system of differences must be the focal point of the analysis because only within such a system can power act. Nursing had (and still has) an important strategic function within psychiatry and the question of how power functions is more a question of strategy in psychiatric practice. In order to demonstrate the hierarchical position of nurses and their role in psychiatry, "deputy head nurse" Oskar Stöbe argued in an article published in 1933 that nurses should consider themselves a member of a family, in which the psychiatrist is the father, the nurse the mother, and the patient the child.

> If we imagine ourselves in all situations as a mother then we will often act in the way we normally would. It goes without saying that the mother *wants to educate the uneducated children*. With beating? Never, she would leave that to the father and therefore proceed with good advice and good examples. She knows from her own youth that children (we want to call the patients like this) are capricious and stubborn [and] often they become naughty. Perhaps they learned it in the street and think they can boast about this. The good mother will not get mean or nervous with her children. She tries, *and if it gets too hard alone, with the advice of the father*, find the right distraction or clarification [of this behaviour]. If the child spits in the mother's face because of a fever during a severe pneumonia, she will not get angry. She will even not go away. She knows that the mental (*seelisch*) functions of her child are not normal. If we really and sincerely try to understand this mother role then, after just one week, life on the ward

---

21 Ludwig Scholz, *Leitfaden für Irrenpfleger* (Halle a.d. Saale: Carl Marhold, 1920), 68–69.
22 Georg Roos, "Beziehung des Krankenpflegers zum Arzt," *Geisteskrankenpflege. Monatsschrift für Geisteskranken- und Krankenpflege* 41, no. 12 (1937): 181.

will be different compared to the current situation in which the maxim prevails that the nurse must be always the stronger of the two.[23]

Stöbe emphasized that nurses were the educator of their patients. The nurses' notes from Friedrichsberg illustrate that the main task of the nurses actually was to provide a kind of long term education based on discipline. Nevertheless, Stöbe demonstrated the idea of "strategic power distribution," because it is the psychiatrist as father figure who constituted the center of the power distribution. All the power was arranged around this figure, but the "family" could only function through the interplay of the father and the mother, or in other words, psychiatric practice was characterized by the same kind of strategic power distribution as was found in so-called traditional families. The nurse, whom Stöbe portrayed as a good mother who was "always cleanly dressed and [who did] not rub perfume into her hair twice a day instead of combing it," was the educator with traditional female attributes such as "goodness, affection, self-mastery, cleanliness, and discipline." It was the nurse who influenced the behaviour of the patient, not necessarily with physical violence but with a more subtle form of manipulation that was able to reach the patient in his or her innermost core. According to Stöbe, physical violence was necessary only if prescribed by the psychiatrist.

This passage highlights the entire rationale behind psychiatric nursing. It is important to understand that perceiving patients as children implied that their development stopped at one point in their lives, that madness thus became a kind of developmental standstill or retardation.[24] Regarding patients as children left them with few rights of their own, and they were seen as needing correction by the nurse, as mother, who knew "how afflicted her children [were] from this suffering." The conclusions reached by Stöbe reflected the basic tenet of psychiatric nursing at this time: "Congenital or acquired, she [the mother/nurse] sees it as her greatest obligation to correct what can possibly still be corrected."[25]

Anna Maria Buller Becomes Dangerous and the War Against the Madness Continues

The psychiatrists' notes on Buller resume on 8 April 1931 after a month's interruption.

---

23 Oskar Stöbe, "Hilfsmittel in der praktischen Geisteskrankenpflge," *Geisteskrankenpflege. Monatsschrift für Geisteskranken- und Krankenpflege* 37, no. 6 (1933): 93. [Emphasis in original].
24 Michel Foucault, *Les Anormaux. Cours au Collège de France. 1974–1975*, eds. François Ewald et al (France: Seuil/Gallimard, 1999).
25 Ibid., 93.

> A little better. Eats spontaneously. But otherwise still very resistant and blocked (unapproachable). If pat. talks at all, speaks only with her mother. Often unprovoked agitation.[26]

This record began with the psychiatrist noting that Buller ate "spontaneously," the same remark made in his last entry, which points out once again that time can disappear in the medical file. This is the same mechanism that will lead to Buller's later "invisibility" over long periods of time. Since Buller remained resistant and unapproachable, however, the idea that she was "a little better" was likely more related to her nutritional status. The use of the term "spontaneous" is interesting because it implied that a personal action arose or proceded entirely from a natural impulse. This word gave the impression that Buller was reacting favourably to the intensive efforts used by the nurses to try to persuade her to eat, an impression strengthened by the following "but otherwise" that suggested her educational nutrition program had been successful even if the nurses had failed to improve her mental state. And indeed, the nurses' notes from March 1931 could be read as a detailed description of a nutrition training program. Nevertheless, it seems as if the psychiatrists were confident that Buller's eating problem was solved, which might also explain their more frequent entries in the medical file until May about other aspects of her treatment.

However, the "unmotivated agitations" noted at the end of this entry became a focus in subsequent notes from both the psychiatrists and nurses, and introduced the idea that Buller's actions were posing increased danger to nurses and other patients.

On the same day as the psychiatrist's last entry, the nurses' noted that

> 8.4.31: Morning: At lunch time pat. ate only a cup of soup. (Kl.)
> 8.4.31: Aftern.: Pat. did not eat anything for dinner. Pat. was very resistant and noisy while walking in the garden. Suddenly she threw herself on the ground and screamed and cried so that her entire body trembled. (Schi.) H.[27]

Apart from the mechanisms at play already analyzed above, also noteworthy here between these two sets of notes is the psychiatrist's borrowing of the word "resistant" from the nurses. Usually a term only employed by the nurses, the word contained an active dimension that seemed to oppose the former emphasis on Buller's apathetic and catatonic state. To resist something implies that something exists against which resistance is possible; in this case, Buller was appearing to resist asylum regulations. However, the recording of Buller's noisy resistance while out walking around in the garden suggested not only that a

---

26 PR, FMR, PN.
27 PR, FMR, NN.

certain behaviour or code of conduct was expected of garden users, but also that these kinds of detailed observations could end up in the nursing notes.

Nevertheless, as both psychiatrists' and nurses' notes demonstrate, the content of the reports begin to shift away from a focus on Buller's catatonic state to her resistance and unpredictability. We can see three phases in this development. In the beginning she was described as being in a catatonic state, not interacting with her surroundings and refusing to eat. The intermediary phase, which continued through her transfer to House 16, maintained a focus on her "apathetic and withdrawn" state and her refusal to eat, although at times she was reported as being restless and agitated. From April 1931 on, the focus shifted once more and Buller was described as resistant and aggressive. These descriptions fit exactly into the frame of the admitting diagnosis, following even its sequence through "catatonic clinical picture. Negativism (refuses any food consumption, completely withdrawn). Temporary states of agitation with hallucinations."

The tendency towards increased reporting of unpredictability and signs of danger can be seen in the entries following 8 April. On 13 to 15 April, the psychiatrist wrote that

> 13.4. Wants to leave the room, verbally abuses the nurses, spits. Resistant. Hits nurses and other patients.
>
> 14.4. Runs around naked, spits and strikes out. Often calls out the name Anita. Shouts: "You horrible women, you are all bad, the animals all cry for me, you pigeon catchers. Lord Jesus you are the best."
>
> 15.4. <u>Obviously hallucinates, shouts: "oh, oh, that damned woman is coming again, that whore" while spitting in her bed. Strikes against the safety boards.</u>
>
> 17.4. Still very agitated, spits, scolds: "this woman is coming again, this miser; Anita come here, now I am kicking my father to death." Must be tube fed.[28]

This new focus of the reports, which transformed Buller into a violent and unpredictable person, was accompanied by continuous note taking and observation. Until the end of April, the psychiatrists took notes nearly every single day. The note from April 15 is underlined, a procedure that occurred otherwise only in the nurses' notes, and it is noteworthy that the content of this sentence reappeared in the medical decision-making on Buller's sterilization process in 1935, more than four years later.

Once again we can see how the psychiatrist based his note on information obtained from nursing observations.

---

28 PR, FMR, PN.

9.4.31: Morning: Patient only ate a little. Otherwise, patient is unchanged (Kli)

9.4.31:Aftern: Patient ate some zwieback and drank a cup of cocoa in the evening. After the meal, pat. suddenly got up, went to the window, lashed out against the frame and shouted, I must get out of here. Open up.(K. Spi.)

10.4.31: Morning: Pat. got a feeding.(Sch.)

11.4.31: Morning: Drank 1.5 cup milk. (Sch.)

12.4.31; Morning: Pat. had 1 cup of cocoa. Drank 1 cup of milk and 1 cup of soup. Apart from this pat. is unchanged. (Kl.)
Aftern.: Pat. unchanged. (Lü.)

13.4.31: Morning: Pat. drank 1 cup of milk, 1 cup of soup. (Kl.)
13.4.: Pat. jumped out of bed at 1.00 a.m., ran to the door noisily and screamed. When pat. was taken back to bed she insulted the nurse saying: " bitch with the red cross, you Satan." Pat. spat at the nurse, scratched her and tried to bite her. Pat. was very resistant. After the injection, the patient got up again, went to the bathroom, said then, "Oh I feel so sick to my stomach." Lay down flat on the floor, was persuaded to get up, went to the dormitory and lay down in patient Kuscher's bed, propped herself with both feet against the bed, so that it was very difficult to get her out. At 2:00 a.m. patient fell asleep again. This disruption woke up all the other patients. (Wa.) H.

14.4.31: Morning: Patient very agitated and noisy, could not be held in bed, tried over and over to leave the room. When holding her back she would lash out, bite and spit. She also lashed out and spat at her fellow patients. When her mother came, she screamed loudly and cried at first, did not eat in her mother's company either. (No.)
14.4.31: Aftern.: Pat. very noisy and agitated, ran around the room nakedly [sic], showed her tongue, lashed out, insulted and spat at the nurse, threw everything out of the bed, wet the bed. When patient was handed over [sic] dinner, she knocked the food out of the nurse's hand, and threw it in the room, after dinner patient demanded water, but had only a few sips and tried again, to throw the cup. <u>Pat. often called the name Anita.</u> (Schi.)
14.4.31: Night: Pat. did not sleep, took off the shirt, threw it in the room, lay in bed naked for the entire night, often came up, muttered to herself quietly, when patient was covered the same always threw back the bedding then turned from one side to the other restlessly. (Wa.) H.

15.4.31: Morning: Pat. is noisy and agitated, threw her bread and the cup containing coffee through the room, complained loudly. "You horrible women, you are all bad. Schubert is my grandfather. The animals all cry for me, you pigeon catchers. Lord Jesus, you are the best, mother, come here. Oh, it is getting worse." Pat. stood high up in bed and said loudly "Lüdewicka here I am come to me," then lay down again crying. Pat. did not eat anything. (Kli.)
15.4.31: Aftern.: Until the next shift started, pat. was very loud and agitated, hit and insulted her mother, tried to tear apart her mother's dress shouting: "You are also such a mean woman!" Pat. sits in bed naked for the entire afternoon, tears apart her shirts, or runs around the dormitory like this; lies down in patient Kuscher's her [sic] bed and holds on to the pat. so tightly that the same can hardly be freed. For tea time, pat.

demands coffee, when handed she knocked the coffee into the nurse's face and threw the cup against the window. Pat. makes loud speeches all the time, it is horrible, "I can't take it anymore, this is the last filth! Oh, oh that damned woman is coming again, that whore; spits in her bed," smears herself with mucus or spits on the floor. "Herta! Come here, August Buller, it is your fault. Jesus! Christ, you are the best! Plutas, come here!" Pat. continuously strikes against the safety boards.(Schi.)

16.4.31: Aftern.: Pat. still unchanged very loud and agitated. Pat. didn't eat anything, was fed.(Schi.) *(H)*.

17.4.31: Morning: Pat. was loud and agitated, threw her lunch on patient Buller's her [*sic*] bed stood up high in bed, pointed at patient Fe. and said "Tante Minna, I am here. The dear good aunt Liesbeth never have I had anything to eat. Mother, this is Lina, this horrible woman. I don't like her." Patient had a cup of milk in the morning. (Kli.)
17.4.31: Aftern.: Pat. very noisy and agitated, repeatedly stood up in bed naked or lay down in patient Buller's bed, spat, insulted, "here comes this woman again, this miser. Anita come here, I am kicking my father to death." Patient did not eat, got a feeding. (Schi.) *H*.[29]

The first sentence of the psychiatrist's note from 13 April ("Wants to leave the room, verbally abuses the nurses, spits") originated from the nurse's note from the night shift, although it is somewhat surprising that the psychiatrist reported an event that obviously occurred after his recording of it. This might well be an indication that the psychiatrists did not always record their notes on the date noted in the file, something that can be traced in other records as well. Still, the psychiatrist's note was once more composed of elements derived from the nurses' observations and once more, he appeared to impose on it a slightly different meaning by seeming to imply that Buller's actions were propelled by an overall drive to leave her room, whereas the nurses were describing just one specific event. Similarly, while the nurses attached Buller's abuse of them to the moment when they tried to take her back to bed, the psychiatrist seemed to suggest that Buller's overall behavior was senseless and "resistant." And although he stated in his note of 13 April that Buller hit the nurses and other patients, that action did not appear in the nurses' notes until the following day. Other interplays between the two sets of notes took place in a manner similar to that previously analyzed.

More interesting at this point, however, is the fact that the nurses' notes changed significantly in character. Previously the nurses seemed only to be gathering evidence on Buller's madness and verifying the admitting diagnosis, but now they were actively intervening in order to correct Buller's behaviour – something that was pointed out especially with the injection Buller received as a consequence of her resistance on 13 April. From this point on, the nurses' notes

---

29 PR, FMR, NN.

can be read as a diary of the therapy (or education) that Buller received. And since a kind of endless fight began between the nurses equipped with delegated power from the psychiatrists on one side, and Buller and the power of her madness on the other, the notes read more and more like war reports.

As the notes from April illustrate, the nurses believed that they were already fighting a sinister, unleashed power that they felt needed restraining. Buller appeared the symbol of complete madness. Foucault called this the "secret of the madness" because for him, madness consisted of a wrong perception of reality that tried to force its own understanding of reality on its surroundings. Foucault in both his lectures and book on madness indicated that Descartes decisively defined the modern idea of madness because he discriminated between madness and reason. Weygandt, the medical director of Friedrichsberg, used the text of Descartes to explain his understanding of madness.[30] Weygandt assumed in his text that "illusions and hallucinations sometimes occurred even in mentally sound persons, as, for example, in Descartes, who reported on particular optical and acoustical hallucinations (*Sinnestäuschungen*)." According to Weygandt, the criteria for "these so-called alert hallucinations (*Wachhalluzination*) is that the person concerned recognizes them as something alien....The dream is a web of false perceptions (*Trugwahrnehmungen*)....It only becomes suspicious that this is a psychosis if the hallucinating person takes them for real and loses the ability to criticise them."[31]

Foucault estimated that Descartes' writing was the decisive text in which madness became the absolute "other" of reason. The causes of lunacy could not be determined but a lunatic could be identified without any doubt because he or she was different. In his text *Meditationes*, Descartes tried to find a unique factor that enabled him to distinguish his dreams from madness. "In the face of these maniacs who imagine themselves 'to be jars or made out of glass,'" Descartes immediately knew that he was not like them: "They were out of their minds."[32] In his lecture on 14 November 1973, Foucault took up this text again. He wrote:

> If you refer then to the texts of Descartes, where it is a question of madmen who take themselves for kings, you notice that the two examples Descartes gives of madness are "taking oneself for a king" or believing one "has a body made of glass." In truth for Descartes and generally [Recording: we can say] for all those who spoke about madness

---

30 Wilhelm Weygandt, "Die ersten Zeichen der Geisteskrankheiten," *Die Heilkunde. Monatsschrift für practische Medicin*, no. 1 (1905): 2–10; Michel Foucault, *Psychiatric Power. Lectures at the Collège de France, 1973–74*, eds. Jaques Langrange et al, trans. Graham Burchell (New York: Palgrave Mc Millan, 2006); Foucault, *Abnormal. Lectures at the Collège de France 1974–1975*, eds. Arnold I. Davidson et al, trans. Graham Burchell (USA: Picador, 2003); Foucault, *Les Anormaux. Cours au Collège de France. 1974–1975*.
31 Weygandt, "Die ersten Zeichen der Geisteskrankheiten," 2.
32 Foucault, *Wahnsinn und Gesellschaft*, 177.

up until the end of the eighteenth century, "taking oneself for a king," or believing one has "a body made out of glass," was excactly the same thing, that is to say they were absolutely identical types of error, which immediately contradicted the most elementary facts of sensation. "Taking oneself for a king," "believing that one has a body of glass," was, quite simply, typical of madness as error.[33]

Nevertheless, the conviction of the lunatic that he or she was a king "is the true secret of madness," because a delirium, an illusion, or an hallucination, etc. is analyzed as a conviction of being a king, "whether the content of his delirium is supposing that he [sic] exercises royal power, or, to the contrary, he believes himself to be ruined, persecuted, and rejected by the whole of humanity." For the psychiatrist in the early years of psychiatry (Foucault called it "proto-psychiatric practice")

> [t]he fact of imposing this belief, of asserting it against every proof to the contrary, even putting it forward against medical knowledge, wanting to impose it on the doctor and, ultimately, on the whole asylum, thus asserting it against every other form of certainty or knowledge, constitutes a way of believing that one is a king. Whether you believe yourself to be a king or believe that you are wretched, wanting to impose this certainty as a kind of tyranny on all those around you basically amounts to "believing one is a king"; it is this that makes all madness a kind of belief rooted in the fact that one is king of the world.[34]

Being mad was "was to seize power in one's head." The real problem for psychiatry therefore was the question of how to persuade someone otherwise who believed herself to be a king. In the early 1940s, psychiatrist Heinrich Stadelmann described the mentally ill person as someone who "[was at home] in a different world than the normal thinking person," which did not mean that mentally ill persons possess other "mental qualities than those one could find in mentally healthy persons." As Stadelmann continued, "If the mental condition of the sick person *deviates from the norm* to such an extent that...*healthy opposing points of view cannot find adjusting entrance*, how than can psychotherapy have a favourable impact and how can nursing be beneficial in psychotherapy?"[35]

This problematic was emphasized by Bleuler too, who described vividly the characteristics of "negativistic schizophrenia" with which Buller had been diagnosed.

> When the sick person should get up, they want to stay in bed; if they should stay in bed, they want to get up. They neither want to dress nor do they want to undress, nor comply

---

33 Foucault, *Psychiatric Power*, 27.
34 Ibid., 28.
35 Heinrich Stadelmann, "Psychotherapie bei der Geisteskrankenpflege," *Geisteskrankenpflege. Monatsschrift für Geisteskranken- und Krankenpflege* 46, no. 61 (1942): 62–63. [emphasis mine].

with an order or act according to the asylum's rules, neither come to eat, nor get down from the table; if they can do all these actions beyond the claimed time or if they can somehow do it against the will of those surrounding, they will do it. They are not going to use the toilet spontaneously if they are accompanied, they withhold their excrement in order later to soil their beds or their clothes. They eat the soup with a fork or with a dessert spoon, the dessert with a tablespoon. Many resist with might and main (*Leibeskräften*) against any influences, often with agitated insulting and swiping…It can develop into a real harassment (*Chicanose*), into an active desire to always annoy in a provocative manner those surrounding them.[36]

This definition of "madness" was important in two ways. First of all, it implied that madness could only be explained by its opposition to what counted as "normal." Madness could not be related straightforwardly to an organic cause nor could it be detected in specific brain damage, but rather was detectable only in behaviour. This aspect has already been touched on in the previous analysis of the admission ceremony and the role of the psychiatrist in deciding what behavior counts as abnormal. What counted as "normal" could only be defined through distinguishing "abnormal behavior," or, in other words, reason can only be defined against its opposite; "we are not like them and that is why we are normal." Only by collecting evidence for madness can reason be defined. Nurses and psychiatrists concentrated on demonstrating the insane nature of Buller's behaviour, because in doing so, they constructed themselves as "normal."

Secondly, Bleuler's remarks highlighted that the "lunatic" could not be convinced by logic, "one cannot forget that it is very rare to persuade the sick person to back down through logic itself." The only possibility of influencing madness was through "purposeful education," especially for the chronic cases who are, "for the most part to be trained to normal behaviour and work."[37] Nurse Heinrich Becker specified that the function of nursing was "to find out in all patients how they are best to be disposed." But in order to be able to do so, the nurse had to "try to infiltrate the trains of thoughts or peculiarities of the sick persons, and when he succeeds, to act out of this knowledge."[38] Becker believed in the specific characteristic of nurses' power "to infiltrate the train of thought" of the sick person in order to influence his or her internal behaviour, describing what Foucault called the disciplinary power of psychiatry that confronts the "sovereign power" of the mad and leads to an endless struggle.

The file on Buller demonstrated that the medical and nursing personnel demonstrated an increasing awareness of behaviour that they considered dan-

---

36 Eugen Bleuler, *Lehrbuch der Psychiatrie*, eds. Manfred Bleuler and Josef Berze (Berlin: Springer-Verlag, 1943), 312.
37 Ibid., 313
38 Heinrich Becker, "Der Umgang mit widerstrebenden Kranken," *Geisteskrankenpflege. Monatsschrift für Geisteskranken- und Krankenpflege* 40, no. 8 (1936): 117.

gerous, a factor found not only in Buller's record but in most of the other medical files analyzed for this project.[39] Using terms like "suddenly" made the outbursts of violence seemed unanticipated. The nurses' notes made this danger visible and illustrated that therapy against this violence was the practice of asylum rules – the nursing domain in which nurses employed a multitude of disciplinary techniques from persuasion to physical and chemical restraints.

It was discussed earlier that the nurses' notes, in conjunction with fever charts, medication plans, weight tables, and nutrition plans, etc., organized a complete takeover of Buller's life, registering and influencing every bodily function. Eating to excretion were all functions targeted by their particular interventions. Even the tube feeding itself became a disciplinary means, since before Buller was forcefully fed, the nurses tried to feed her or convince her to eat by herself. All in all, more than 200 nurses' notes referred to the tactics employed to convince Buller to eat one way or the other. Nurse Becker, however, had recommended against force feedings, because one mostly "achieves the opposite, namely an ever-increasing persistence in refusing to eat. [Only after] one has unsuccessfully offered food from time to time…should one conduct an emergency tube feeding."[40]

In dealing with Buller's eating disorder a whole range of nursing interventions were used. For example, tube feeding was prescribed in February twice a day but at the same time, the nurses tried to get her to eat on her own. On 26 February Buller ate a little at each meal, obviously not actively resisting and therefore not receiving a tube feeding that day. The next day, however, she actively refused food and was force fed. It was thus not only the question of Buller eating, but that she ate at the asylum's official mealtimes. In the months to come when Buller wanted to eat again, she decided to eat at any time of the day and even took food from other patients, which again became a problem for the nurses.

From mid-April 1931 on, however, the recording of Buller's refusal to eat changed slightly. On 10 April, Buller was tube fed but at this time, tube feeding had no longer been prescribed by the psychiatrist but rather depended on the judgment of the nurses whether or not they considered her food intake suffi-

---

39 Many files described how patients deemed "dangerous" were targeting with numerous combinations of medications and endured isolation and other shock therapies. Most were eventually killed.To mention just some of the more voluminous medical records: Staatsarchiv Hansestadt Hamburg 352-8-7, Staatskrankenanstalt Langenhorn, Abl.1-1995, Krankenakte 13986. The female patient of this record was admitted the first time in 1916 and killed in 1943 in Hadamar. She was diagnosed with Dementia praecox and later with schizophrenia. Even though nursing notes exist only from the years from 1928 to 1931, they highlight that no medical therapy took place but that the patient became the target of severe sanctions such as isolation and injections based on her perceived increasing dangerousness. Similar mediacl records: 10243; 26752; 23536; 2312; 23856; 27846; 16292; 22694; 23548.
40 Becker, "Der Umgang mit widerstrebenden Kranken," 118.

cient. Nevertheless, the decision for Buller to be tube fed also depended on her behaviour in the asylum. In House 10, Buller had received a tube feeding twice a day (according to the fever chart), but in House 16, it was much more flexible. On some days she had one tube feeding, but on 18 March, the systematic recording of the tube feedings broke off completely. It seems that a calculated and continuous alteration took place between offering Buller food, talking to her in order to convince her to eat, forcing her to eat, and forcing a tube feeding when she refused everything else. Tube feedings also had an educational dimension. Up until 10 April Buller had escaped forced feedings because she had fed herself, or at least had allowed the nurses to feed her. On that day, however, she did receive a tube feeding and the only thing that had changed in the nurses' notes was the description of Buller's behaviour. The next time she received a tube feeding was on 16 and 17 April, even though she had eaten almost nothing for a week. In the first case, Buller received a tube feeding after only one refusal to eat dinner, but in the second case, she was forced fed only after refusing food for several days. The decision to tube feed also apparently depended on the behaviour that was noted in the record; the more aggressive Buller became, the more likely it was that she would be tube fed. The eating problem accompanied the nurses' notes throughout the next months of Buller's stay and every time the nurses considered that Buller resisted eating, they intervened. For example, a nurse noted on 21 May that "Pat. ate very little this evening, spat everything out again, was very resistant when being fed."

Being fed implied some violence – the nurses were determined to feed her despite resistance. But the nurses had more than force or coercion in their repertoire; rather they tried to convince Buller to eat or else they tried to influence her through her mother, because she seemed to be particularly successful in convincing her daughter to eat. These attempts Becker described as "[infiltrating] the train of thought" of the sick person in order to influence behavior from the "interior." As mentioned previously, Becker believed that forcing sick people to eat would only increase their resistance to eating, although tube feeding could be used when all else failed.[41] Nurse Philipp Seibert urged nurses to encourage sick persons who believed that food was poisoned or forbidden to eat. "A warm word often helps in case of resistant sick persons and those in a bad mood."[42] As Bleuler described his strategy, "sometimes detours can be taken through which one can entice patients to eat; thus some of them will take food on the sly if food is left around for them."[43]

---

41 Ibid., 117.
42 Philipp Seibert, "Zur Pflege Geisteskranker," *Geisteskrankenpflege. Monatsschrift für Geisteskranken- und Krankenpflege* 44, no. 12 (1940): 151.
43 Eugen Bleuler, *Lehrbuch der Psychiatrie* (Berlin: Springer, 1923), 166.

However, Bleuler advocated tube feeding if all else had failed, stating that the patient should be placed in a lying or sitting position in such a manner that a fight was impossible. With the tube fixed correctly through the nose, the nurses were to pour in a mixture of milk and eggs. This procedure obviously required a certain amount of force, because sufficient personal were needed in order to firmly restrain the patient while threading the tube, especially since it could very easily be introduced into the respiratory tract. However, this kind of force was not directed personally against the patient – not aimed to take revenge – but rather it was a kind of "clinical" violence characterized by the calculated employment of force necessary to correct a certain behaviour. It was a kind of "mute power" that used only as much force as was necessary to convince the patient that resistance would be useless. A similar situation occurred on 13 April when Buller was given an injection after noisily jumping out of bed at night and insulting and assaulting the nurse when she tried to put her back.[44] Administering the injection in this case was a disciplinary means to get Buller to stay in bed and to stop her disturbance but it was described in neutral words and without any resentment. The injection was thus just a logical consequence of Buller's behaviour.

The "feeding strategy" was unsuccessful, for Buller lost more and more weight; the weight table showed that she weighed only 41.5 kg at the end of April 1931. Nevertheless, on another level, it did seem to work, because from the end of April 1931 on the nurses began to report more frequently that Buller ate too much, ate food that was not hers, and began to eat at times outside the regular mealtimes. For example on 28 April, she refused her own bread at dinner "but took it away from other patients and bit immediately into it. Did the same with the beverage."[45] On 6 June, she "was in a good mood. In the evening, she got out of bed all the time, took away patient M's chocolate."[46] And on 22 June the nurses noted that "Pat. got up a lot. Got cake out of her bedside table, started eating. When the remaining cake was taken from her, she demanded it back and got up again."[47] So even though it was obviously becoming more of a problem that Buller did not eat according to asylum rules, she was eating "spontaneously." This was a declared aim of therapy, and as the administrative chief inspector (*Verwaltungs Oberinspektor*) Sieben summarized, "the arousal and strengthening of the sick person's 'will to be cured' (*Heilungswillen*), the personal collaboration of the sick person with the physician and nurses, and a prudent and

---

44 PR, FMR, NN.
45 Ibid.
46 Ibid.
47 Ibid.

comprehensive attitude of the patient towards his suffering and his surrounding, can and must be achieved in the hospital."[48]

Disciplinary power thus had a productive dimension; it could not be reduced solely to oppression and negation but rather it influenced individuals profoundly, simultaneously producing them, or as Foucault described it, transforming the "somatic singularity"[49] into a subject and an individual in the first place.[50] The term "somatic singularity" is used as a kind of placeholder to indicate that the subject existed "pre-discursively" as a physiological body but achieved its subject status and its individuality only within the discourses that constructed it. This mechanism will be analyzed in more detail at the end of this chapter.

The nurses' notes also described an ongoing educational process meant to influence Buller to eat in the prescribed manner. The note from 22 June demonstrated that the nurses intervened when Buller behaved in an illegitimate manner and began to eat at night. The nurse reacted by taking away her cake, which in return provoked Buller. This action was exactly what was meant by an educational intervention; as nurse Seibert wrote, "all mentally ill persons are to be educated to tidy conduct and engagement."[51]

Education was not limited to the problem of eating but rather was the core of what could be called psychotherapy at that time. As has been emphasized several times, nurses took control over most of Buller's bodily functions. But also discussed has been that the takeover of control went beyond the mere physical body, but this was only indirectly mentioned in the nurses' notes. As previously noted, continuous bed rest could only be perceived because the bed was very often the point of reference for the description of Buller's behaviour; in other words, we only know about the rule of continuous bed rest because of the frequent reference to the bed in nursing descriptions of Buller's negative behaviour. Even after Buller was transferred to House 16, she spent most of her time on bed rest and was even washed and dressed by the nurses. On 17 March, the nurse on duty noted that "Pat. slept quietly, very resistant when she was washed."[52] The manner in which this observation was made demonstrated that this "washing" was not a single instance but rather part of the daily routine. The reason why the washing of Buller was noted this day was because she resisted. (Perhaps, since the night

---

48 Verwaltungs-Oberinspektor Sieben, "Erziehungsfragen bei dem Krankenhausaufenthalt," *Zeitschrift für das gesamte Krankenhauswesen*, no. 23 (1938): 65.
49 Foucault, *Psychiatric Power*, 46–58.
50 Hubert L. Dreyfus and Paul Rabinow, eds., *Michel Foucault : Beyond Structuralism and Hermeneutics* (Brighton: Harvester, 1982); Judith Butler, "Gender Regulations," in *Undoing Gender* (New York: Routledge, 2004), 40–56.
51 Seibert, *Zur Pflege Geisteskranker*, 152.
52 PR, FMR, NN.

nurse wrote the note, it was because she was being washed very early in the morning.) Nursing notes relating to washing can be found during the first couple of months, as, for example, on 31 May, "in the evening, patient let herself be washed and went to bed quietly."[53] Once again, we understand from this note that washing was a nursing routine that took place at least twice a day, as did dressing. For example, on 17 May, one nurse wrote that "in the evening, patient resisted being dressed in her nightshirt, went to bed naked, was quiet,"[54] and on May 28, Buller "screamed when getting dressed."[55] First, these notes affirm that they were written for those working in the asylum and therefore needed to convey only information important for the accomplishment of everyday work and, second, that they were only understandable against the backdrop of what I call "background knowledge," because every nurse working in Friedrichsberg certainly did know that patients were on bed rest and that it was a nursing task to wash and dress them at least twice a day.

Nevertheless, these duties also implied a restriction on any "free space," because patients could not decide for themselves whether or not they wanted to get washed and dressed. In the previously mentioned nurses' textbook, nurses were admonished that patients who were unclean in clothing and body demanded the "indefatigable attention of the nurse" to clean them.[56] Again, these nursing interventions are performed on the patient's body, with the washing and dressing done at prescribed times in a prescribed manner with specified clothing (because patients had to wear institutional clothing and in Buller's case, usually nightshirts). "Sick persons who are prone to tear [their clothes], to undress, or to twist off buttons [were to] receive so-called closure shirts (*Scließkleider*) or suits made out of 'untearable' material in some asylums."[57] However, increasingly limited and controlled "free space" for patients automatically implied that resistance would occur, because its restriction meant that nearly any behaviour appeared to be resistant, thus becoming even more evidence for a patient's madness. As already mentioned also, "barrier boards" used to prevent patients from getting out of bed provoked attempts to climb out or beat against these boards, behaviour also deemed resistant. Measures employed to restrain madness apparently also served to inflame it.

The nurses' reports can often be read as struggles to educate Buller. Although the notes only report on everyday minor occurrences in the asylum, they nevertheless highlight the rationale behind the nurses' continuous micro-interventions. For example, on 14 April, one nurse wrote that "pat. very agitated and

---

53 PR, FMR, NN.
54 PR, FMR, NN.
55 PR, FMR, NN.
56 Scholz, *Leitfaden für Irrenpfleger*, 73.
57 Ibid., 75.

noisy, could not be held in bed, tried over and over to leave the room. When holding her back she would lash out, bite and spit."[58] On 28 May 28, she "soiled herself and wet the bed" and screamed "when the nurse tried to dress her."[59] And again, on 15 July, she undressed completely in the garden and "went jogging, very resistant to put on the dress again."[60]

These examples emphasize the everyday struggles between the nurses and Buller. The largest part of the nurses' interventions in 1931 consisted of continuous and patient correction of her erratic behaviour. This would change, however, in the years to come, as the disciplinary means became more and more severe. Even in 1931, there were indications that the nurses could deliberately tighten their war against the madness by drawing on the large repertoire at their disposal.

One way to discipline patients was to transfer them to another house with a stricter control system where there were fewer possibilities for distraction, or to place them in a ward where they would be under constant surveillance. From mid-April on, Buller was more and more described as "completely" mad – no realm of her life seemed to be exempt from madness. She was hallucinating, was unpredictable in her behaviour, and aggressive with the nurses and other patients. The psychiatrist perceived Buller as a child, writing about her on 4 May that she "climbs about everywhere, is very untidy, often runs around naked. Extremely infantile behaviour, in between times again unapproachable, negativistic."[61] This description of her was still within the diagnostic frame of schizophrenia but was supplemented by the childish dimension of Buller's behaviour. In mid-May, she was transferred to House 14.

> 12.5. Pat. was transferred from House 16 to here, behaved calmly. Played with a ball for a short period of time, then threw it away, and stood around with a melancholic expression on her face. When her mother gave her some bread, she took a bite and then threw it away. In the evening, patient danced to a few beats of some music with a smiling expression on her face and then suddenly stopped, closed her eyes and made a sad face. In the evening, pat. ate well without having to be encouraged, milk had to be given to her. (Oi.)[62]

It is noteworthy that the nurse's notes from House 14 are very detailed, and furthermore, that they read like a continuation of Buller's history. This continuation is once more made possible by the medical record, because the concentration on her eating behaviour demonstrated that the nurse was aware of

---

58 PR, FMR, NN.
59 PR, FMR, NN.
60 PR, FMR, NN.
61 PR, FMR, PN.
62 PR, FMR, NN.

Buller's problems from the previous house, again strengthening the thesis that the record intervened in asylum interactions. For example, on 18 May the psychiatrist wrote that

> 18.5. All in all a little more orderly. Keeps busy for a short period of time, then runs around in the garden again, laughs, is being silly. Because she tried to climb over the garden fence, she was transferred to House 14 on 12.5. In the morning while getting up she mentions: "What shall I, I am dead, I cannot live on one leg."[63]

Again, the information in the psychiatrist's note is derived from the nurses' written observations His reference to her "climbing over the garden fence" – an event that happened in another house one week before he wrote his note, highlights once more how the record enabled one to "travel back" in the patient's history. Even the fact that he judged Buller's behaviour as "a little more orderly," though he was seeing her for the first time, demonstrates the power of the record. But the fact that Buller was transferred at all, because she broke a rule, illustrates that transfers within the asylum were not motivated by diagnostic considerations but rather by disciplinary rationalities.

Buller was transferred because it was felt that she could be kept under better control in House 14. During May and June, however, the nurses wrote irregularly, recording their observations only if it seemed that something noteworthy had occurred in Buller's behaviour. The psychiatrists, too, rarely took notes more than two or three times a month, since the nurses were responsible for Buller's care and "education." Not only was the physical space divided in House 14, the time lapses between the documentation on her introduced another form of division, at this point, a division by time.

> 4.6.31: At times, patient was very disobedient, spat at other pat. and threw stones at pat. Gü., had to be taken to the noisy room.
> 4.6.31: Aftern: Patient threw stones at the inspector. Patient was quite lively all afternoon, could not be persuaded to lie down in the lawn chair, often got up at night. (St.) H.
>
> 5.6.31:Pat. had to be brought back to the room temporarily because she threw pebbles all the time and spat. (Gr.)
>
> 6.6.31: Aftern: Patient sang and danced around the garden, was in a good mood. In the evening, she got out of bed all the time, took away patient M.'s chocolate. (St.)
>
> 10.6.31: Patient was very restless, took off her socks and shoes all the time, took away needlework, book or things like that from other pat. Patient had to be taken to the noisy ward again. Later often out of bed. (St.) H.

---

63 PR, FMR, PN.

15.6.31: Morning: In the garden, patient took off her dress and undergarment and went jogging, very resistant to put on the dress again. (Me.)

15.6.31: All afternoon, patient was very lively, jumped on benches and tables, ran around with her dress pulled up, tried to pick branches from bushes and spat all the time. (Sch.) H.[64]

As these notes suggest, Buller was transferred internally in House 14 for rule violations. Each time she became too noisy or too "resistant" she was put in either the "noisy room" or the observation ward, which prevented her from using the garden or circulating freely on the ward. On 4 June the nurse used the term "disobedient" because it characterized exactly what nursing interventions were about: to educate the patient to become obedient. Transferring patients to the noisy room against their will was possible only by force. In the Langenhorn nursing school textbook the procedure was described as follows: "in order to avert a tussle (*Balgerei*) a couple of [male] nurses should be ready on hand; the sick person generally discerns that resistance is futile and complies. In case that he [the sick person] still resists, no rules can be designated how he could be handled gently. It is practical if the [male] nurses arrange beforehand which part of the body each one should catch."[65] The use of force should be reduced to a minimum and should be applied strategically but the scenario should be such that the patient acknowledges that resistance is futile.

House 14 seemed to be set up for the purpose of applying many different types of disciplinary means. "Work therapy" was one means, and it was a nursing task to teach patients how to work, as was noted on 27 July when "pat. was encouraged to do some needlework but wasn't of much use. Wound the wool around the needles and played horse with it, at times talking incoherently and senselessly."[66] (See Figure 17) The nurses supervised this work and intervened in cases of misbehaviour when, for example, on 18 May when the nurse observed that "Pat. was very restless, knotted up her needlework, when patient was called, she said: 'You bitch, I am absolutely not obliged to be here.'"[67]

Because many notes related to Buller's behavior in the garden, they suggest that a secure space outside the building existed that too was highly controlled, since the nurses were able to observe everything that was going on and to intervene if necessary. For example, on 18 May "at noon in the garden, pat. hit pat. La. with her belt; when she was stopped for doing it, she said 'I am allowed to do that.'"[68] Even though the patients at times felt unobserved, they were under scrutiny. On 4 July, one nurse wrote that "until 10 am, patient was very restless,

---

64 PR, FMR, NN.
65 Scholz, *Leitfaden für Irrenpfleger*, 75–76.
66 PR, FMR, NN.
67 PR, FMR, NN.
68 PR, FMR, NN.

climbed up the tree, as soon as patient felt unobserved, she'd climb into the basement, she also sat down in the garden, collected stones, had a bowel movement. When the nurse paid attention to her, patient was friendly and obedient."[69]

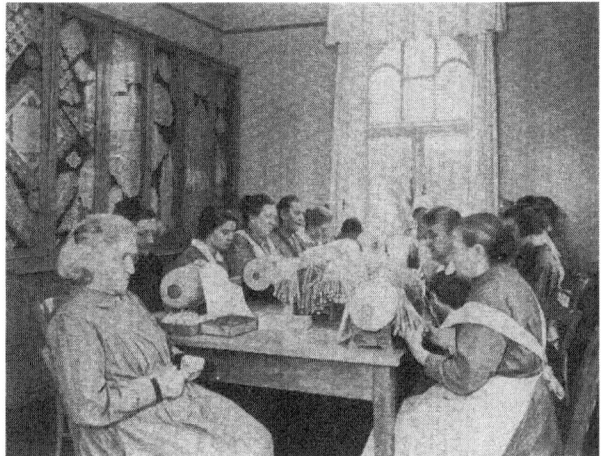

Figure 17: Sewing room in Friedrichsberg, c. 1928.[70]

However, the disciplinary repertoire of the nurses was broader than the use of violence and oppression. At times they appeared sympathetic to their patients. For example, on 12 May, Buller "played with a ball for a short period of time, then threw it away, and stood around with a melancholic expression on her face."[71] Deacon Wilhelm Thielmann believed that the relevance of playing games in psychiatric practice – that the main task of nurses and psychiatrists – was to motivate sick persons to undertake serious activities during the day and then to allow them to have "leisure time after work."[72] Games were a means to awaken the "stupid ones and idiots. Even if is difficult one must always try." Games enabled moving the "aimless, volatile activities of a schizophrenic in an orderly direction,"[73] which accelerated their process of adaptation. However "the day was to be primarily reserved for the work." It was only the evenings that should be "filled with all kinds of board games, card games, and parlor games...[and] music should be cultivated as well as readings." Nevertheless games should remain games and they should not lead to quarrels. "Only one person can win in

---

69 PR, FMR, NN.
70 Weygandt, *Die Staatskrankenanstalt Friedrichsberg*, 193.
71 PR, FMR, NN.
72 Wilhelm Thielmann, "Das Spiel und der Kranke," *Geisteskrankenpflege. Monatsschrift für Geisteskranken- und Krankenpflege* 41, no. 10 (1937): 183.
73 Ibid., 184.

the game [and] that must always be emphasized." Games were meant to socialize patients into orderly behavior, both in the game and in other parts of asylum life, without them being aware of it. Playing games was just another strategic tool used to influence the patient to accept the reality of the asylum.

Again the role of the nurses must be emphasized. The break in the psychiatrists' reports between February and March 1931, when the nurses continued to record their observations, is highly suggestive that the nurses had a great deal of autonomy. The psychiatrists wrote notes only on the rare occasion during this period, and thus the nurses appeared to have had a relatively long free period in which to interact with their patients. And because all information written by the psychiatrists continued to be derived from the nurses' notes, the nurses thus occupied a very powerful position. It was they who ultimately defined what became a part of the psychiatrists' reports and therefore it was they who defined the "image" of the patient that developed within the record. It was their written observations that identified targets for interventions, thus initiating further interventions, as in the case of Buller's transfer to House 14 in the first place in reaction to her attempt to climb over the fence, which they had recorded in the notes.

Enforcing the asylum's reality

This analysis has demonstrated so far that the asylum regulations formed a backdrop to the nurses' notes and that many of the nursing observations were a succession of recorded rule violations. Again, in September 1931.

> 2.9.31: The patient does not obey the nurses. She always gets what she wants. (Fb)

> 4.9.31: Patient is always very lively, talks all the time about her trips and that she had been to India. Is always very full of herself, says that she has had wonderful skin, but now her face was full of pimples. In the evening patient often talks with patient Jü., when she is told to be quiet she always talks back in a cheeky way and is still not quiet but thinks she must have the last word. Patient is always hard working and wants to please. (F. He.) H.[74]

Every daily entry referred to a hidden rule, and the last quote especially demonstrated that the nurses evaluated Buller's behaviour according to her capacity to submit – the reason why the nurses talked so often about her behaviour as "quiet," "reluctant," "noisy," or "struggling against," etc. The "wish to please" alone was not sufficient. However, it was only against the backdrop of asylum regulation that these observations could be made in the first place. According to

---

74 PR, FMR, NN.

Foucault, the objectified medical gaze, as the fundamental condition for the constitution of medical knowledge, requires a certain order and a particular distribution of bodies, gestures, behaviour, and discourses in space and time.[75] Only within such a regulated distribution can the medical gaze find its object. Distribution is enabled by the disciplinary order. Simultaneously, this disciplinary order is the condition for a durable cure of the mad because the transformation of the sick person into somebody who ceases to be sick is only possible within this regulated dissemination of power. The reality of the asylum is traversed by a complete power dissymmetry that is bound to a medical instance. This medical instance is endowed with an infinite power against which resistance is futile. The medical instance functions first of all as power and only thereafter can it function as knowledge. This is the reason why Buller was transferred within the asylum according to her behaviour and not according to a specific diagnosis or nosography. This is similar for the treatments of other patients because in all the records used for this analysis, individual treatments are characterized by the same "psychotherapy" independently from patient diagnosis (see also Endnote 39). The only differences in treatments can be found in the medications administered but the psychotherapy as such was always the same. This is to say that the psychiatric asylum cannot be considered as an institution that functions according to specific rules, but rather it is a field that is polarized by an essential power dissymmetry that is physically constituted even in the body of the psychiatrist. That is the deeper meaning of Bleuler's assumption quoted earlier –"that it is very rare to persuade the sick person to back down through logic itself, but rather the appearance of the one who applies the logic," or the bodily appearance of the psychiatrist that is important.

However the power of the psychiatrist was distributed in a system of differences. Around the psychiatrist was grouped a series of "intermediary" groups, one of which was the nurses, and the other, technologies. According to Foucault, the psychiatric asylum is a "curing dispositif" or a "curing machine" in which the actions of the physician constitute an absolute body within the institution, the rules, and the buildings. It is a kind of uniform body in which the walls, the rooms, the instruments, the nurses, the wards, and the psychiatrists are elements with different functions but with a common and most important purpose of achieving a particular effect through their interplay. It is striking that in the medical record under study here, nothing points to it being led by an anatomic-pathological discourse or a kind of nosography. In the final analysis it seems as if psychiatric practice did not act in accordance with a theory but rather was composed of maneuvers, tactics, actions, and reactions. In brief, psychiatric

---

75 Foucault, *Le pouvoir psychiatrique. Cours au collège de France. 1973–1974.*

practice appeared as a tactical corpus and strategic ensemble and this seems to be all that could be reported in the notes.[76]

This disciplinary space of the psychiatric asylum is further characterized by the fact that nurses and psychiatrists were "masters of reality." The notes demonstrate that nurses especially had to provide the idea of "reality" so strongly in order to seize and penetrate the madness to make it "disappear." Under the authority of the psychiatrists, nurses became the supplementary force enabling reality to force itself onto the madness or, conversely, to prevent the madness from withdrawing from reality. Nurses appeared as an intensifying factor of the real. They were agents of a superior power of the real through which the real was forced onto the madness in the name of a power that claimed truth based on medical knowledge.[77] This enforcement of reality was based on the dispositif of psychiatry that enabled it to conduct and govern the madness. The superior power of the real is enabled by the interplay of different variables: the disciplinary power asymmetry, the imperative use of language, and the enforcement of a statuary identity in which the sick person must recognize himself or herself. The desire to find a way out of madness implied acknowledging this medical power as all powerful, renouncing the omnipotence of madness, and accepting the documentary-biographical identity. The latter will be analyzed in more detail in the next section. Thus, the instruments employed by psychiatry in order to dominate madness become simultaneously the criteria for recovery. Foucault called this the "tautology of psychiatry" because, on the one hand, the asylum forcibly awards reality and, on the other hand, simultaneously represents reality as pure power, a reality that is intensified through medical and nursing functions.[78] In other words, the medical-nursing power-knowledge complex has no other function than being the agent of reality itself. To construct reality as superior power is enabled by the fact that this reality is reproduced within the asylum. On the one hand, the asylum is nearly completely cut off from the outside world; it is a specific world that remains completely under the control of a medical power (that defines itself by competency in medical knowledge). On the other hand, asylums must remind patients of everyday life as much as possible, with similarities to workshops and prisons. It seemed as if Buller could only resist by fighting the nurses, wetting the bed, undressing, or tearing her own shirt; in the years to come she even begin to self-injure. That these actions were forms of resistance is demonstrated by the fact that they can be found in most of the analyzed records. However, as further analysis will highlight, disciplinary means became so strong in the years to come that finally, the dis-

---

76 Foucault, *Le pouvoir psychiatrique*, 125.
77 Foucault, *Le pouvoir psychiatrique*, 131.
78 Ibid., 165.

ciplinary power of the psychiatrist turned into an absolute sovereign power and, in the end, enabled Buller's assassination.

As already mentioned above, the written reports were of particular importance for enforcing psychiatric reality on patients. Within Buller's medical file, a documentary-biographical identity evolved that subjectified the "somatic singularity" (as earlier defined). This mechanism will be analyzed in the next section.

The Record, the Script, the Dispositif[79], and the Subject

The analysis has so far suggested that psychiatric practice can only be understood if one considers the complex interplay of multiple actors. One mechanism not yet analyzed in depth is the significance of the record for the subjectification of the patients. The interconnections between different inscriptions and different technologies highlight one mode by which human beings are made subjects. According to Foucault, this mode can be described as an objectification through "dividing practices," meaning that the "subject is either divided inside himself or divided from others...[a process] that objectifies him."[80] The architecture of the modern asylum, for example, enabled the separation of mentally ill persons in such a way that it allowed for the control and the discipline of the insane. It was understood that the insane could be arranged geographically according to the perceived danger of their conduct, their ability to work, their ability to disturb asylum routine, or their gender, and rooms were constructed to enable wide-ranging surveillance of these patients. Asylum architecture was guided by the desire to closely regulate the behaviour of the mentally ill, an aspect that will be developed further later.

It was only within the modern asylum, which designated a specific space for the care of the insane, that the idea of the "insane" emerged in the first place. Subjectivity does not exist prior to discourse but is constructed through discourse, and modes of subjectification are always embedded in power relations, which cannot be analyzed, according to Foucault, on a legal model or by asking questions such as "What legitimates power?"[81] It is not so much a question of

---

79 In this book the French pronounciation of Dispositif is used in order to highlight that the term is part of Foucaults' theoretical approach. Whereas the term dispositive in English has multiple connotations, the term dispositif has a very specific relevance to Foucault's take on power, knowledge and subjectivity.
80 Michel Foucault, "The Subject and Power." In *Michel Foucault: Beyond Structuralism and Hermeneutics*, edited by Hubert L. Dreyfus and Paul Rabinow (Chicago: University of Chicago Press, 1983), 208.
81 Ibid., 209.

"such and such" institution of power, or group, or elite, or class, but rather a technique, a form of power. This form of power applies itself to immediate everyday life which categorizes the individual, marks him [sic], imposes a law of truth on him which he must recognize and which others have to recognize in him. It is a form of power which makes individuals subjects. There are two meanings of the word subject: subject to someone else by control and dependence, and the other, tied to his own identity by a conscience or self-knowledge. Both meanings suggest a form of power which subjugates and makes subject to.[82]

Based on Foucault's concept of subjectification and regulation as a twofold process, the process described above is a form of subject construction. According to Foucault, regulatory power "not only acts upon a preexisting subject but also shapes and forms that subject" and even disciplinary power has productive effects. For example, even though the nurses forced Buller to eat, she, at times, did eat. Power is not only coercive but also has a kind of beneficial effect. However, "to become subject to a regulation is also to become subjectified by it," or in other words, a subject is brought into being through the act of regulation.[83]

As already demonstrated in several instances, psychiatric practice targets complete possession of the body and an all-embracing control, both of which are connected to the written recording of observations. As a disciplinary power, psychiatric practice with its characteristic form of hierarchical continuum required the use of writing in order to register everything about a patient – everything that the patient did and what he or she talked about. The medical record enabled nurses to pass along information from the bottom-up and the documents, because they were written, allowed all information to be accessible at any time. Written documents therefore enabled and assured permanent visibility. It was also a method of centralizing information and of coordinating different levels within disciplinary systems. Graphing bodily functions allowed a direct and continuous relationship between writing and body to evolve. The visibility of the body and the permanency of the writing were not detachable from each other and produced the effect of what Foucault called, a "schematized and centralized individualization,"[84] centralized because all information regarding the patient was collected in a record that was entirely controlled and inspected by the medical director (or his representative).

The bodies, the gestures, the behaviours, and the discourses are all encircled by a web of writing, which registers, codes, and schematizes. However, the continuous visibility of the body through graphing enabled a further important effect by triggering an immediate reaction of disciplinary power. This effect was

---

82 Ibid., 212.
83 Butler, "Gender Regulations," 41.
84 Foucault, *Le pouvoir psychiatrique*, 53.

already analyzed in the section on the interplay between different inscriptions, which enabled the perception of something that had not yet been materialized or became visible only through inscriptions, as, for example, Buller's bladder infection or her eating disorder. This capacity inherent in documenting was also demonstrated at the times when Buller became too excited and received "prophylactic" sedatives. Uninterrupted documentation enabled interventions to take place from the first moment of translation on the chart, virtually from the first sign or gesture on. The previous section that dealt with nurses' notes as war reports demonstrated the continuous concern of the nurses to document Buller's behaviour in such detail that it enabled them to intervene as quickly as possible when she behaved in certain ways. The least glimmer of a change in her mood, for example, could result in the nurses transferring her prophylactically to the "noisy room." This prophylactic intervention illustrates a further significant characteristic of disciplinary power because its aim is to enable intervention at a point of time when conduct is still virtual and only just about to be realized. The intervention takes place before the act itself, something that is only possible because of the complex interplay among surveillance, reward, punishment, and pressure, or, in short, through "infra-judiciary" forms of intervention.[85]

Disciplinary power thus establishes a permanent pressure that is not only directed towards committed actions and their subsequent damage, but also toward the potential of such behaviour. Before any gesture is carried out its precursor must be identified to enable disciplinary power to intervene before the behaviour, the body, the gesture, or the discourse actually comes into existence. This dimension that is concerned with virtual possibility, the disposition, or the volition, can be characterized as "the soul."[86] Foucault called this interplay the "panoptical principle" (the ability to see anyone anytime) that consists of the following aspects: first, the occupation of the time, the life, and the body of the individual; second, a centralized individualisation based on writing; and third, this principle also contains the possibility for continuous penalization that targets a virtual behaviour and that goes beyond the body to project something like the "psyche." This is to say, interventions first and foremost constitute the psyche that is being "treated" in the asylum.

This interrelation between punishment, script, and technologies will be analyzed in more detail in the notes of the years from 1936 to 1938 and in 1940, where it will be demonstrated once again how multiple technologies were able to transform Buller profoundly. But as these notes also highlight, deviant conduct was punished but conduct evaluated as "normal" was rewarded. The construction of the asylum helped to materialize these principles of disciplinary

---

85 Ibid.
86 Ibid.

power since different asylum spaces and the spatial organization of the wards were constructed according to levels of punishment and reward.

As suggested earlier, "normal" behaviour was rewarded by allowing patients certain liberties such as "free" circulation on the ward or access to the garden. Especially in Langenhorn, the amount of food to which one was entitled depended on work performance, based on the logic that patients who were motivated to work could expect more and better food. This aspect had a decisive impact on the chances of survival in Langenhorn during the Nazi regime and more particularly, during the Second World War, because only those patients not accommodated in "secured houses" had a chance to organize supplementary food outside the houses.[87] Discipline thus functioned not only by oppressing behaviour considered undesirable but also by provoking or constituting behaviour considered desirable through continuous punishment and education (e.g. stimulating the desire to work in order to get better food).

However, the main effect of the disciplinary power was the profound re-creation of the relationship between the somatic singularity, the subject, and the individual. It is again Foucault who analyzed the impact of this mechanism in detail and the following section tries to grasp some of his central ideas, because it enables us to more fully understand the rationale behind the documentary corpus of the record.

According to Foucault, sovereign power is characterized by specific ceremonies and procedures that create the process of individualization from the top down, and it is the sovereign who is the most individualized element in this system. Disciplinary systems, however, are characterized by the fact that the individualizing function disappears from the top. Those who are charged to direct the dispositif (in the case of the psychiatric asylum it is the medical director) are not important as individuals but only in their function. This function could be accomplished by a particular person, but it could in principal be carried out by anybody.[88] This was demonstrated in the analysis above when the nurses intervened in order to correct "misbehaviour," they did so only in their function as nurses and not for personal revenge. I call this aspect the "anonymous power" of the nurses, because violence was justified only insofar as it enabled the education of the patient; it was simply a strategic consideration

---

87 Michael Wunder, *Euthanasie in den letzten Kriegsjahren. Die Jahre 1944 und 1945 in der Heil- und Pflegeanstalt Hamburg Langenhorn*; Böhme, *1893–1993 100 Jahre Allgemeines Krankenhaus Ochsenzoll*; Klaus Böhme and Uwe Lohalm, eds. *Wege in den Tod. Hamburgs Anstalt Langenhorn und die Euthanasie in der Zeit des Nationalsozialismus*, Forum Zeitgeschichte ed. Vol. 2 (Cloppenburg: Ergebnisse Verlag, 1993); Götz Aly, "Medicine against the Useless," in *Cleansing the Fatherland: Nazi Medicine and Racial Hygiene*, eds. Götz Aly, Peter Chroust and Christian Pross (Baltimore and London: Johns Hopkins University Press, 1994), 22–99.
88 Foucault, *Psychiatric Power*.

and not bound to a specific person. Foucault described this theoretical aspect as the democratic principle of the Panopticum, because even those who assume responsibility within this disciplinary system are themselves only part of a bigger system that controls them and in which they are disciplined themselves.[89]

In contrast to a system of sovereign power, disciplinary power implies a strong individualization "from below." Unlike in systems of sovereign power, in which the somatic singularity exists as a non-subjectified body, in systems of disciplinary power, the somatic singularity becomes subjectified: its body, its gestures, its place, its movements, its force, its lifetime, and its discourses. Disciplinary power thus constitutes this mode of subjectivity. Discipline is a power technique through which the subject mode is placed on and aligned with the somatic singularity, making "the body" into an individual. The most fundamental characteristic of disciplinary power is that it produces subordinated bodies by enforcing the subjectvity onto the body. Disciplinary power produces these bodies and distributes these bodies in a specific manner and thereby acts as an individualizing agent only through the fact that individuals are nothing more than these subordinated bodies. The activities are bound to the system of surveillance-script (or, in other words, through a panoptic system) that projects a "psyche" as the backdrop or origin of the somatic singularity and implements the idea of normal as the obligatory principle in order to divide and normalize all the individuals constituted by this system.

Disciplinary power enforces the subject mode onto the somatic singularity through the combination of the sustained gaze, the script, the mechanism of endless minor penalties, the projection of a psyche, and finally, the subdivision of normal-abnormal. All these aspects together make up the disciplined individual and what can be described as an "individual" is finally nothing else than something to which political power can connect. What we call an individual, according to Foucault, is nothing other than the result of the amalgamation of the somatic singularity with political power. Discipline is the final, capillary form of power that constitutes the individual as its target, its partner, and its counterpart in relations of power. This is to say that the individual is neither antecedent to the subject function nor to the projection of a psyche nor to the normalizing instances. On the contrary, it was only because the somatic singularity became the carrier of the subject function that something like the concept of individual could appear within the political system. Only by encircling the body with endless surveillance, endless writing, and virtual penalization, with its subsequent subordination, could something like the individual be constituted. Only because the normalizing instance distributes and excludes those "body-psyches" in a particular manner is the in-

---

89 Michel Foucault, *Überwachen und Strafen. Die Geburt des Gefägnisses*, trans. Walter Seitter (Frankfurt a.M.: Suhrkamp, 1994).

dividual characterized. Due to the fact that the body was subjectified, which means that the subject mode was fixed on it, and because it was psychologized and normalized, something like the individual appeared. From this moment on it was possible to talk about the individual as an object of scientific inquiry.[90]

Fixing the subject function onto Anna Maria Buller

At the beginning of this analysis I contended that the documented biography in Buller's medical record had a wider aim than the simple reporting of particular events that occurred during her stay in the asylum. The admission ritual was the first step towards fixing a documentary identity onto individuals because, as I outlined in its analysis, it forced individuals to recognize themselves in their documentary histories and in the documented events that took place during their stay in the asylum. For this reason, psychiatrists regularly repeated interrogations and asked questions about events that they knew about only because they were reported in the nurses' notes. With the foregoing theoretical considerations in mind, it becomes easier to understand the importance of an interrogation that was carried out just before Buller was discharged from Friedrichsberg in 1931. Two versions of this interrogation exist; one was written by the nurses and one by the psychiatrist. On 4 September 1931, the psychiatrist wrote:

> 4.9.31: Improved a lot lately. Eats a lot now and gained a lot of weight. At the ward cheerful, again busy with something. Talks a lot, seeks contact with other patients. During doctor's visit trusting behaviour.
>
> Explor. [Exploration] Walks in happily, shakes hands, Takes an interest in the room. Did not have the feeling she was ill during the recent time.
> (Why didn't you eat?) I don't know; I couldn't eat.
> (Why didn't you speak?) I couldn't; I didn't feel like saying something; I was like without consciousness, like numb.
> (Why always naked?) I really don't know the answer to that
> (Hearing voices?) Yes I am sure I have heard those; let me think; I heard music, all the time. I heard the music Frederic the Great has written. I heard clearly.
> (Have you been to India?) Oh yes, sure. I have written books about it. Yes, beautiful flowers, nice trees, flags
> (Also spoken?) As far as I know I have spoken also. With the birds that carry rubbish bins. As far as I know we took the ship Ambrades.
> (When?) That was not long ago. I've just come back now. (But she is not quite sure about this,) But it all seems to me like a dream. It appears so unreal. I also don't know what those East Indians look like. (Shortly after she is more certain again) I was in Jokohama too; as far as I know I was there. The city is 200x bigger than Germany"

---

90 Foucault, *Le pouvoir psychiatrique*, 21–39

(Were you really there?) Yes, nobody believes me. It doesn't really matter; maybe I just read about it.

Talks about all this willingly and happily. Good mood. Very childish way of being.[91]

Two days earlier, the nurses had written:

> 2.9. To the doctor's question if the patient remembered that she had been tube fed, the patient replied smilingly "yes." Why not eaten? "I didn't like it." Patient used to run around the room naked a lot. To that patient replied: "but it is nice to run around like that when the sun is shining." [Asked] if patient wasn't ashamed to run around like this, it is not nice of a young girl, she promptly answered: "Ach, why, when it is so warm." To further questions concerning the trip to India, if patient had really been there with Mr. He., patient laughed and answered affirmatively, after further investigations about the trip patient admitted that it had all been made up. Patient behaves in an infantile/childish manner and laughs all the time. *H.*[92]

Because the interrogation that took place on 4 September 1941 was pertinent for Buller's further "career," it was a decisive day for her. Following this interrogation Buller was granted leave for a couple of weeks and then discharged from the asylum. The reason for her discharge must be searched for in the final interrogation and the statements Buller made in the course of the interrogation. For the first time in the whole record, this minute of the interrogation provides a more or less detailed report on Buller's response to questioning and the stand that she took regarding her madness. From the perspective of the analysis outlined to this point, it is also significant because Buller "acknowledged" her madness by recognizing herself in the documented biography of the record. The documentation thus comes full circle: what began with the admission ritual is determined by the final interrogation.

Before a discussion of the theoretical implications of this interrogation, some particularities of the content should be highlighted. Two versions of the interrogation exist and it is unclear if these versions refer to the same interrogation or if two took place. Buller had been transferred to the house in which this interrogation took place just 13 days prior, meaning that Buller was personally known to the new team of psychiatrists and nurses for only a couple of weeks. All questions asked were related to events that happened in the past, events that the nurses and doctor could not have witnessed firsthand. These events were only knowable to them because they were documented in the record, again illustrating the mechanism analyzed in detail above. The record is a biographical corpus from which a patient's history could be reconstructed. The comment about her improved disposition and her weight gain was gleaned from in-

---

91 PR, FMR, PN.
92 PR, FMR, NN.

formation contained in Buller's record, because the assessment of her ingestion especially referred to events that took place at the beginning of Buller's admission and in the other houses. Buller's weight gain could only be known by comparing the different entries in the weight table (according to the table Buller put on 10 kg of weight). The depiction of her behaviour differed significantly from the admission ritual; whereas at the beginning she was perceived as catatonic, negativistic (refuses any food consumption), and completely withdrawn. Now she was described by the psychiatrists as "cheerful, busy with something, talking a lot, and even seeking contact with other patients," although she was still portrayed as childish. Despite this dramatic turnaround, however, the vocabulary used by the psychiatrists clearly indicated that they believed Buller was still mad. For example, the term "cheerfully" implied that her behaviour was somehow inappropriate, and describing her as talking a lot suggested that she was "overshooting" in her attempts to overcome her previously non-talkative state. Although "shaking hands" implied a certain trust in her relationship with the psychiatrist, this type of unobtrusive behaviour strengthened the physician's impression that she had no insight into her illness. He believed that Buller was still mad and that her behaviour had merely changed from being dangerous and negativistic to harmless and childish.

Between the nurse's note and that written by the psychiatrist, there is a slight difference in the manner in how Buller's answers are reported. In response to the question concerning Buller's previous refusal of food, the psychiatrist recorded that she "couldn't eat," while the nurse noted Buller had not liked the food. Although the psychiatrist seemed to suggest that Buller's reluctance to take any food was somehow "unmotivated," the nurse's note demonstrated that Buller justified her behaviour because she did not like the food. But what must also be emphasized at this point is that the nurse's note explicitly mentioned that the questions were related to the documented behaviour.

During this interrogation, it was also revealed that Buller believed she had travelled to India, something that had never before been mentioned in either set of notes. Many drawings and writings produced by Buller were found in an envelope at the back of her medical file, as well as a kind of travel diary in which she wrote about her travels to India and described the fauna of the country. (See Figures 18 – 24) These drawings point out that Buller was unwittingly involved in proving her madness, an aspect that was true for all the records analyzed in this analysis. Letters, drawings and any other object that could somehow be related to the madness of the patient and that could be used as evidence for the diagnosis were kept in the records.

The interrogation followed the same format as already analyzed in detail for the admission ritual: the psychiatrist asked the questions and the patient had to answer them. Apart from the fact that both this interrogation and the admission ritual were demonstrations of power of psychiatric practice, and more precisely, the psychiatrist, they differ in some key aspects. The admission ritual focussed first and foremost on the constitution of a mental illness and sought to find its beginnings in early childhood. In this interrogation, the psychiatrist based his questions directly on the record's documented events, and the sequence of the interrogation followed exactly that found in the medical file. This clearly demonstrates what is meant by fixing a documentary identity onto individuals and, consequently, forcing individuals to recognize themselves in their documentary histories and in the documented events that took place during their stay in the asylum. The final aim of this interrogation was to convince Buller to admit that "yes, it was me described in these events and that yes, I am mentally ill and therefore need the therapy, the psychiatrist, and the asylum."

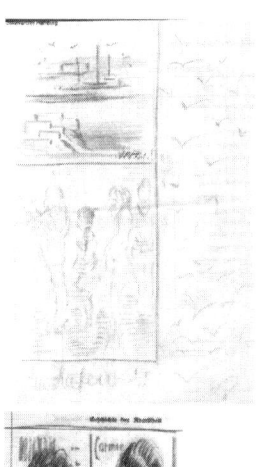

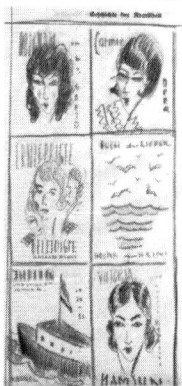

Figure 18, 19 and 20: Drawings and travel diary of Buller's virtual travels to India. At the left are pictures of Naples, and of her departure from Hamburg. In the middle is a kind of botanic description of an exotic flower. The remaining drawings are from 1931. Patient record 28338.

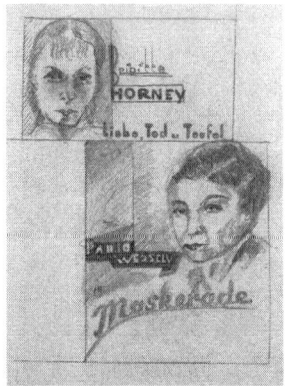 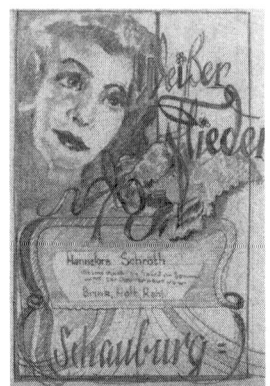

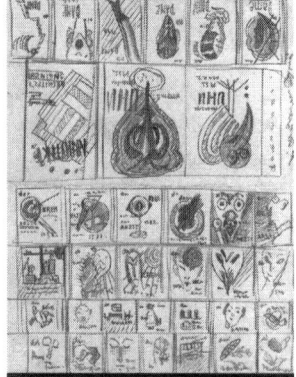

Figure 21, 22 and 23: The remaining drawings are from 1931.

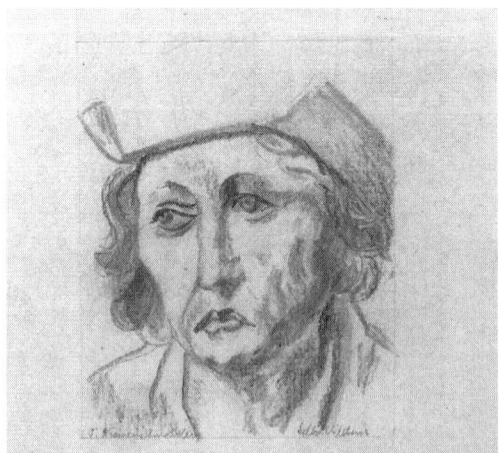

Figure 24: Self-portrait (no date). Patient record 28338.

Psychiatry interpellates Buller as subject

This analysis has arrived at a crucial point, because the mechanism roughly described as the fixation of the subject function onto the somatic singularity is central to psychiatric practice and utterly relevant to understand the assassinations of sick persons. It is therefore necessary to theoretically elaborate this mechanism in more detail and one approach that seems promising is Althusser's investigation of ideology and subjectification.[93] The central claim of Althusser's theory is that ideology

> "acts" or "functions" in such a way that it "recruits" subjects among individuals (it recruits them all), or "transforms" individuals into subjects (it transforms them all) by that very precise operation which I have called interpellation or hailing, and which can be imagined along the lines of the most commonplace everyday police (or other) hailing: "Hey, you there."
>
> Assuming that the theoretical scene I have imagined takes place in the street, the hailed individual will turn round. By this one-hundred-and-eighty-degree physical conversion, he becomes a subject. Why? Because he has recognized that the hail was "really" addressed to him, that "it was really him who was hailed" (and not someone else).[94]

Althusser used the term individual here with the same intent with which Foucault used "somatic singularity" as defined earlier, namely as a kind of placeholder. Althusser staged a social scene that was both "punitive and reduced, for the call [was] made by an officer of 'the Law,' and this officer [was] cast as singular and speaking. This scene was meant to be exemplary and allegorical, implying that "it never [needed] to happen for its effectivity to be presumed."[95] Interpellation is a certain way of staging the call, "where the call, as staged, becomes deliteralized in the course of its exposition, and is figured as a demand of an ideology (or better, ideologies) to align with the ideology."[96] It is a turning around to face the ideology and an entrance into the language of self-description – hence "Here I am."

Before continuing with the analysis of subjectification, one must grasp the significance of Althusser's concept of ideology. Stuart Hall pointed out that Althusser had developed the concept of ideology in his earlier writings and that the definition in these writings was broader and more "elaborated" than the one

---

93 Louis Althusser, "Ideology and Ideological State Apparatuses: Notes Towards an Investigation," in *Lenin and Philosophy and Other Essays* (New York: Monthly Review Press, 2001), 85–126.
94 Ibid., 118.
95 Judith Butler, *The Psychic Life of Power: Theories in Subjection* (Stanford: Stanford University Press, 1997), 106.
96 Ibid., 107.

he used later.[97] According to Hall, Althusser defined ideologies as "systems of representation – composed of concepts, ideas, myths, and images – in which men [and women] live their imaginary relation to the real conditions of existence."[98] By defining ideologies as "systems of representation," Althusser characterized them as essentially discursive and semiotic. In Hall's words, "*systems of representation* are the systems of meaning through which *we represent the world to ourselves and to one another.* It acknowledges that ideological knowledge is the result of specific practices" or in other words, specific practices are involved in the production of meaning. This is to say that every social practice is constituted within the interplay of meaning and representation and thus meaning or ideas materialize in social practices. Hall formulated this interrelation as "there is no social practice outside of ideology. However, this does not mean that, because all social practices are within the discursive, there is nothing to social practice but discourse."[99]

This interrelation between social practices and the materialization of certain rationalities or ideas forms the central thesis of my analysis so far. Psychiatry as analyzed in this book can only be comprehended as a complex interplay between psychiatric practice understood as materialized discourses and psychiatric discourses understood as a result of psychiatric practice. Buller's medical record is thus the result of a process of the production of meaning and the tool of representation par excellence, which is to say that psychiatric practice can be defined as an apparatus. To use Althusser's term, the psychiatric asylum is an "ideological state apparatus" that produces the representations in which psychiatric patients live. It is important to emphasize that it is not possible to bring ideology to an end and simply live the real. "We always need systems through which we represent what the real is to ourselves and to others."[100] This is to say, that we always use a variety of systems of representations in order to experience, interpret, and "make sense of" the conditions of our existence.

> It follows that ideology can always define the same so-called object or objective condition in the real world differently. There is 'no necessary correspondence' between the conditions of a social relation or practice and the number of different ways in which it can be represented. It does not follow that, as some Neo-Kantians in discourse theory have assumed, because we cannot know or experience a social relation except 'within

---

97 Stuart Hall, "Signification, Representation, Ideology: Althusser and the Post-Structuralist Debates," in *Critical Studies in Mass Communication*, eds. R. K. Avery and D. Eason (New York: The Guilford Press, 1991), 88–113; Althusser, "Ideology and Ideological State Apparatuses," 85–126.
98 Hall, "Signification, Representation, Ideology," 101.
99 Ibid.
100 Ibid. 102.

ideology,' therefore it has no existence independent of the machinery of representation...[101]

One experiences the world within systems of representation and this experience is the result of codes of intelligibility and schemes of interpretation, as demonstrated in my analysis for Buller's case record. The analysis of this record highlights the fact that what is represented in the record was the result of schemes of interpretations, and what was "experienced" by nurses and psychiatrists was bound up in their codes of intelligibility. As Hall stated, "consequently, there is no experience outside of the categories of representation or ideology."[102] This relationship between the conditions of social conditions and the manner in which they are experienced is what Althusser called "imaginary" in his definition of ideology cited above. This returns us to the original question of "how it is that subjects recognize themselves in ideologies," or as Hall put it "How is the relationship between individual subjects and the positionalities of a particular ideological discourse constructed?"[103]

In order to answer this question it is helpful to consult Althusser's definition of the interrelationship between ideologies and the category of the subject. "I say: the category of the subject is constitutive of all ideology, but at the same time and immediately I add that the category of the subject is only constitutive of all ideology insofar as all ideology has the function (which defines it) of "constituting" concrete individuals as subjects. In the interaction of this double constitution exists the functioning of all ideology, ideology being nothing but its functioning in the material forms of existence of that functioning."[104]

This definition not only implies that we are always already subjects but also that we constantly practice rituals of ideological recognition, which guarantee for us that "we are indeed concrete, individual, distinguishable and (naturally) irreplaceable subjects."[105] This sentence describes exactly the functioning of the interrogation in psychiatry. I already mentioned that one decisive aim of psychiatry is to fix the subject function onto the somatic singularity and that the interrogation of the patient targets, among other things, the need for the patient to recognize himself or herself in the schematized and centralized biography of the documentation. However, the sentence also highlights that some of the basic positioning of somatic singularities (or individuals) in language are constituted through unconscious processes in the psychoanalytical sense, at the early stages of formation. These processes are already operating in early infancy "making

---

101 Ibid.
102 Ibid., 103.
103 Ibid., 104.
104 Althusser, "Ideology and Ideological State Apparatuses," 116.
105 Ibid., 117.

possible the formation of relations with others and the outside world."¹⁰⁶ To illustrate the power of ideology to constitute subjects, Althusser used the example of the divine voice that names, and in naming, brings its subjects into being. As philosopher Judith Butler explained,

> Baptism exemplifies the linguistic means by which the subject is compelled into social being. God names "Peter," and this address establishes God as the origin of Peter, the name remains attached to Peter permanently by virtue of the implied and continuous presence in the name of the one who names him. Within the terms of Althusser's examples, however, this naming cannot be accomplished without a certain readiness or anticipatory desire on the part of the one addressed. To the extent that the naming is an address, there is an addressee prior to the address; but given that the address is a name which creates what it names, there appears no "Peter" without the name "Peter."¹⁰⁷

Social ideologies operate in an analogous way, according to Althusser. Setting aside that in using the divine voice, "Althusser inadvertently assimilates social interpellation to the divine performative," the parallel to psychiatric interrogation is striking. I want to broaden his perspective to include the psychiatrist's voice hailing the psychiatric patient in unfolding the biography of the record: "You are mentally ill."

In requesting Buller to recognize herself in the reported events of the record, the psychiatrist interpellates Buller. Nevertheless, the analysis above highlights that this naming cannot be accomplished without a certain readiness or anticipatory desire on the part of the one addressed. Only if Buller recognized herself in these events and turned her face towards the psychiatrist's power that hailed her, and only by admitting "yes it is really me who is described in these events," was the naming successful.

> In this sense, as a prior and essential condition of the formation of the subject, there is a certain readiness to be compelled by the authoritative interpellation, a readiness which suggests that one is, as it were, already in relation to the voice before the response, already implicated in the terms of the animating misrecognition by an authority to which one subsequently yields. Or perhaps one has already yielded before one turns around, and that turning is merely a sign of an inevitable submission by which one is established as a subject positioned in language as a possible addressee.¹⁰⁸

Again, this kind of analysis can be paralleled to the psychiatric interrogation, because the focus of the interrogation is to expose Buller's readiness to be compelled by the authoritative interpellation. Her turning was a sign of the inevitable submission to psychiatric power by which Buller was established as a psychiatric subject positioned in language, and it was the pre-condition for her

---

106 Hall, "Signification, Representation, Ideology," 104.
107 Butler, *The Psychic Life of Power,* 111.
108 Ibid., 111–112.

to be released from the asylum. This is the mechanism that decided whether or not Buller could be considered incorrigible. In cases in which patients did not recognize themselves as individuals in the documented events in their record, their prospects of being "cured" were poor. In Buller's case, it was the last part of the interrogation that was of particular significance. When she confessed that "nobody believes me. It doesn't really matter; maybe I just read about it," it was the first time that she had acknowledged that she might be wrong. At the end of her 1931 admission, we clearly see this "readiness to be compelled by the authoritative interpellation" of the psychiatrist, and therefore Buller received permission first to spend a couple of weeks with her parents, and then was allowed a full discharge from the asylum, only to be re-admitted two months later in 1932.

After her last interrogation that included Buller's confession, a wondrous transformation took place in the psychiatrist's notes. In the last line of his note he stated that she talked "about all this willingly and happily. Good mood. Very childish way of being," which was a continuation of the reports of the last weeks. But although the patient was portrayed as a good-natured and somewhat feeble-minded child, all aspects of excitement and aggression had vanished from the reports, and she appeared ready for discharge. Following her return from a one-day leave, the psychiatrist noted on 16 September that she "[w]as home for 1 day. Much more lively than before the disease, when she was calm and withdrawn. All three – she and her sisters – were childish and infantile for their age, according to the mother."[109] Stating that Buller was livelier than ever before meant that he had obtained information from the admission ritual, the only place it had been recorded that Buller had been withdrawn in her youth. He connected the information obtained from her mother during the admission interrogation with the current condition of the patient, in effect closing the circle with the suggestion that the amelioration of the patient's condition was due to therapy and the result of psychiatric knowledge. Now he constructed a new narrative: the patient was childish in behavior because all of her siblings had developed the same way.

It should be emphasized, however, that a subject becomes a subject only by entering the normativity of language; according to Butler, the "rules precede and orchestrate the very formation of the subject."[110] But entering into language has its price because the subject is differentiated against the "unspeakable"; the production of the "unspeakable" is the pre-condition for the subject formation. Along with Lacan, Butler argued that a "bar" exists in political life that marks the

---

109 PR, FMR, PN.
110 Butler, Judith, *Excitable Speech. A Politics of the Performative* (London: Routledge, 1997), 135.

point where the question of being able to speak is a condition of the subject's survival. Butler calls this "foreclosure" because it is prior to speech and is a reiterated effect of a structure. This means that the subject is performatively produced as a result of the "primary cut."[111] And again, this is the theoretical formulation for what happened in the interrogation. Nevertheless, this theoretical claim has wide-reaching consequences, because it implies that the somatic singularity that is not able to enter into language automatically drops back into the "unspeakable." If it becomes impossible to be differentiated against the unspeakable then one is excluded from the realm of the visible and reduced to a "bare life."[112] If this happens, the disciplinary power of the psychiatrist transforms into a sovereign power. In front of this power the subject is neither living nor is it really dead. According to Foucault, it is the sovereign who can decide if the subject has the right to live or if the subject must die. However, the right of the sovereign is only realized at the moment when the sovereign is about to kill the subject, the reason why Foucault called it the right of the sword. This is what happened with Buller in the years to come.[113]

The moralizing dimension

The nurses' descriptions of Buller's behaviour throughout her stay in the asylum contained a moral and gendered dimension. This was especially clear in the repeated descriptions of both Buller's inclination to run around in the nude and in her tendency to be incontinent. The nurses were disgusted by this behaviour and judged that Buller's behaviour was intentional and meant to provoke. Buller's aggressive behaviour and her unwillingness to participate in doing housework or needlework were also seen as unwomanly. The latter will be analyzed in more detail during the discussion of Buller's 1940 admission.

Between April and September of 1931, the notes described in detail how often and when Buller was incontinent, particularly in June when the accumulating instances of incontinence were perceived as intentional misbehaviour. For example, the nurse noted on 17 June that "patient wet bed, even though she was taken to the bathroom,"[114] and in the night of the same day "patient wet bed right after 10 o'clock, got up a lot and sat up in bed."[115] Although the first nurse emphasized that

---

111 Ibid., 138.
112 Giorgio Agamben, *Homo Sacer: Sovereign Power and Bare Life*, trans. D. Heller-Roazen (Stanford, California: Stanford University Press, 1998).
113 Michel Foucault, *Il faut défendre la société. Cours au College de France. 1976.* (France: Gallimard Seuil, 1997), 214.
114 PR, FMR, NN.
115 PR, FMR, NN.

Buller intentionally wet the bed, the second note linked her incontinence to her resistant behaviour in general. One day later the nurse reported that Buller had removed her clothes in the garden and "[tried to] run around naked. In the room, patient wet the bed + was very lively."[116] Similar instances took place on 22 June, 1 July, and again on 18 July, when Buller "wet the bed" and was "very noisy and disturbing."[117] The fact that the nurses spent so much time and energy in counting and describing the situations in which Buller wet herself (or her bed) seems to indicate that this behavior was particularly disgusting to them. According to the notes, they spent a great deal of time washing and dressing her again. Patients apparently had few forms of resistance besides their excrement – reports of sudden incontinence can be found in many of the records consulted. Foucault found that these actions had a particular relevance for psychiatry because against the sovereign power of madness, which used excrement as an ultimate form of resistance, the disciplinary power of psychiatry, represented by the nurses, intervened to restrain, undress, and clean the patient, thus producing the patient's body as "clean and true."[118] Once again, the functioning of disciplinary power was demonstrated through even these minor details.

Another aspect that was often described in detail in the nurses' notes, both in Buller's record and in others, was the aspect of nudity. Although other behaviors were described in broad terms such as "restless" or "lively," nudity was often described in every detail. That the nurses considered Buller's tendency to run around naked as shameless was especially clear in their final interrogation report. As the nurse revealed, she did not consider it "nice" for young girls to run around in the nude, placing a moral judgement on Buller's actions. The nurse linked Buller's undressing to other behaviours that they considered shameless, such as using coarse language, spitting, or beating other patients, giving the impression that she behaved more like an animal than a woman. On June 16, for example, Buller "took off her dress and undergarment and went jogging, very resistant to put on the dress again." In the afternoon of that same day, she "was very lively, jumped on benches and tables, ran around with her dress pulled up, tried to pick branches from bushes and spat all the time."[119] On 17 August, "[t]owards the evening, [she] became very lively, refused to put on a shirt. Used coarse language."[120] Again, on 25 August, she "was very lively, jumped around the garden, dug on the grass, denuded the upper part of her body to let the sun shine on it."[121]

---

116 PR, FMR, NN.
117 PR, FMR, NN.
118 Foucault, *Le pouvoir psychiatrique*, 27.
119 PR, FMR, NN.
120 PR, FMR, NN.
121 PR, FMR, NN.

This day-to-day information that became part of the official record is not understandable without knowledge of the improvised but "normal" rules and theories utilized by nurses and psychiatrists, which were still supplemented by "common sense or folk typifications."[122] In other words, the nurses and psychiatrists had to map their observations onto medically relevant categories to justify their interventions, but they also combined this information with a kind of tacit knowledge that they received. This is to say, their observations and notes were influenced by knowledge of the world that appeared to them to be "deceitfully natural" or embodied knowledge.[123]

That the nurses had an exact conception (embodied knowledge) about what it meant to behave as a "good woman" is illustrated in their notes. For example, most of the time, the nurses registered only how aggressive Buller had been, even against her own mother. For example, they noted on April 15 that Buller had been "very loud and agitated, hit and insulted her mother, tried to tear apart her mother's dress shouting: 'You are also such a mean woman!'"[124] During visiting hours on April 19, however, she "was at times lively, especially talking to a young aunt of hers. At times, lay down or bedded herself in her aunt's arms, had her eyes closed almost all the time."[125] Apart from the fact that both of these notes demonstrate the nurses' meticulous surveillance of Buller, the latter comment was the first time during her admission that a positive anecdote was recorded. "[Bedding] herself in her aunt's arms" was an obvious reaching out for human contact, a searching made even more positive, in the eyes of the nurses, because it was to a close family member. The nurses judged this kind of behaviour positively because it fit with their moral standpoint – their embodied normativity – whereas her aggressive behaviour was thought to be abnormal and judged accordingly. It is also noteworthy that after the positive description of Buller's conduct her name was used for the first time in the nurses' notes.

However, Buller's life of suffering did not come to an end in 1931; in contrast the described incidents were nothing less than the introduction of an intensification of war against Buller's insanity in the years to come. One year later, in 1932, Anna Maria Buller was once again admitted to the Friedrichsberg asylum and the following chapter continues with her second admission and Buller's slow but steady way into death at Hadamar.

---

122 Aaron V. Cicourel, "Police Practices and Official Records," in *Ethnomethodology: Selected Readings*, ed. Roy Turner (Middlesex, England: Penguin Education, 1975), 85–95.
123 Hannelore Bublitz, "Täuschend natürlich. Zur Dynamik gesellschaftlicher Automatismen, ihrer Ereignishaftigkeit und strukturbildenden Kraft," in *Automatismen*, eds. Hannelore Bublitz and others (München: Wilhelm Fink, 2010), 153–171.
124 PR, FMR, NN.
125 PR, FMR, NN.

Chapter 6: The Intensification of the War against the Madness: Buller's Subsequent Admissions (1932–1943)

The psychiatric dispositif

Nearly nine months after her discharge from Friedrichsberg, Anna Maria Buller was once again admitted to the asylum on 13 July 1932. The administrative record (*Personalakte*) from the Langenhorn asylum contains a small typewritten informal paper, obviously a carbon paper from an official report and signed by a physician. This small paper was very powerful because it enabled the compulsory hospitalization of Buller. Dated 13 July, it contained only one sentence: "Anna Buller must immediately be admitted to the asylum of Friedrichsberg because of a sudden emerging insanity. Signed Dr. Fuchs." Dr. Fuchs was the public medical officer who obviously did not possess any information about Buller's former admission to Friedrichsberg, because from his perspective her illness was sudden. Nonetheless, when she actually entered the asylum, his diagnosis was subsumed under Buller's previous biographical corpus and this new admission became nothing more than the continuation of her history that had begun in 1931. For someone not in possession of her record, Buller's insanity attack was a sudden irruption, but for someone who knew her history, it was a logical continuation of her diagnosis and an expected decline in her mental state. Once again the record preserves a biography that can at any time be reread and reused.

This second admission differed from the first one only because Buller was forcibly committed. The same administrative process took place as previously analyzed; an admission sheet was completed from which it is apparent that Buller arrived with a group transport. Similarly too, the nurses were the first persons in the asylum with whom Buller had contact; although she arrived in the evening she did not see any psychiatrist until the next day.

> 13–14.7: Night: New admission. Pat. came in the room singing loudly, very wild behaviour in bed, impossible to hold patient down. Pat. got an injection which slowly showed an effect. Pat. screamed "God, take me in I have sinned too seriously," said the

"Our Father," screamed again "the apple, it is the apple's fault, oh heaven how the women are bad, everywhere they want to be popular." Pat. alternately cried and laughed, pulls out hair. (A. Ei.)

Morning: Pat. was very noisy in the morning, raved about the room and screamed, kicked the nurse with her feet when touched, got an injection, calmed down a little, did not eat. At 9AM patient was out of bed again, walked around the room restlessly, knocked on doors, said "Open up, give me my stuff, I must leave. Yak, yak, you bitch you animal, I'd prefer a snake any time." Then patient reached for the nurse's hands and said: "I am sorry. I did you injustice," and cried. Shortly after patient became very restless, climbed up on the windowsill and screamed the "Our Father" out of the window for half an hour. With the help of a second nurse, she was taken down, knelt on the floor, folded her hands, "Lord help me we have not deserved the water." Patient screamed for one hour, another injection. Fell asleep half an hour later. Pat. tore apart her shirt, did not eat. (Tu.)

Afternoon: After 4 PM, pat. is very noisy, sings, prays and quotes the Bible. Throws herself on the floor cries heavily. Becomes even louder, runs through the room with clenched fists, climbs on the windowsill and screams towards the garden. Transferred to Hs. 8 (S. K. Lu.)[1]

At first glance these descriptions closely resemble Buller's first admission in 1931. According to the notes she was completely trapped in her madness – the nurses were describing a succession of insane events. This time, however, Buller's "misbehaviour" was punished or corrected directly by injections or by force. Although she had received an injection shortly after her first admission to Friedrichsberg, it was more of a "preventive" intervention. This time the injection was clearly related to the apparent impossibility of controlling her wild behaviour. The next morning, after she "raved about the room and screamed, kicked the nurse with her feet when touched, she received an injection that calmed [her] down a little bit"– again clearly a reaction to Buller's behaviour. Continuing to scream "for one hour" she received another in a short space of time, and both of these were also noted on the fever chart as Morphium-Scopolamine injections. Furthermore, Buller climbing on the windowsill and screaming out the window had also happened exactly in the same manner one year earlier, but this time the disciplinary power reacted with more insistence with the use of chemical means to calm her. Even more surprising was her transfer to another house after just one day in Friedrichsberg, where before it had taken a week before she was transferred. In 1931 it had seemed as if the time on the admission ward was used to underline her admission diagnosis, but this time the diagnosis was already verified because it was part of the record. Both the

---

1 Staatsarchiv Hansestadt Hamburg 352 – 8-7, Staatskrankenanstalt Langenhorn, Abl.1 – 1995, Krankenakte 28338 (hereafter Patient Record (PR), Friedrichsberg Medical Records Section (hereafter FMR), psychiatric notes (hereafter PN).

immediate employment of chemical restraint and the rapid transfer to House 8 (See Figure 25 and 26) demonstrate that this time there was no question of assessing Buller's behavior but rather she was treated as if she had never left the asylum.

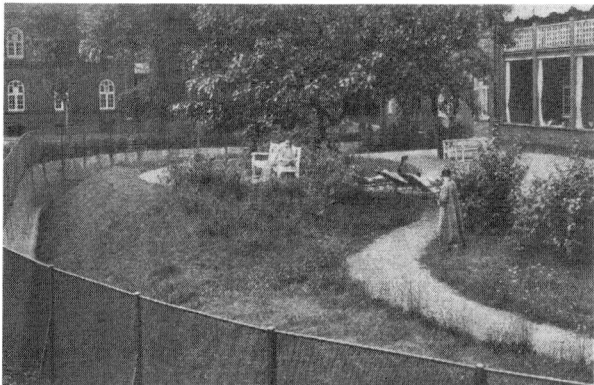

Figure 25: View on the secure House 8, c. 1928. Note the construction of the fences flush to the ground.[2]

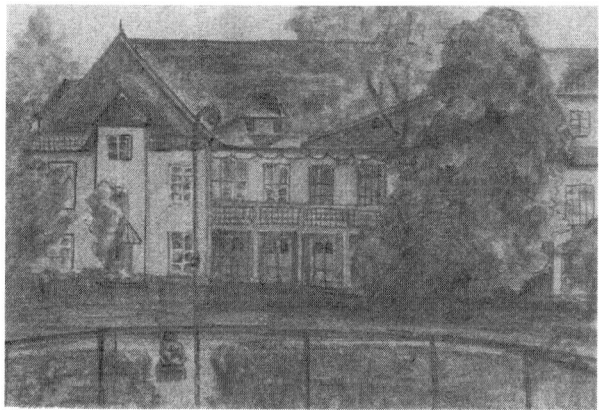

Figure 26: Anna Maria Buller's perspective from House 8. Patient record 28338.

As soon as Buller was admitted a nutrition plan was also laid out, even though any eating problems were not reported. The decision to observe Buller's nutri-

---

2 Wilhelm Weygandt, "Die Staatskrankenanstalt Friedrichsberg", in *Hygiene und soziale Hygiene in Hamburg. Zur neunzigsten Versammlung der deutschen Naturforscher und Ärzte in Hamburg im Jahre 1928* (Hamburg: Hartung Verlag, 1928), 186.

tional intake in detail was based on her "biographic corpus" already in place, underlining the fact that the record preserved a history of its own that was activated at the moment of reading. This is also highlighted in the psychiatrists' notes.

As had happened in 1931, the psychiatrist began by questioning Buller's mother.

> Mother: In the end, she was like before. Just complained about back pain all the time. Yesterday, she suddenly did all the laundry for the mother, packed up. She always wanted to bake. Washed the dishes in the morning as well as in the evening. She had read about natural healing methods. Voices, no, did talk to each other all afternoon. In the evening she suddenly jumped up, opened the window, screamed out of the window "Our Father in Heaven," etc. Could not be held back. Mother tried without success, father came for help. Pulled her back. People had already called the police in the street. Dr Fuchs came right away. She spat, scratched the wall paper etc.[3]

Equipped with this information the psychiatrist then began to question Buller, but this time he possessed not only the information provided by the mother but also that in the record. The interrogation began with a summary of the nurses' night and morning notes.

> 14.7.32 Leaves bed all the time, frightened, restless.

The course of the interrogation differed in some aspects from the one in 1931.

> Orientation. Where lived/ with parents, street: + [symbol for 'positive' which means Buller gave the right answer.]
> Date/ month/ year: +.
> Location here: +
> Why here? Don't know how all this happened.
> Sick?/No
> Agitated?/ Don't know
> Sang last night?/ Well, that's the way it is.
> In a good mood?/ No, not at all, quite the opposite. Most people laugh about the bible.
> Sect?/No.
> What do you mean about the bible/ They take it all so for real and then they don't understand it
> Divulgence of God's will/ Maybe. I preached aloud in front of the window
> Visions, figures?/No
> Heard voices, God's voice?/ No. Don't know
> Paranoia, remote influence (control), observation?/ No
> Workplace?/ 2 years apprenticeship with Arthmann Poolstr. Art Store Learned writing (print). Left because of illness
> What illness?/ Don't know. First Barmbek. hospital.

---

3 PR, FMR, PN.

When?/ 1930, no 1929. No 1931. Until October in hospital. Then quit job. I was here before. In the mental department. Once in house 16, then house 14.
Doctor?/ Dr. Badt.
Why were you here?/ Back then I always thought they wanted to poison me. Veronal that was.
Who: they?/ My Mother. But I didn't believe it later anymore I also always talked about that.
Any complaints now?/ Nothing.
Memory?/ not so good anymore before I could always remember everything
What did you do now, at home?/ I helped cleaning.
What done in spare time?/ went for walks a lot.
Girlfriend or boyfriend?/ Girlfriend yes. Boyfriend never. No interest in that.
Why supposedly sad?/ Avoids answer.
Why are you sighing?/ It is so horrible.
I don't know how it happened that I have a STD[sexually transmitted disease].[one of the previous questions of the Ref had been have you ever had an STD?
Why did you come to Barmbek before?/ I was too agitated, had such a feeling of being frightened.
Starting again: It is so horrible, this disease. Is it going to go away again?

This interrogation is very similar to the one at the end of Buller's hospitalization in 1931. The psychiatrist was not at all interested in Buller talking freely about herself but rather confined her to answering only the questions he asked. He is thus asking questions drawn from Buller's biography, using the information he already possessed from his earlier questioning of the mother and from the record. The questions were aimed to assess how far Buller was able to recognize herself in the biography contained in the record.

This interrogation highlights once again the mechanisms analyzed earlier. However, this interrogation is distinguished from the earlier one in 1931 because now there was little interest in obtaining information about the early signs of madness, the family history, or the hereditary aspects of Buller's madness. All this information was already part of the record and therefore it was unnecessary to ask again unless it was useful to see if Buller gave right answers. Over the course of the interrogation Buller began to actualize her symptoms through the psychiatrist's prodding about her "hallucinations." As discussed earlier, the purpose of the interrogation was to reduce the illness to its "main symptom," not only to make the subject acknowledge this absolute core but also to effectively actualize it during the interrogation. Actualization happened either by means of a patient's confession like "yes, I hear voices," because in that moment the symptoms would be fixed to the individual in the form of a first-person statement, or by the provocation of a crisis, for example, by triggering hallucinations. In the course of this interrogation, the psychiatrist reported that Buller

> [s]uddenly touches her body in a hectic gesture: "It is such a strange feeling. It is so horrible, it is not my fault. That is what people say that it is my fault that I'm sick." ....
> Interrupts herself again "It is so unfair, it is not my fault. Can't one do anything about it? What if I'm pregnant? (Touches her body again) It is such a strange feeling in my stomach. Something is moving as well. It feels so strange. My body (belly) became bigger too."
> .... Do you have the feeling of something strange (foreign) in your body?
> Very relieved. Yes, that is the feeling. If I have a STD, I am going to infect everybody, or?
> You get a rash, don't you?
> Do you have a STD?/ Yes, I don't know how it is. And with the child, awful. What can one do about it?
> Is that all only an idea of yours?/ No, I don't think so.
> Hypnosis, electrification, remote influence/ No
> Suddenly starts crying hard. It is so awful.(Calms down fast)
> Since when that feeling/ Only since today

Acknowledging their madness meant that patients also admitted that they were actually ill, in need of a physician and interment. These were the kinds of patients for whom psychiatric asylums were built.

The psychiatrist returned later to conduct a physical exam.

> A little later, when she is examined again she is very agitated and says to the nurse on duty, she could be in trouble. Leaves bed all the time, tends to go in beds of other patients. When addressed during the doctor's visit, she runs off negatively. Frightened, restless, can be settled. Quite strong Idées fixes
> (Believes to be pregnant, STD the latter less intense) absorbed by her idées fixes (that's why only superficial replies to questions from other areas);
> For example she recalls year of her time in Barmbek hospital. First as 1929, then 1930, then 1931.) Sometimes superficial- depressive, then childish, jolly and silly [läppisch]. No optical or acoustic hallucinations. No "remote control" feeling. Superficial "relationship ideas" ("That is what people say," s.above.)
> Physical examination: Is very agitated when to be examined again. Prays loudly the "Our Father" with her hands lifted. Says to the doctor, "you must work hard but not the devil's stuff with dance and art." Lifts her hand to hit the Ref [stands for referee], cannot be examined. Recognizes the doctor as such, though.[4]

The psychiatrist assessed Buller's inability to recall correctly the year of her admission to Barmbek as a sign of her being absorbed by her "idées fixes." However, the words that he used to describe Buller – "sometimes superficial – depressive, then childish, jolly and silly [läppisch]" – is suggestive of the dehumanizing language psychiatrists employed after the Nazis came to power and especially after the official start of "*Aktion T4* in 1939."[5] While the use of these

---

4 PR, FMR, PN.
5 Klaus Böhme and Uwe Lohalm, eds. *Wege in den Tod. Hamburgs Anstalt Langenhorn und die Euthanasie in der Zeit des Nationalsozialismus*, Forum Zeitgeschichte ed. Vol. 2. (Cloppen-

terms in records may have grown during the Nazi regime, in this record, the dehumanizing process through language was already in use long before. As well, Buller recognizing her doctor "as such" was similar to an earlier nursing observation from 1931, when Buller "called the doctor and nurses to come to her [and] called their names."[6] In many records, it seemed to be important to psychiatrists that patients recognized them, since to do so meant acknowledging their superiority within the hierarchical structure of the asylum.

The psychiatrist noted that Buller had been "very agitated although being in a good mood most of the time, which does change very much. Reacts strangely when talked to. Screams, sings in foreign, or made up language. Too noisy for House 10. House 8 downstairs." His remarks highlight once again how the space of the asylum was effectively divided between those considered curable or incurable, quiet or agitated, compliant or resistant, or between those able to work or and those who were not, or those who needed punishment and those who did not, or between those patients who had to be observed continuously and those who needed only minimal supervision or even none at all. Asylum space was segmented by these variables and not by patient diagnoses of illness.

Nonetheless, the most significant aspect of Buller's move to House 8 was her "disappearance" in the record. From 14 July 1932, the date of her transfer, the nurses interrupted their note taking for more than three months. Although there is the possibility that their notes have been lost, it is somewhat suspicious that they stopped precisely on the day Buller was transferred to House 8 and were only resumed on the day she was transferred to another house. Furthermore, the fever chart, the nutrition plan, other nursing forms, as well as Buller's drawings, are still part of the record, making it unlikely that only the nursing notes were lost. Simultaneously the psychiatrists wrote only rarely, and no longer did their notes contain any differentiated information, strengthening the thesis that the nurses' notes were indeed interrupted and not lost, since the psychiatrists depended on them to write their own.

As had happened in 1931, Buller received Digitalis, but now as daily medication. As well, this drug was often combined with Morphium-Scopolamine injections and given up to four times a day. She also received an enema every second day. The following few lines from the psychiatrists are all that remain of the next three months of Buller's life in Friedrichsberg's House 8.

15.7.32: Continuous bath
16.7.32: Continuous bath; injection; does not eat well
17.7.32: Sits outside the bathtub; cries; prays the "Our Father"
18.7.32: Pat. Eh. (Ingeborg) touched her on her neck to examine her;

burg: Ergebnisse Verlag, 1993), 43–49; Klaus Böhme, ed. *1893–1993 100 Jahre Allgemeines Krankenhaus Ochsenzoll.* (Hamburg: Sozialtherapiezentrum des AK Ochsenzoll, 1993).
6 PR FMR NN.

pat. defends herself. A few long scratch marks on her neck.
1.8.32: Continues to be agitated.
6.8.32: Later on a little calmer. Kept clothes on.
31.8.32: At times, out of bed.
12.9.32: Occasionally washes (the floor?); then naked again and continuous bathing
10.10.32: Still very agitated.[7]

The style of these notes suggests that they might have been written in one day. Although they will not be analyzed in any detail, some differences do exist to those from 1931. First of all, they were apparently not aimed at outlining Buller's behaviour in any detail; her condition had already been described exhaustively in both the psychiatric summary and the nursing notes. Buller seemed to be nothing more than an aggressive untouchable lunatic. With more of an emphasis on lab reports, they are more a depiction of how "treatment" was succeeding rather than a construction of her biography. And while the nurses' notes from 1931 revealed the different means used to "educate" Buller, this more recent writing on her is more a listing of the chemical and physical means employed to correct her behaviour. Against the lack of nursing notes, Buller disappeared in the record; House 8 appeared to be a kind of "collection tank" for asylum residue.

With the rendering of her invisibility, Buller lost her "status as a subject," or was de-subjectivized, both aspects of Foucault's "dispositif." In discourse theory, dispositif can be defined as the "material and ideational infrastructure" of discursive formations, comprising a "package of measures, systems of rules, and artefacts through which discourses are (re)produced and effects are constituted."[8] Foucault broadened this understanding, however, defining dispositif as a "heterogeneous ensemble" of differential elements like discourses, institutions, architectures, regulated decisions, laws, etc., – the spoken as well as the non-spoken. However, the dispositif is not simply the sum of these elements but rather it enables a focus on the network that can be established between these elements.[9] Discursive and non-discursive elements connect to strategies that are the effects of specific power relations and at any given historical moment the dispositif had as its major function the ability to respond to an emergency. The dispositif therefore has a dominant strategic function;[10] this is to say that the

---

7 PR FMR PN.
8 Reiner Keller, *Wissenssoziologische Diskursanalyse. Grundlegung eines Forschungsprogramms* (Wiesbaden: VS Verlag, 2005), 230.
9 Michel Foucault, "Le jeu de Michel Foucault," in *Dits et Ecrits*, eds. Michel Foucault and others, Vol. 3 (Paris: Gallimard, 1994), 299.
10 Ibid.

dispositif is a kind of operator in order to deal with and to resolve problematic social questions.

Gilles Deleuze pointed to the relationship between words and things and demonstrated Foucault's definition through describing dispositifs as composed of different lines. To analyze a dispositif means to follow these different lines or dimensions in order to form a kind of map. Deleuze says that the "the first dimension of a dispositif, or those which Foucault addresses first, are the curves of visibility and the curves of enunciation. Dispositifs are like the machines of Raymond Roussel as Foucault analyzes them: these are machines to make see and make speak."[11] According to this definition, each dispositif has its own "regime of light" (*régime de lumière*) a particular manner of how the light falls, "becomes blurred, and spreads throughout, distributing the visible and the invisible, giving rise to or making the object disappear; the object which would not exist without it."[12] A dispositif acts in part by determining what we can see and say in a certain historical configuration of forces.

This description of a dispositif helps to explain Buller's disappearance in House 8, since it has the ability to illuminate certain elements or somatic singularities, making some visible and others invisible. It is as if the light was turned away from Buller and she sank into the darkness of the asylum. As already analyzed in detail in the first part, the dispositif shed light on Buller as a mentally ill person– the result of Buller's subjectification process in the record. This is to say that even within the asylum something like a "zone of normality" existed, and the continuum between normality and abnormality was a decisive characteristic of disciplinary power. Within a disciplinary dispositif, every element occupies a defined place, for example, some elements give orders whereas others receive orders. As already discussed in some detail above, disciplinary systems classify, organize into a hierarchy, observe, etc. but the point at which these systems are in danger of breaking down is an encounter with somebody who cannot be classified, who escapes surveillance, and who cannot be integrated into the system. These are the residue – the irreducible, the non-classifiable, and the non-assimilable. Even within the asylum, which was already the collecting tank for the "residue of the residue," "zones of normality" were erected for those able to subordinate themselves and to acknowledge the reality of the asylum. However, those who did not acknowledge the asylum's reality and who were continuously resistant could disappear into the invisible zones of psychiatric practice.

---

11 Gilles Deleuze, "Qu'est-ce qu'un dispositif?" in *Michel Foucault philosophe. Rencontre internationale Paris, 9,10,11 Janvier 1988* (Paris: Éditions du Seuil, 1989), 186. [translation mine].
12 Ibid.

Apart from the "*régimes de lumière*" that exist in every dispositif, there is also a regime of enunciations (*régime des énoncés*). Deleuze emphasizd this perceptual but also onto-creative aspect, describing the curves of enunciation that he says are "not subjects and not objects, but the regimes which must be defined for the visible and the sayable, with their derivations, with their transformations, their mutations."[13]

Thirdly, a dispositif is composed of "lines of force," which intersect with the other two dimensions. This curve of power is produced in every relation between one point to another and it passes through the whole space of the dispositif. Invisible and nameless, it is closely intermingled with the other lines, however detachable.[14] In other words, this is the dimension of power that is linked to specific knowledge, as analyzed earlier in detail.

The "line of subjectification" of a dispositif defines a process or a production of subjects; subjectivity is enabled and produced within the constraints of the dispositif.[15] It is a kind of vanishing line. The Self is neither knowledge nor power. It is a process of individualization that acts on groups or persons and results from established power relations such as those in constituted knowledge: it is a kind of surplus value.[16]

According to Deleuze, the dispositif is a heterogeneous, dynamic and a moving configuration. He calls it a "multilinear ensemble" and emphasizes the dishomogeneity and disequilibrum of these lines. Philosopher Jeffrey Bussolini emphasized in an article that "similar to the language of forces that Foucault uses," Deleuze notes that "each line is broken, submitted to variations of direction, changing tack and slipping, submitted to derivations." He uses almost physical language to describe this interplay of forces and ongoing movement and interaction between the lines. Because of this, Deleuze maintains that in Foucault's thought "Knowledge, Power, Subjectivity have no contours once and for all, but are chains of variables which fight between themselves."[17]

The current analysis has tried to trace these different lines of the psychiatric dispositif. The first part concentrated on the aspect of the subjectification and the decisive role of the record in this process. Over the course of this analysis it has become clear that these processes can only be analyzed if one considers the power structure in psychiatric practice and its importance for the individualization process in the record. In the course of the analysis it was highlighted that the psychiatric dispositif not only constitutes subjects but is able to

---

13 Ibid.
14 Ibid., 186.
15 Ibid., 187.
16 Ibid.
17 Jeffrey Bussolini, "What is a Dispositive?" *Foucault Studies* 10 (2010): 100 http://rauli.cbs.dk/index.php/foucault-studies/article/viewFile/3120/3294 (accessed 10 January 2011).

"turn the light away from certain subjects" and thereby de-subjectify them, because they seem to disappear in the record. This process will be analyzed in more detail below.

However, the above quote from the psychiatrist's note demonstrates once more the war against madness and the importance of integrating the "line of force" in the analysis. As already mentioned above, the notes were a successive description of Buller's misbehaviour and the means used to correct it – namely continuous baths (see Figure 27) and injections as read on the fever chart. These interventions were used independently of an individual diagnosis because they were used in all cases of disobedient and resistant patients, as all the records used for this analysis highlight. Again, neither continuous baths nor Morphine-Scopolamine injections were guided by a nosography or kind of medical-theoretical knowledge, but rather were used as techniques of discipline. Bleuler explained the benefit of continuous baths in the therapy of "agitated" patients.

> [B]aths at nearly or full body temperate are an important tool for anxious patients and sometimes for those with depressions. Excitement is calmed down in the bath; a fatigue [that occurs] without decreasing the psychic or physical abilities lets the sick person become better accessible. But even in cases in which the bath is not so successful, the mild bath (35 to 36 degrees C) is an excellent place to stay for sick persons, because it keeps them continuously busy in a manner that is riskless for them, other people, and for surrounding objects.[18]

This description emphasizes that the continuous bath was part of a directive system, since interventions of this kind were awkward for patients and were utilized as a kind of punishment. As will be discussed later, Buller was "treated" with different "shock therapies" and injections, as a way to apply discipline in the asylum to the body. Although the role of morphine apparently was to calm the patient's nervous system, it was, in fact, quite simply the extension of the asylum regime, the regime of discipline, inside the patient's body; it was to ensure the calm that was prescribed within the asylum and to extend this calm into the patient's body.[19] Once again, the asylum psychiatrist did not act solely on medical knowledge but redefined psychiatric theory through actual practice.

---

18 Eugen Bleuler, *Lehrbuch der Psychiatrie* (Berlin: Springer, 1923), 165.
19 Michel Foucault, *Le pouvoir psychiatrique. Cours au collège de France. 1973–1974*, eds. François Ewald et al, Hautes études ed. (France: Seuil/Gallimard, 2003), 178.

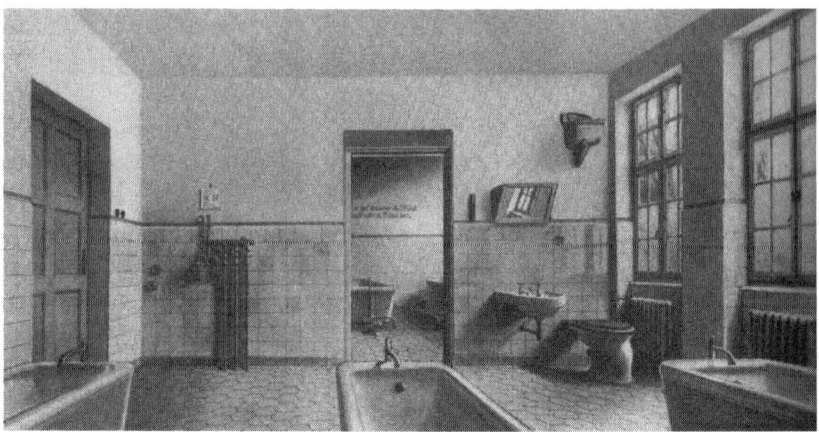

Figure 27: One of the halls for continuous baths in Friedrichsberg, House 30, c. 1928.[20]

On 3 November Buller was transferred back to House 10, and the nurses' notes resumed again. They were condensed, however, and like the psychiatrist's notes, were little more than a listing of disrobing behaviours on Buller's part and the nurses' subsequent interventions. Nevertheless, only the psychiatrists mention the regular application of continuous baths. From 27 November to 7 December 1932, the nurses' notes are as follows:

24.11: Pat. presents nothing special. (O.)
Night: Pat. insulted loudly, got an injection. (H.)
27.11: Pat. is lively, a lot out of the bed, is annoyed. (O.)
Night: Pat. insulted and sung loudly, got an injection. (H.)
28.11: Pat. was more quiet. (O.)
Night: Pat. became loud, got an injection, slept. (M.)
29.11: Pat. ran around loudly, shouting and insulting. (E.)
Afternoon: Pat. behaved more quietly during the afternoon. (O.)
30.11: Pat. is at times loud, talked very much, got an injection. (O.)
Night: Pat. slept. (E.).
2.12: Pat. behaved quietly. (O.)
Night: Pat. slept. (E.)
3.12: Pat. browsed in newspapers. (E.)
Night: Pat. slept with interruptions, became loud, got an injection. (E)
4.12: Pat. all the time out of bed. (E.).
Night: Pat. became lively, got an injection.(H.)
5.12: Pat. fairly quiet. (O.)
Night: Pat. slept. (E.)

---

20 Weygandt, *Die Staatskrankenanstalt Friedrichsberg*, 194.

6.12: Pat. quiet, good appetite. (O.)
Night: Pat. slept. (H.)[21]

Even though the nurses resumed their note taking it was obvious that these notes differ significantly in content from the notes taken in 1931. Buller's activities are effectively reduced in these notes to animal-like behaviour, with seemingly nothing "human" to be found in her conduct. The only course open to the nurses was to somehow to try to get her under control. Every time she exhibited signs of disobedience – even though her behaviour had not yet materialized and was still in a "space of possibility" or a virtual state in the process of becoming – they intervened with injections. The strategy – or therapy – appeared to be "working," as Buller became more and more helpless.

13.12: Pat. is often out of the bed, standing around in the room, does not know what she wants. Wets herself 2 times. (H.)
14.12: Pat. often out of the bed, goes to the toilet and didn't do anything, wets herself later. (H.)
14.–15.12: Pat. was disturbing, got an injection. (O)
15.12: Pat. often out of the bed and ran around helplessly in the
room. (H.).[22]

Buller had never before been described as "helpless" or not knowing what she wanted. In 1920, authors Alfred Hoche and Karl Binding called this the development of "an empty human shell." The nurses' notes break off on 17 December and, after almost six months at Friedrichsberg, Buller was transferred to Langenhorn on 20 January 1933. In her last months at Friedrichsberg, the psychiatrists reported on Buller

5.11.32: A lot of continuous baths.
30.11.32: Helps washing the floor in the morning.
25.12.32: Drawings. Continuous bath. Scopol. Morph. Inj. –
20.1.33: Transferred to Langenhorn – Agitation – Schizophrenia.
(Dr. K.)[23]

Buller's First Admission to the Asylum of Langenhorn

The fact that Buller was transferred to Langenhorn after being described as "helpless" and as somehow empty illustrated the function of the Langenhorn asylum. All the records used in this analysis were cases that had been transferred from Friedrichsberg to Langenhorn and in all of them the same pattern can be

---

21 PR FMR NN.
22 PR FMR NN.
23 PR FMR PN.

discerned. Most patients were transferred at the moment that they were perceived as chronic and hopeless. When no change in their condition was expected after a course of "therapy," they were transferred to Langenhorn.

The Friedrichsberg medical record was always sent with the patient to Langenhorn, making it available for analysis in this book. The medical records used in Langenhorn were similar to those in Friedrichsberg but also contained an administrative record. Although the psychiatrists used similar forms, the nurses' notes differed in many respects from Friedrichsberg. Whereas the nurse's notes in Friedrichsberg were written on printed forms entitled "nursing reports," the nurses' notes at Langenhorn were written on ordinary writing paper, which became an official document with simply the handwritten title of "nursing notes." Apart from the title and the first entry, which were written in ink (indicating that the head nurse entered the data), they were written in pencil. (See Figure 28) The first entry always contained descriptions of the admission situation and the routine measurements of weight, length, body temperature, etc. The material appearance of these sheets of paper imparted a kind of impermanency; the writing appeared scribbled down, and neither the nurses' initials nor any underlining can be found. Their construction also made it difficult for nurses to write long descriptions because every sheet of paper had to be laid out, which was a time-consuming procedure. Nevertheless, other forms for nursing notes existed, comparable to those used in Friedrichsberg, but these were found only in records of patients directly admitted to Langenhorn. For the patients transferred from Friedrichsberg, the nurses used only the formless sheets of papers above described, the reason being that their notes were taken only for the first couple of days in Langenhorn. In Buller's case, they appeared for the first ten days of her stay at the new asylum.

These notes served first to decide in which house a patient should be accommodated, and thus they were taken at very close intervals. Every shift had to make a report and note the exact time of entries. The reason is, I believe, that the nurses were discovering whether or not a patient was suicidal or aggressive, and thus the notes functioned as proof of observation. Both the nurses' notes and the medical record in general were a source for continual and retrospective inspection of the adequacy of the staff's action. The record consists, according to ethnographer Harold Garfinkel, "of procedures and consequences of clinical activities as a medico-legal enterprise."[24] It makes public "what really happened" for supervisors, colleagues, and officials. Every note that became part of the record constituted a social event and was made with the awareness that it might be used later.

---

24 Harold Garfinkel, "Good Organizational Reasons for 'Bad' Clinic Records," in *Studies in Ethnomethodology* (Cambridge: Polity Press, 2010): 198.

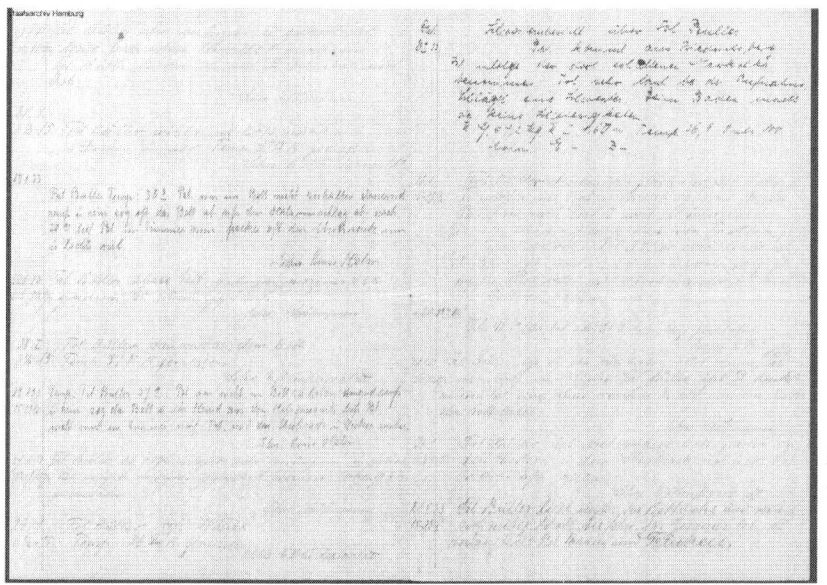

Figure 28: Nursing reports from Langenhorn. Patient record 28338.

As had happened in Friedrichsberg, the nurses admitted Buller; not until five days after her arrival was she examined by a psychiatrist. On admission, Buller was still sedated, although she soon woke up. "Pat. comes from Friedrichsberg. Due to the narcotic she received there, patient is dizzy. Is very noisy during admission. Hits a nurse. No problems when bathing her."[25] The subsequent report was a direct continuation of the notes in Friedrichsberg.

> 20.1. 33: 11:30: Miss Buller immediately soils her bed and the floor and demands food all the time. Pat. had to go to room 11 because she always carried around the bedding and was hit by Mrs. A. Miss Buller says she is 18 years old and used to work as a drawing instructor. Patient says a lot of confused things and cannot be kept in bed.

Here all the elements are assembled that will accompany Buller throughout her stay in Langenhorn. She is again depicted as being completely mad – and the "dirtiness" that came from her soiling the bed and floor reinforced a kind of animal-like behaviour. Room 11 was the isolation cell where Buller spent much of her time and from where the nurses reported on her over the next few days.

---

25 Staatsarchiv Hansestadt Hamburg 352 – 8-7, Staatskrankenanstalt Langenhorn, Abl.1 – 1995, Krankenakte 28338 (hereafter Patient Record (PR), Langenhorn Medical Records Section (hereafter LMR), nursing notes (hereafter NN).

8 – 11:30p.m..: Miss Buller slept after 8:30PM. (E.)

21.1.33: 11:30p.m.–7:30a.m.: Miss Buller sat on the floor without her shirt on and smeared urine. Miss Buller eats and drinks on her own. Pat. went to wash herself and stayed in bed afterwards covered with her duvet. (N. P)

6:30a.m.–3p.m.: Miss Buller spends a lot of time out of bed and keeps on packing and moving her bedding and the sac of straw, often demands food. (N. S)

3 – 11:30 p.m.: Miss Buller is under her bedding and keeps quiet. Whenever the nurse enters the room patient demands food and something to drink. Has a good appetite. Slept till 11:30PM. (N. S)

22.1.33: 11:30p.m.–7:30a.m.: Miss Buller spent a quiet night. In the morning patient was led away, but still wetted herself. Miss Buller ate and drank on her own but demanded more and more food. N. P.)

6:30a.m.–3p.m.: Miss Buller kept on packing her bedding and soiled her room. Patient often demands food. (N. W.)

23.1.33: [no time specification] Miss Buller is always out of bed and keeps packing and moving her bedding and the sack of straw back and forth. Patient is very restless and untidy. (N.H.)

24.1.33:11:30 p.m.–7:30 a.m.: Miss Buller had a quiet night. In the morning she smeared herself with urine. Miss Buller is very untidy. (N. P.)

6:30 a.m.–3 p.m.: Miss Buller had a continuous bath treatment, Pat. went calmly into the bathtub and at times spoke insultingly and vulgarly. While eating, pat. behaved very unmannerly and spat out a lot of food. (N. K.)

3 p.m.– 11:30 p.m.: Miss Buller took a continuous bath and at times sang very loudly, spat a lot. After 9:30PM patient was calm, fell asleep. (N.H.)

References to "packing her bedding" or to a "sack of straw" indicate the usual bedding in an isolation cell. Dr. Buder, a senior psychiatrist at the Winnetal asylum, described an isolation cell as a "bald room with solid, lockable, often doubled doors, with secured windows made of thick glass, without furniture, at the most a makeshift bed on the floor."[26] Buller's behaviour, however, was paradoxically enabled by her segregation. Sitting on the floor without her shirt on and smearing urine was only possible because she was not disturbing other patients or the ward routine, and thus the isolation room provoked the very behaviour against which psychiatric practice fought. As Buder noted as early as 1918, if accommodation in a "single" room continued over a longer period of time, certain drawbacks occurred.

> The sick persons neglect themselves [*verwahrlosen*] and run wild more and more; they become soiled, smear themselves and the single room with their excretions [*Ausleerungen*] throw their feces on the ceiling or at the faces of the physician and the nurses;

---

26 Dr. Buder, "Über das Alleinlegen," *Die Irrenpflege. Monatsschrift für Irren- und Krankenpflege* 22 (1918), 2.

they tear their shirt and bedsheets, waste the food...Finally one can try to lock the sick persons in the cell naked and to give them nothing more than goose grass so that they cannot tear anything.[27]

Nevertheless, Buder emphasized the necessity of isolation cells for particular patients to render them harmless – those with a "criminal disposition," who are "under the influence of hallucinations and misperceptions and therefore can become dangerous for their surroundings," or "the group of the degenerated [*Entartete*] or notorious criminals who try to plot against the physicians or the staff."[28] Despite recognizing the value of isolation cells, he nevertheless believed that continuous baths, even at night, reduced the need for them, thus acknowledging that both segregation and enforced bathing were more disciplinary than therapeutic. For Buller, the cell as well took the place of the morphine-scopolomine injections that she had endured in Friederichsberg. The war against her madness continued with all means possible.

The psychiatrist's admission examination was based on the record from Friedrichsberg and also on the nursing notes from Langenhorn.

> For the report of the physical examination, see Friedrichsberg report.
> There haven't been any changes. Patient gives the impression of a demented schizophrenia. Catatonic symptoms, suddenly impulsively agitated, tears apart sacks filled with straw, has to be isolated. Catatonic rigidity, negativism, very untidy must be cared for.
> 25.1.33. Always answers in a silly [*läppisch*], infantile way, suddenly a loud laughter, suddenly lashes out, tears down curtains.

Fully aware of her record from Friedrichsberg, the psychiatrist could assess Buller for any behavioural changes, illustrating how the documentary biography and patient history could "travel" wherever needed. In Latour's words, the record was an "immutable mobile," which accounts for its power.[29] It enabled readers to "travel" through past events in order to actualize them in the present. Based on the history in the record and the nurses' notes from Langenhorn, the psychiatrist labelled Buller with "demented schizophrenia," officially categorizing her as a hopeless case. The rest of the admission report was simply a listing of the diagnostic terms already used in the first admission diagnosis in 1931.

However, once at Langenhorn, Buller seemed to have disappeared into a zone of invisibility. Although she spent nearly three years there, the psychiatrist's notes fit into two pages and the nurses' notes broke off completely at the end of January. For example, the entire psychiatric record from 1934, in which Buller

---

27 Ibid., 7.
28 Ibid., 6.
29 Bruno Latour, "Visualisation and Cognition: Thinking with Eyes and Hands." *Knowledge and Society* no. 6 (1986): 1–40.

appeared to be little more than a bundle of instinctual reactions, consists of the following:

> 10.1.34: Always very noisy, completely unapproachable. Continuous bathing treatment necessary.
> 4.3.34: Very agitated. Does not speak. Tears apart clothes.
> 5.6.34: Agitated most of the time. Spits. Has to be isolated often.
> 3.9.34: Same condition. For a short period of time quiet and orderly, then agitated again.
> 5.12.34: Pulls her hair, tears apart clothes.

Bare Life

As philosopher Gorgio Agamben theorized, Buller was thus reduced to a "bare life."[30] Agamben's analysis is useful in thinking about the rendering of Buller as invisible. As has been repeatedly emphasized throughout this book, psychiatric practice must be analyzed as a form of disciplinary power that aimed to influence and transform patients at their very core. This practice was arranged around the absolute power of the psychiatrist and could only function because it was a hierarchical power distribution in which the nurses had a definite strategic function. One important characteristic of this anonymous power (anonymous because it is a form of power that intervenes without emotions and is independent from the person who has it) is that it subjectifies the somatic singularities in its reach by constructing a centralized identity and attaching this identity onto the somatic singularity. However, in Buller's records, as well as in all the other records that are part of this research, we find at some point the exact opposite operation, which appears to be a paradox: specific patients were suddenly de-subjectified and disappeared into a zone of indifference. In these zones it seemed as if anything was possible, because the little information that we have on these zones illuminates a severe intensification in the use of coercive means.

Using Agamben's theoretical approach, it becomes possible to conceptualize the "zones of invisibility" as zones of banishment or "zones of exception." In these zones the patient is held in a "relation of exception [which is an] extreme form of relation by which something is included solely through its exclusion."[31] This again is exactly what happened to Buller and other patients in Langenhorn because they were abandoned by psychiatric practice but simultaneously, it maintained control over their lives and even intensified corporeal interventions.

---

30 Giorgio Agamben, *State of Exception*, trans. Kevin Attel (Chicago: University of Chicago Press, 2005); Giorgio Agamben, *Homo Sacer: Sovereign Power and Bare Life*, trans. Daniel Heller-Roazen (Stanford, California: Stanford University Press, 1998), 15.
31 Agamben, *Homo Sacer: Sovereign Power and Bare Life*, 18.

Furthermore, as discussed earlier, from the end of the 1930s on, Langenhorn transferred thousands of patients to other asylums around Hamburg where most were killed. It seems as if in Langenhorn certain areas existed that could be described as "zones of exception" but these other asylums were nothing but "zones of exception." Barely any information exists about what was going on in these asylums.

Agamben believed that the present was a catastrophic endpoint of a political tradition that had its origins in Grecian antiquity and which culminated in the Nazi extermination camps. For him, sovereign power was at the core of biopolitics, and modern age does not mark a break with the occidental tradition (or the traditions in the Western world) but merely generalizes and radicalizes what was there originally.[32] The production of a biopolitical body was the original purpose of sovereign power, whose inclusion into the political community was only possible, if, at the same time, there were humans for whom the status of legal subjects was denied.

According to Agamben, it is necessary to examine the exception to understand the functioning of sovereign power, because it is in the exception that the nature of state authority will be revealed. Agamben explored the "states of exception," where a sovereign state declares a time or a place that the rule of law can be suspended in the name of self-defense or national security.[33] The sovereign decision over the exception is contained in the original juridical structure and principle in the Western World and is actualized through the declaration of the state of exception. The sovereign, who has the legal power to suspend the law, puts himself legally outside of the law; this is the paradox of sovereignty. The moment a sovereign declares the state of exception, he does so by declaring that there is no existence outside the law. "I, the sovereign, who is outside of the law, declare that there is nothing outside of the law."[34] The most prominent characteristic of the exception is that what is excluded in the exception is not, on account of being excluded, absolutely without relation to the rule.[35] What is excluded maintains itself in relation to the rule. "In this sense, the exception is truly, according to its etymological root, *taken outside (ex-capere)*, and not just excluded."[36] The exception is not brought into being by an interdiction, but rather by means of a suspension of the juridical order.

According to Agamben, the act of banishment is the purpose of exception,

---

32 Thomas Lemke, "Die politische Ökonomie des Lebens – Biopolitik und Rassismus bei Michel Foucault und Gorgio Agamben," http://www.thomaslemkeweBullerde/publikationen/Die%20politische%20%D6konomie%20des%20Lebens%20ll.pdf (accessed 12/07, 2007).
33 Paul Rabinow and Nikolas Rose, "Biopower Today," *BioSocieties*, no. 1 (2006): 195–217.
34 Agamben, *Homo Sacer: Sovereign Power and Bare Life*, 15.
35 Ibid., 17.
36 Ibid., 18 [original emphasis].

which means that the banished are abandoned by the law. The original power of the law contains within it the possibility of abandoning life but through this act, the law maintains control over life. Sovereignty then, becomes the point where it is impossible to distinguish between law and violence; it is the threshold where violence transforms into law and law transforms into violence, and at the same time, it is the threshold where nature and culture become indistinguishable. That is what characterizes sovereignty. For Agamben, the leading political differences since Grecian Antiquity have not been between friend and enemy, but the chasm between bare life (*zoé*) and the political existence (*bios*), or in other words, between natural existence and the legal entity of human. Agamben used the term *homo sacer*, a figure from Roman law, to describe a human who could be killed without punishment because he had been banished from the legal political community and reduced to the status of a physical existence. Whilst even a criminal had the right to reclaim certain legal protection, the *homo sacer* was completely without it. Once one was excluded from the legal community, one could not be prosecuted nor become a religious sacrifice. "Neither completely living nor completely recognized as dead, the *homo sacer* was a sort of "living dead," one who did not have even the elementary right to die like a human."[37] A structural analogy exists between the sovereign exception and the *homo sacer*, in that they are two symmetrical extremes within the logic of sovereignty. A sovereign has the power to declare any person a *homo sacer*, but compared to a *homo sacer*, everybody could be a sovereign.

The state of exception was not an invention of totalitarian governments but rather developed from a democratic-revolutionary tradition.[38] Every democratic constitution contains the possibility of declaring a state of exception.

Bare Life and the Camp

Concentration camps were one attempt to make this structure visible. For Agamben, the camp and not the prison was the original structure of the law or *nomos*. The laws of prison administration are created by the legal system, but the camp is ruled by martial law. It is not possible to analyze the camp in the same way that Foucault did with asylums and prisons because the camp is the absolute exception and completely different from either of them. The camp is the "hidden matrix" of political space.

Agamben defined the camp as a space without legal subjects (*bios*); in the

---

37 Lemke, "Die politische Ökonomie des Lebens – Biopolitik und Rassismus bei Michel Foucault und Gorgio Agamben," 18.
38 Agamben, *State of Exception*.

camp only "bare life" (*zoé*) existed. The paradigmatic figure of the camp is *der Muselmann*,[39] a being from whom humiliation, horror, and fear has taken away all consciousness and all personality as to make him absolutely apathetic and degraded.[40] These people were not only excluded from the political and social context they once belonged to, but they also no longer belonged to the world of humankind, not even to the precarious world of the camp detainees who had ceased to recognize them. They remained mute and absolutely alone.[41]

Critical Remarks

Before I continue to use some aspects of Agamben's theoretical consideration for my analysis, I want to highlight some pertinent limitations and misconceptions of his approach. Agamben's approach was criticized by a multitude of scholars.[42] One of the main critiques focused on his notion of continuity, which proceeded from a fundamental continuity of biopolitical mechanisms whose foundation he

---

39 Primo Levi, *Les naufragés et les rescapés. Quarante ans après Auschwitz* (France: Arcades Gallimard, 2008); Primo Levi, *Si c'est un homme* (France: Julliard, 2008); David Rousset, *Les Jours de notre mort* (Paris: Hachette Littératures, 2008); Rousset, *L'univers Concentrationnaire* (France: Les Éditions de minuit, 2005).
40 Agamben, *Homo Sacer: Sovereign Power and Bare Life*, 185.
41 Ibid.
42 Bernard Aspe and Muriel Combes, "Retour sur le camp comme paradigme biopolitique," *Multitudes* 1, no. 1 (2001): 29–44; Judith Butler, "Indefinite Detention," in *Precarious Life: The Powers of Mourning and Violence* (London, New York: Verso, 2004); Judith Butler and Gayatri Chakravorty Spivak, *Who Sings the Nation-State? Language, Politics, Belonging* (New York: Seagull Books, 2007); Rainer M. Kiesow, "Ius sacrum. Gorgio Agamben und das nackte Recht," http://magazines.documenta.de/attachment/000000778.pdf (accessed 12/27, 2007); Thomas Lemke, *Bio-Politics: An Advanced Introduction* (New York: New York University Press, 2011); Thomas Lemke, Susanne Krasmann and Ulrich Bröckling, "Gouvernementalität, Neoliberalismus und Selbsttechnologien. Eine Einleitung," in *Gouvernementalität der Gegenwart. Studien zur Ökonomisierung des Sozialen*, eds. Thomas Lemke, Susanne Krasmann and Ulrich Bröckling (Frankfurt a.M.: Suhrkamp, 2000), 7–40; Thomas Lemke, *Eine Kritik der politischen Vernunf. Foucaults Analyse der modernen Gouvernementalität* (Hamburg: Argument, 1997); Lemke, *Die politische Ökonomie des Lebens – Biopolitik und Rassismus bei Michel Foucault und Gorgio Agamben*, 18; Toni Negri, "Le monstre politique. Vie nue et puissance," *Multitudes* 3, no. 33 (2008): 37–52; Rabinow and Rose, *Biopower Today*, 195–217; Paul Rabinow, *French DNA* (Chicago: University of Chicago Press, 1999); Nikolas Rose, *The Politics of Life Itself: Biomedicine, Power, and Subjectivity in the Twenty-First Century* (USA: Princeton University Press, 2007); Katherina Zakravsky, "'Homo Sacer' and the Consequences: Two Remarks on Holocaust Commemoration and 'Bare Life' in Contemporary Art," http://magazines.documenta.de/attachment/000000778.pdf (accessed 12/27, 2007).; Katherina Zakravsky, "Zur Kritik des "nackten Lebens"," http://platform.factlink.net/fsDownload/Katherina%20Zakravsky-Enthuellungen.Zur%20Kritik%20des%20nackten%20Lebens.pdf?forumid=336&v=1&id=235172 (accessed 07/07, 2009).

found in the logic of sovereignty. He found a historical caesura in the modern era because "bare life," formerly on the margins of political existence, increasingly shifted into the center of the political domain. Biopolitics therefore followed thanatopolitical rationalities and strategies. These assumptions were criticized by philosophers Paul Rabinow and Nikolas Rose, among others, who argued that exceptional forms of biopower can lead, "especially in conditions of absolutist dictatorship and when combined with certain technical resources, to a murderous 'thanatopolitics' – a politics of death,"[43] but that biopower in contemporary states takes a different form. This critique coincides with my perspective developed in chapter 2, in which I tried to demonstrate that even under National Socialism, health policy cannot be reduced to thanatopolitic but must rather be analyzed as a complex interplay of different rationalities in order to govern the health of the population. Sociologist Thomas Lemke contended that Agamben's notion of continuity between a "biopolitics situated in antiquity and the present is unconvincing" because the term "life" as it is used "in antiquity and modernity has little but a name in common, and this is so because "life" is an especially modern concept."[44] Again, this is an important aspect discussed in chapter 2 as well. Only with the emergence of modern biology did the idea appear that life follows its own autonomous laws and is an area of study in its own right. The idea of hereditary dangers for a population, for example, was based on theories about degeneration and Darwin's theory of evolution. Seen from this perspective, biopolitcs is a historical phenomenon that cannot be separated from the development of modern states, the emergence of the humanities, and capitalist relations of production. "Without the bio-political project's necessary placement within a historical-social context, "bare life" becomes an abstraction whose complex conditions of emergence must remain as obscure as its political implications."[45]

However, I want to concentrate my critical remarks on two other aspects that are more closely related to the results of my analysis. Agamben conceives the "camp" as a line that divides bare life (*zoé*) and political existence (*bios*). The "camp" appears as kind of border or "as a kind of line without extension or dimension that reduces the question to an either-or."[46] Therefore, he is drawing on a distinction pointed out by Hannah Arendt in *The Human Condition*. Arendt's notion of a *bios* that is not yet a *bios politikon* is based on Aristotle's definition of the quality that sets humankind off from other living beings. This

---

43 Rabinow and Rose, *Biopower Today*, 195; Lemke, *Bio-Politics: An Advanced Introduction*, 5; Lemke, "Die politische Ökonomie des Lebens – Biopolitik und Rassismus bei Michel Foucault und Gorgio Agamben," 18.
44 Lemke, *Bio-Politics: An Advanced Introduction*, 62.
45 Ibid., 63.
46 Ibid., 59.

quality is found "in their moral and legal community, in that supplement of political life, and is intimately linked to language, which elevates humans above the level of animal existence."[47] Queer theorist and philosopher Judith Butler emphasized that many critical questions must be posed, "but one surely has to do with how a population is cast out of the polis and into bare life, conceived as unprotected exposure to state violence. Can life ever be considered "bare"? And has not life been already entered into the political field in ways that are clearly irreversible?"[48]

These questions touch the core of my analysis, because what I tried to demonstrate throughout chapters 3 to 5 was how Anna Maria Buller was subjectified by the disciplinary power of psychiatric practice and how the different technologies constructed her identity. My analysis so far has emphasized how gradations and valuations within the "bare life" of psychiatric patients emerged. Psychiatric practice arranges the subjects produced by psychiatry according to a norm and qualifies life as "higher" or "lower," as "descending" or "ascending." This was the reason why interrogations were carried out regularly and this was the main objective in taking notes. According to this kind of analysis, discipline and training were crucial aspects of psychiatric practice, and psychiatry as such was meant to normalize and standardize life. All these aspects are not central to Agamben's thinking, instead, death as the establishment and materialization of a boundary is.

The effort to establish an exclusionary logic depends upon the depoliticization of life. Butler asserted further that Agamben's recourse to Arendt's *Human Condition*

> is all the more curious here since it relies on Aristotle's notions of biology, suggesting not only that contemporary science is irrelevant to the matter of thinking in the sphere of the political but incapacitating any vocabulary that might explicitly address all that falls under the rubric of the politics of life.[49]

This aspect is also in the center of philosopher Toni Negri, whose critique emphasized that it is necessary to differentiate between different forms of "bare life." The "bare life" of the inmates in the concentration camps is different to the bare life of those who are fighting against their own exclusion. To confound these different forms of "bare life" is a mystification.[50]

The second problem with Agamben's analysis consists in its concentration on the state and centralized forms of regulations. In the course of my analysis I criticized in chapter 2 approaches that tried to reduce the killings of sick persons

---

47 Rabinow, *French DNA*, 15.
48 Butler and Spivak, *Who Sings the Nation-State?*, 37.
49 Ibid., 38.
50 Negri, "Le monstre politique," 39.

to the strategy of a central state apparatus. As Rabinow and Rose emphasized, biopolitics is based on "one or more truth discourses about the 'vital' character of living human beings, and an array of authorities considered competent to speak that truth."[51] In my description of the history of the Langenhorn asylum I emphasized the struggle of the psychiatrists and medical directors to gain absolute control. The medical director's claim for power rested in his position as head of the asylum. From 1941 on psychiatrists and nurses decided, independently from state apparatuses, who they considered as "life unworthy of living." The killings carried out before and after the Nazi regime were never centrally planned or carried out by state apparatuses.

Another problem is with Agamben's notion of *"bios"* of a person, because it is only linked to its political status. By "political" here is meant membership in the ranks of citizenship. Butler rightly asked if this move does not "precisely place an unacceptable juridical restriction on the political?" and answers her question as follows:

> After all, if to be "bare life" is to be exposed to power, then power is still on the outside of that life, however brutally it imposes itself, and life is metaphysically still secured from the domain of the political. We can argue that the very problem is that life has become separated from the political (i.e. conditions of citizenship), but that formulation presumes that politics and life join only and always on the question of citizenship and, so, restricts the entire domain of bio-power in which questions of life and death are determined by other means. But the most important point here is that we understand the jettisoned life, the one both expelled and contained, as saturated with power precisely at the moment in which it is deprived of citizenship. To describe this doubled sense of the "state" through recourse to a notion of "power" that includes and exceeds the matter of the rights of citizens, and to see how state power instrumentalizes the criteria of citizenship to produce and paralyze a population in its dispossession.[52]

However, Agamben suggested that the state of exception is not only the origin of politics but also its very purpose and definition. Therefore, he "reduces politics to the production of *homines sacri*, which must be regarded as unproductive, for "bare life" is created only to be oppressed and killed." Agamben dismisses the fact that biopolitic cannot be reduced to the simple extermination of "bare life." Psychiatric practice and the killings of sick persons were aimed to improve the health of the population and to improve its hereditary quality. Thomas Lemke called this the "bioeconomic imperative" and emphasized that biopolitics is "essentially a political economy of life."[53]

Nevertheless, I find Agamben's distinction *bios/zoé* illuminating without

---

51 Rabinow and Rose, "Biopower Today," 197.
52 Butler and Spivak, *Who Sings the Nation-State?* 39–40.
53 Lemke, *Bio-Politics: An Advanced Introduction*, 60.

adopting his "diagnosis of Western history as a growing biopolitical nightmare."[54] His description of the camp seems especially helpful to better understand how zones of exception were erected and maintained within psychiatric asylums. Furthermore, Agamben's approach enables one to understand the peculiar symbiosis between the psychiatrist, supported by the nurse, and the jurist.

The Psychiatric Asylum as a Camp

As mentioned above, the *Muselmann* in the concentration camps was excluded from the world of humankind and even the camp detainees had ceased to recognize him/her – the *Muselmann* was absolutely alone. During 1932, Anna Maria Buller, too, was increasingly described as helpless and disoriented, a condition that became more pronounced in her later admissions from 1940 to1943 and which eventually led to her killing. Dorothea Buck, a survivor of the psychiatric system, described her experience of exclusion.

> In 1936, 71 years ago – at the age of just 19, I went through the most inhuman experience of my life in a psychiatric institution, against which even being buried alive during the 2nd World War paled into insignificance. I experienced the psychiatric system as being so inhuman, because nobody spoke with us. A person cannot be more devalued than to be considered unworthy or incapable of conversation.[55]

As Agamben stated, what is excluded in the camp, and, according to my perspective, in the psychiatric hospital, is included through its own exclusion. Both the camp and the psychiatric hospital were "a hybrid of law and fact in which the two terms have become indistinguishable."[56] Both the camp and the psychiatric hospital were characterized by the fact that their inhabitants "were stripped of every political status and wholly reduced to bare life."[57] The camp and the hospital became biopolitical spaces, "in which power confront[ed] nothing but pure life, without any mediation."[58]

However, Agamben notes that the question of "how crimes of such an atrocity could be committed against human beings" is often posed.[59] This question is the

---

54 Rabinow, *French DNA*, 16.
55 Dorothea Buck, "70 Years of Coercion in German Psychiatric Institutions, Experienced and Witnessed," http://www.bpe-online.de/1/buck-wpa-2007-e.pdf (accessed 04/10, 2011).
56 Agamben, *Homo Sacer: Sovereign Power and Bare Life*, 170.
57 Ibid., 171.
58 Ibid.
59 Ibid.

starting point of many historical studies in nursing as well.[60] Nevertheless, I concur with Agamben that it would be

> more useful to investigate carefully the juridical procedures and deployments of power by which human beings could be so completely deprived of their rights and prerogatives that no act committed against them could appear any longer as crime. (At this point, in fact, everything had truly become possible).[61]

In the case of the killing of patients during the Nazi regime, the sovereign established a symbiosis not only with the jurist but also with the physician, supported by the nurse. Alfred Hoche, a specialist in criminal law, and Karl Binding, a physician specializing in ethics, attempted to legitimate in 1920 the extermination of "life unworthy life." Binding's concept of "life unworthy life" and "mercy death" reappeared in the Nazi regime. Masked as a humanitarian problem – against the background of a new biopolitical determination of the National Socialist state – the sovereign power practiced the power of decision over "bare life." "Life unworthy life" was not an ethical but rather a political term because it allowed for the possibility of a person being able to detach the bare life (*zoé*) from *bios* in another person.

The National Socialist government never adopted a law regarding its "euthanasia" program; it was simply based on a secret decree that never gained legal force. All physicians and nurses involved in this program were thus in a doubtful judicial position; it was a state of exception. The sovereign decision over "bare life" shifted away from political motivation and entered an ambivalent terrain wherein the sovereign and the physician, along with the nurse, began changing places. The precondition for these killings was that all murdered persons were judged as already having been excluded from the political community. They

---

60 Susan Benedict, Arthur Caplan and Traute Lafrenz Page, "Duty and 'Euthanasia': The Nurses of Meseritz-Obrawalde," *Nursing Ethics* 14, no. 6 (November 2007): 781–794; Benedict and Georges, *Nurses and the Sterilization Experiments of Auschwitz: A Postmodernist Perspective*, 277–288; Susan Benedict, "Killing while Caring: The Nurses of Hadamar," *Issues in Mental Health Nursing* 24, no. 1 (Jan-Feb 2003): 59–79; Susan Benedict, "The Nadir of Nursing: Nurse-Perpetrators of the Ravensbrück Concentration Camp." *Nursing History Review*, 11 (2003): 129–146.; Susan Benedict and Jochen Kuhla. "Nurses' Participation in the Euthanasia Programs of Nazi Germany." *Western Journal of Nursing Research*, 21, no. 2 (Apr, 1999): 246–263.; Maria Berghs, Bernadette Dierckx de Casterlé and Chris Gastmans, "Practices of Responsibility and Nurses during the Euthanasia Programs of Nazi Germany: A Discussion Paper," *International Journal of Nursing Studies* 44, no. 5 (July 2007): 845–854.; Barbara Brush, "Nursing Care and Context in Theresienstadt." *Western Journal of Nursing Research* 26, no. 8 (Dec, 2004): 860–871.; Bronwyn Rebekah McFarland-Icke, *Nurses in Nazi Germany : Moral Choice in History*; Hilde Steppe, "Nursing in the Third Reich", *History of Nursing Society Journal* 3, no. 4 (1991): 21–37.; Hilde Steppe, "Nursing in Nazi Germany." *Western Journal of Nursing Research* 14, no. 6 (1992): 744.; Hilde Steppe, *Krankenpflege im Nationalsozialismus* (Frankfurt a.M.: Mabuse, 2001).
61 Agamben, *Homo Sacer: Sovereign Power and Bare Life*, 171.

were living in a borderland between life and death, between interior and exterior, where they were nothing more than bare life. They were reduced to *homines sacri* and in this "no man's land," the physician, nurse, and scientist were acting where, in former times, only the sovereign could act.

As already mentioned over the course of the analysis, the nurses carried out all interventions. Thus, they controlled these zones of exception and, therefore, it can be concluded that they claimed sovereignty. As the sovereign stands above the law, so is bare life outside the scope of the law, but at the same time, a part of it. In psychiatric practice, nurses and psychiatrists had control over life and death of their patients, even to the point of deciding who could be recognized as human.

This, then, was the actual mechanism that enabled the killing of patients, and it was a mechanism that existed as an integral part of psychiatric practice and not as an invention of the Nazi regime. This transformation of the psychiatrist from a representative of disciplinary power into a sovereign was central to the very core of psychiatric practice. Psychiatry could not exist without it and it is the reason why the killings did not come to a stop after WWII. In Germany, psychiatrists and nurses did actually assassinate sick persons but in many ways, these persons were dead long before. Foucault emphasized that killing someone is not simply the physical extermination of the other but that there are also indirect forms of murder: "the fact of exposing someone to death, increasing the risk of death for some people, or, quite simply, political death, expulsion, rejection, and so on."[62]

Buller's forced sterilization or the psychiatrist becomes a judge

This changing of places between the jurist and the ambiguous figure of the sovereign psychiatrist is particularly clear in the decision to sterilize Buller in 1935. By 22 October 1935, Buller had been in Langerhorn nearly three years. At this time, the psychiatrist noted that the "Sterilization report written. Continuing sudden alternation between calm and agitated phases."[63]

This report, which had a strong impact on Buller's future, was a consequence of the "Law for the Prevention of Genetically Diseased Offspring."

(1) Any person suffering from a hereditary disease may be rendered incapable of procreation by means of a surgical operation (sterilization), if the experience of medical science shows that it is highly probable that his descendants would suffer from

---

62 Foucault, *Society must be Defended*, 256.
63 Staatsarchiv Hansestadt Hamburg 352-8-7, Staatskrankenanstalt Langenhorn, Abl.1-1995, Krankenakte 28338 (hereafter Patient Record (PR), Langenhorn Administrative Records Section (hereafter LAR).

some serious physical or mental hereditary defect.
(2) For the purposes of this law, any person will be considered as hereditarily diseased who is suffering from any one of the following diseases:

(1) Congenital Mental Deficiency
(2) Schizophrenia
(3) Manic-Depressive Insanity
(4) Hereditary Epilepsy
(5) Hereditary Chorea (Huntington's)
(6) Hereditary Blindness
(7) Hereditary Deafness
(8) Any severe hereditary deformity

(3) Any person suffering from severe alcoholism may be also rendered incapable of procreation.

The law was enacted on 14 July 1933 and in force on January 1934. The decision to sterilize was assigned to the "Genetic Health Courts," consisting of a judge, a medical officer, and a medical practitioner, "which shall decide at its own discretion after considering the results of the whole proceedings and the evidence tendered." The decision of the court could be appealed to a "Higher Genetic Health Court," but if the appeal failed, the sterilization was to be carried out with the law specifying that the "use of force [was] permissible."[64] In reality, physicians made decisions on their own to sterilize patients, with the judge involved only to make sure that legal obligations were respected in the process. These Genetic Health Courts held their meetings in asylums.[65]

The note in Buller's record from 22 October was only the peak of a process that had begun in April 1934. The administrative record contains a typewritten copy of a remarkable letter that was obviously sent to court.

Langenhorn, 9.4.1934
The sterilization of the patient Anna Maria Buller residing with her parents in...- Hamburg is necessary, according to the law for the prevention of hereditarily diseased offspring. In order to carry out this surgical operation the consent of a legal representative would be necessary. The mother who could assume the trusteeship and could

---

[64] *The Law for the Prevention Hereditarily Diseased Offspring*, (1935):, http://www.facinghistorycampus.org/campus/rm.nsf/0/81C67 A69F8081 A5885257037005E9C6 A (accessed 07 January 2009).

[65] During my archival research I found a file entitled "Sterilizations. Individual cases. 1934–1940, 1941" that contains a large number of lists with the dates of the court sessions in Langenhorn. From this list one can see that the sessions were limited to fifteen minutes per case. This file contains also a large number of transport lists, because Langenhorn was designated to issue sterilization reports for persons who were not hospitalized. These persons were required to be admitted for a period of six weeks in order to be observed by the psychiatrist. Staatsarchiv Hansestadt Hamburg 352–8-7 Staatskrankenanstalt Langenhorn 134, [SArHH 352–8-7 Langenh 134], "Sterilisationen. Einzelfälle. 1934–1940, 1941."

apply for the sterilization refuses to do so. This is the reason why an official trustee is requested. Signed: Dr. H., department physician

As this letter demonstrates, the psychiatrist knew that Buller would be sterilized a year and a half before the sterilization report was officially submitted. The whole process was nothing more than a formality, since the decision had already been made by the psychiatrist. The mother's resistance was simply a problem to be solved by the appointment of an official trustee, although who this was could not be determined from the file. Moreover, this letter was written just three months after the law took effect.

The administrative file also contained a letter written by her father, in which he stated that the condition of his daughter had improved and that he planned to take her home. He requested Langenhorn to transfer her back to Friedrichsberg, emphasizing that he paid 30 Marks every months and therefore thought that he had the right to claim this service. It is somewhat surprising, however, that her father judged Buller's illness improved since the few notes in her file suggest only that her condition continued to be disastrous.

Buller's administrative record contains two handwritten drafts as well as a typewritten carbon copy of the final sterilization report, which is identical with the second handwritten draft. The medical files typically contain just the typewritten copy of the report that was submitted to the court, but in Buller's case, the two drafts imply that the report was the result of much work – work that was normally not visible in the final version. The two drafts differ in some aspects and highlight what Latour called "thinking with eyes and hands," suggesting that "hard facts" do not solely exist in theory but rather were also crafted through the act of writing. As the different drafts showed, how Buller was perceived in the final version of the sterilization report was not something that was just observed but had to be constructed carefully. Latour called this aspect the necessary "craftsmanship" that one had to master to convince others. It was a "strategy of deflation" because written notes and diagrams conflated complex data into a two-dimensional image on paper. Writing and drawing were "both material and mundane, since they [were] so practical, so modest, so pervasive, so close to hands and eyes that they [escaped] attention."[66] In order to be convincing, the document had to be constructed in such a manner that it could "muster on the spot the largest number of well aligned and faithful allies," which is to say, it had to align all the "hard facts" from nurses' and psychiatrists' notes, former examination reports, laboratory results, photography, etc. that that had the potential to intervene in the decision-making. These inscriptions were thus not

---

66 Latour, "Visualisation and Cognition," 3; Bruno Latour, "The Powers of Association," in *Power, Action, and Belief: A New Sociology of Knowledge*, ed. John Law, Sociological Review Monograph 32 ed. (London: Routledge and Kegan Paul, 1986), 45–70.

only visualizations but also mobilizations, because they were able to convince those who could not "observe" Buller themselves. Latour described this necessity as having "to invent objects which have the properties of being mobile but also immutable, presentable, readable and combinable with one another."[67] All of these factors applied to the sterilization report and the record, since they were both mobile – they were sent to the court, exchanged among different asylums, and could be read everywhere – with its text remaining stable independent of its readers.

The court requested that the medical record stand as evidence. At the same time, the sterilization report "governed from a distance" because of its construction as a questionnaire that asked only for predetermined information. This document not only determined how Buller would be defined but it also standardized the terms that could be employed in order to complete the questionnaire, even if the same categories were used for years.

The six-page sterilization questionnaire resembled the construction of the admission ritual. The first page collected demographic information while the second was concerned with the patient's family history. In the first draft on Buller, the mother supplied all the information, including the fact that the maternal grandfather had used alcohol well into his old age – a fact that had never before been revealed in any of Buller's previous admission records. It was deleted in the final draft of the sterilization report, likely because it could not be used as evidence for a hereditary load. However, its appearance suggests that the psychiatrist was searching for any indication that could be used as evidence of Buller's "hereditary dangerousness." The third page of the questionnaire recorded the patient's own history. In the first draft again, it was noted that as a child, Buller had often moaned with abdominal pain although no cause could be found – something that had been only marginally noted in her first admission ritual in 1931. The ability of the record to conserve information over the years to be used in different contexts was also clear when the psychiatrist repeated the symptoms noted on her first admission to Friedrichsberg; he wrote that she had been stuporous, aggressive, and negativistic, and refused food necessitating tube feeding. The fourth and fifth pages of the questionnaire were devoted to the physical and mental condition of the patient. They demonstrate how years of confinement in the asylum could be compressed into a short, simple summary. Buller's mental state was described as "stump," and the psychiatrist wrote that she showed "severe states of excitation" and undertook violent attacks against both the nurses and her relatives. He also noted that she threw food and smeared her feces – although he reported that she also periodically lapsed into a catatonic state. According to her medical file, however, Buller had only attacked her

---

67 Bruno Latour, "Visualisation and Cognition," 6.

mother in 1931, and only once in 1933 did the nurses report that she had attacked them and this information was never recorded in the psychiatrist's report. Similarly, they reported only once that she had thrown her dishes and food. In this draft, the psychiatrist was obviously constructing a new narrative from a new combination of elements derived from the medical file. The sixth page of the questionnaire asked for her diagnosis, which was given as "schizophrenia," and the psychiatrist justified the request for sterilization on her "occasional catatonic states." He also warned that her "severe annoyance" might make surgery and her first treatment difficult.

The second draft and the subsequent final version differ in some significant ways from the first. This time the psychiatrist who completed the questionnaire had meticulously studied the record. For example, a sister, who had been mentioned only once in the entire record – at Buller's first admission in 1931 – replaced the grandfather. And where the first draft mentioned Buller's suffering from abdominal pain in her childhood, the final version referred to her 1931 admission when the admitting psychiatrist reported her broken nose. Again, although this information appeared only once in the record, it is noteworthy that it reappeared more than four years later in the sterilization report. The final version also recorded more details from 1931, such as her school career and her lack of interest in men. Perhaps more importantly, the psychiatrist avoided the previous list of medical terms for a larger but vivid explanation of her symptoms, perhaps in order to allow a non-medical person like the judge to better understand the situation. He argued that "the diagnosis [resulted] from a progression. In the past [she exhibited] delusional ideas (now [she] barely talks)." He went on to write that

> Buller was admitted to the AK [general hospital] Barmbek from 10.2.–18.2.31 and then transferred to Friedrichsberg due to agitations and was diagnosed with schizophrenia. In Barmbek she was periodically very agitated, was in a state of anxiousness, looked around wide-eyed, very afraid. Most of the time she did not talk and refused food. During the admission in Friedrichsberg she was noisy and lashed out. Nighttime very restless, periodically agitated. [She believed that] she should be decapitated because she did wrong. Periodically stuporous. Lay lethargic in the bed. Refused nutrition. During the last admission to Friedrichberg anxious, restless, on the run from her bed. Delusional ideas (thought she was pregnant, suffering from venereal diseases).
> Miss Buller is <u>not</u> legally competent.
> Signed Dr. H (department physician)

Once again Buller's medical history was re-written, since all the elements contained in this summary were derived from psychiatrists' notes from Friedrichsberg over a four-year period. Surprisingly, the psychiatrist never mentioned Langenhorn despite Buller spending nearly three years in the asylum, the greater part of her hospital career. It is even more astonishing since Langenhorn "specialized" in observing patients for sterilization reports. I think this detail can only be explained because no traces of Buller existed in Langenhorn; nothing had been reported on her because she was living in the "zone of exception" and was reduced to a kind of living death.

Buller's medical file assumed another far-reaching role in the sterilization process. The administrative record contains letters addressed from the court to Buller, strongly suggesting that they never made it to her house in the asylum for her to read. Every letter was also signed only by the medical director and not by her, as would have been the prescribed procedure.

The court decision and a document entitled "decline of legal means" are the most important documents. On 25 November 1935 the "Genetic Health Court" decided that Buller must be sterilized. Psychiatrists had examined her and applied for her sterilization, and now physicians were again acting as judges in determining the accuracy of her examination and the application for sterilization. The asylum had transformed into a court and the patient became the accused. According to the written court decision, Buller was not represented by a lawyer, and since the final decision was contained in her file, she never saw it. Buller also received the "decline of legal means," which informed her that she had a right to object to the decision. Glued over the original text, which told her that she had one month to reply in writing to the court registry, was a modified version that gave her only 14 days. The letter was sealed and signed and therefore endowed with legal power. Another letter for her arrived four days later from the gynaecological hospital Finkenau, informing her that her surgery would take place on the exact day the "new" objection period ended and that the police had the power to enforce this order if need be. This virtual procedure illustrates dramatically what is meant by "the judge and the physician changing places."

A document claiming that Buller had been properly informed about the nature of her sterilization surgery was also found in her file. Buller had allegedly received a handout on her planned sterilization, although this "informed consent" was signed by the same psychiatrist who had written the sterilization report one day before the report had been submitted and one month before the court decision. Buller's sterilization had been decided long before her case went through the legal process.

Soon after the surgery, Buller was discharged from hospital on the insistence of her mother. In a letter dated 16 December 1934, three days after Buller's surgery, her mother wrote:

> In possession of your letter from the 12th of this month I was informed that my daughter Anna was transferred to the gynecological clinic Finkenau in order to perform an operation. Now I want to ask for the permission to bring my daughter home from the Finkenau as soon as she will be healthy.
> Heil Hitler
> J. Buller

Buller's mother was apparently informed about her daughter's surgery only after she had been transferred to Finkenau and thus it is highly unlikely that she ever knew about the letters in Buller's file. The approval for her surgery had come from the same psychiatrist who had been responsible for the entire process. Buller herself seemed to realize what had occurred. In a kind of diary that was also found in her file, she wrote:

> 1935. Langenhorn. Discharged on the 12th December 1935. From here to the Finkenau, on Saturday the 13, operated (sterilized) 25. December 1st visit. On the 29th discharge. New Year's Eve party at home. At New Year walk. (See Figure 29)

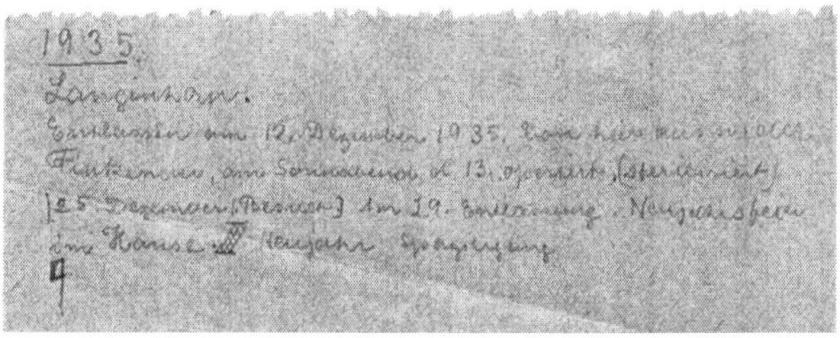

Figure 29: Anna Maria Buller's original "diary." Patient record 28338.

From this time forward, the fact that Buller was sterilized was marked in red everywhere, including on the cover of her file, so that it became the first thing that caught the reader's eye. The sterilization itself thereby became strong evidence for Buller's severe mental illness and for her being a hereditary danger.

Admission 1936

On 10 February 1936, Buller was committed to Friedrichsberg once again, although the medical officer this time remarked that she might be transferred to Langenhorn later. Her diagnosis was a logical continuation of her earlier admissions: "old schizophrenic with distinct defect symptoms; psychic desolation."[68] Buller was once again placed in House 8, where the psychiatrists used

---
68 PR LMR PN.

terms like "dumb facial expression,"[69] "wrinkled face [*Faltengesicht*],"[70] "mutistic," and "autistic,"[71] to describe her. Although this admission closely resembled the one in 1932, she experienced an increased number of bodily disciplinary interventions, especially by chemical means. Buller received so many injections in combination with other sedatives like Paraldehyde, that the nurses had to construct a handwritten "medication plan" in order not to lose track of these ongoing medications. (See Figure 30).

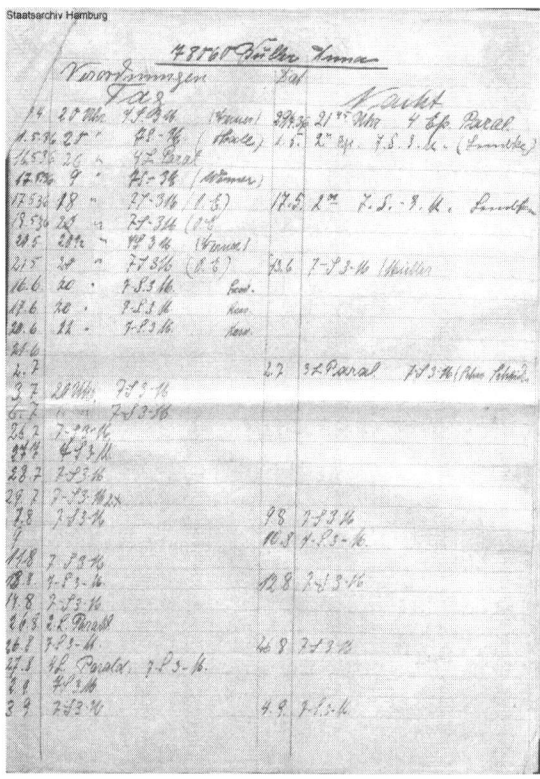

Figure 30: Medication plan from April to September 1936. Patient record 28338.

Even then, it is possible that Buller received more injections that those recorded, especially in situations where she seemed to be particularly resistant.

In September 1936, Buller was again transferred to Langenhorn where again

---

69 Staatsarchiv Hansestadt Hamburg 352–8-7 Staatskrankenanstalt Langenhorn Abl.1–1995, [SArHH 352–8-7 Langenh 1–1995], Krankenakte 28338.
70 Ibid.
71 Ibid.

she was kept in an isolation cell most of the time. The psychiatrist noted on 23 September 1936 that she "[has] to be kept [*gehalten werden*] in the cell since she attacked other patients in her state of dementia. She runs around in the cell at times agitated, gesticulates, talks incomprehensibly to herself, must be fed, experiences her surroundings without any reaction."[72] It is significant that the psychiatrist used the verb *gehalten werden* that refers usually to keeping animals.

One of Buller's drawings remaining in her medical record is remarkable because it illustrates the disciplinary distribution of space in House 8. (See Figure 31).

Buller moved between the isolation cell, the room with three beds, and the room with ten beds. The drawing demonstrates what is meant by the asylum walls being one with the psychiatrist's body, because the patients knew at any time what would happen if they misbehaved by the arrangement of the rooms. According to the seriousness of their misbehaviour, the different rooms enabled diverse forms of punishment, which ranged from continuous baths through confinement in the isolation cell. Buller drew the bed in the isolation cell in black, indicating that she saw herself kept in this cell.

At Langenhorn, Buller was even being given non-approved medication in an illegal experiment, again pointing out that that she had lost any legal status and was vegetating in a zone of "bare life" in which anything was possible. As the psychiatrist wrote on 4 November 1937, Buller "has taken Eugenocym for a couple of months (by request of the mother) without success."[73]

The method of continuous baths or "cold wet sheet packs" was used extensively in Friedrichsberg and Langenhorn and was mentioned frequently in the other records used in this book. Her situation could best be described by Dorothea Buck:

> How were we given rest? With buckets of cold water poured over our heads, with long-duration baths in a tub covered with canvas with a stiffed high collar in which my neck was fixed for 23 hours, from one doctor's ward-round to the next, with the "cold wet sheet packs" and with sedating injections of paraldehyde. In the case of the "cold wet sheet packs" one could be wrapped into them so tightly that one could no longer move at all. Due to the body temperature the sheets would become first warm and then hot. I would cry out in rage at this senseless restraint in these hot sheets.[74]

Buller was discharged home on 31 March 1938, not because the psychiatrists thought she should be but because Buller's parents intervened in favour of their daughter. The admission record, which contains the correspondence between

---

72 Ibid.
73 Ibid.
74 Dorothea Buck, "70 Years of Coercion."

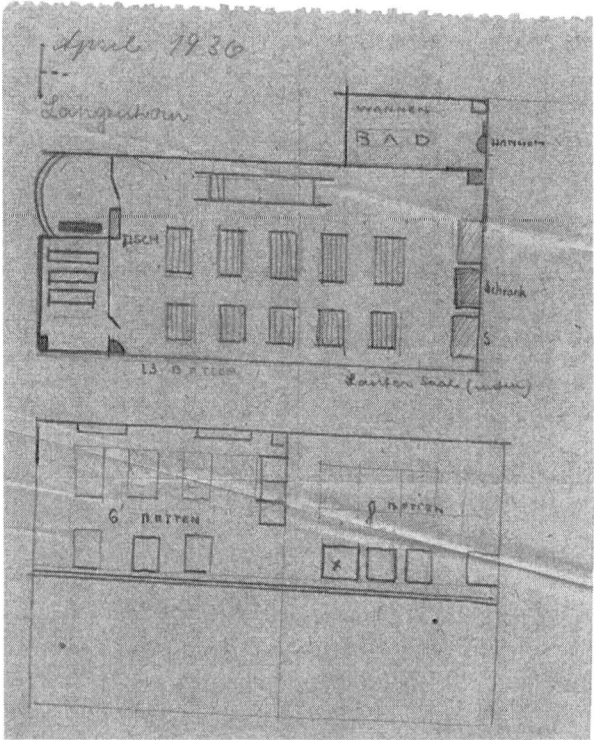

Figure 31: Anna Maria Buller's drawing of House 8. Translation: *Wannen Bad*: continuous bath; *Schrank*: cabinet; *Lauter Saal (unten)*: noisy hall (downstairs); *Betten*: beds; *Tisch*: table [the nurses' table]. Patient record 28338.

her father and Langenhorn, suggest that the father's demands had been ignored for months until the psychiatrist finally granted a one-month leave. During this leave, Buller's father believed that his daughter had clearly improved and asked for her complete discharge, which was approved by the medical director. It appears that without the insistence of her family, Buller would not have been discharged.

Admission 1940

Buller's admission in 1940 to the Clinic for Psychiatric and Nervous Diseases at Eppendorf, which was the new name of the psychiatric asylum at the University of Hamburg after Friedrichsberg was closed down, is worth analyzing in some detail. Not only was she killed in 1943 after her subsequent transfer back to Langenhorn, but her therapy also took a radical twist at this time. To begin with, her diagnosis in Eilbektal (the abbreviated designation of the new psychiatric asylum) differed from those given earlier. Buller was now somewhat surprisingly diagnosed with "Dementia praecox," a term derived from Kraeppelin's nosography. Her previous diagnoses of schizophrenia had been based on Bleuler's nomenclature, demonstrating once again that psychiatric practice was not guided by a particular medical nosography but rather could be perceived as a distribution of disciplinary power aimed at transforming the patient to his or her very core. Dementia praecox, under Kraeppelin's nosography, led to a process of stupefaction that was irreversible, whereas Bleuler's term of schizophrenia did not necessarily lead to stupefaction. The former implied that no curing was possible and that it was an irreversible process. One month before Buller was transferred to Langenhorn her diagnosis changed again to "hebephrenic," although on the date of her transfer, she was returned to a "schizophrenic," albeit "schizophrenic final state."

On the day of this admission and under her modified diagnosis, Buller was placed again in House 8. Similar to the earlier 1936 admission, the nurses laid out a medication plan in order to record the multiple Morphine-Scopolamine injections and Paraldehyde that she received. However, a new drug was introduced on 26 February: Cardiazol.

> 26.4.40: Pat. often outside the bed, food must be administered. Got Cardiazol, pat. stayed in bed, was quiet. (Nurse O.)
> Night: Pat. did not sleep until 2AM. Got Paraldehyde, slept immediately after this. (Ka.)
>
> 27.4.40: Pat. got Cardiazol, stood up in bed, got often out of the bed. Stands helplessly around. (Nurse O.)

Furthermore, Cardiazol treatment was combined with an "Insulin deep coma" therapy.

According to procedures in the asylum in Friedrichsberg, Cardiazol treatment, which was meant to induce seizures in patients, was to follow a precise scheme of two shocks per week at intervals of two to three days. Buller's Cardiazol injections started on 26 April 1940 with the usual dose for women but this was considered ineffective and the injections were repeated one day later with a slightly larger amount, eventually leading to a seizure. From then on, the nurses reported only from time to time on her Cardiazol injections, and the psychiatrist did not mention them until 12 June, more than two months after they began. The medication plan in Buller's case, however, shows that no regular schedule was employed. (See Figure 32, 33, 34 and 35) She received these injections on an irregular basis; in June, for example, she was given seven while in July, she received none. The Cardiazol injections were combined with insulin injections from 6 May to 16 May 1940. Nowhere in the record were the Cardiazol injections defined as a "therapy," whereas the insulin injections explicitly were.

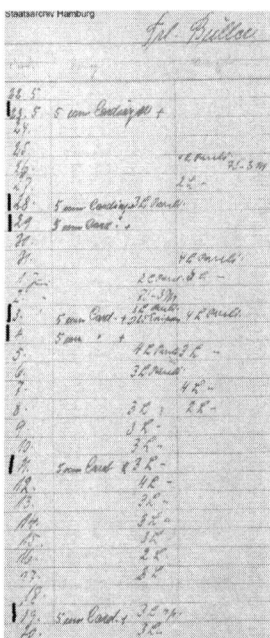

Figure 32 and 33: Insulin injection plan and Cardiazol injections April – June 1940. The Cardiazol injections are marked with a dash, the Insulin injection with a dot. Patient record 18338.

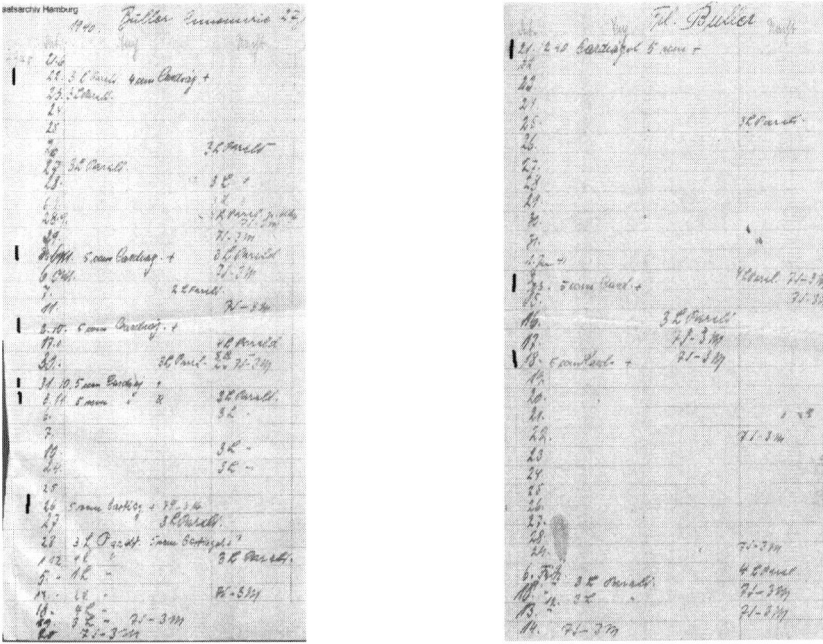

Figure 34 and 35: Medication plan June 1940 – February 1941. Patient record 18338.

Comparing the medication plan with the nurses' notes and the descriptions of Buller's behaviour, it is clear that the Cardiazol injections were used as a disciplinary measure against what the nurses (and through them, the physicians) deemed bad behaviour. On 29 October 1940, the nurses wrote

> 29.10.40: Pat. [patient] is very inhibited, stands around and must be
> urged to eat. (Nurse O.)
> Aftern. [Afternoon]: Pat. was very blocked. In the evening beat another patient with her slipper. Cried a little. Got Paral[dehyde].
> Night: Restless, often out of bed, disturbs other sick persons,
> pinched them. (Inj.) [Morphine Scopolamine]

> 31.10.: Pat. was restless in the morning, ran around crying, got Cardiazol |, became quiet afterwards. (Nurse O).

Between 24 and 28 November, Buller received both Paraldehyde and Cardiazol at least once and was also strapped to the bed several times for her restlessness. The entry on the afternoon of 28 November demonstrated well the aim of "treatment" and the type of behaviour that the nurses desired. During the periods that Anna Maria Buller seemed to "behave well," according to the nurses' perceptions, she received no Cardiazol injections. Cardiazol was only applied when nurses and psychiatrists estimated her behaviour as disruptive.

25.11. Night:Pat. [patient] stood always in front of the window, slept after she received Paral [Paraldehyd]. Pat. ran around sobbing, came into the belt.(Nurse O.)

26.11. Pat. got Cardiazol. Was very restless, always out of the bed, talked quietly to herself.
Aftern. The same

27.11. Pat. was very restless, was put into the belt.
Aftern. Pat. was very excited during visiting hours, transferred to ward #13. (Nurse L.)

28.11. Pat. got Cardiazol, very restless. Aftern. The same. (Nurse S.)
Aftern. Pat. nice and orderly, [did] housework, [laughed] And[answered] questions." (Nurse S.)
Morning: Pat. helps with sewing.

30.11. Pat. was nice and friendly.

By January 1941, Buller had received Cardiazol injections, however irregularly, for nearly one year. Within a psychiatric dispositive, even medications that were initially prescribed according to a certain conception of the etiology of mental illness or its organic correlations were re-utilized in a directive system. As one psychiatrist reported, a "young schizophrenic male patient" had been "threatened by his physician [that he would] get [Cardiazol], the 'shaking treatment,' (accompanied by a demonstration of it), if he [did] not soon wake up, get peppier and work faster and with more interest. Immediately he [began to defend himself against [Cardiazol]], worked with more zest, looked brighter, and when he saw his doctor approaching he busied himself where he could not be overlooked."[75]

Shock Treatments and Psychiatric Practice

Cardiazol had never been used before in Anna Maria Buller's case but was part of what Bleuler called "the active therapy" that complemented the "educational therapy of schizophrenia,"[76] or what was called psychotherapy at the time.[77] Cardiazol shock therapy – intravenous injections of pentamethylentetrazol, a camphor-like substance used to provoke an epileptic seizure – was introduced by neuropathologist and neurologist Lazlo (Ladislaus) Meduna in 1934, and from June 1936 on, insulin and Cardiazol shock therapies were carried out at Frie-

---

75 L. Kerschbaumer, "Spontaneous Reactions to Metrazol Therapy," *Journal of Nervous and Mental Disease* 98 (1943): 394.
76 Bleuler, *Lehrbuch der Psychiatrie*, 330.
77 Carl Schneider, *Behandlung und Verhütung der Geisteskrankheiten. Allgemeine Erfahrungen, Grundsätze Technik Biologie.* (Berlin: Julius Springer, 1939).

drichsberg. In the US, Metrazol/Cardiazol therapy was introduced in 1937,[78] and in Canada, at the Ontario hospital in Hamilton in September 1938.[79] Meduna's theory was that genuine epilepsy rarely occurred in combination with schizophrenia, creating what he called a "biological antagonism" between these two diseases. Because the two diseases were mutually exclusive, he contended that synthetically provoking artificial epileptic seizures should positively influence schizophrenia. However, this theory was immediately challenged. As an international debate highlights, practitioners like military psychiatrist Hirsch Gordon identified 50 different shock therapy theories.[80] Psychiatric journals published an overwhelming number of studies that tried to discover the exact mode of action and the impact of different shock therapies on patients' behaviour, but they were less interested in finding theoretical underpinnings for the causes for schizophrenia and how shock therapies influenced them.

American psychiatrist Louis H. Cohen emphasized that the Cardiazol procedure was relatively simple, economical, and did not involve restraint. Whereas all conventional forms of treatment, such as continuous baths, packs, seclusion and chemical sedation, were effective only during the period that they were applied, shock therapies appeared to last longer over time. Cohen stated that even after the treatment discontinued "most patients remain[ed] quiet and cooperative" and many of them "for the first time in years, [were] capable of doing productive work." Cardiazol therefore was considered one solution for administrative problems concerning the handling of "chronically disturbed patients."[81] Another American psychiatrist summarized that the duration of the illness was shortened and that "some of the others [patients who could not be discharged] became better hospital citizens."[82] Even if patients remained unchanged, most of them improved regarding their over-activity, aggressiveness, and destructiveness. "Necessary sedation has been diminished to practically nil."[83] These considerations were also sometimes closely related to eugenic arguments. For example, Professor H. Mouttet explained at an international conference of the Swiss Psychiatric Association in Münsingen that was devoted to measures for the treatment of schizophrenia: "We officers of the state who are

---

78 H. O. Colomb and G. L. Wadsworth, "An Analysis of Results in the Metrazol Shock Therapy of Schizophrenia," *Journal of Nervous and Mental Disease* 93, no. 1 (1941): 53–62.
79 J. A. Cummins, "Metrazol Shock Therapy Administered in the General Hospital," *Canadian Medical Association Journal* 50 (1944): 420–421.
80 Hirsch L. Gordon, "Fifty Shock Therapy Theories," *The Military Surgeon* 102–103 (1948), 397–401.
81 Louis H. Cohen, "The Early Effects of Metrazol Therapy in Chronic Psychiotic Over-Activity," *American Journal of Psychiatry* 95 (1938), 228.
82 Colomb and Wadsworth, "An Analysis of Results in the Metrazol Shock Therapy of Schizophrenia," 58.
83 Cohen, "The Early Effects of Metrazol Therapy in Chronic Psychotic Over-Activity," 332.

concerned with prosperity, the health and the well-being of our fellow citizens expect from you the transformation of useless human beings into individuals useful to society."[84] Leading psychiatrists like Carl Schneider in Germany emphasized on the one hand the necessity "to furnish the new times with new humans" and underlined, on the other hand, the connection between curing and devastation.[85] "Psychiatric patients should receive intensive "biological" therapy, but if they were incurable and could not be integrated into society, they lost their reason for existence in the biological sense as well."[86]

No consensus existed as to how exactly the therapy should be carried out and for how long. Higher doses of the drug were to be administered within a couple of minutes if any seizure occurred, but if no seizure could be provoked, further injections were to be held until the following day. According to Bleuler, who followed Meduna's recommendations, patients would ideally receive two shocks per week – 15 to 20 in all.[87] But a look at the international literature shows that the suggestions regarding the duration of the course and the frequency of injections were quite arbitrary.[88] Sometimes the injections were given daily,[89] sometimes every second day.[90]

Psychiatrists usually gave the intravenous injections. Because patients often vomited, they were fasting, and were placed in bed in a particular way. To reduce the risk of injuries, a piece of rubber hose was inserted between their teeth to prevent them biting their tongue.[91] As was the case with epileptic seizures in general, induced seizures also left patients unconscious, although they often suffered dislocations of joints, bone fractures, and other surgical complications. Ten to fifteen seconds after the injection, a so-called pre-paroxysmal phase occurred that was characterized by a short interval of coughing, which watchers stated was "followed by [an interval] usually lasting not more than ten seconds during which the patient [made] thrashing movements and [flailed] his arms

---

84 H. Mouttet, "The Treatment of Schizophrenia Insulin Shock, Cardiazol, Sleep Treatment," *American Journal of Psychiatry* 94, no. suppl. (1938): 3.
85 Schneider, *Behandlung und Verhütung der Geisteskrankheiten*.
86 Maike Rotzoll and Gerrit Hohendorff, "Krankenmord im Dienst des Fortschritts? Der Heidelberger Psychiater Carl Schneider als Gehirnforscher und "Therapeutischer Idealist","" *Der Nervenarzt* 83, no. 3 (2012): 317.
87 Bleuler, *Lehrbuch der Psychiatrie*, 331.
88 Louis H. Cohen, "Observations on the Convulsant Treatment of Schizophrenia with Metrazol," *The New England Journal of Medecine* 218, no. 24 (1938): 1004.
89 Cohen, "The Early Effects of Metrazol Therapy in Chronic Psychotic Over-Activity," 327–333
90 Eugene Ziskind, "Memory Defects during Metrazol Therapy," *Archives of Neurology and Psychiatry* 45, no. 2 (1941): 223–234.
91 Harold Widenmeyer Dr., "Die Insulin- und Cardiazolschockbehandlung der Schizophrenen," *Geisteskrankenpflege. Monatsschrift für Geisteskranken- und Krankenpflege* 41, no. 12 (1937): 161–165.

and legs about, his facial expression closely resembling terror."[92] The assistant physician at the Illenau asylum in Germany explained that "most sick persons oppose the Cardiazol treatment, because in the short interval that lasts only several seconds ... [they] experience a displeasing feeling, especially in the cardiac region, that can bring on a mortal fear. Nevertheless, it is just a misperception that is not based on a real specific danger."[93]

This "misperception" is worth analyzing in more detail. Psychiatrists generally agreed on the fact that the fear provoked in patients during the therapies (especially in the case of Cardiazol shock therapy) had an impact on the outcome of the treatments. They disagreed only to what extent. From 1937 to 1939, a large number of studies carried out in U. S. asylums tried to determine the impact of fear in shock therapies, for example, by artificially provoking prolonged sequences of fear that lasted sometimes up to three hours. Cohen described the fear experienced by patients as a "threat to the self which arises out of the experiences of impending catastrophe."[94] Humbert & Friedemann described this feeling as a "falling into non-existence" which invoked in the patient "the primitive complex of the association of life-death ... that appeared to have cumulative effects."[95]

Psychiatrists who studied the impact of fear agreed on the fact that the "animal-like expression of fear" was a sign of a kind of fear articulated at a lower biological level, and they differentiated this kind of fear from that consciously expressed by patients, which often led them to resist treatment. As two researchers asserted, a patient "suddenly and in the course of a few seconds after the injection of [Cardiazol] receives a terrific assault upon his entire economy including [his] consciousness and his instinct of self-preservation. He almost dies but does not."[96] Schilder described this condition as a "threat of annihilation and death and indeed during the epileptic fit and the following coma the patient comes very near to death."[97] The patient is "dead for a minute or so in an average attack. He goes through a terrifying experience of which he is aware, in active consciousness or in a subconscious state, only for a short time." The fear of impending death is "probably more real than that of the angina patient."[98] This

---

92 Cohen," Observations on the Convulsant Treatment of Schizophrenia with Metrazol," 1004.
93 Widenmeyer, "Die Insulin- und Cardiazolschockbehandlung der Schizophrenen," 163.
94 Louis H. Cohen, "The Therapeutic Significance of Fear in the Metrazol Treatment of Schizophrenia," *American Journal of Psychiatry* 95 (1939): 1349–1357.
95 F. Humbert and A. Friedemann, "Critique and Indications of Treatments in Schizophrenia," *American Journal of Psychiatry* 94, no. 2 (1938): 180.
96 Samuel N. Clark and Frank Garm Norbury, "A Possible Role of the Element of Fear in Metrazol Therapy," *Diseases of the Nervous System* 2, no. 6 (1941): 197.
97 Paul Schilder, "Notes on the Psychology of Metrazol Treatment of Schizophrenia," *The Journal of Nervous and Mental Disease* 89, no. 2 (1939): 142.
98 Clark and Norbury, "A Possible Role of the Element of Fear in Metrazol Therapy," 197.

profound fear on a "lower biological level" was only experienced if it was followed by seizures. However, it was possible to produce a less profound kind of fear by provoking "abortive seizures," which occurred if the dose of Cardiazol was too low or if it was injected too slowly. Patients clearly remembered the fear brought on by these abortive seizures, leading to the speculation that injection of lower levels of the drug or too slowly had the potential to be used deliberately. Cohen regarded shock therapies as "the twentieth-century variety of shock treatments of the past, in which fear [was] instilled [for a] therapeutic purpose."[99]

This suspicion is pertinent in Anna Maria Buller's case, because the medication plan clearly indicates that in the course of her treatment "single shot injections" became more frequent. For some of these injections she successfully experienced a seizure (in these cases, a + sign is marked beside the entry) but some injections obviously did not provoke seizures. According to standard procedures, in these cases the injections had to be repeated until a seizure occurred (or the injections had to be resumed on the next day) but in Buller's case, this did not happen. It seems as if the rationale behind these single injections was to discipline specific behaviour that the nurses reported in order to obtain permission from the psychiatrist for another injection.

As was the case for Anna Maria Buller, Cardiazol therapy was often combined with insulin shock therapy. The addition of insulin, which had been developed by Manfred Sakel in the 1930s, was based on the theory that insulin antagonized the neuronal effects of products of the adrenal system that were considered the physiological cause of the patient's illness. Insulin shock therapy was employed on a grand scale in Hamburg and elsewhere. The former medical director of Friedrichsberg, Prof. Dr. Hans Bürger-Prinz, emphasized after the end of the Second World War that a quarter of the patient beds had been reserved for insulin shock treatments, or 80 beds out of 320.[100] The insulin units were mostly the sole responsibility of nurses,[101] who administered not only the insulin but also the glucose via a nasal tube.[102]

"Deep insulin coma therapy" was extremely rigorous. Comas were induced

---

99 Cohen, "The Therapeutic Significance of Fear in the Metrazol Treatment of Schizophrenia,"1349.
100 Angelika Ebbinghaus, "Kostensenkung, "Aktive Therapie" und Vernichtung. Konsequenzen für das Anstaltswesen," in *Heilen und Vernichten im Mustergau Hamburg. Bevölkerungs- und Gesundheitspolitik im Dritten Reich*, eds. Angelika Ebbinghaus, Heidrun Kaupen-Haas and Karl Heinz Roth (Hamburg: Konkret Literatur Verlag, 1984), 141.
101 Jean-Noël Missa, *Naissance de la psychiatrie biologique: Histoire des traitements des maladies mentales au XX. siècle* (Paris: Presse Universitaire de France, 2006).
102 Enge, "Aufgaben des Pflegepersonals bei der Insulinschock- und der Cardiazol- bzw. Azomankrampf-Behandlung," *Geisteskrankenpflege. Monatsschrift für Geisteskranken- und Krankenpflege* 44, no. 11 (1941): 134–136.

on five or six mornings a week. Typically, the "therapy" began with an initial dose of 10 – 15 units of insulin with a daily increase of 5 – 10 units until the patient showed a severe hypoglycemia. Treatment continued until there was a satisfactory psychiatric response or until 50 – 60 comas had been induced. In Anna Maria Buller's case the "therapy" started with 30 units and with a daily increase of 10 units, reaching up to 100 units on the ninth day.

Hypoglycemia made patients extremely restless and liable to major convulsions.[103] Comas were terminated by administration of glucose via a nasal tube or through intravenous injection. Patients required continuous nursing supervision for the rest of the day since they were liable to experience hypoglycemic "after-shocks" and a doctor had to be immediately available.

Bürger-Prinz pointed out that patients experienced these periods of "forced unconsciousness in slow motion," which caused "panicky anxiety states in them."[104] Cardiazol shock provoked a profound fear of death in the patient, but insulin coma therapy was literally a death threat. Although American psychiatrist Jellife asserted that the hypoglycemic death threat was unique. "Genetically considered, it may be thought of as a very primordial, primitive and massive type of threat which strikes at the very initial stages of life" since "carbohydrates were among the first energy transforming substances creating life."[105] Insulin coma therapy produced, similarly to Cardiazol shock therapy, a reaction on a deep and profound level but "the death threat is a much more vital one coming from this direction than from almost any other." The death threat experienced by the "withdrawal of glycogen forces a definite withdrawal of libido from the aggressive, hostile anal, oral and other negativistic behavior patterns"[106] because it strikes at the initial stages of life.

Shock therapies were enthusiastically received in Germany and abroad. An overwhelming number of case studies were published that demonstrated astonishing results for patients who had successfully recovered from schizophrenia. It must be emphasized that psychiatrists referred only to "remissions" of patients, not to cures. As mentioned above, Bleuler considered schizophrenia to be a "heredodegeneration" even though he admitted that no medically sound idea existed for its causes.[107] From this perspective, the course of the illness could

---

103 Kingsley Jones, "Insulin Coma Therapy in Schizophrenia," *Journal of the Royal Society of Medicine* 93 (2000): 147 – 149.
104 Bürger-Prinz as cited in: Ebbinghaus, *Kostensenkung, "Aktive Therapie" und Vernichtung. Konsequenzen für das Anstaltswesen*, 141.
105 Smith Ely Jelliffe, "Discussion Paper Presented at the Section of Neurology and Psychiatry, New York, Academy of Medicine, and the New York Neurological Society. Joint Meeting, January 12, 1937," *Journal of Nervous and Mental Disease* 85, no. 5 (1937): 577.
106 Ibid., 577 – 578.
107 Bleuler, *Lehrbuch der Psychiatrie*, 326 – 327.

be influenced only through psychotherapy, meaning that patients could be educated but not really cured. Psychiatrists internationally thus tried to define the success of therapies through classification of patient behaviour. L.v. Angyal and K. Gyárfás distinguished four forms of "remission": "complete (A), good (B), social (C), and none (0)" People with complete remission,

> can be considered those cases who attained complete insight into their illness regarding their pathological experiences, hallucinations, etc. and who are able carry out their work and who are also considered by those around them as completely cured, psychic healthy people.[108]

The definition of good remission is exactly the same criterion for patient recovery as was discussed regarding the final interrogation. The defining mechanism of the final interview was the questioning by the psychiatrist and the acknowledgement of the patient that the centralized identity in the record was really him or her. From this perspective, Cardiazol shock therapy became a means to achieve this confession, and as the statement above highlights, it can be defined as introducing the psychiatrist's will into the body of the patient.

To reduce the purpose of shock therapies to produce only more manageable patients, however, is too simplistic. As the quote from Angyal & Gyárfás highlights, patients who were considered in complete remission had complete insight into their illness. Solomon et al. described in his case study how patients who were "hostile to questioning" about their mental illness before shock treatment exhibited "a cooperative cordial attitude towards" the psychiatrist after they recovered.[109] They were able to give an "objective outlook and an apparently adequate rationalization" of their problems.[110] The authors defined "psychologic resistance" as a "hostile, angry, disputing attitude towards the examiner."[111] Starks carried out interviews on the subjective experiences of patients receiving insulin and Cardiazol therapy. As one patient stated, "Before the treatment, I was in a little world by myself, having bad feelings. After I got the treatment, I felt rather the reality [became more aware of his surrounding]." Another patient admitted that he had been mentally ill, that he had "imagined things that didn't exist in reality." After the treatment "my mind began to look at things realisti-

---

108 L. v.Angyal and K. Gyárfás, "Über die Cardiazol-Krampfbehandlung der Schizophrenie," *Archiv für Psychiatrie* 106 (1937): 2.
109 Alfred P. Solomon, Chester W. Darrow and Melvin Blaurock, "Blood Pressure and Palmar Sweat (Galvanic) Responses of Psychotic Patients before and After Insulin and Metrazol Therapy: A Physiologic Study of 'Resistant' and Cooperative Attitudes," *Psychosomatic Medicine* 1, no. 1 (1939): 125.
110 Colomb and Wadsworth, "An Analysis of Results in the Metrazol Shock Therapy of Schizophrenia," 57–58.
111 Solomon, Darrow and Blaurock, "Blood Pressure and Palmar Sweat (Galvanic) Responses of Psychotic Patients," 120.

cally again. It made me very reasonable, very rational, and [able to] think clearly."[112] In contrast, a patient who did not "change" through the treatment "admitted only what she wished to admit, often answering one question by asking another. The patient made no attempt to use the interview to gain insight into her problems."[113] From this perspective, shock therapy became a means to achieve these confessions, and could be defined as introducing the psychiatrist's will into the body of the patient.

Psychiatrists acknowledged that the effects of Cardiazol and insulin were "deeper than the effects of what we call psychic influence. The treatment is an organic treatment reflected in psychological attitudes." The psychosis was not forgotten "but the individual changed his emotional attitude."[114] This was especially true in cases of "degenerative schizophrenia" (classical dementia praecox) in which the "psychotherapeutic influence is forcibly limited to superficial re-education." These cases that were considered hopeless appeared to be "responsive to shock treatment either by insulin or by Cardiazol."[115]

Shock therapies in general thus had a very specific effect on patients, because they not only changed the way they communicated verbally but also how they acted in front of psychiatrists and nurses. Kerschbaumer described these changes as "a positive transference" leading to a "close patient-physician relationship," where, for example, "some male patients [saw] in the woman-psychiatrist a sweetheart, wife, beloved sister or mother-substitute."[116] This "close patient-physician relationship" seemed to be a consequence of extreme fear because patients appeared to almost cling to their rescuers.[117] Schilder noted that after a fit, a patient "experiences ... a slow revival of his interest in the world and an enormous feeling of relief in which he grasps for any contact offered to him."[118] In this final stage of shock treatment the patient perceived psychiatrists and nurses as rescuers and tried to establish close contact with them.

Nurses thus conducted patients systematically into a "twilight state" between life and death but it is obvious from the nurses' notes that they were only concerned in recording patient behavior, as they did for Anna Maria Buller.

---

112 Hamlin A. Starks, "Subjective Experiences in Patients Incident to Insulin and Metrazol Therapy," *Psychiatric Quaterly* 12, no. 4 (1938): 703.
113 Solomon, Darrow and Blaurock, "Blood Pressure and Palmar Sweat (Galvanic) Responses of Psychotic Patients," 131.
114 Schilder, "Notes on the Psychology of Metrazol Treatment of Schizophrenia," 143.
115 Bleuler, *Lehrbuch der Psychiatrie*, 345.
116 Kerschbaumer, "Spontaneous Reactions to Metrazol Therapy," 390.
117 Ibid., 395.
118 Schilder, "Notes on the Psychology of Metrazol Treatment of Schizophrenia," 142.

15.5. Afternoon: Pat. got Insulin. Pat. walked around nude. Was drowsy. Must be urged to eat. Ate well then. (Nurse H.)
Night: Slept . (Nurse M.)

16.5.Pat. got Insulin. Is always out of the bed. (Nurse M.)
Afternoon: Pat. removed her shirt, walked around.
Night: Slept till morning. (Nurse K.)

17.5.Got Cardiazol (+ ['seizure']) afterwards unchanged. (Nurse L.)
Night: unchanged

18.5.Pat. got Cardiazol. Afterwards quiet. Vomited a bit. (Nurse M.)
Afternoon: Pat. was quiet. (Nurse O.)[119]

Death threats provoked though shock therapies were not only imagined by the patients but deaths themselves were very real, as was reported in all the medical literature of that time. Historian Angelika Ebbinghaus presumed that the increase in the mortality rate in Friedrichsberg was due partly to the new "active" therapies. According to her research, patients were already dying from these shock therapies long before the beginning of the planned and systematic assassination of patients under the Nazi regime. (See Table 5) While the table indicates that the number of admitted patients did not double between 1936 and 1941, the number of deaths more than tripled in the same period of time.

Table 5: Number of treated patients and number of patients who died in Eilbektal, the asylum at the University of Hamburg.[120]

Year	Number of patients treated in the asylum of the University of Hamburg	Number of deaths in the asylum of the University of Hamburg
1936	1333	85
1937	1990	142
1938	2196	154
1939	2516	188
1940	2113	235
1941	2391	290

The example of Anna Maria Buller highlights the fact that shock therapy was a technique that contained within it the whole rationale of psychiatric practice, that of forcing the reality of the asylum onto the individual. In Anna Maria B.'s

---

119 Staatsarchiv Hansestadt Hamburg 352–8-7, Staatskrankenanstalt Langenhorn, Abl.1– 1995, Krankenakte 28338.
120 Angelika Ebbinghaus, "Kostensenkung, 'Aktive Therapie' und Vernichtung. Konsequenzen für das Anstaltswesen," in *Heilen und Vernichten im Mustergau Hamburg. Bevölkerungs- und Gesundheitspolitik im Dritten Reich*, eds. Angelika Ebbinghaus, Heidrun Kaupen-Haas and Karl Heinz Roth (Hamburg: Konkret Literatur Verlag, 1984), 143.

case, for example, Cardiazol and insulin coma therapy was combined with the usual Morphine-Scopolamine injections, with Paraldehyde, often given via enema in order to increase the sedative effects, and a whole array of other disciplinary interventions. All these interventions were aimed to correct her behaviour and the nurses' notes focused primarily on potential changes in her behavior. As the notes pointed out, Buller was considered a chronic case that became increasingly disoriented: "Sitting around and does not know what to do" or "Pat. sits at one place with her head down for hours." On 20 February 1941 the psychiatrist noted that "she was completely unchanged and negativistic in character." She remained alternately stuporous and excited, out of touch with her surroundings, and "must be strapped down." As a consequence, Buller was diagnosed as "schizophrenic final state." This state might also have been due partly to the extensive use of Cardiazol and other medications, since Ziskind reported on memory defects that ressemble Korsakoff syndrome in patients who had received this drug.[121] These findings coincide with the findings of Platner and Müller who reported Korsakoff syndrome[122] as a complication of shock therapy of both insulin coma and Cardiazol shock therapies.[123] Ziskind argued that these symptoms were significant, because "they are readily recognized as being due to the treatment and not part of the original disease." He further emphasized that shock therapy augmented memory defects in patients depending on the duration of treatment and the spacing of convulsions.[124]

Seen against the backdrop of these findings it does not seem to be an exaggeration to assume that psychiatrists and nurses actively contributed to the "final state" of Anna Maria B. The nurses' and psychiatrists' notes resembled what psychiatrist Alfred Hoche termed as descriptions of the "mentally dead."[125]

I used the metaphor of "war against madness" in order to describe what happened to Anna Maria Buller. This military vocabulary is not an exaggeration

---

121 Ziskind, "Memory Defects during Metrazol Therapy," 230.
122 "Korsakoff's syndrome is a brain disorder usually associated with heavy alcohol consumption over a long period. Historically it has also been called 'Korsakoff's psychosis,' although this can be confusing, as there are no true psychotic symptoms in the medical sense. Sometimes it is referred to as 'alcohol amnestic syndrome' – amnestic meaning loss of memory – although in rare cases alcohol is not the cause. Although Korsakoff's syndrome is not strictly speaking a dementia, people with the condition experience loss of short-term memory." Alzheimer Society, "What is Korsakoff's Syndrome?" http://alzheimers.org.uk/site/scripts/documents_info.php?documentID=98 (accessed 07/23, 2012).
123 P. Platner, "Korsakoff Syndrome after Insuline and Metrazol Treatment of Schizophrenia," *Zeitschrift für die gesamte Neurologie und Psychiatrie* 162 (1938): 728–735.; M. Müller, "Insulin Therapy of Schizophrenia," *American Journal of Psychiatry* 94, no. supl. (1938): 5–15.
124 Ziskind, "Memory Defects during Metrazol Therapy," 230.
125 Karl Binding and Alfred Hoche, *Die Freigabe der Vernichtung lebensunwerten Lebens. Ihr Maß und ihre Form (1920)* (Berlin: Berliner Wissenschaftsverlag, 2006).

but rather a precise description of the rationale behind the deployment of shock treatments in psychiatry. During the international conference of the Swiss Psychiatric Association in Münsingen in 1937 mentioned above the founder of the hypoglycemic insulin convulsant therapy of schizophrenia, Manfred Sakel, used military vocabulary to describe the interplay between epileptic seizures and hypoglycemic coma. "The epileptic attack is the artillery [and] the hypoglycemia is the infantry in the battle against the disease. According to military theory, the artillery never conquers and occupies hostile territory. It can only open the way for the infantry." The restoration of normality needs very subtle means able to reach the damaged parts and the finest mental processes in order to restore larger clarity in the mental and emotional spheres.[126]

Even if patients were not killed in this war at the Hamburg University asylum, they certainly arrived in Langenhorn in a much-reduced bodily condition.[127]

Last Transfer to Langenhorn

Once again, Buller was sent back to Langenhorn on 9 March 1941, where she immediately received Morphine-Scopolamine injections and Paraldehyde. The psychiatrist saw Buller for the first time on 10 March 1941 and described her as completely apathetic. His final remark – "Completely unapproachable. Completely autistic. Always opposing in negativistic manner" – was derived from the nurses' notes.

---

126 Manfred Sakel, "The Nature and Origin of Hypoglycemic Treatment of Psychosis," *The American Journal of Psychiatry* 94, no. suppl. (1938): 25.
127 That the psychiatrists and nurses consciously accepted that their patients would be harmed is seen particularly in the case of Richard Rudolf Heinrich A., who was admitted 6 May 1936 to Langenhorn after spending only four days in Friedrichsberg. A. was admitted with the diagnosis "progressive paralysis" and treated with countless medications. Even though he was not treated with a shock therapy (although he even received Cardiazol in the course of his endless therapies) he became the target of another kind of "active" therapy. The handling of the medications in this case is paradigmatic. His martyrdom began in 1936 with a Malaria-tertiana therapy that was stopped because he had a circulatory collapse. Even though he showed serious symptoms of cardiac insufficiency, he was treated further with a Bismogel-therapy (1936), followed by a Pyrifer therapy to which Cardiazol injections were added. The first three "medications" were used to provoke high fevers in patients to fight against syphilis, a cause of progressive dementia, and which A. had been diagnosed with, but Cardiazol was typically reserved for shock therapies in cases of schizophrenia. In August 1936 another Pyrifer therapy was started and was repeated in 1937. In 1938 a malaria therapy was again begun but stopped due to cardiac complications. It is obvious that A. was treated with therapies that had serious health hazards even for healthy patients, and A. received them even though the psychiatrists knew about his cardiac situation. Staatsarchiv Hansestadt Hamburg 352–8-7, Staatskrankenanstalt Langenhorn, Abl.1–1995, Krankenakte 23121.

On 10 March the nurses' daily notes broke off, as happened before. Nevertheless, Buller's medical file contains small sheets of seemingly scrap paper with random, widely spaced documentation, as well as other kinds of summarized notes – papers that had not been produced for any of her earlier admissions. The first of these papers is a report from 25 March 1941.

> 25.3.41: Buller, Miss Annamaria. Pat. is very restless, moves her bedding/ covers around a lot, rattles the wooden bed rails, spits, attacks the nurses, is in every way unapproachable. Pat. hallucinates, talks to herself all the time, cries and accuses herself, "I am Jesus, have hung on the cross," and so on. Pat. does not eat well, makes little balls made of bread and throws them. Pat. must be taken away.
> 25.3.41: 11/2p.m.: Pat. is very restless often tries to attack the nurse, cries quietly, was given sleeping medicine. (S.)
>
> 30.3.41: Pat. still very restless, talks to herself in a very excited, lively way, cries a lot, is tormented a lot. Pat. is out of bed often, attacks patients and spits, Pat. was especially agitated during and after visiting time. (N. A.)

Three months later, the note from 25 March reappeared in the psychiatrist's summary.

> 26.6.41: Is very restless, moves her bedding around a lot, spits, attacks the nurses and other patients. Hallucinates, lively monologues. Cries and accuses "I am Jesus, have hung on the cross and so on!" Poor eater. Must get enemas. During visits autistic as well.

Once again the psychiatrist has combined events in a new fashion and it is not readily apparent that he has used the nurses' notes written three months ago. It appears that the nurses recorded their observations mainly just before the psychiatrist did his rounds, which in Buller's case happened between two and five times per year. Buller had nearly completely disappeared and became once again the "living dead."

The psychiatrist wrote his assessment of Buller on "Reporting form 1," a questionnaire in line with *Aktion T4*. (See Figure 36). The capturing and selection of the victims for the centrally planned killing (see chapter one) took place through a nationwide dispatching of report sheets (*Meldebogen T4*), documents that had to be completed by each asylum and submitted to two psychiatric reviewers and a supervising psychiatric expert. They were to identify patients hospitalized for more than five years, or who were categorized as schizophrenic, "feeble-minded," epileptic, or in the final stages of neurological disease – all those who were not able to work or able to do only "mechanical work." Included in this list were all mentally ill persons charged with criminal offences, as well as non-German patients who were to be divided by race. Identification of these people was thus made under the following selection criteria: "heritability," "incurability," "productivity," "anti-socialness," and "race affiliation."

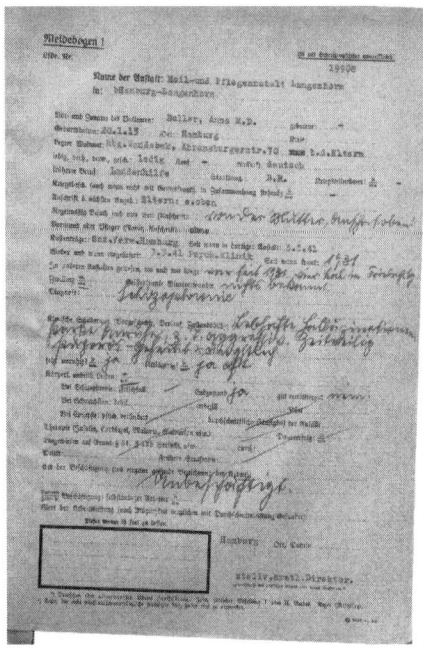

Figure 36: Anna Maria Buller's completed report sheet 1 (Meldebogen 1) of Aktion T4. Patient record 28338.

Although the form insisted that it "Must be completed with typewriter!" only the administrative part was; the rest was handwritten, and was thus likely a draft of the form that was finally sent on to Berlin. As was the case for the sterilization report, the form prescribed the type of information to be entered, limiting it to specific terms and a small space. This form is therefore another example of the ability of documents to "govern at distance." The handwritten answers on her form are written here in italics.

> Has been in other institutions, where and for how long: *was in Friedrichsberg four times since 1931*
> Twin: *no*
> Mental illness in (blood)relatives/family: *not known*
> Diagnosis: *Schizophrenia*
> Clinical description(history, progression of illness, current condition): *vivid hallucinations, very restless, at times aggressive, at times stuporous-shy & timid.*
> Very restless: *yes* bedridden? *Yes, yes often.*
> Incurable physical diseases: *no*
> Final condition: *yes* diminishing: *no*
> Kind of work (detailed description of work): *Not working.*

This report provides another example of the continuous rewriting of Buller's history, since the terms used compressed more than ten years of asylum confinements. Simultaneously, it also officially confirmed that Buller was a hopeless case. Nothing new was added to her biography but it allowed her whole life to be displayed on one page. In the end, it is not clear if the form was actually mailed to Berlin, because *Aktion T4* was officially ended in August 1941.

Anna Maria Buller's way into death

Only six nursing notes and five psychiatrist's notes exist from 1942, and they are mostly reiterations of the same story. In October 1942, she was diagnosed with tuberculosis of the bone after a large abscess was drained. Transfer to Sahlenburg, an institution specializing in the treatment of patients with tuberculosis, was ruled out because of her "psychological condition." She was sent back to Langenhorn, where her long term prognosis was deemed "very uncertain, specifically because of the poor general condition the patient is in and because of her difficult eating habits," a clear indication that even the surgeon judged Buller's life as worth nothing

However, her parents understood the impact of this diagnosis. Her father wrote the following letter to the medical director of Langenhorn.

> Filled with great concern for the health of my daughter Anna Maria Buller (House 4) I allow myself to ask if there isn't anything that can be done to keep her alive.
> Anna Maria is such a talented and hard-working person when she is healthy that one can say her life is worth living and is productive. I would be happy to pay any extra cost that might occur in connection with special treatment.
> Would it be possible to send my daughter to a specialized clinic for respiratory diseases? If this is not possible, could you at least give her some whole milk and provide her with healthier food. Other patients with tuberculosis also get milk. She did not have this disease when she was admitted to your clinic so the disease should still be in its beginning state and should be curable with good food and fresh air.
> I am looking forward to your reply.
> With German regards,
> J. Buller

This letter is interesting from two perspectives. First, although Buller's father was implicitly criticizing the treatment in Langenhorn, he wrote somewhat defensively, seemingly aware that the letter would become part of the medical record and read by the medical director, as holder of absolute power and with the potential to use it against the patient. These letters thus cannot be read as undistorted historical documents. Second, it is clear that the parents knew what this diagnosis meant for their daughter. By referring to her productivity and thus worthy life when she was healthy was a way of using the logic of Nazi propaganda in an attempt to save the life of his daughter. It was a counterargument to the claim (particularly to authors like Hoche and Binding) that mentally ill persons were considered wasters of national wealth. The medical director, however, refused the father's requests for better treatment and nutrition for his daughter, arguing that the parents had to pay for these extra expenses themselves which the father had offered to do. From this time on Buller's father paid 1.50RM (approximately 36 cents at that time) out of pocket, more than one-fourth of the whole boarding wages.

The nurses' notes break off once more and are resumed only three months later just before the psychiatrist made his next rounds on 17 February 1943. The nurses wrote that Buller remained "noisy and agitated" and that she "received package in which she didn't stay calmly," package meaning the cold wet sheet packs in which patients were tightly wrapped. The reference to "package" highlights once again the importance of background knowledge in the use of terms that were not self-explanatory.

In the final note in Buller's record, recorded on 20 June 1943, the nurse wrote that Buller was "disoriented and very confused, mistakes people." She was "very agitated and loud, lashed out," hitting the head nurse on her back, after which she was confined to a single room. This last note might have been the trigger for the decision to transfer Buller to Hadamar, where she was sent five days later.

Hadamar was one of six "gas-killing facilities" that had been used under the centrally organized *Aktion T4*, which from January 1940 to August 1941 had sent patients to its gas chambers. Relatives had received falsified "consolatory letters" (*Trostbriefe*), which were constructed in a sophisticated system of utmost secrecy and which suggested that the sick persons had been released from their suffering. Even though *Aktion T4* was officially ended in 1941, these hospitals continued to serve as killing facilities for psychiatric patients who continued to arrive in a reduced physical conditions and who were then killed by medications (especially through injections of Luminal) or through neglect and starvation. Patients often received a diagnosis of some life-threatening condition before their death was announced. Sometimes patients were already dead and buried in the hospital's own cemetery before their relatives received notice. Hadamar even possessed its own registry office to issue official death certificates.

As discussed earlier head nurses made the decisions to transfer patients to the other asylums. For someone like Buller who was already living in the "zone of exception," any incident could become a reason for transfer. On 5 July 1943, Buller had apparently come "down with intestinal catarrh and heart failure." On that day the senior psychiatrist wrote the following letter to her parents.

> Your daughter Anna has developed the condition of enteritis. The progression of the illness indicates that it is the result of a tubercular process. As a consequence of its fast

progression and the patient's irregular food consumption the patient's physical condition has weakened considerably. Due to the bad mental condition the patient is in, a deterioration of her general condition is possible. Visits are permitted. 5/7.43 H.

Buller, however, died the next day, her death attributed to "enteritis colitis."

Horrorism

Hannah Arendt, in her book *Origins of Totalitarianism,* presented a perspective on the atrocities committed by nurses and psychiatrists which can be read from a biopolitical standpoint. Focusing on concentration and extermination camps, she argued that victims were randomly chosen and "even without being accused, declared unfit to live." Extending this analysis to sick persons in asylums, she wrote that

> Freedom in this system has not only dwindled down to its last and apparently still indestructible guarantee, the possibility of suicide, but has lost its distinctive mark because the consequences of its exercise are shared with completely innocent people. If Hitler had had the time to realize his dream of a German Health Bill, the man suffering from a lung disease would have been subject to the same fate as a Communist in the early and a Jew in the later years of Nazi regime.[128]

The concentration and extermination camps served not only as extermination machines but also as laboratories for experiments of all kind, especially medical experiments. Citing Adolf Hitler, Arendt presented the path to total domination, which for him could only happen

> if each and every person can be reduced to a never changing identity of reactions, so that every one of these bundles can be exchanged at random for any other. The problem is to fabricate something that does not exist, namely, a kind of human species resembling other animal species whose only "freedom" would consist in "preserving the species."[129]

According to Arendt, under scientifically controlled conditions, the camps were to eliminate spontaneity as an expression of human behaviour and to transform "the human personality into a mere thing, into something that even animals are not."[130] The camp was an experiment in total domination, transforming humans into "uncomplaining animals," and thus into "the true central institution of totalitarian power."[131] The horror of the concentration camps can never be fully

---

128 Hannah Arendt, *The Origins of Totalitarianism* (New York: Harcourt Brace Jovanovich, 1994), 433..
129 Ibid., 438 [Hitler, as cited in Arendt].
130 Ibid.
131 Ibid., 438–439.

reported "for the very reason that the survivor returns to the world of the living, which makes it impossible for him to believe fully in his own past experiences. It is as though he had a story to tell from another planet, for the status of the inmates in the world of the living, where nobody is supposed to know if they are alive or dead, is such that it is as though they had never been born."[132]

The camps were economically useless and even when shortages of building material and rolling stock appeared in the midst of war, the Nazis "set up enormous, costly extermination factories and transported millions of people back and forth."[133] Arendt's description of the extermination camps can be applied, on a smaller scale, to psychiatric asylums. The techniques of killing were developed and deployed in the asylums, even after the official end of *Aktion T4*, with some personnel moving into the extermination camps. Arendt goes even further than Agamben, however, because to her it was not only a question of distinguishing between *bios* and *zoé*, as in Agamben, but that the significance of "death" and "life" was decided on an ontological criterion. For Arendt, according to Adriana Cavaerero, horror had to do with the human condition.

> It consists precisely in the perversion of a living and a dying that, in the Lager [camp], are no longer such, because they concern a living being understood as 'a specimen of the animal-species man' in which the uniqueness of every human being, and hence the necessarily unique dimension of life that concludes with death, has been annihilated.[134]

From this perspective, horror "has to do with the *killing of uniqueness*" and consists "in an attack on the *ontological material* that transforms unique beings into a mass of superfluous beings." The murder of these actively produced beings is, according to Arendt, "as impersonal as the squashing of a gnat."[135] This analysis has highlighted many of the mechanisms and methods employed to transform "unique beings into a mass of superfluous beings." What remained at the end were "ghastly marionettes with human faces"[136] that had nothing more of the human about them.

As was shown in Buller's case, this was often a lengthy process, one which often began long before the Nazis gained power. Arendt described these "ghastly marionettes," these specimens "of the animal-species man," as automatons who behaved like the dogs in Pavlov's experiment. But, as Cavarero emphasized, this

> [i]s not an example of the canine species observed in its natural behavior but rather a dog of a perverted kind. The "ghastly marionettes" are indeed perverted with respect to

---

132 Ibid., 444.
133 Ibid., 445.
134 Adriana Cavarero, *Horrorism. Naming Contemporary Violence* (New York: Columbia University Press, 2009), 43.
135 Arendt, *The Origins of Totalitarianism*, 433 [emphasis mine].
136 Ibid., 455.

the natural spontaneity that is rooted in the uniqueness of every human being: they are the result of a systematic destruction of the human being that the laboratory of the Lager carries out in order to demonstrate "that everything is possible."[137]

To my mind, this is an exact description of what happened in the "zone of exception" within asylums. It is not enough to concentrate just on the killings that took place during the "euthanasia" action under the Nazi regime. In order to understand the role of nurses in these atrocious crimes, one has to carefully analyze how nurses themselves produced these "ghastly marionettes."

---

137 Cavarero, *Horrorism*, 45.

Chapter 7: Conclusion

The aim of this book was to highlight the role of nurses in the killing of psychiatric patients during the time of the Nazi regime, through an analysis of patient records obtained from two psychiatric hospitals in Hamburg. The research hypothesis was that scientific discourses of that time, found within medical textbooks and nursing journals, shaped the recordings of nurses and psychiatrists on the patients' files. This research focused on deciphering the interrelationships between these discourses and the patient notes in order to demonstrate that what was written in the notes was not dependent on the individual "author," but rather was the product of scientific classifications and discourses, and, as a result, nurses and psychiatrists perceived their patients as having a life not worth living.

When the data collection and analysis of the records was initiated, it quickly became evident that the research was significantly more complex than originally thought. First of all, it became clear that there were ongoing suspicions among historians that patients were being killed in German psychiatric hospitals from the end of the First World War until after the end of the Second – thus, both before and after the Nazi regime. The reason for these killings must be searched for within the field of psychiatric practice. My research supports the theory that the killing of patients did not occur solely due to Nazi ideology but rather was founded on what can be referred to as "the whole realm of psychiatric practice" in the late nineteenth and early twentieth century. Second, many techniques to "treat" patients, ranging from enforced bed rest, isolation cells, continuous baths, to medications etc., were noted in the records. The deployment of these techniques suggests that psychiatric practice somehow actively produced individual lives that asylum personnel considered not worth living. In order to understand the mechanisms that enabled the killing of psychiatric patients, it was necessary to analyze in detail the meaning and role of these techniques in psychiatric practice. Third, to understand how the killings were enabled necessitated examining not only scientific discourses in psychiatry in vogue in the early twentieth century but also actual asylum psychiatric practice.

The functioning of the asylum can only be understood by analyzing psychiatric practice as a strategic interplay of political technologies aimed at establishing a kind of reality that was forced onto patients. As such, the analysis had to be broadened in order to grasp this strategic interplay. Some records were several hundred pages long but others were very short and concise. While patients remained in hospital for various lengths of time, some "constructed" in these records endured a hospital "career" that spanned several decades. The record, and consequently the act of note taking to develop the record, therefore had specific relevance to the field of psychiatry and to the treatment of patients. Psychiatric personnel reported their observations in them but patients' very identities were constructed through these records.

My findings suggest that psychiatric practice was a mechanism of "normalization" that continually attempted to classify what was considered normal behaviour and what was not, and who was deemed curable and who was not. The two hospitals that are the focus of my analysis can be distinguished by the fact that Friedrichsberg (asylum of the University of Hamburg and the admission clinic for Hamburg) was responsible for the "curable" patients, whereas Langenhorn (a long-term asylum) admitted those considered "hopeless." Though the files used in my analysis were obtained from Langenhorn, the medical histories from Friedrichsberg are part of these records. Within these asylums, zones were erected to contain patients who were classified as being unworthy of living; persons who were already classified as socially dead before they were physically killed. My analysis highlights how these zones were constructed and how patients "disappeared" into what I have termed spaces of exception.

The psychiatric asylum was just part of a psychiatric practice that could best be described as a disciplinary practice. This practice was based on a power structure that hierarchically placed the psychiatrist at the top. The nurses, as the delegated representatives of the psychiatrist's power, were strategically positioned "beneath" the patient, because only from this position was it feasible for them to understand the patient in every detail and to influence his or her behaviour in depth. Psychiatric practice (termed a practice and not a discourse because the asylum cannot be understood by scientific discourses alone) was characterized by this disciplinary power, because it was an anonymous power that aimed to influence the conduct of the patient. Nurses played a crucial role in this practice, as they were able to reach out and influence the patients' innermost thoughts and behaviours. The problem, however, was that scientific knowledge had no considerable impact on psychiatric practice itself. For example, patient treatment remained the same regardless of individual diagnoses. Therapy always aimed to influence patients' behaviour and the means employed to treat them were always the same. Irrespective of any psychiatric theory (if such a theory existed), the practice of psychiatry continued to construct a strategic power field within the asylum.

The strategic power distribution of psychiatric practice intervened to correct and influence certain behaviours of the insane. It was not related to a specific person but rather performed through a complex interplay of different actors. As a result, the asylum became a space where a kind of war took place between the disciplinary power of psychiatry (representing the "absolute will" of the psychiatrist) and the absolute power of the mentally ill – absolute because patients tried to force their reality onto their surroundings, for example, by claiming that "somebody is talking to me." By imposing their own "rules," patients opposed the "reality of the asylum."

This "war" led to a paradoxical situation wherein psychiatric practice tried to anticipate certain behaviours or to intervene before they occured, yet at the same time, it provoked these same behaviours. To analyze this strategic power field means grasping the intricate connections between a myriad of "technologies of power" that are directed onto the body of the patient and are aimed at profoundly transforming him or her. The asylum can thus be perceived as a kind of machine and psychiatric practice as a complex interplay between discourses, technologies, architecture, institutions – in other words, a dispositif. Apart from attempting to intrude the will of the psychiatrist into the patient, the dispositif installs certain lines of visibility, which is to say that within a dispositif only those aspects upon which the dispositif sheds light are visible. The question of what becomes visible or not within the dispositif is bound up with technologies of power, which allow an understanding of how knowledge is inscribed within the practical exercise of power, authority, and rule. The focus of such an analysis includes what a specific form of knowledge does and makes possible, and how it operates in relation to organized regimes of institutional practices and practical rationalities. A specific knowledge shapes particular ways of representing, seeing, acting, and intervening. Within networks, power is more or less the result of the successful coordination or alignment of different actors. Technical objects define and distribute roles to humans and non-humans and are linked to inscription devices of various sorts that include checklists, codes, records, and official documents. One of these inscriptions is the record that is constructed as a kind of "container of evidence" to support the insanity of the patient, but I argued that the record had more far reaching effects. My analysis highlights, for example, how the record constructed the identity of the patient and became the only reliable source of her biography. When Anna Maria Buller ceased to talk altogether, the record spoke in her place. The record not only represented the patient, but it also distributed specific roles to the nurses, psychiatrists, administrators, and so on. Furthermore, it initiated further action, intervening, for example, in her sterilization process and in the selection of her for murdering.

Technology approaches the forces of the body and the aptitudes and capabilities of individuals in order to shape their behaviour. It is invested with a strategic rationality that seeks to subsume the patient's conduct to the requirements of psychiatry, to introduce the will of the psychiatrist into the patient's core. The success of these interventions was determined by their ability to influence patient behaviour. Every time Buller behaved in a certain way that the nurses deemed illegitimate, they intervened with a whole range of specific devices that included patient restraints, isolation cells, and continuous baths. Even the shock therapies and medications used were first and foremost aimed at converting her behaviour, as the notes clearly indicated. This analysis highlights how this strategic interplay between different actors resulted in the production of patients as "empty shells" that could justifiably be murdered. At this point the analysis used the theoretical insights of Gorgio Agamben and his concept of "bare life." Even though some aspects of his approach were challenged by the results of this empirical research, his idea of "zones of exceptions" is helpful for comprehending how patients literally disappeared not only in the record but also became invisible in the asylum. Using Agamben's theoretical approach makes it possible to conceptualize the "zones of invisibility" as zones of banishment or "zones of exception." Anna Maria Buller and other patients in Langenhorn were abandoned by psychiatric practice but simultaneously, it maintained control over their lives and even intensified corporeal interventions.

The technologies mentioned above often produced effects that were not completely calculated. When Buller was incarcerated in an isolation cell for long periods of time, she began to talk to herself, threw her excrement, and started to destroy the mattress on which she had to sleep. Her isolation was meant to prevent her from disturbing the routine of the ward but it also had the consequence of bringing out a panoply of symptoms, demonstrating that technologies employed within psychiatric practice often produced behaviours later treated as deviant.

The medical record played an active, constitutive role because it shaped and maintained the patient's trajectory in the asylum and was involved in the construction of hierarchical relations between patients and psychiatrists, and psychiatrists and nurses. The record functioned as a "mediator" because it mediated the relations that acted and worked through it, transforming social interaction.

The medical record was activated through the practice of reading and writing. These practices, in which the record was turned to, leafed through, read, used for jotting, communicated through or dispatched, formed a crucial part of the sociotechnical organization of medical work. Without these practices, the record would lack relevance. These activities allowed it to have its mediating role in the organization. The psychiatrist could only be a psychiatrist, nurses could only be nurses, and the patient could only be diagnosed as mentally ill on the condition that this interrelation of people and paperwork existed. As previously described above, psychiatric practice was a complete appropriation of the patient's body and implied its complete control of it. The act of writing the record was a necessary precondition in allowing this appropriation of his or her body. Without the record, the discipline of psychiatry could not produce evidence; the writing of the record enabled information on "everything" that transpired and "everything" that the individual did to be transferred from the bottom up. Furthermore, these written records enabled information to be accessible at any time and hence assured the principle of the permanent visibility of the disciplinary system.

It is, of course, inaccurate to state that these scripts captured everything – every action and observation of the patient – because information was selectively compiled and included in the record. Not everything was noted because the space in the record was limited and the recorded information had to be written in such a manner that it was useable in the workspace. Since the written information became evidence of the madness of the patient, how the psychiatrists and nurses depicted this insanity depended on the descriptive categories they selected and employed in the record (and these categories were derived from scientific discourses). Information from diverse sources was constantly compressed into short statements of "what really happened" and summarized into "what was the case." The psychiatrists condensed the information gathered from tests, patients, their relatives, nurses, and previous entries, to create a concise statement of the relevant "problems" and their histories. The patient's history was thus selectively re-written. Detailed descriptions were lost within pages and were no longer considered factual. They were summarized in one sentence, and later, in one word, as was the case in the re-formulation of Buller's case history in the sterilization process and later in the *Meldebogen* T4.

This ongoing re-summarizing also contributed to the construction of narratives in which the ambiguities, the ad hoc and fluid character of the medical work, were lost. This restructuring was required to produce an account supporting specific actions or enabling effective communication of what was going on. This reconstruction work can be seen in the medical examination form for Buller's sterilization in 1935, the discharge letter from Eppendorf in 1942, as well as in the *Meldebogen* T4. Almost every sentence of these reports reflected a history of repeated reconstructive work.

Documents possess the ability to coordinate different levels within a disciplinary system and by "objectifying" information, they govern complex disciplinary systems. Documentary reality evolves and significantly affects the patient's situation in the asylum. For example, the *Meldebogen* T4 was specially designed as a kind of checklist to identify patients who were destined to be killed. Completing this report pronounced a verdict, thus making the form performative. A court proceeding was necessary to decide on Buller's sterilization. The asylum was transformed into a courtroom and the psychiatrist became simultaneously the expert witness, judge, and executioner. This process was a virtual process because all the correspondence between the court, the patient, and her family took place in the record; it became a Kafkaesque process because Buller was not informed of what was going on, and the sentence was executed without providing her the opportunity to intervene.

Through the writing of the documents, a direct and continuous relation between the script and the patient's body was established. The visibility of the patient's body and the permanence of the script cannot be separated, an effect that could be called a schematized and centralized individualization. It is only through the record that the "somatic singularity" becomes an individual, and the biography that evolves becomes the history of the individual. The patient's body, gestures, behaviours, and discourses are surrounded by a script-tissue (a graphic plasma) that records, codes, and schematizes. This centralized individualization is of crucial significance for psychiatric practice, because the "insane" have to recognize themselves within their written biographies. They must acknowledge that the events reported in their own records really happened, and only if they are capable of recognizing themselves do they have a chance of being "cured." The mechanisms of this "identity construction" correspond to Althusser's explanation of the constitution of subjects. Only at the moment that a somatic singularity is hailed by the power, and in turn, reacts to it, does it become a subject.

The analysis also demonstrated that the making of the text in the record proceeded through different stages. First of all, the nurses noted their observations according to descriptive categories that they had learned during their training. Second, the psychiatrists reformulated the nurses' notes according to their own diagnostic pattern, and seemingly followed from the nurses' notes as if they were based inductively on "what really happened." All of the work that the nurses invested in their own notes (especially the utilization of different technologies) was invisible in those written by the psychiatrists. Third, the psychiatrists' notes become part of other official documents that led to further interventions (for example the *Meldebogen* T4).

Based on this understanding, the crucial point of my analysis is the following: if it is correct that the somatic singularity becomes an individual only through the fact that notes are taken and written down, then this implies that if the note taking stops, the individual ceases to be a subject and falls into a zone of indifference. The patient's identity breaks down, because the patient no longer exists within the documentation. If these patients cease to exist in the record, then this implies that anything could be done with them, because they are socially dead – reduced to their "bare life." From a certain moment on, after some patients were transferred to Langenhorn, they seemed to disappear from the record. They existed only in the psychiatrists' notes, often taken irregularly, and in the administration record. In sum, patients like Anna Maria Buller disappeared from the record, and then physically disappeared through their murders. Nonetheless, we must never forget that patients' intense suffering during their stay in the asylum was real and it must be acknowledged.

Finally, some important limitations of the present book must be emphasized. Two elements of the record were only barely mentioned in the analysis. The first was the photographs that the psychiatrists took throughout Anna Maria Buller's multiple admissions to the asylums and which constitute the book cover (see Appendix 2). These photographs deserve a detailed study of their own since they were "immutable mobiles" as defined in chapter 3, and made the madness visible at a glance. Also part of her record is the collection of drawings she did, only some of which were able to be mentioned. Psychiatrists, as "art critics," labeled these drawings as "degenerate art" and thus they became more visible evidence of Buller's madness. They, too, need an analysis of their own. The drawings are contained in the Appendix. Another more serious limitation of this book must be mentioned. More detailed research is needed to confirm the hypothesis of this study that the reasons for the patients' murders after 1945 must be searched for in psychiatric practice as such. The suspicions that patients were killed by applying shock therapies and other medical interventions and that some patients were systematically deprived of sufficient nutrition especially must be analyzed in more depth. Further research should also be conducted on files from different periods of time, especially the period after the end of the Second World War.

Although this book was supported by information gleaned from other patient records, it focused primarily on one medical file. Thus, there are obvious limitations on its ability to claim that the results can be generalized. To widen its scope, more systematic analysis could be carried out to understand the differences and similarities within different German asylums in the same time period as this book. Finally, studies of medical files from different countries and institutional settings, particularly in psychiatric practices, could provide an international perspective on the role and function of both the record itself and nurses' contributions to it.

Nonetheless, the strength of this book lies in its demonstration of how fruitful a detailed analysis of one medical record can be. The Nazi regime carries certain kinds of perceptions; it is viewed as a particularly brutal era but also one that is in the past. This kind of analysis, however, has implications for nurses and nursing practice that reach into the present. It sheds light on how concepts of norms and the idea of normalization – as a subconscious part of everyday medical practice – are transcribed onto the written record. It describes how the written record – and the role that nurses play in its construction – has real power to shape the identity of patients, with potentially devastating consequences for them. Since the medical record continues to be the prime form of communication about patients and their treatment, it is my belief that nurses need to understand the power of the record throughout history.

Although the reader may well feel that the "unmaking" of Anna Maria Buller was barbarian (continuous baths, drug treatments, etc), barbarism continues to exist – in a different way but based on similar underlying mechanisms. Record keeping, for example, is still an important task and few health care professionals are aware of the scope and consequences of their reporting. This aspect becomes even more pertinent as the use of electronic Patient Data Management Systems increases and extends the active role played by the collection of patient data in creating specific subjectivities and patient identities within hospitals. Furthermore, long term care facilities, psychiatric hospitals, and other institutions continue to be places where the idea of bare life exists, making this ability of record keeping of crucial importance not only for contemporary nursing but also for medicine and other health care professions. Insights from this research provide useful inspiration for an ethics of vulnerability in health care.

Appendix

Appendix 1 – Drawings

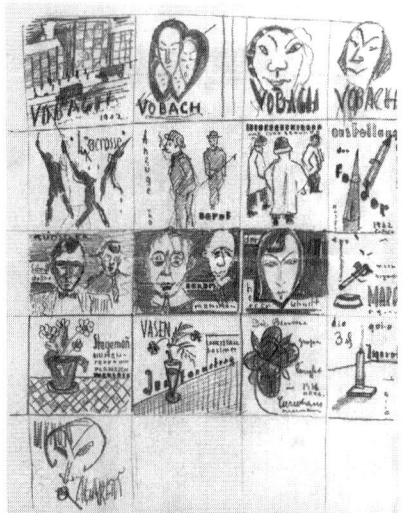
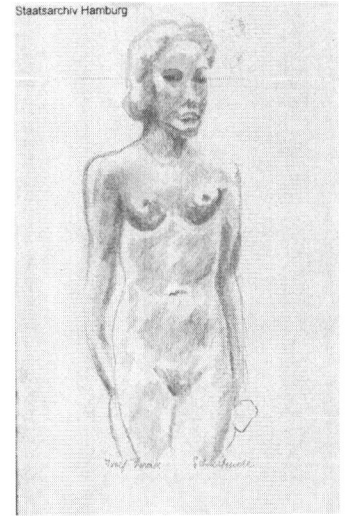
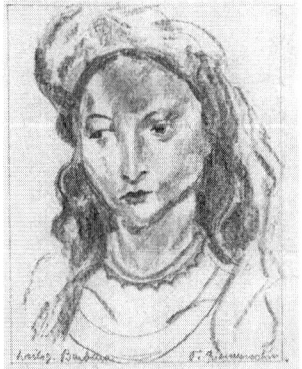
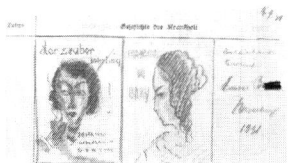

Figure 37, 38, 39 and 40: Some of Anna Maria Buller's drawings.

Appendix 2 – Admission Photographies of Anna Maria Buller

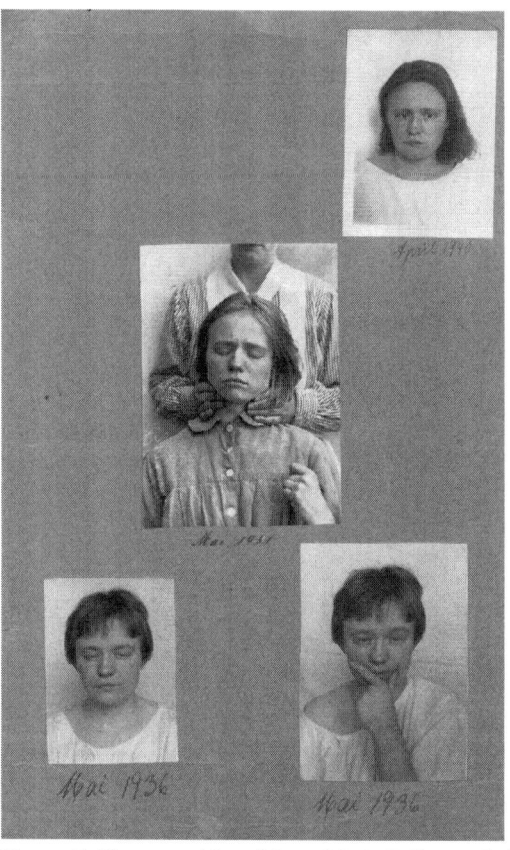

Figure 41: Photographies of Anna Maria Buller made by the psychiatrists, with the year specifications.

Bibliography

Primary Sources

A. State Archives of Hamburg (Staatsarchiv Hansestadt Hamburg)

A.1 State Asylum Langenhorn (Staatskrankenanstalt Langenhorn) 352–8-7

Patient Records: Transfer from Langenhorn to State archive 1 – 1995

Anna Maria B.	28338
Martha M. O. A.	13986
Elisabeth E. A. F.	10243
Richard R. H. A.	23121
Alwine K.	26752
Martha E. A.	16292
Werner A. F. R., Dr.	22694
Henriette A.	23548
Heinrich M.	27846
Erika W.	23856
Karl W. E. B.	23536

Administrative Records: 352–8-7 Transfer from Langenhorn to State archive 2 – 1995

Construction, Enlargement, Organisation of the Asylum (Errichtung, Erweiterung, Organisation der Anstalt):

1909–1916	File 8
1913, 1925, 1927	File 9
1925–1928	File 12
Considerations about a Transformation of the Asylum into a Care Facility under the control of the Social Services as Mean of Cost Savings (Erwägungen über die Umwandlung der Anstalt in eine Pflegeanstalt der Wohlfahrstbehörde aus Kostenersparnisgründen)	File 15

Diverse Affairs of the Asylum (Diverse Anstaltsangelegenheiten):
  Quaterly Reports from 1899 to 1920 Annual Reports (fragmentary) from   File 16a
  1906 to 1931, 1937, 1938. (Quartalsberichte für 1899 bis 1920
  (unvollständig) Jahresberichte für 1906 bis 1931, 1937, 1938.)

Inspection Protocols of the Commission for the Regulation of the Service for the Insane 1900–1936.	File 17
Other Reports (Andere Berichte)	File 110

Sterilizations (Sterilisationen)

Individual Cases (Einzelfälle) 1934–1940, 1941	File 134
Annual Statistics (Jahresstatistiken) 1893–1924 (fragmentary)	File 139
The Right to Complain of Sick Persons and their Relatives (Beschwerderecht der Kranken und deren Angehörigen) 1901–1920, 1922	File 147
Nurses. Education. Pflegepersonal. Establishment of the Nursing School. (Ausbildung. Eröffnung der Irrenpflegeschule)	File 46

A.2   Provincial Government of the City of Hamburg, Health Authority: 352–3

Medical Council II	File L1d Volume 1
	File L1d Volume 2
	File L5 Volume 3

A.3   Higher Education II File Gb11 Volume 1

A.4   Public Prosecutor's Department Hamburg (Staatsanwaltschaft Hamburg) File Number: 147 Js 58/67

Bill of Indictment (Anklageschrift) against Lensch and Dr. Struve	File 147 Js 58/67
Special Volumes (Sonderbände), Volume 1 and 2	Pages 1–350
Supplementary Files: Report for the Prosecutor by Josef Radzicki	Pages 3315–3419

Secondary Sources

Adams, Mark Buller, ed. The Wellborn Science: Eugenics in Germany, France, Brazil, and Russia. New York/Oxford: Oxford University Press, 1990.
Agamben, Giorgio. Ausnahmezustand. Frankfurt a.M.: Suhrkamp, 2004.
–. Homo sacer. Die Souveränität der Macht und das nackte Leben. Frankfurt a.M.: Suhrkamp, 2002.
–. Homo Sacer: Sovereign Power and Bare Life. Translated by D. Heller-Roazen. Stanford, California: Stanford University Press, 1998.
–. State of Exception. Chicago: University of Chicago Press, 2005.
Althusser, Louis. "Ideology and Ideological State Apparatuses: Notes Towards an Investigation." In Lenin and Philosophy and Other Essays, 85–126. New York: Monthly Review Press, 2001.

Aly, Götz. "Medicine against the Useless." In Cleansing the Fatherland. Nazi Medicine and Racial Hygiene, edited by Götz Aly, Peter Chroust and Christian Pross, 22–99. Baltimore: Johns Hopkins University Press, 1994.
–. Medizin gegen Unbrauchbare, in Aussonderung und Tod. Die klinische Hinrichtung der Unbrauchbaren, edited by Götz Aly, Angelika Ebbinghaus, Matthias Hamann, Friedemann Pfäfflin, Gerd Preissler, Beiträge zur nationalsozialistischen Gesundheits- und Sozialpolitik: 1 ed., 9–74. Berlin: Rotbuch Verlag.
Aly, Götz and Karl Heinz Roth. Die restlose Erfassung. Volkszählen, Identifizieren, Aussondern im Nationalsozialismus. Farnkfurt a.M.: Fischer, 2005.
Alzheimer Society. "What is Korsakoff's Syndrome?" accessed 07/23, 2012, http://alzheimers.org.uk/site/scripts/documents_info.php?documentID=98.
Amtsblatt, Public Law 152, (1904): 915.
Arendt, Hannah. The Origins of Totalitarianism. New York: Harcourt Brace Jovanovich, 1994.
Arnold, Doris. "Pflege und Macht. Der Beitrag Foucaults." In Pflege-Räume, Macht und Alltag, edited by Sabine Braunschweig, 155–164. Zürich: Chronos, 2006.
Aspe, Bernard, & Combes, Muriel. "Retour sur le camp comme paradigme biopolitique." Multitudes 1, no. 1 (2001): 29–44.
Atkinson, Paul. The Clinical Experience: The Construction and Reconstruction of Medical Reality. Farnborough: Gower, 1981.
Austin, John L. Zur Theorie der Sprechakte (How to do things with words). Stuttgart: Reclam, 2002.
Bajohr, Frank and Michael Wildt, eds. Volksgemeinschaft. Neue Forschungen zur Gesellschaft des Nationalsozialismus. Frankfurt a.M.: Fischer, 2009.
Barker, Phil and Gary Rolfe. "Psychiatric Nursing: Living with the Legacy of the Holocaust." Journal of Psychiatric and Mental Health Nursing 9 (2002): 365–375.
Becker, Heinrich. Der Umgang mit widerstrebenden Kranken. Geisteskrankenpflege. Monatsschrift für Geisteskranken- und Krankenpflege, 40, no. 8 (1936): 116–118.
Benedict, Susan. "Killing while Caring: The Nurses of Hadamar." Issues in Mental Health Nursing 24, no. 1 (Jan-Feb 2003): 59–79.
–. "The Nadir of Nursing: Nurse-Perpetrators of the Ravensbrück Concentration Camp." Nursing History Review 1 (2003): 129–146.
Benedict, Susan, Arthur Caplan, and Traute Lafrenz Page. "Duty and 'Euthanasia': The Nurses of Meseritz-Obrawalde." Nursing Ethics 14, no. 6 (Nov. 2007): 781–794.
Benedict, Susan and Jane M. Georges. "Nurses and the Sterilization Experiments of Auschwitz: A Postmodernist Perspective." Nursing Inquiry 13, no. 4 (Dec. 2006): 277–288.
Benedict, Susan and Jochen Kuhla. "Nurses' Participation in the Euthanasia Programs of Nazi Germany." Western Journal of Nursing Research 21, no. 2 (Apr. 1999): 246–263.
Berg, Marc. "Practices of Reading and Writing: The Constitutive Role of the Patient Record in Medical Work." Sociology of Health and Illness 18, no. 4 (1996): 499–524.
Berghs, Maria, Bernadette Dierckx de Casterlé, and Chris Gastmans. "Practices of Responsibility and Nurses during the Euthanasia Programs of Nazi Germany: A Discussion Paper." International Journal of Nursing Studies 44, no. 5 (July 2007): 845–854.
Binding, Karl and Alfred Hoche. Die Freigabe der Vernichtung lebensunwerten Lebens. Ihr Maß und ihre Form (1920). Berlin: Berliner Wissenschaftsverlag, 2006.

Black, Edwin. IBM und der Holocaust. Die Verstrickung des Weltkonzerns in die Verbrechen der Nazis. München: Ullstein, 2002.
Bleuler, Eugen. Lehrbuch der Psychiatrie, edited by Manfred Bleuler, Josef Berze. Berlin: Springer-Verlag, 1943.
– . Lehrbuch der Psychiatrie. Berlin: Springer, 1923.
Böhme, Klaus, ed. 1893 – 1993 100 Jahre Allgemeines Krankenhaus Ochsenzoll. Hamburg: Sozialtherapiezentrum des AK Ochsenzoll, 1993.
Böhme, Klaus and Uwe Lohalm, eds. Wege in den Tod. Hamburgs Anstalt Langenhorn und die Euthanasie in der Zeit des Nationalsozialismus. Forum Zeitgeschichte ed. Vol. 2. Cloppenburg: Ergebnisse Verlag, 1993.
Breiding, Birgit. Die braunen Schwestern. Ideologie, Struktur, Funktion einer nationalsozialistischen Elite. Stuttgart: Franz Steiner Verlag, 1998.
Brown, Wendy. Regulating Aversion. Tolerance in the Age of Identity and Empire. Princeton: Princeton University Press, 2008.
Brush, Barbara L. "Nursing Care and Context in Theresienstadt." Western Journal of Nursing Research 26, no. 8 (Dec. 2004): 860 – 871.
Bublitz, Hannelore. Diskurs. Einsichten – Vielsichten ed. Bielefeld: transcript, 2003.
–. "Täuschend natürlich. Zur Dynamik gesellschaftlicher Automatismen, ihrer Ereignishaftigkeit und strukturbildenden Kraft." In Automatismen, ed. by Hannelore Bublitz, Roman Marek, Christina L. Steinmann and Hartmut Winkler, 153 – 171. München: Wilhelm Fink, 2010.
Buck, Dorothea. "70 Years of Coercion in German Psychiatric Institutions, Experienced and Witnessed." http://www.bpe-online.de/1/buck-wpa-2007-e.pdf, accessed 04/10, 2011
Buder, Dr. Über das Alleinlegen. Die Irrenpflege. Monatsschrift für Irren- und Krankenpflege 22 (1918): 2 – 12.
Burleigh, Michael. Death and Deliverance: "Euthanasia" in Germany c 1900 – 1945. Cambridge, England: Cambridge University Press, 1994.
Bussolini, Jeffrey. "What is a Dispositive?" Foucault Studies 10 (2010): 85 – 107.
Butler, Judith. Excitable Speech. A Politics of the Performative. London: Routledge, 1997.
–. "Gender Regulations." In Undoing Gender, 40 – 56. New York: Routledge, 2004.
–. "Indefinite Detention." In Precarious Life: The Powers of Mourning and Violence, 51 – 100. London, New York: Verso, 2004.
–. The Psychic Life of Power: Theories in Subjection. Stanford: Stanford University Press, 1997.
Butler, Judith and Gayatri Chakravorty Spivak. Who Sings the Nation-State?: Language, Politics, Belonging. London ; New York: Seagull Books, 2007.
Castel, Robert. The Regulation of Madness: The Origins of Incarceration in France. Great Britain: University of California Press, 1988.
Cavarero, Adriana. Horrorism. Naming Contemporary Violence. New York: Columbia University Press, 2009.
Cicourel, Aaron V. "Police Practices and Official Records." In Ethnomethodology. Selected Readings, ed. Roy Turner, 85 – 95. Middlesex, England: Penguin Education, 1975.
Clark, Samuel N. and Frank Garm Norbury. "A Possible Role of the Element of Fear in Metrazol Therapy." Diseases of the Nervous System 2, no. 6 (1941): 196 – 198.

Cohen, Louis H. "The Early Effects of Metrazol Therapy in Chronic Psychotic Over-Activity." American Journal of Psychiatry 95 (1938): 327–333.

–. "Observations on the Convulsant Treatment of Schizophrenia with Metrazol." The New England Journal of Medicine 218, no. 24 (1938): 1002–1007.

–. "The Therapeutic Significance of Fear in the Metrazol Treatment of Schizophrenia." American Journal of Psychiatry 95 (1939): 1349–1357.

Colomb, H. O. and G. L. Wadsworth. "An Analysis of Results in the Metrazol Shock Therapy of Schizophrenia." Journal of Nervous and Mental Disease 93, no. 1 (1941): 53–62.

Cummins, J. A. "Metrazol Shock Therapy Administered in the General Hospital." Canadian Medical Association Journal 50 (1944): 420–421.

Dean, Michael. "Putting the Technological into Government." History of the Human Sciences 9, no. 3 (1996): 47–68.

Deleuze, Gilles. "Qu'est-ce qu'un dispositif?" In Michel Foucault philosophe. Rencontre internationale Paris, 9,10,11 Janvier 1988, 185–194. Paris: Éditions du Seuil, 1989.

Delius, Peter. Das Ende von Strecknitz: Die Lübecker Heilanstalt und ihre Auflösung 1941: Ein Beitrag zur Sozialgeschichte der Psychiatrie im Nationalsozialismus. Kiel: Malik-Verlag, 1988.

Dreyfus, Hubert L. and Paul Rabinow, eds. Michel Foucault: Beyond Structuralism and Hermeneutics. Brighton: Harvester, 1982.

Ebbinghaus, Angelika. "Kostensenkung, 'Aktive Therapie' und Vernichtung. Konsequenzen für das Anstaltswesen." In Heilen und Vernichten im Mustergau Hamburg. Bevölkerungs- und Gesundheitspolitik im Dritten Reich, eds. Angelika Ebbinghaus, Heidrun Kaupen-Haas and Karl Heinz Roth, 136–146. Hamburg: Konkret Literatur Verlag, 1984.

Ebbinghaus, Angelika, Heidrun Kaupen-Haas, and Karl Heinz Roth. Heilen und Vernichten im Mustergau Hamburg. Bevölkerungspolitik im Dritten Reich. Hamburg: Konkret Literatur Verlag, 1984.

Enge, Dr. "Aufgaben des Pflegepersonals bei der Insulinschock- und der Cardiazol- bzw. Azomankrampf-Behandlung." Geisteskrankenpflege. Monatsschrift für Geisteskranken- und Krankenpflege 44, no. 11 (1941): 134–136.

–. "Beobachtungsberichte des Pflegepersonals" Geisteskrankenpflege. Monatsschrift für Geisteskranken- und Krankenpflege 37, no. 1 (1933): 113–115.

–. "Krankheitsfeststellung durch bloße Betrachtung" Geisteskrankenpflege. Monatsschrift für Geisteskranken- und Krankenpflege 40, no. 9 (1936):129–138.

–. "Die Vorgeschichte (Anamnese) und ihre Bedeutung für die Krankheitsfeststellung (Diagnose)." Geisteskrankenpflege. Monatsschrift für Geisteskranken- und Krankenpflege 37, no. 6 (1933): 87–90.

Faulstich, Heinz. Hungersterben in der Psychiatrie 1914–1949. Mit einer Topographie der NS-Psychiatrie. Freiburg im Breisgau: Lambertus, 1998.

–. "Die Zahl der 'Euthanasie'-Opfer." In "Euthanasie" und die aktuelle Sterbehilfe-Debatte. Die historischen Hintergründe medizinischer Ethik, eds. Andreas Frewer and Clemens Eickhoff, 218–234. Frankfurt, New York: Campus, 2000.

Foth, Thomas. "Nurses, Medical Records and the Killing of Sick Persons before, during and After the Nazi Regime in Germany." Nursing Inquiry March 7 (2012): Doi: 10.1111/j.1440-1800.2012.00596.x.

–. "Regieren durch Akten. Die Funktion der Patient Innenakten bei den Krankenmorden während des NS-Faschismus." In Strukturentstehung durch Verflechtung. Akteur-Netzwerktheorie(n) und Automatismen, eds. Hannelore Bublitz, Tobias Conradi and Florian Mühe, 219–235. München: Wilhelm Fink, 2011.
Foucault, Michel. Abnormal. Lectures at the Collège De France 1974–1975. Trans. Graham Burchell, eds. Arnold I. Davidson, Valerio Marchetti, Antonello Salomoni, François Ewald and Ewald Fontana. USA: Picador, 2003.
–. Geschichte der Gouvernementalität I. Sicherheit, Territorien, Bevölkerung. Trans. Claudia Brede-Konersmann and Jürgen Schröder, ed. Michel Sennelart, Frankfurt a.M.: Suhrkamp, 2004.
–. L'archéologie du savoir. France: Gallimard, 2008.
–. Les Anormaux. Cours au Collège de France. 1974–1975. Hautes études, eds. François Ewald, Alessandro Fontana, Valerio Marchetti and Antonella Salomoni Seuil/Gallimard, 1999.
–. Il faut défendre la société. Cours au College de France. 1976. France: Gallimard Seuil, 1997.
–. "Governmentality." In Power: Essentials Works of Foucault 1954–1984, ed. James D. Faubion, 201–222. London: Penguin Books, 1994.
–. "Le jeu de Michel Foucault." In Dits et Ecrits, eds. Michel Foucault, Daniel Defert, François Ewald and Jacques Lagrange. Vol. 3. Paris: Gallimard, 1994.
–. Le pouvoir psychiatrique. Cours au collège de France. 1973–1974, Hautes études, eds. François Ewald, Alessandro Fontana and Jacques Lagrange. France: Seuil/Gallimard, 2003.
–. Madness and Civilization: A History of Insanity in the Age of Reason. Trans. Richard Howard. New York: Vintage Books, 1973.
–. "Panopticism." In Discipline & Punish: The Birth of the Prison. Trans. Alan Sheridan, 195–228. USA: Vintage Books, 1995.
–. Psychiatric Power: Lectures at the Collège De France, 1973–74. Translated by Graham Burchell, edited by Jaques Langrange, Arnold I. Davidson, François Ewald and Alessandro Fontana. New York: Palgrave Mac Millan, 2006.
–. Sécurité, Territoire, Population. Cours au Collège de France. 1977–1978. France: Gallimard Seuil, 2004.
–. Society must be Defended: Lectures at the Collège De France 1975–1976, eds. Mauro Bertani, Alessandro Fontana and François Ewald. New York: Picador, 2003.
–. "The Subject and Power." In Michel Foucault: Beyond Structuralism and Hermeneutics, eds. Hubert L. Dreyfus and Paul Rabinow, 208–226. Chicago: University of Chicago Press, 1983.
–. Überwachen und Strafen. Die Geburt des Gefägnisses. Frankfurt a.M.: Suhrkamp, 1994.
–. Wahnsinn und Gesellschaft. Frankfurt a.M.: Suhrkamp, 1969.
Friedlander, Henry. The Origins of Nazi Genocide: From Euthanasia to the Final Solution. Chapel Hill: University of North Carolina Press, 1995.
Friedrich, Norbert. "Christentum und Krankenpflege-Einige historische Anmerkungen." In Quellen zur Geschichte der Krankenpflege, ed. Sylvelin Hähner-Rombach, 43–58. Frankfurt am Main: Mabuse-Verlag, 2008.
Fürstler, Gerhard and Peter Malina. "Ich tat nur meinen Dienst." Zur Geschichte der Krankenpflege in Österreich in der NS-Zeit. Wien: Facultas, 2004.

Gaida, Ulrike. "Eugenik im Deutschen Reich und im Nationalsozialismus." In Quellen zur Geschichte der Krankenpflege. Mit Einführungen und Kommentaren, ed. Sylvelyn Hähner-Rombach, 531–543. Frankfurt a.M.: Mabuse, 2008.

–. Zwischen Pflegen und Töten. Krankenschwestern im Nationalsozialismus. Einführung und Quellen für Unterricht und Selbststudium. Frankfurt a.M.: Mabuse, 2006.

Garfinkel, Harold. "Good Organizational Reasons for 'Bad' Clinic Records." In Studies in Ethnomethodology, Harold Garfinkel, 186–207. Cambridge: Polity Press, 2010.

Gellately, Robert. Backing Hitler: Consent and Coercion in Nazi Germany. New York: Oxford University Press, 2009.

–. "Denunciation as a Subject of Historical Research." In Denunciation in the 20th Century, ed. Inge Marszolek, 16–29. Kölln: Quantum, 2001.

Goffman, Erving. Asylums: Essays on the Social Situation of Mental Patients and Other Inmates. New York: Doubleday and Co., 1961.

Gooding, David. "Putting Agency Back into Experiment." In Science as Practice and Culture, ed. Andrew Pickering, 63–112. Chicago: University of Chicago Press, 1992.

Gordon, Hirsch L. "Fifty Shock Therapy Theories." The Military Surgeon 102–103 (1948): 397–401.

Hacking, Ian. "Biopower and the Avalanche of Printed Numbers." Humanities in Society Band 5 (1982): 279–295.

–. "Making Up People." In Reconstructing Individualism: Autonomy, Individuality, and Self in Western Thought, eds. Thomas C. Heller, Morton Sosna and David E. Wellbery, 222–237. Stanford: Stanford University Press, 1986.

Hall, Stuart. "Signification, Representation, Ideology: Althusser and the Post-Structuralist Debates." In Critical Studies in Mass Communication, eds. R. K. Avery and D. Eason, 88–113. New York: The Guilford Press, 1991.

Harms, Ingo. "Krankenmord in der Heil- und Pflegeanstalt Wehnen – Forschungsprobleme." In NS-"Euthanasie" und lokaler Krankenmord in Oldenburg, Klingenmünster und Sachsen. Erinnerungskultur und Betroffenenperspektive: Berichte des Arbeitskreises Band 6, ed. Arbeitskreis zur Erforschung der nationalsozialistischen "Euthanasie" und Zwangssterilisation, 25–42. Münster: Klemm und Oelschläger, 2011.

–. 'Wat mööt wi hier smachten…' Hungertod und 'Euthanasie' in der Heil- und Pflegeanstalt Wehnen im 'Dritten Reich'. Oldenburg: Druck & Verlagscooperative GmbH, 1996.

Hinrichs, Ullrich. "Über Dauerschlafbehandlung mit Scopolamin-Paraldehyd bei Geisteskranken." Zeitschrift für die gesamte Neurologie und Psychiatrie 105, no. 1 (1926): 623–633.

Hohendorf, Gerrit. "Ideengeschichte und Realgeschichte der nationalsozialistischen "Euthanasie" im Überblick." In "Das Vergessen der Vernichtung ist Teil der Vernichtung selbst" Lebensgeschichten von Opfern der nationalsozialistischen "Euthanasie", eds. Petra Fuchs, Maike Rotzoll, Ulrich Müller, Paul Richter and Gerrit Hohendorf, 36–52. Göttingen: Wallstein Verlag, 2008.

Hohendorf, Gerrit, Maike Rotzoll, Paul Richter, Walter Eckart, and Christian Mundt. "Die Opfer der nationalsozialistischen "Euthanasie-Aktion T4". Erste Ergebniss eines Projektes zur Erschließung von Krankenakten getöteter Patienten im Bundesarchiv Berlin." Der Nervenarzt 73, no.11 (2002): 1065–1074.

Holmes, Dave. "Police and Pastoral Power: Governmentality and Correctional Forensic Psychiatric Nursing." Nursing Inquiry 9, no. 2 (2002): 84–92.

Holmes, Dave and Denise Gastaldo. "Nursing as Means of Governmentality." Journal of Advanced Nursing 38, no. 6 (2002): 557–565.

Hoskins, Sylvia A. "Nurses and National Socialism – a Moral Dilemma: One Historical Example of a Route to Euthanasia." Nursing Ethics 12, no. 1 (Jan. 2005): 79–91.

Humbert, F. and A. Friedemann. "Critique and Indications of Treatments in Schizophrenia." American Journal of Psychiatry 94, no. 2 (1938): 174–183.

Jaroszewski, Zdzislaw, ed. Die Ermordung der Geisteskranken in Polen 1939–1945. Warszawa: Wydawnictwo Naukowne PWN, 1993.

Jelliffe, Smith Ely. "Discussion Paper Presented at the Section of Neurology and Psychiatry, New York, Academy of Medicine, and the New York Neurological Society. Joint Meeting, January 12, 1937." Journal of Nervous and Mental Disease 85, no. 5 (1937): 575–578

Johnson, Terry. "Governmentality and the Institutionalization of Expertise." In Health Professions and the State in Europe, eds. Terry Johnson, Gerald Larkin, and Mike Saks, 7–24. London: Routledge, 1995.

Jones, Kingsley. "Insulin Coma Therapy in Schizophrenia." Journal of the Royal Society of Medicine 93 (2000): 147–149.

Kaiser, Jochen-Christoph. "Konfessionelle Wohlfahrtspflege im Nationalsozialismus. Caritas und Innere Mission." In Caritas und Diakonie in der NS-Zeit. Beispiele aus Niedersachsen, ed. Hans Otte, 45–61. Hildesheim: Olms, 2001.

Kankeleit, Dr. Was kosten die Minderwertigen den Staat? Hamburger Anzeiger 21, no. 12 (1925): 10.

Keller, Reiner. Wissenssoziologische Diskursanalyse. Grundlegung eines Forschungsprogramms. Wiesbaden: VS Verlag, 2005.

Kerschbaumer, L. "Spontaneous Reactions to Metrazol Therapy." Journal of Nervous and Mental Disease 98 (1943): 390–395.

Kiesow, Rainer M. "Ius sacrum. Gorgio Agamben und das nackte Recht," http://magazines.documenta.de/attachment/000000778.pdf., accessed 27 December 2007.

Klee, Ernst. "Euthanasie" im NS-Staat. Die "Vernichtung lebensunwerten Lebens". Frankfurt a.M.: Fischer, 2009.

Kraepelin, Emil. Psychiatrie: Ein Lehrbuch für Studierende und Ärzte. Vol. 2, Klinische Psychiatrie. Leipzig: Barth, 1922.

Kreutzer, Susanne. "'Before, We Were Always There-Now, Everything is Separate': On Nursing Reforms in Western Germany." Nursing History Review 16 (2008): 180–200.

–. "Die Einheit von Leibes- und Seelenpflege als Kern des tradierten christlichen Pflegeverständnisses." In Transformationen pflegerischen Handelns. Institutionelle Kontexte und soziale Praxis vom 19. bis 21. Jahrhundert, ed. Susanne Kreutzer, 109–130. Göttingen: V&R unipress, Universität Osnabrück, 2010a.

–. "Fragmentierung der Pflege. Umbrüche pflegerischen Handelns in den 1960er Jahren." In Transformationen pflegerischen Handelns, ed. Susanne Kreutzer, 109–130. Göttingen: V&R unipress, Universität Osnabrück, 2010b.

–. "Nursing Body and Soul in the Parish: Lutheran Deaconess Motherhouses in Germany and the United States." Nursing History Review 18 (2010): 134–150.

Kreßin, Arthur. Das allgemeine Krankenhaus Langenhorn in Hamburg: 1950. Hamburg: Wöll, 1950.

Kühl, Stefan. Die Internationale der Rassisten. Aufstieg und Niedergang der internationalen Bewegung für Eugenik und Rassenhygiene im 20. Jahrhundert. Frankfurt a.M.: Campus, 1997.
–. The Nazi Connection: Eugenics, American Racism, and German National Socialism. New York: Oxford University Press, 1994.
Kwan, Patrick and Martin J. Brodie. "Phenobarbital for the Treatment of Epilepsy in the 21st Century: A Critical Review." Epilepsia (2004), Wiley Online Library, http://onlinelibrary.wiley.com.proxy.biBulleruottawa.ca/doi/10.1111/j.0013-9580.2004.12704.x/full, accessed 24 December 2011.
Latour, Bruno. "The Powers of Association." In Power, Action, and Belief: A New Sociology of Knowledge, ed. John Law. Sociological Review Monograph, 32 ed. London: Routledge and Kegan Paul, 1986.
–. "Technology is Society made Durable." In A Sociology of Monsters: Essays on Power, Technology and Domination, ed. John Law, 103–131. London: Routledge, 1991.
–. "Pragmatogonies. A Mythical Account of how Humans and Nonhumans Swap Properties." American Behavioral Scientist 37, no. 6 (1994): 791–808.
–. Reassembling the Social: An Introduction to Actor-Network-Theory. New York: Oxford University Press, 2005.
–. Science in Action. Cambridge: Harvard University Press, 2003.
–. "Visualisation and Cognition: Thinking with Eyes and Hands." Knowledge and Society no. 6 (1986): 1–40.
–. We have Never Been Modern. Cambridge, Massachusetts: Harvard University Press, 2002.
Latour, Bruno and Steve Woolgar. Laboratory Life: The Construction of Scientific Facts. Princeton: Princeton University Press, 1986.
Law, John. "Notes on the Theory of the Actor Network: Ordering, Strategy and Heterogeneity." Centre for Science Studies, Lancaster University, http://www.lancs.ac.uk/fass/sociology/papers/law-notes-on-ant.pdf, accessed 24 January 2012.
Lemke, Thomas. Bio-Politics: An Advanced Introduction. New York: New York University Press, 2011.
–. Eine Kritik der politischen Vernunf. Foucaults Analyse der modernen Gouvernementalität. Hamburg: Argument, 1997.
–. "Die politische Ökonomie des Lebens – Biopolitik und Rassismus bei Michel Foucault und Gorgio Agamben," http://www.thomaslemkeweBullerde/publikationen/Die%20politische%20%D6konomie%20des%20Lebens%20ll.pdf, accessed 7 December 2007.
Lemke, Thomas, Susanne Krasmann, and Ulrich Bröckling. "Gouvernementalität, Neoliberalismus und Selbsttechnologien. Eine Einleitung." In Gouvernementalität der Gegenwart. Studien zur Ökonomisierung des Sozialen, eds. Thomas Lemke, Susanne Krasmann and Ulrich Bröckling, 7–40. Frankfurt a.M.: Suhrkamp, 2000.
Lessing, Michael Buller. Handbuch der praktischen Arzneimittellehre. Für Studierende, praktische Aerzte, Physicats-Aerzte und Apotheker, 6. ed. Vol. 2. Berlin: Verlag von Albert Förstner, 1851.
Levi, Primo. Les naufragés et les rescapés. Quarante ans après Auschwitz. France: Arcades Gallimard, 2008a.
–. Si c'est un homme. France: Julliard, 2008b.
Link, Jürgen. "Diskursanalyse unter besonderer Berücksichtigung von Interdiskurs und

Kollektivsymbolik." In Handbuch Sozialwissenschaftliche Diskursanalyse 1: Theorien und Methoden, eds. Reiner Keller, Andreas Hirseland and Werner Schneider. Vol. 1, 407–430. Opladen: VS Verlag, 2006.

–. "Dispositiv und Interdiskurs. Mit Überlegungen zum 'Dreieck' Foucault-Bourdieu-Luhmann." In Foucault in den Kulturwissenschaften, eds. Clemens Kammler and Rolf Parr, 219–238. Heidelberg: Synchron, 2007.

–. Versuch über den Normalismus. Wie Normalität produziert wird. Göttingen: Vandenhoeck und Ruprecht, 2006.

–. "Warum Diskurse nicht von personalen Subjekten 'ausgehandelt' werden. Von der Diskurs- zur Interdiskurstheorie." In Die diskursive Konstruktion der Wirklichkeit. Zum Verhältnis von Wissenssoziologie und Diskursforschung, eds. Reiner Keller, Andreas Hirseland, Werner Schneider and Willy Viehöver, 77–99. Konstanz: UvK, 2005.

Lüdtke, Alf. "Alltagsgeschichte: Stand der Diskussion und Perspektiven." In Alltag in der Pflege – Wie machten sich Pflegende bemerkbar? Beiträge des 8. Internationalen Kongresses zur Geschichte der Pflege 2008, eds. Andrea Thiekötter, Heinrich Recken, Manuela Schoska and Eva-Maria Ulmer, 13–26. 2009.

McFarland-Icke, Bronwyn R. Nurses in Nazi Germany: Moral Choice in History. Princeton: Princeton University Press, 1999.

Miller, Peter. "Accounting as Social and Institutional Practice: An Introduction." In Accounting as Social and Institutional Practice, eds. Anthony G. Hopwood and Peter Miller, 1–39. Cambridge: Cambridge University Press, 1994.

Missa, Jean-Noël. Naissance de la psychiatrie biologique: Histoire des traitements des maladies mentales au XX. Siècle. Paris: Presses Universitaires de France, 2006.

Mouttet, H. "The Treatment of Schizophrenia: Insulin Shock, Cardiazol, Sleep Treatment." American Journal of Psychiatry 94, suppl. (1938): 1–5.

Müller, M. "Insulin Therapy of Schizophrenia." American Journal of Psychiatry 94, suppl. (1938): 5–15.

Müller, Ulrich. "Metamorphosen: Krankenakten als Quellen für Lebensgeschichten." In "Das Vergessen der Vernichtung ist Teil der Vernichtung selbst" Lebengeschichten von Opfern der nationalsozialistischen "Euthanasie", eds. Petra Fuchs, Maike Rotzoll, Ulrich Müller, Paul Richter and Gerrit Hohendorf, 80–96. Göttingen: Wallstein, 2007.

Negri, Toni. "Le monstre politique. Vie nue et puissance." Multitudes 3, no. 33 (2008): 37–52.

Neuberger, Theodor Dr. "Die Irrenanstalt Langenhorn." In Deutsche Hei-und Pflegeanstalten für psychisch Kranke in Wort und Bild, ed. Johannes Bresler, 310–323. Halle: Marhold, 1910.

Nolte, Karen. "Pflege von Leib und Seele: Krankenpflege in Armutsvierteln des 19. Jahrhunderts." In Alltag in der Krankenpflege: Geschichte und Gegenwart/Everyday Nursing Life: Past and Present, ed. Sylvelyn Hähner-Rombach, 53–82. Stuttgart: Franz Steiner, 2009.

–. "Pflege von Sterbenden im 19. Jahrhundert. Eine ethikgeschichtliche Annäherung." In Transformationen pflegerischen Handelns. Instituionelle Kontexte und soziale Praxis vom 19. bis 21. Jahrhundert, ed. Susanne Kreutzer, 87–107. Göttingen: V&R unipress, Universität Osnabrück, 2010.

–. "Telling the Painful Truth: Nurses and Physicians in the Nineteenth Century." Nursing History Review 16 (2008): 115–134.

Platner, P. "Korsakoff Syndrome after Insulin and Metrazol Treatment of Schizophrenia." Zeitschrift für die gesamte Neurologie und Psychiatrie 162 (1938): 728–735.
Prior, Lindsay. Using Documents in Social Research. London: Sage, 2008.
Prior, Lindsay. "The Architecture of the Hospital: A Study of Spatial Organization and Medical Knowledge." The British Journal of Sociology 39, no. 1 (March 1988): 86–113.
Proctor, Robert. Racial Hygiene: Medicine under the Nazis. Cambridge: Harvard University Press, 1988.
Rabinow, Paul. French DNA. Chicago: University of Chicago Press, 1999.
Rabinow, Paul and Nikolas Rose. "Biopower Today." BioSocieties 1 (2006): 195–217.
Reich, Warren T. "The Care-Based Ethic of Nazi Medicine and the Moral Importance of what we Care about." American Journal of Bioethics 1, no. 1 (2001): 64–74.
Reichsausschuß für Volksgesundheitsdienst. "Krankenpflegelehrbuch." (1939).
Riepenhausen, Josef. "Azoman-Therapie-symptomatisch und 'ätiologisch'". Psychiatrisch-neurologische Wochenschrift 43, no. 23 (1941): 233–252.
Riesenberger, Dieter. Das Deutsche Rote Kreuz. Eine Geschichte 1864–1990. Paderborn: Schöningh, 2002.
Roelcke, Volker. "The Establishment of Psychiatric Genetics in Germany, Great Britain and the USA, circa 1910–1960: To the Inseparable History of Eugenics and Human Genetics." Acta Historica Leopoldina 48, no. 48 (2007): 173–190.
–. "Mentalities and Sterilization Laws in Europe during the 1930: Eugenics, Genetics, and Politics in a Historic Context." Der Nervenarzt 73, no. 11 (Nov. 2002): 1019–1030.
–. "Zeitgeist und Erbgesundheitsgesetzgebung im Europa der 1930er Jahre. Eugenik, Genetik und Politik im historischen Kontext." Der Nervenarz 73 (2002): 1019–1029.
Roelcke, Volker, & Gerrit Hohendorf. "Akten der "Euthanasie"-Aktion T4 gefunden." Vierteljahreshefte für Zeitgeschichte 41, no. 3 (1993): 479–481.
Roos, Georg. "Beziehung des Krankenpflegers zum Arzt." Geisteskrankpflege. Monatsschrift für Geisteskranken-und Krankenpflege 41, no. 12 (1937): 180–181.
Rose, Nikolas. Powers of Freedom: Reframing Political Thought. Cambridge: Cambridge University Press, 2005.
–. "Numbers." In Powers of Freedom: Reframing Political Thought, ed. Nikolas Rose, 197–232. Cambridge: Cambridge University Press, 2005.
–. The Politics of Life Itself: Biomedicine, Power, and Subjectivity in the Twenty-First Century. Princeton: Princeton University Press, 2007.
Rose, Wolfgang. "Der dezentrale Krankenmord. 'Euthanasie' durch Medikamente und Nahrungsentzug." In Tödliche Medizin. Rassenwahn im Nationalsozialismus, ed. Stiftung Jüdisches Museum, 100–107. Berlin: Wallstein Verlag, 2009.
Rotzoll, Maike and Gerrit Hohendorff. "Krankenmord im Dienst des Fortschritts? Der Heidelberger Psychiater Carl Schneider als Gehirnforscher und 'Therapeutischer Idealist'." Der Nervenarzt 83, no. 3 (2012): 311–320.
Rotzoll, Maike, Petra Fuchs, Paul Richter, and Gerrit Hohendorf. "Die Nationalsozialistische 'Euthanasieaktion T4.' Historische Forschung, Individuelle Lebensgeschichten Und Erinnerungskultur." Der Nervenarzt 81 (2010): 1326–1332.
Rotzoll, Maike, Gerrit Hohendorf, Petra Fuchs, Paul Richter, Christoph Mundt, and Wolfgang U. Eckart, eds. Die nationalsozialistische "Euthanasie"-Aktion "T4" und ihre Opfer. Geschichte und ethische Konsequenzen für die Gegenwart. Paderborn: Schöning, 2010.

Rousset, David. Les Jours de notre mort. Paris: Hachette Littératures, 2008.

–. L'univers Concentrationnaire. France: Les Éditions de minuit, 2005.

Sakel, Manfred. "The Nature and Origin of Hypoglycemic Treatment of Psychosis." The American Journal of Psychiatry 94, suppl. (1938): 24–40.

Schäfer, Gerhard Dr. "Über einige Aufgaben des Arztes bei der Durchführung des Gesetzes zur Verhütung erbkranken Nachwuchses." Ärzteblatt für Hamburg und Schleswig Holstein 1, no. 15) 1934: 136–137.

Schäfer, Gerhard Dr. and Rudolf Birkenstock. "Staatskrankenanstalt Langenhorn." In Hygiene und soziale Hygiene in Hamburg. Zur neunzigsten Versammlung der deutschen Naturforscher und Ärzte in Hamburg im Jahre 1928, ed. Gesundheitsbehörde Hamburg, 198–208. Hamburg: Paul Hartung Verlag, 1928.

Schilder, Paul. "Notes on the Psychology of Metrazol Treatment of Schizophrenia." The Journal of Nervous and Mental Disease 89, no. 2 (1939): 133–144.

Schmidbauer, Marianne. Vom Lazaruskreuz zur Pflege aktuell: Professionalisierungsdiskurse in der deutschen Krankenpflege 1903–2000. Königstein/Taunus: Ulrike Helmer Verlag, 2002.

Schmidt, Jutta. Beruf Schwester: Mutterhausdiakonie im 19. Jahrhundert. Farnakfurt am Main: Campus, 1998.

Schmuhl, Hans-Walter. Rassenhygiene, Nationalsozialismus, Euthanasie-Von der Verhütung zur Vernichtung "lebensunwerten Lebens" 1890–1945. Kritische Studien zur Geschichtswissenschaft 75 ed. Göttingen: Vandenhoeck und Ruprecht, 1987.

–. "Ärzte in Konfessionellen Kranken- und Pflegeanstalten 1908–1957." In Beruf und Religion im 19. und 20. Jahrhundert, eds. Frank-Michael Kuhlemann and Hans-Walther Schmuhl, 176–194. Stuttgart: Kohlhammer, 2003.

Schneider, Carl. Behandlung und Verhütung der Geisteskrankheiten. Allgemeine Erfahrungen, Grundsätze Technik Biologie. Berlin: Julius Springer, 1939.

Schneider, Silke. "Diskurse in der Diktatur? Überlegungen zu einer Analyse des Nationalsozialismus mit Foucault." In Foucault: Diskursanalyse der Politik. Eine Einführung, eds. Brigitte Kerchner and Silke Schneider, 123–144. Wiesbaden: VS Verlag, 2006.

Scholz, Ludwig. Leitfaden für Irrenpfleger. Halle a.d. Saale: Carl Marhold, 1904.

Scholz, Ludwig. Leitfaden für Irrenpfleger. Halle a.d. Saale: Carl Marhold, 1920.

Schoska, Manuela. "Pflegerische Verantwortung in der Zeit des Nationalsozialismus – eine Analyse von Aspekten der Verantwortlichkeit im pflegerischen Berufsalltag." In Alltag in der Pflege-Wie machten sich Pflegende bemerkbar? Beiträge des 8. Internationalen Kongresses zur Geschichte der Pflege 2008, eds. Andrea Thiekötter, Heinrich Recken, Manuela Schoska and Eva-Maria Ulmer, 245–259. Frankfurt am Main: Mabuse-Verlag, 2009.

Schweikhardt, Christoph. "'Der Stosstrupp 1937/38 rückt in Würzburg ein!' Eine Fallstudie zur Ausbildung einer NS-Krankenschwester am dortigen Luitpoldkrankenhaus." Historia Hospitalium 22 (2000/2001): 103–136.

–. "Krankenpflege im Nationalsozialismus." In Quellen zur Geschichte der Krankenpflege. Mit Einführungen und Kommentaren, ed. Sylvelyn Hähner-Rombach, 554–564. Frankfurt a.M.: Mabuse, 2008.

Seibert, Philipp. "Zur Pflege Geisteskranker." Geisteskrankenpflege. Monatsschrift für Geisteskranken-und Krankenpflege 44, no. 12 (1940): 149–153.

Shear, M. K. and M. Sacks. "Digitalis Delirium: Psychiatric Considerations." International Journal of Psychiatry Medicine 8, no. 4 (1977–1978): 371–381.
Sieben. "Erziehungsfragen bei dem Krankenhausaufenthalt." Zeitschrift für das gesamte Krankenhauswesen 23 (1938): 62–67.
Smith, Dorothy E. Institutional Ethnography: A Sociology for People. Oxford: Alta Mira Press, 2005.
–. "'K. is Mentally Ill': The Anatomy of a Factual Account." Sociology 12 (1978): 23–53.
–. "The Social Construction of Documentary Reality." Sociological Inquiry 44, no. 4 (1974): 257–268.
–. "Textually Mediated Social Organization." International Social Science Journal 36, no. 1 (1984): 59–76.
–. Writing the Social. Critique, Theory, and Investigations. Toronto: University of Toronto Press, 2004.
Smith, George W. "Policing the Gay Community: An Inquiry into Textually Mediated Social Relations." International Journal of the Sociology of Law 16 (1988): 163–183.
Solomon, Alfred P., Chester W. Darrow, and Melvin Blaurock. "Blood Pressure and Palmar Sweat (Galvanic) Responses of Psychotic Patients before and after Insulin and Metrazol Therapy: A Physiologic Study of 'Resistant' and Cooperative Attitudes." Psychosomatic Medicine 1, no. 1 (1939): 118–137.
Stadelmann, Heinrich. "Psychotherapie bei der Geisteskrankenpflege." Geisteskrankenpflege. Monatsschrift für Geisteskranken-und Krankenpflege 46, no. 61 (1942): 66.
Starks, Hamlin A. "Subjective Experiences in Patients Incident to Insulin and Metrazol Therapy." Psychiatric Quaterly 12, no. 4 (1938): 699–709.
Steppe, Hilde. '…Dem Kranken zum Troste und dem Judenthum zur Ehre…'. Frankfurt am Main: Mabuse, 2006.
–. Krankenpflege im Nationalsozialismus. Frankfurt a.M.: Mabuse, 2001.
–. "Das Selbstverständnis der Krankenpflege in ihrer historischen Entwicklung." Pflege 13 (2000): 77–83.
–. "Nursing in Nazi Germany." Western Journal of Nursing Research 14, no. 6 (1992): 744.
–. "Nursing in the Third Reich." History of Nursing Society Journal 3, no. 4 (1991): 21–37.
Steppe, Hilde and Eva-Maria Ulmer. "Ich war von jeher mit Leib und Seele gerne Pflegerin." Über die Beteiligung von Krankenschwestern an den 'Euthanasie'-Aktionen in Meseritz-Obrawalde. Frankfurt a.M.: Prisma, 2001.
Sticker, Anna. Agnes Karll. Die Reformerin der deutschen Krankenpflege. Ein Wegweiser für Heute Zu ihrem 50. Todestag. Stuttgart: Aussaat, 1984.
–. Die Entstehung der neuzeitlichen Krankenpflege. Deutsche Quellenstücke aus der ersten Hälfte des 19. Jahrhunderts. Stuttgart: Kohlhammer, 1960.
–. Friederike Fliedner und die Anfänge der Frauendiakonie. Ein Quellenbuch. Neukirchen/Vluyn: Neukirchener Verlag, 1961.
Stöbe, Oskar. "Hilfsmittel in der praktischen Geisteskrankenpflge." Geisteskrankenpflege. Monatsschrift für Geisteskranken-und Krankenpflege 37, no. 6 (1933): 92–93.
Süß, Winfried. Der "Volkskörper" im Krieg. Gesundheitspolitik, Gesundheitsverhältnisse und Krankenmord im nationalsozialistischen Deutschland 1939–1945. Studien zur Zeitgeschichte. 65th ed. München: Oldenbourg, 2003

Thielmann, Wilhelm. "Das Spiel und der Kranke." Geisteskrankenpflege. Monatsschrift für Geisteskranken-und Krankenpflege 41, no. 10 (1937): 183–185.

v. Angyal, L., K Gyárfás. "Über die Cardiazol-Krampfbehandlung der Schizophrenie" Archiv für Psychiatrie 106 (1937): 1–12.

Waldschmidt, A., A. Klein, M. Tamayo Korte, and S. Dalman-Eken. " Diskurs im Alltag-Alltag im Diskurs: Ein Beitrag zur empirisch begründeten Methodologie sozialwissenschaftlicher Diskursforschung [69 Absätze]." Forum Qualitative Sozialforschung / Forum: Qualitative Social Research 8, no. 2 (2007): http://www.qualitative-research.net/index.php/fqs/article/view/251/554, accessed 28 September 2012.

Weber, Hannes. "Luminal und Luminal-Exanthem." Klinische Wochenzeitschrift 20, no.1 (1922): 998–999.

Weingart, Peter. "Eugenics – Medical Or Social Science?" Science in Context 8, no. 1 (Spring, 1995): 197–207.

Weingart, Peter, Kurt Bayertz, and Jürgen Kroll, eds. Rasse, Blut und Gene. Geschichte der Eugenik und Rassenhygiene in Deutschland. Frankfurt a.M.: Suhrkamp, 1992.

Weygandt, Wilhelm. "Die Ersten Zeichen der Geisteskrankheiten." Die Heilkunde. Monatsschrift für practische Medicin no. 1 (1905): 2–10.

–. Forensische Psychiatrie. II. Teil. Sachverständigentätigkeit, ed. Vereinigung wissenschaftlicher Verleger. Sammlung Göschen ed. Berlin, Leipzig: de Gruyter & Co, 1922.

Weygandt, Wilhelm, ed. Die Staatskrankenanstalt Friedrichsberg. Hygiene und soziale Hygiene in Hamburg. Zur neunzigsten Versammlung der deutschen Naturforscher und Ärzte in Hamburg im Jahre 1928, ed. Gesundheitsbehörde Hamburg. Hamburg: Paul Hartung Verlag, 1928.

Widenmeyer, Harold. "Die Insulin- und Cardiazolschockbehandlung der Schizophrenen." Geisteskrankenpflege. Monatsschrift für Geisteskranken-und Krankenpflege 41, no. 12 (1937): 161–165.

Wildt, Michael. Volksgemeinschaft als Selbstermächtigung. Hamburg: Hamburger Edition, 2007.

Winkler, Ulrike and Gerrit Hohendorff. "Nun ist Mogiljow frei von Verrückten. Die Ermordung der PsychiatriepatientInnen in Mogilew 1941/42." In Krieg und Psychiatrie 1914–1950, eds. Babette Quinkert, Philipp Rauh and Ulrike Winkler. Beiträge zur Geschichte des Nationalsozialismus 26 ed. Göttingen: Wallstein, 2010.

Witetzki, H. "Über die Anwendung und Verabreichung von Arzneimitteln bei Geisteskranken." Geisteskrankenpflege. Monatsschrift für Geisteskranken-und Krankenpflege 38, no. 3 (1934): 92–96.

Wunder, Michael. "Die Auflösung von Friedrichsberg – Hintergründe und Folgen." Hamburger Ärzteblatt 44 (1990): 128–131.

–. Euthanasie in den letzten Kriegsjahren. Die Jahre 1944 und 1945 in der Heil- und Pflegeanstalt Hamburg Langenhorn, eds. Rolf Winau, Heinz Müller-Dietz. Abhandlungen zur Geschichte der Medizin und der Naturwissenschaften ed. Vol. 65. Husum: Matthiesen, 1992.

Zakravsky, Katherina. "'Homo Sacer' and the Consequences. Two Remarks on Holocaust Commemoration and 'Bare Life' in Contemporary Art." http://magazines.documenta.de/attachment/000000778.pdf, accessed 27 December 2007.

–. "Zur Kritik des 'nackten Lebens'," http://platform.factlink.net/fsDownload/Katherina

%20Zakravsky-Enthuellungen.Zur%20Kritik%20des%20nackten%20Lebens.pdf?forumid=336&v=1&id=235172, accessed 7 July 2009.

Ziskind, Eugene. "Memory Defects during Metrazol Therapy." Archives of Neurology and Psychiatry 45, no. 2 (1941): 223–234.

e

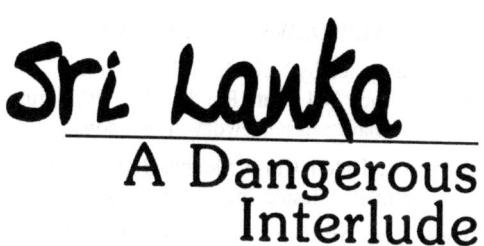
Sri Lanka
A Dangerous Interlude

Apratim Mukarji

NEW DAWN PRESS, INC.
USA• UK• INDIA

NEW DAWN PRESS GROUP
Published by New Dawn Press Group
New Dawn Press, Inc., 244 South Randall Rd # 90, Elgin, IL 60123
e-mail: sales@newdawnpress.com

New Dawn Press, 2 Tintern Close, Slough, Berkshire, SL1-2TB, UK
e-mail: salesuk@newdawnpress.org

New Dawn Press (An Imprint of Sterling Publishers (P) Ltd)
A-59, Okhla Industrial Area, Phase-II, New Delhi-110020, India
e-mail: info@sterlingpublishers.com
www.sterlingpublishers.com

Sri Lanka: A Dangerous Interlude
© 2005, Apratim Mukarji
ISBN 1 84557 530 X

All rights are reserved. No part of this publication may be reproduced, stored in a retrieval system or transmitted, in any form or by any means, mechanical, photocopying, recording or otherwise, without prior written permission of the publisher.

PRINTED IN INDIA

Dedicated to my wife Ena who shares many happy and sad memories of Sri Lanka

and

to the people of Sri Lanka who deserve peace and not war.

Contents

	Introduction	ix
1.	Frozen Peace Melting?	1
2.	Karuna's Revolt	38
3.	Is LTTE a Liberation Movement?	70
4.	Sri Lanka and India	100
5.	Colombo Continues to Miss Out	131
6.	Somebodys vs. Nobodys	159
	Epilogue: Tsunami and Dialogue	186
	Postscript to Epilogue	212
	Appendix	219
	Glossary	283
	Index	284

Introduction

War and peace stood still in Sri Lanka in October, 2004. The stillness lying heavy as tension was generated by a prolonged deadlock in the peace process with the government and the Liberation Tigers not yet prepared to return to negotiations. The ceasefire almost miraculously held on, heightening anxiety in the international community over the continuing inability of the two players to break out of the impasse and start talking to each other. As the eternally feuding Sinhalese leaders of the two main southern political parties continued to thrust and parry at each other, the Tamil rebels who were also terrorists visited European capitals in search of sympathy and understanding for their cause.

The Sri Lankan situation offered many opportunities to study and analyse the unscheduled, longish break in a peace process which had got going famously between the ceasefire agreement of 22 February, 2002, the holding of the first round of talks at the Rose Garden, Sattahip, Thailand, during 16-18 September, 2002, followed by three more rounds of talks, and then the unilateral withdrawal of the Liberation Tigers of Tamil Eelam (LTTE) from the talks on 22 April, 2003.

A big change had, however, occurred in the interregnum since the sudden halt to the talks; a new government had taken charge in Colombo in April, 2004, run by the very people who had led a sustained and high-velocity campaign against the manner in which the previous government, run by the United National Front, carried on the peace dialogue with the LTTE.

One of the first commitments made by the United People's Front Alliance government was towards the peace process, affirming that it would abide by it and by the ceasefire agreement.[1] Soon, president

Chandrika Bandaranaike Kumaratunga started making appeals to the LTTE to return to negotiation. On its part, the latter reciprocated the gesture but stuck to its demand that it would rejoin talks only if its Interim Self Governing Authority (ISGA) proposals, submitted on 31 October, 2003, formed the basis for negotiation. That these declarations of commitment to the peace process were not cynical camouflages for contrary intentions was amply proved in the intervening months as the ceasefire was maintained and there was absolutely no indication that either side was preparing a clandestine return to fighting.

Despite this reasonably positive approach to the peace process by both the Sri Lankan state and the Tamil rebels, the stalemate in negotiations continued. Apart from the installation of a new government in power, another major change from the previous period took place. "Col." Karuna, the most successful rebel commander, broke away from the LTTE on 3 March, 2004, in a surprise move, momentarily causing apprehensions in various quarters that the unexpected and significant development might affect the peace process adversely.

The sensational defection was soon followed by the breakout of a fierce campaign of attrition unleashed by the LTTE aimed at obliterating the challenge to its monolithic image from Karuna in the quickest time possible. Seven months later, killings and reprisal killings continued to fill newspaper headlines, with panicked pleas by the international community to stop them lest the fragile peace process was eventually derailed.

This book records all these developments and seeks to analyse and understand them with a view to appreciate the nature, causes and consequences of the ethnic strife. But, above all, it proposes to analyse the contradictions that seem to have bedevilled the Sri Lankan peace process. This exercise also seeks to probe the roles being played by the two principal players in the conflict, the Sri Lankan state and the LTTE, in the search for peace.

As the following chapters will reveal, the conclusions that emerge from this study of the Sri Lankan peace process bring little credit to the Sri Lankan state which is liable to be held largely responsible for the seemingly intractable situation the country and its people face today. The conclusions should not prove unique to perceptive observers of modern Sri Lanka, for they draw heavily upon established facts and authoritative analyses done by capable scholars, politicians, diplomats and journalists with first-hand knowledge of the complexities of the Tamil question. The uniqueness of this study, however, derives from its objectivity and ability to judge events, actions and words in the correct perspective.

This book proceeds to examine the issues at hand through the prism of a set of questions which are fundamental to an understanding of the Sri Lankan situation. These are – at the end of 2004, the LTTE stood fully identified as a terrorist organisation, run in a fascist style, holding a sizeable population in its thrall. Why was it then incumbent upon the legitimate and internationally recognised Sri Lankan government to enter into a dialogue with it? If it was true that the Sri Lankan government was responsible for upholding the sovereignty, territorial integrity and unity of the country, why was it apparently unable to ensure that the people living in the LTTE-held territory in northeastern Sri Lanka were freed from the shackles imposed by the Tamil Tigers? Why was it that the state was incapable of protecting its citizens from the wrath of the rebels even in the relative security of Colombo?

Answers to these questions are liable to lead one to a conclusion which would be unpalatable to the Sri Lankan state but which would also be truthful and, therefore, unavoidable. The things have come to a pass principally because over the years the state has failed repeatedly to establish its writ over large tracts of the country. As a consequence of these recurring failures, the state has come to be perceived as a weak and dithering entity, of which liberty could be taken by unscrupulous and adventurous groups.

As the following chapters seek to establish, this unflattering image of the Sri Lankan state came to be as a result of a traditionally fractured and pathologically heterogeneous leadership of the majority Sinhalese-Buddhist community, which had preferred to drown all the national woes in a bitter, never-ending game of one-upmanship rather than to face them straightaway and try to settle them honestly.

As many scholars and journalists have done before, even a cursory look at the origins of the Tamil militancy establishes that a proper and sagacious handling of the grievances of the main minority community could have prevented militancy from usurping the leadership of the community. In the formative years of the young republic, the Tamils of the northeastern Sri Lanka displayed enough forbearance to go by constitutionality and legality in order to get their grievances redressed.

Political militancy and armed insurrection crept in and eventually won the day only because the Sinhalese-Buddhist community which ran each government of the post-independence period not only did not stop with ignoring the Tamils but also took conscious steps to humiliate and brutalise a largely peaceful and obedient population.

The southern leadership also took recourse to plain cheating in order to deprive the Tamils of natural justice, with even prime ministers breaking their solemn promises at will. These unwise acts of omission and commission were gradually accompanied by bloody riots let loose upon the Tamils, in which hundreds of lives were lost and scores of valuable residential and business properties destroyed and looted. The earliest internally displaced Tamils were of circa 1956. Since then for nearly fifty years on, Sri Lankan Tamils have had good reasons to feel uncertain and scared about their future in their country.

If the Sinhalese-run state had failed to restore the Tamils' confidence, the latter received a crueller treatment from the Tamil rebels who thrived at continuing bloody encounters with security forces. The survival and growth of the LTTE came to depend on military adventurism practised assiduously by the Colombo-run state machinery. The Tigers succeeded in equating their own survival with that of the civilian population and thus came to project themselves as the saviours of the Tamils. It was this successful manipulation of political, social and economic conditions prevailing in the northeast that had led to the situation today when the state was obliged to acknowledge the pre-eminence of the LTTE as the sole representatives of the Sri Lankan Tamils.

As a perceptive Tamil analyst sees it, the LTTE's emphasis on a monolithic unity of the Tamil community is a consequence of its

Introduction XIII

attempt to invent a new Tamil identity, where the basis of political programmes and alliances are of an ethnically essentialist character. This becomes necessary because the classical identity would not have accommodated ethnic exclusivism and resultant self-imposed isolation. In this framework, political identity is directly derived from one's ethnic identity. Class, caste, gender, individual aspirations, and broader social issues are relegated to the periphery.[2]

The LTTE invented a new Tamil identity by simultaneously drawing upon and denying history. This identity claims to be tied to history on the basis of language, region and tradition. But the Tigers are anti-historical because they are committed to denying that the Tamil identity also includes a history of co-existence with other communities (Jaffna Tamils continue to lament to this day the exodus of Sinhalese bakers from the peninsula in the wake of the first "eelam" war; "Nobody can bake like them, " is the time-honoured refrain). The denial of pluralism among communities is only a step away from the denial of pluralism within a community. Thus, one implication of this invented Tamil identity (through ethnic essentialism) is that the Tigers have to deny and eliminate real or potential differences of opinion and interests among the Tamils.

This particular analysis appears to have penetrated right inside the Tamil psyche, both of the people and of the Liberation Tigers, and offers a most plausible explanation of the eventual alienation of the Muslims of the northeast from the Tamils, a legacy of which is found in today's Sri Lanka where as government-LTTE parleys continue off and on, the Muslims grow increasingly nervous about life under a Tigers dispensation in the near future.[3]

It is pertinent in this context to analyse the LTTE's demand for a Tamil homeland in the northeast and a permanent merger of the northern and eastern provinces. Both the demands are steadfastly opposed and denied by the majority community as also by the Muslim community. As we see later in this book, the colonisation policy so consciously pursued by the successive Sri Lankan governments succeeded in bringing about a significant demographic change in the eastern province where all the three communities now share an equal weightage though a Tamil predominance was at one time self-evident.

The colonisation policy was no doubt born of malevolence than any other sentiment, and the Tamils' resentment of it was equally appreciable. But, judging by what happened to the Sinhalese in the north and to the Muslims in the east (in the latter's case, the persecution continues to this day), it would be appropriate to conclude that one bulwark against an eventual LTTE fascist rule in the northeast could well be the relocation of the Sinhalese in the east.

There is sufficient ground to theorise that the inability or deliberate design of the Sinhalese leadership to respond positively to the political aspirations of the Tamil community and the LTTE's ascendancy as the sole representatives of the community acted in tandem, for a recounting of the developments in recent years of a search for a political settlement of the ethnic conflict shows that each Sinhalese failure or denial was matched by one more step forward of the Liberation Tigers. The LTTE could pull through such coups because the majority of governmental efforts at a political solution were insincere and calculated more in terms of electoral gains than Tamil aspirations.

At the same time, as the following chapters record, the rebels were astute enough to be able to sabotage whatever genuine efforts at reconciliation and settlement were attempted. The peace initiative undertaken by Kumaratunga during 1994-95 illustrates this aspect very well indeed. The LTTE's success in thwarting her move was so comprehensive that till this day, she continues to be portrayed as the worst of the enemies of the Tamil community while in reality she is the very opposite.

A comparative analysis of Kumaratunga during her first year in power and in subsequent years and especially since the Wickramasinghe government came into being illustrates how the change in her public image (in the Tamil perception) has served to bolster the LTTE's case for continuing belligerency. Ever since she worked to ease the Wickramasinghe government out of office, dissolved parliament and saw her own alliance form the present government, the Tigers have worked overtime to show her in the worst possible light. The reason for this is her tough stand against allowing the Tigers have the leeway in peace negotiations, her unabated campaign during the Wickramasinghe regime which even threatened to disturb the

Introduction

facilitators, Norway, at one point and, presently, her lack of decision to resume negotiations on the basis of the ISGA proposals.

A degree of alarm is also discernible in the LTTE's pronouncements about the president ever since an impression began to gather ground, in the last quarter of 2004, that the state was accelerating defence tie-ups with major countries. The Indo-Sri Lanka defence act, which was just one step away from implementation in October, appeared to have disturbed the Tigers as much as the steadily expanding defence cooperation with the United States.

At the end of October, 2004, India and the United States were perceived by the Tigers as begetters of potential danger. Following the finalisation of the draft India-Sri Lanka pact, LTTE political adviser Anton Balasingham was quoted by the Voice of Tigers radio saying that the proposed agreement would tilt the military balance between the government forces and the Liberation Tigers and strain the already fragile peace process.[4]

Significantly, the objection to the defence agreement came not only from the LTTE but also from unaffiliated sections of the Tamil community. A commentator in the popular *Sunday Virakesari* went to the extent of accusing India of fishing in the troubled waters of Sri Lanka in order to establish its economic and military hegemony over the country. He predicted that once the ethnic conflict was resolved, Sri Lankans would have to jointly fight a long and destructive war against India. In a front page editorial, *Thinakkural* said that India would have to clarify whether the pact was aimed at scuttling the Tamils' struggle for substantial autonomy based on their right to self-determination. It pointed out that successive governments in Colombo had desired to use India in order to crush the legitimate struggle of Sri Lankan Tamils.

An unnamed LTTE source was quoted in a news report saying that the Liberation Tigers were concerned about the growing political, financial and military influence of the United States in Sri Lanka. It said that though the LTTE itself continued to be diplomatically mute about its worry, it had let out a steady barrage against the perceived threat through the means of media reports and comments and academic discourses.[5]

The report pointed out that in Sri Lanka, not a week would pass without a Tamil newspaper lambasting the United States for supporting the Sri Lankan government's case at the expense of the Tamils. Tamil journalists, whether writing in English or Tamil, would routinely note with alarm the manner in which the Americans would flex their muscles through well-publicised visits of military officials to the country. The Tamil media would carry extensive articles on the way the Americans had exploited internal conflicts in various Third World countries in order to gain a foothold there. The writings would exhort the Tamils to be wary about the possible consequences of a growing American presence in the country for their liberation movement.

The report quoted an LTTE supporter writing in a pro-rebel website, www.tamilcanadian.com (2 October, 2004) that "In the late 1960's, Indonesia witnessed a ruthless murder campaign culminating in the emergence of the Suharto dictatorship. Nearly one million civilians were killed in the bloodbath, mainly members of Indonesia's communist party. The United States played an odious role during this barbaric episode, which reportedly involved discrete US funding of the death squads that were responsible for the killings."

The LTTE's objection to the India-Sri Lanka defence pact on the grounds that it would destroy the military balance between the two sides and thus threaten the already fragile peace process is noteworthy because it betrays two separate concerns of the rebels. As far as military strength is concerned, government forces clearly enjoy a superiority which the rebels can never aspire to match. The issue of a so-called military balance appears to be more of a ploy to register a strong protest at a development which cannot be stopped but can be resented. Similarly, the peace process cannot be perceived to be affected in any manner by the state seeking stronger military strength (which does not appear to be the case in hand, since the bare outlines of the agreement available at the time of writing indicated that only a framework seemed to be being put on an already existing relationship between the two countries with no implication that India would actually come to defend Sri Lanka in case of a breakout of war with the Tamil rebels) because the process does not preclude the state from doing so. Besides, the state, which is a legal and constitutional entity,

Introduction XVII

cannot be subjected to any stipulation under the provisions of the ceasefire agreement not to pursue greater military capability as it is its function to constantly upgrade the security of the country and its people. The LTTE's objection to Sri Lanka obtaining larger military prowess (granted that, that indeed is the case with the government) is, therefore, more of an academic exercise than a serious and sustainable protest.

More importantly, the chorus of Tamil protests is aimed at establishing that the pact would encourage fresh aggression against the community. The outlines of the agreement available indicate that India is far from assuming such a policy. In fact, the Indian policy remains exactly what it was, to provide assistance to enable the Sri Lankan state to perform its various constitutional functions, and nothing else.

Nevertheless, the rebels' discomfiture undoubtedly stems from estimable implications of the state's growing security relationships with the regional power, India, and the global power, the United States. Later in this book, mention is made of the very substantial military assistance being provided by the United States to Sri Lankan forces the initial results of which are already available. Similarly, an active cooperation with the Indian navy is certain to bring valuable dividends to the Sri Lankan navy in dealing with possible future transgressions by the rebels. To that extent, the LTTE cannot help being alarmed by the development.

Forceful expressions of concern in this regard, however, raise a pertinent question: how serious are the Liberation Tigers in pursuing peace? As a primarily military force, it is but natural for the LTTE to be ever alert regarding future clashes with security forces and the southern media constantly speculate on its clandestine strength advancement recourses. A big question, however, looms over the frequently aired allegation, in which even the Sri Lankan state has participated, that the rebels are fortifying themselves in the Trincomalee harbour area and that the security of the harbour is under threat. As this book records, the allegation has been confirmed by the naval chief, who should be regarded as the last authority on the issue. Further respectability was lent to the charge when the visiting Indian navy chief Admiral Arun Prakash said in Colombo, that there "is some concern that it (the harbour) should not fall into the wrong hands. It seems to me that at the moment the LTTE is closely bearing down on Trincomalee."

A recent report of the Sri Lanka Monitoring Mission (SLMM), however, leads one to entertain doubts about the authenticity of the allegation. The media reported on 24 October, 2004, that the SLMM, in its latest report, had denied the existence of any LTTE military build-up around the harbour. They quoted SLMM spokesman Oskar Solnes saying that the ceasefire monitors had not found any indication of such a build-up in the area and that all the rebel installations the SLMM had visited during its investigation were situated "well within the LTTE-controlled area." The SLMM report certainly appears to demolish the very basis of the allegation voiced, among others, by navy chief Daya Sandagiri.[6]

The eminent Sri Lankan bureaucrat Bradman Weerakoon, who was intimately associated with various governments from the early 1950's onward and specifically with the rehabilitation and developmental work in the northeast since the ceasefire agreement came into existence, told the author, "A lot of nonsense is being said these days about the LTTE building up bases in the Trincomalee harbour region. Till recently, I was associated with the peace process and I can say with first-hand knowledge that nothing of the sort is being done by the LTTE."[7]

The peace process has been marked by an unseemly assault on the functioning of the SLMM and on the Norwegian facilitators by both the government and the rebels. The president in particular has been noticeably severe in her criticisms of their roles though she also took pains at times to appreciate the facilitators; in effect, the presidential accusations amounted to charging the SLMM in particular of indirectly facilitating the LTTE's perceived and proven acts of defying the ceasefire agreement. There have been noisy demonstrations in Colombo against the Norwegians. On 20 September, 2004, protesters left the body of a murdered Tamil politician in front of the Norwegian embassy. News reports said that the casket contained the remains of Thambithurai Sivakumaran, an activist of the pro-

Introduction XIX

government Eelam People's Democratic Party, who was killed allegedly by the LTTE on 18 September. A few days later, the state-run Sri Lankan Broadcasting Corporation chose to highlight a news item which could only be construed as a deliberate attempt to instil doubts about Norway's credibility in the minds of Sri Lankans. That professionally indelicate story cited unnamed expatiate organisations from India, the Philippines and Sri Lanka as having condemned Norway for being hypocritical in castigating suicide bombings in Iraq but not elsewhere. *The Hindu*, an Indian newspaper read widely in Sri Lanka, said in an editorial in its 26 October, 2004, issue (Delhi edition), "As the facilitator of the peace process, it is time for Norway to play its part sincerely and effectively in bringing the LTTE back to the table without further delay." The implication is that the facilitator is not playing its role satisfactorily.

The Sinhalese ire against the Norwegians is in fact linked with a popular impression that the international community as a whole has failed the Sri Lankan state in shoring up adequate support and, in contrast, betraying sympathy for the rebels. It is in the context of this widely shared perception that it is important to listen to a well-known social activist, Jehan Perera, who counters that contrary to the popular belief, the international community has been actually playing a corrective role, helping to remove the imbalances that are creeping into the peace process from time to time.[8]

Perera says that after the signing of the ceasefire agreement, the majority of the international community treated the LTTE in a very positive manner as they seemed to be impressed with the rebels, who were hitherto notorious for being one of the deadliest militant organisations in the world and had at last turned towards a political process of conflict resolution.

"Thereafter, the emphasis of the international community appeared to be a desire to engage with the LTTE by giving them economic aid and exposure visits rather than to criticise them. This has resulted in a widespread perception in Sri Lanka that the international community is biased towards the LTTE, " he says. The Norwegian facilitators, in particular, have been accused of being biased towards the LTTE. In truth, however, as the facilitator, Norway has played the vitally important role engaging closely with the LTTE, building up confidence and preparing the LTTE for dealing with the political process.

The SLMM has also been perceived as partial towards the rebels and ineffective. This has been on account of its inability to stop the LTTE from violating provisions of the ceasefire agreement (the records establish that the ceasefire provisions have been violated as many as 2,439 times by the LTTE against 111 times violations by the government). Perera says the problem is that the LTTE has openly refused to heed the rulings of the SLMM.

What is the way out? While unhappy Sri Lankans have suggested that the SLMM personnel should be changed, Perera says that a solution would be to strengthen the role of the international monitors. He, however, points out that this would only be possible if both the government and the rebels agree to a strengthened role for the SLMM. As long as the present hiatus lasts, such an agreement is unlikely to materialise.

In this context, a recent speech of the German ambassador in Sri Lanka Juergen Weerth appears to have attracted considerable attention. Speaking on the occasion of the German day of unity, the ambassador defended Norway's role as a facilitator strongly, noting that he did not agree with those who sought to blame the Norwegians for the present problems in the peace process. He said something which Sri Lankans do not appear to appreciate. He said, "The responsibility for the future of your country lies in your hands or still is in the hands of the political elite and your people, and failure is their collective failing. We should, therefore, be grateful to the Norwegians for their role as facilitator and never blame them for the lack of progress in the peace process." He pointed out that there was a need to recognise and appreciate a simple fact, namely, that though peace talks between the government and the LTTE had been suspended for nearly 19 months, no previous ceasefire had lasted more than three months. This has been achieved despite widespread pessimism in Sri Lanka on the onset of the ceasefire, predicting LTTE attacks on government forces within the first three months (revised later to six months).

As will be noted later in this book, the true achievement in Sri Lanka is the duration of the ceasefire, and there is little doubt that

Introduction XXI

this has been possible largely because of the sustained and patient handling of the situation by the international community, and particularly by the two countries intimately connected with the peace process, Norway as the facilitator and Japan as the largest donor. As recorded in the present volume, despite the fact that there is no forward movement towards a resumption of talks, the peace process has continued amid repeated assurances by the two adversaries about their resolve to stick to the ceasefire, which they have till now honoured. This clearly leaves the onus of actually restarting the dialogue with the government and the LTTE; neither can deny that the international community has already shown enough perseverance to cajole them to return to negotiations.

This book also deals extensively with the intimate relationship between the issues involving the deadlocked peace dialogue and Sri Lankan politics, a factor which complicates, rather than facilitates, the peace process. When the peace process started, the Wickramasinghe government was never armed with an unstinted support from the president and parliament; as a matter of fact, sections within the ruling United National Front became uncertain and uneasy about the contours of the process as the opposition parties celebrated a rising crescendo of Sinhalese-Buddhist criticism of the 'concessions' the government was perceived to be giving away to an 'unscrupulous' LTTE, the latter allegedly helped by the facilitator. The government's apparent recalcitrance in attempts to keep the president at bay, which is not explained satisfactorily to this day and which in turn exacerbated Kumaratunga's assertiveness, led ultimately to a demoralising climax by first neutering it through the takeover of three vital ministries and then the dissolution of parliament.

Kumaratunga's calculation in going for a snap general election could only have been an intense desire to do away with the irritant of the Wickramasinghe government and to better the electoral prospects of her own party, Sri Lanka Freedom Party (SLFP). At the time the election were announced, the UNF had no reason to apprehend a debacle. Yet, that was exactly what happened, catching it by surprise; but far less encouraging was the performance of the SLFP which actually lost in as many as seventeen seats, with its tally declining from 77 in the previous parliament to sixty. The elections, however, brought unexpected cheers to the SLFP's main ally, the Janatha Vimukthi Peramuna (JVP) which soared from sixteen seats to forty seats in the new parliament. What could have been Kumaratunga's expectation from forging the alliance with the JVP which was and remains to this day deadly set against any peace deal with the LTTE and definitely not on the basis of the ISGA proposals? Her obvious miscalculation was that an electoral alliance with the JVP would help her party regain some of its lost constituencies. In the event, the JVP not only gained spectacularly but, significantly, it beat the SLFP to the preference lists in several electoral districts. On the other hand, the old workers' parties, the Lanka Sama Samaj Party and the Communist Party, the SLFP's other allies which could have brought some positive thinking in the alliance (United People's Freedom Alliance) and which had been losing popular appeal steadily, fared worse in the 2004 elections. Thus, once the new parliament and government were formed, Kumaratunga was increasingly called upon to mount a much more difficult campaign in favour of restarting negotiations with the LTTE than would otherwise have been the case.

Writing a few days after the 2 April, 2004, general election, K Ratnayake commented, "The JVP's inclusion in government for the first time can only heighten political tensions. Despite the UPFA's claims that it will abide by the ceasefire and restart talks with the LTTE, the JVP's hostility to any concessions to the Tamil minority threatens to scuttle the 'peace process' and plunge the country back into civil war. For months, its speakers have been denouncing the UNF for betraying the country in negotiations with the LTTE."[9]

Apart from producing a government which continues to be sharply divided over the issue of resuming dialogue with the rebels, the general election also ended up with sharpening divisiveness in Sri Lankan electoral politics on communal lines, which again deflects from, rather than helps, a political settlement of the ethnic conflict. Apart from the JVP, two other parties performed creditably, the Tamil National Alliance (TNA) which with twenty-two MPs has since turned out to be a strong defender and advocate of the LTTE and the ISGA proposals and has in fact embarked upon a campaign to popularise the federal concept. The other party to have gained is the Jathika Hela Urumaya (JHU), an extremist Sinhalese-Buddhist party which fielded Buddhist monks in the polls and is now nine-MP-strong. Thus, while the SLFP and the UNF or UNP walk the middle path, supporting the peace process and desiring a return to negotiations with the Tigers, the JVP and the JHU are carrying on a fierce campaign against a dialogue based on the ISGA proposals and the TNA, at the other end, is busy explaining away the sins of the LTTE and putting up a strong advocacy for the rebels' causes. Incidentally, the JHU has also gone to the length of demanding that Sri Lanka be declared a theocratic state.

As was foreseen by perceptive observers at the time of the general election, Kumaratunga's virulent campaign against the conduct of the peace process by the UNF government resulted not only in whipping up the Sinhalese-Buddhist antipathy towards a political settlement of the ethnic strife and thus strengthening the JVP and the JHU but also weakened her own party. The SLFP panicked over losing traditional constituencies of the Sinhalese-Buddhists to the two ultra-nationalist parties and split at the time. The party has since recovered its aplomb to some extent and continues to be worried over the steady inroads being made by the JVP in its vote bank. As a result, out of both a fear of further electoral losses and a disaffection towards the LTTE, the SLFP remains hostile to the ISGA proposals.

It is this highly inhospitable environment for the government and the ruling coalition to initiate negotiations with the rebels that encourages the UNF and Ranil Wickramasinghe to laugh with derision at Kumaratunga's desperate bids to include the opposition in any exercise towards a resumption of peace talks. In a conversation with this author, Wickramasinghe was surprisingly cool about the president's inability to break out of the trap she has worked herself in and initiate a meaningful dialogue with the Liberation Tigers. "But can she persuade the JVP to fall in line with her intention to resume peace talks with the LTTE on the basis of the ISGA proposals, as the Tigers are demanding? Will her government last if she tries to go ahead on her own? A withdrawal by the JVP from the coalition would lead to an immediate fall of the government. Will she risk that much for the sake of restarting talks? We have serious doubts. To her, it was more important to dismiss my government than to ensure that the peace process continued undisturbed. At any count, she would have never condescended to allow my government to reach a successful settlement on the Tamil issue. It was that determination that shaped her policy at the time; she cannot now get out of the mess of her own creation."[10]

That Wickramasinghe's harsh criticism of Kumaratunga's policy has credibility is borne out by the fact that the formation of the UPFA, which required to be registered as a party under Sri Lankan law, was neither preceded nor followed by an agreement on a common minimum programme accommodating an agreed approach to the ethnic question. Since a settlement of the Tamil question acceptable to all sections of Sri Lankan society was and continues to be the single most important problem before the country, it would have been wise to thrash this out before the coalition was formed. But then, since the JVP's extreme position on the issue was well-established and in fact, its election campaign revolved around it, any such attempt to arrive at a common minimum programme for the new government would certainly have collapsed at the very first attempt.

Not surprisingly, the president's explanation of her action in taking over the three ministries of defence, interior and mass communication, suspension of parliament and the call for fresh election found few takers in Sri Lanka. In a typical presentation of the overwhelmingly majority view of her action, Prof G H Peiris, a well-known academic, wrote, "...for those more acutely conscious of Kumaratunga's confrontational style of politics and her constitutional powers as head of state and head of government, her action on 4 November (2003) represented no more than an expected culmination of the escalating power struggle between the virulently hostile national parties, the UNF and Kumaratunga's own Sri Lanka Freedom Party. There could hardly be any doubt that by bringing about a major cabinet reshuffle, what the president wanted more than (anything) else was a political showdown with the prime minister."

The inevitability of the development was emphasised by the fact that the president acted well within her constitutional rights, and Peiris remarked, her show of power was a response to the barely concealed and sustained attempt by the prime minister and his colleagues to bypass her in key decision-making processes.[11]

Introduction XXV

To look at the trial of strength between Sri Lanka's president and prime minister and its consequences from the point of view of the Liberation Tigers, the surprising fact was that there was no prior consultation between the two highest-ranking officials of the republic before the Wickramasinghe government responded to the unilateral ceasefire declared by the rebels on 24 December, 2001. Barely two years earlier, the president had survived a close assassination attempt on her life with a lifelong scar left on her. Nor was there any role assigned to her, also the commander-in-chief of the government forces, in the formulation of the terms and conditions of the memorandum of understanding signed by Wickramasinghe and LTTE leader Velupillai Prabhakaran on 22 February, 2002. The president was again kept out of the actual six rounds of negotiations between the government and the rebels though she maintained at the time that her representative should be included in the government delegation.

In retrospect, one would believe that the LTTE must have drawn immense pleasure out of the spectacle that the openly divided Sri Lankan state offered for view. Going through the litany of the acts of omissions and commissions that the Wickramasinghe government perpetrated during those days, obviously out of an intense desire to keep the president out of the entire peace process, it is scarcely credible that a government could at all behave in such an irresponsible manner. Information available at the time, corroborated later by the president herself, indicated that throughout the negotiations the government maintained a perfunctory manner of briefing the president about the details and, especially, about the 'concessions' that were being granted to the LTTE. This rather unconventional style of the functioning of a state must have confirmed the rebels in their belief that the way out of the dialogue process would turn out to be relatively easy and profitable. The eventual dissolution of parliament, which also led to a virtual dismissal of the Wickramasinghe government, brought extensive disappointment to the Tigers for good reasons.

Kumaratunga got away by dispensing with Wickramasinghe in the most humiliating manner imaginable because she was able to take advantage of a number of facilitating factors. The popularity of the government, which enjoyed the rare privilege of a parliamentary majority, had reached the nadir with prices of essential goods soaring, unemployment reaching record levels, the all-powerful Buddhist clergy finding itself increasingly ignored, the Sinhalese-Buddhists' phobia about an LTTE takeover of the northeast accentuating with fresh bouts of "concessions" being doled out to the "scheming" Tamils, the benefits of the peace process not reaching the people in the south and, as the ultimate folly, an injudicious design to browbeat the Supreme Court by attempting to impeach the chief justice on the eve of settling a crucial constitutional dispute.[12]

It was rather astonishing, therefore, to find the UNF unusually optimistic about its electoral prospects on the eve of the general election. In its view, despite the frequent presidential interventions, it had performed reasonably well while in office, with the economy flourishing, foreign investment promising to be flooding in and, most famously, the peace process including the ceasefire (which almost everybody had expected to collapse within its first three months of existence) was progressing smoothly with an approving nod from the international community now and then. The general secretary of the party, Senarath Kapukotuwa was quoted saying at the time that "we are ready to face an election at any moment. We are confident of victory. The party machinery is fully prepared to face an election." This optimism was apparently shared by political parties supporting the government from within and outside the coalition. As several commentators pointed out at the time, the readiness of the UNF to go for fresh polls and its energetic pursuit of the 19th amendment, which would have prevented the president from dissolving parliament and summoning fresh election, ran counter to each other. If the UNP and its allies were truly prepared to face fresh election, why should they have gone to the length of bringing in the aborted amendment?

Its defeat in the polls, therefore, was a major shock. Yet, an objective analysis of the conditions prevailing in the country at the time the election was announced would have left little room for doubt that the government was in fact highly unpopular. Months after the election, when this author was visiting Sri Lanka, sections of the Sinhalese-Buddhist community narrated woeful tales of growing deprivation in the countryside, the poor visibly getting poorer while large businesses made merry. Unemployment in particular became a truly burning issue, and the JVP jumped on the bandwagon and made its potentially embarrassing promises of a seventy per cent wage rise for government sector workers, restoration of subsidies, a lowering of the cost of living and an end to privatisation. All of these were also the UPFA's election promises none of which has been implemented in the months after the new government came into being. More than the SLFP, however, it is the JVP which is being increasingly called upon to explain its perceived failure to persuade the government carry out the promises, especially the bit about the seventy per cent wage rise in government-run entities.

As Norway the facilitator and Japan the chief donor renewed their efforts to get the talks going, there was little indication in Sri Lanka that a conducive atmosphere would soon be created for such an exercise. On 26 October, 2004, the UNP's media spokesman Prof G L Peiris, who was the chief government negotiator during the talks, announced that his party would take "every possible step" to prevent a reported presidential move to get her tenure extended through holding a referendum because this would be an extra-constitutional means. "The current constitution does not allow a referendum in this regard, " the former constitutional affairs minister said.

Reiterating his party's caveat for accepting the president's invitation to participate in the National Advisory Council for Peace and Reconciliation, he said that the UNP would do so only after the UPFA government resumed peace talks with the Liberation Tigers on the basis of the ISGA proposals. As we have seen, this was sheer politicking since the assumption behind the assurance of support was that the talks would not be resumed due to opposition from the JVP. The government, however, soon moved in to pour cold water on the UNP's enthusiasm to oppose the supposed presidential measure. Information minister Mangala Samaraweera said in Colombo the following day that "the government is not keen on holding Sri Lanka's presidential election in December, 2005, or a referendum to extend the current term." He added that the president had no intention of contesting the presidential election for a third term by resorting to an amended constitution.

If there were no encouraging signs for the government from either the main opposition party or the main ally, the end of October, 2004, also brought in a chilling reminder that the LTTE might suddenly introduce a dangerously uncertain element in the deadlocked peace process. The Tamilnet website quoted LTTE ideologue Anton Balasingham asserting that the Tigers had never given up on the right to secede from Sri Lanka.

Balasingham said that a joint statement issued after a round of discussions with the government, held in Oslo, had been "misunderstood and misinterpreted" to imply that the LTTE had finally abandoned the Tamils' right to external self-determination and secession. "The Liberation Tigers' decision to explore federalism…does not entail an unconditional abandonment of the Tamils' right" to secede from the country. The remarks were quoted by the website from Balasingham's forthcoming book, *War and Peace: Armed Struggle and Peace Efforts of Liberation Tigers.*

While ever since the Oslo Declaration, which Balasingham said was no declaration at all but a mere record of decisions, opinion in Sri Lanka appeared to have concluded that the LTTE had publicly accepted the concept of federalism, the rebels' ideologue sought to clarify what he called the misunderstanding and misinterpretation. If that indeed was the case, it is worthwhile noting that following the Oslo meeting, it was the Norwegian foreign ministry which stated that "the parties agreed to explore a solution founded on the principle of internal self-determination in areas of historical habitation of the Tamil-speaking peoples, based on a federal structure within a united Sri Lanka." But, according to the website, Balasingham had said in his book, "I feel it is necessary to clarify our position on this controversial issue. It must be stated that there was not any specific proclamation titled the 'Oslo Declaration.' The decision to explore federalism was included in the record of decisions at the Oslo talks and signed by the chief negotiators of both (the) delegations and the head of the Norwegian facilitating team." The LTTE, however, continued to operate within the "overall framework of the right to self-determination, with its internal and external aspects." If their demand for regional self-rule was ultimately rejected, Balasingham

Introduction XXIX

emphasised, they would have no alternative but to secede and form an independent state.

As a fresh international initiative was on its way at the end of October, 2004 (Japan's special envoy for the Sri Lankan peace process Yasushi Akashi visited Sri Lanka and held discussions with the political leadership), to revive the deadlocked talks, there were several ways of looking at Balasingham's comments, which at the first glance presented a new challenge to those involved in the peace process. Was Balasingham delivering a threat to the government to fall in line without further dithering and recommence talks on the basis of the ISGA proposals? Was this aimed to arm the international community to mount further pressure on the government to return to the negotiating table on the LTTE's terms? G L Peiris, who had led the Wickramasinghe government's delegation to the peace talks, however, felt that Balasingham was being merely truthful to what the LTTE position had always been and that there was scarcely any element of surprise in his blunt words. "The LTTE's position, as I understand it, was that they would try their utmost to work out with the Sri Lanka government a solution on federal lines. It is true that there was no absolute exclusion of the notion of secession but they did say that that (secession) would be the last resort." It was the LTTE's belief at Oslo that it would not have to fall back on any option other than federalism. "The whole tenor of the discussion (at Oslo) was that it is not necessary to look at options that they would fall back on, if everything failed, because they did not anticipate failure. On the contrary, there was every reason to anticipate progress and that was very much the atmosphere at the talks in Oslo at that time," he told *The Hindu* (30 October, 2004). Incidentally, Peiris managed to convey another impression without using as many words, namely, that the Oslo talks represented a genuine advance towards a political settlement of the ethnic question with both the government and the rebels participating sincerely and that it was only the presidential intervention later that had led to today's deadlock in the peace process.

The government, however, on its side continued to respond diplomatically to the pressure that was building up for a quick start to talks. Samaraweera reiterated on 28 October, 2004, (what he had first said about a fortnight back) that the government had drawn up a new blueprint to convert the ceasefire into lasting peace but insisted that the rebels must resume talks. "We want to take the counter-proposals with us when the discussions begin, " he said. "We are prepared to discuss the Interim Self Governing Authority. It all depends on the (Tigers') response now." In response, the Tigers stuck to their stand that they were prepared to start talking solely on the basis of the ISGA proposals. It was obvious that both the parties had fallen back upon their time-honoured practice of attempting to outwit each other. Since the LTTE had not mended its position in response to the government's stand that talks could be resumed on the basis of the ISGA proposals and its counter-proposals which presumably dealt with what it called the 'core' issues, Colombo preferred to push the ball into the rebels' court with the hope that the latter would be forced to either continue to decline the invitation to talk or succumb to the mounting international pressure to end the deadlock. Similarly, the rebels appeared to have held back with the expectation that the government would finally bow down to international pressure and agree to start talks on the basis of its maximalist proposals, knowing of course well that the JVP would be the last entity to permit the government to traverse that road.

While peace and war thus hung in balance in the autumn of 2004, Sri Lanka appeared to be caught in an uncomfortable vacuum in which everything waited to happen but nothing really did. Even in the midst of frenzied visits by the facilitators and donors, responsible voices expressed an unseemly but realistic degree of pessimism. "Nothing is likely to happen in the next six months, " said interlocutors who should have known better. "The good thing is that neither side wants to be the first to start fighting."

There is, however, one aspect of life in today's Sri Lanka that scarcely gets being talked about, its relatively improved human rights situation. Compared to the earlier two decades, there is a marked improvement in the observance of human rights and in punishment meted out to violators of human rights. Yet, there are nuances in this situation which point towards potential dangers. For instance, the Human Rights Commission of Sri Lanka, essentially a product of the

Introduction

liberal period introduced by Kumaratunga during her first presidentship, feels constrained because of a patently unhelpful and, sometimes decidedly hostile, bureaucracy which seems to feel threatened by the very presence and functioning of the commission and due to the ingrained sense of immunity from the punitive qualities of the rule of law that appears to pervade the security forces, including the police. "...owing to the heavy cuts imposed on the HRC budget in terms of the government's budgetary policy, " the commission said, "(the) HRC was severely constrained ...in carrying out its routine duties such as visiting police stations and this often hampered the commission in performing this deterrent role as efficiently as it would have."

It is with good reason that the Sri Lankan human rights watch body looks with admiration at its Indian counterpart. "We look upon the National Human Rights Commission of India as a role model, " said commission secretary D H Siriwardene. "Our constant endeavour is to be like the Indian commission. We are in close touch with it and try to benefit from its experiences. We believe that the Indian commission is a truly independent body run by people imbued with the highest principles of justice. Its success lies in its ability to persuade the executive to heed its findings and conclusions."[13]

Even though the Sri Lankan state is mandated by law to provide 'adequate' funds for smooth functioning of the Human Rights Commission, a constant funds crunch afflicts it seriously. "The state agencies deliberately choose to ignore budget recommendations, " said Siriwardene. Funds are released at times after the commission threatens the agencies with litigation. "The Paris Principles demand that the human rights commission should enjoy quasi-legal rights but even this is grudged. There are a lot of inadequacies in the present system. Right now, there are approximately 12,000 backlog cases. Besides, there is no system of a proper case assessment. Sadly enough, the commission itself is not attuned to the ground realities." Sources in the commission talked of its commissioners looking upon their appointments as essentially stop-gap arrangements and appearing to be mindful of not antagonising the powers-that-be. All these, they indicated, worked to the detriment of the proper functioning of the human rights commission which was the highest human rights watch body in the country.

On 27 September, 2004, an incident occurred which exposed the contradiction of the insecurity in which the commission was functioning in a seemingly vibrant parliamentary democracy. The officer in charge of the Jaffna office of the commission and a United Nations volunteer were assaulted while they were probing a complaint of torture that had allegedly occurred at the Jaffna police station. Talking about the incident to the Sinhala service of the BBC, Sandeshaya, the commission officer explained that he had sent another officer to enquire about a person who was being tortured at the police station. After reaching the police station, the officer rang up the officer in charge to inform that he was at the police station premises and could hear a man shouting 'ammo', which would imply that someone was in acute pain. The latter officer immediately telephoned the assistant superintendent of police and obtained his permission to go to the police station. The senior police officer also instructed a police officer and a UN volunteer to accompany the HRC official.

According to the interview with the BBC, when the HRC officer and the UN volunteer reached the police station, they found about thirty-five police officers gathered there. These officers started jeering and making abusive statements at them. The HRC officer tried to explain that he and his companion were visiting the police station on duty. Following this, he was pushed around and hit upon his head by the police officers who finally pushed them out of the police station. The torture victim was also taken out and put into a police van. The senior police officer had arrived at the scene by then who was shown the victim being taken away. As the HRC officer insisted that he could identify those who had assaulted him and his companion, the ASP asked all the officers to come out of the police station but only nine out of the thirty-five did so, and the one who had hit the HRC officer was not among them. The HRC officer told the BBC that it was his duty to inspect police stations and investigate allegations of illegal detention and torture. If he could be treated in such a fashion, he wondered what the fate of the common people would be.

Reporting the incident, the Asian Human Rights Commission (AHRC) pointed out that this was the second incident in less than

Introduction XXXIII

three months in which HRC officers had been obstructed or assaulted when attempting to inspect police stations. The first incident was reported from the Payagala police station.[14]

The AHRC called upon the Sri Lankan government to thoroughly investigate the matter and take serious action against the officers concerned. It recommended that the conduct of the ASP also required to be investigated. As any obstruction to public officers in carrying out their duties was a criminal offence, the culprits must be probed and charged. The AHRC called upon the inspector-general of police, the highest ranking police officer in the country, and the National Police Commission as well to investigate and take speedy action in the matter. To its credit, the state had since moved purposefully in the matter and the culprit police officer was identified and proceedings would no doubt have been initiated.

The human rights situation in the Jaffna Peninsula and district has always attracted extraordinary attention because of its unique circumstances, the region having been the cradle of the rise of Tamil militancy and the primary battleground where the civil war was being tenaciously fought. The Sri Lanka commission's annual report pointed out, " The Jaffna region has experienced the ravages of prolonged military combat on a scale and level of intensity not witnessed in other parts of the conflict-affected areas. The impact the armed conflict has, therefore, had on the derogation of human rights has been (the) severest on the Jaffna region and its inhabitants. More than most other areas in the north and east, it has suffered from loss of contact and communication with the rest of the country. The presence of the army on the one hand and the threat from the LTTE and other militant groups on the other hand created conditions which led to the disempowerment of civil society and the erosion of the entire infrastructure that was needed for the protection of human rights. Consequently, most of the institutions and processes that are needed for sustaining an effective human rights regime have been greatly impaired if not altogether destroyed. The renewal and restoration of these processes and institutions and the building of new capacity to meet the challenges that are emerging with the ongoing peace process require a special, concentrated effort on the part of the HRC. The Jaffna region contains the whole gamut of problems relating to human rights violations of diverse groups that have occurred during the war, ranging from the internally displaced, the missing persons, the female-headed households, disabled and conscripted children, refugees returning from abroad, and problems arising out of the ethnic 'cleansing.' The nature of the problems in every area related to human rights is exceedingly complex… The challenges that Jaffna will face as the ongoing peace process matures presents the Human Rights Commission with a unique opportunity to develop such an institution (a regional committee for human rights under section 11b of the HRC Act) and gain the knowledge and experience that would be relevant for the other regions." [15]

The general law and order situation (apart of course from the rising numbers of LTTE-related incidents), if considered in conjunction with this portrayal of the human rights commission's experiences, would not appear to be quite satisfactory. Gang warfares were becoming increasingly familiar incidents throughout the south, including Colombo; contract killings were said to be growing in numbers, and various related incidents indicated that social tensions were creating conditions for further slippage in the rule of law.

At the time the author was visiting Sri Lanka, the curious case of a former soldier R K L G Dingiri Banda was attracting a lot of public attention. The Asian Human Rights Commission said in early September, 2004, that it had received information from Banda on the 'serious' security threat by two unknown men a few days back. Banda was pursuing three cases against two army officers who were presently in the rank of captain; the cases were related to the severe assault on him which took place on 21 February, 2000, at the officers' mess of the Gajaba regiment at Saliyapura. He strongly believed that the two men might have been contracted or mobilised to harm his life due to his complaints against the army captains.

Commenting in this context, the AHRC made a statement which should not be dismissed lightly as it was a severe indictment of the law and order situation in Sri Lanka. "The rate of assassinations in Sri Lanka is very high and intimidation of complainants and witnesses is also very common," it said. "Under these circumstances, urgent action is required to pressure the government of Sri Lanka to provide immediate and adequate protection to Banda without delay. In particular, there is more reason to provide such protection to the victim as the opponents are powerful persons in the Sri Lankan army."[16]

A still more trenchant criticism of the law and order situation was made by the AHRC later in the same month. It said that Sri Lanka's bar association should defend the independence and credibility of its profession by taking active part in maintaining the rule of law and curbing the growing crime problem. It said that the bar association should speak out against those 'unprofessional and unscrupulous' practices of law enforcement to protect the rights of innocent people as well as of lawyers. "We are aware, " the AHRC said, "of enormous dissatisfaction that many lawyers from around Sri Lanka are experiencing about the strong impediments that have come their way for practising their profession in an independent and fearless manner. We urge that your organisation take up these matters in a credible way so that the others will find courage to get more involved in such matters and to build a strong public support for the elimination of crime." The AHRC found it 'rather strange' that professional bodies and courts did not notice the fact that more than 40, 000 fingerprints remained unchecked over the past ten years due to a lack of computers. "Often this incapacity results in the search for innocent persons to be substituted for actual criminals whom such (law-enforcement) officers cannot identify. The studies of hundreds of innocent torture victims demonstrate this fact, " it said.

One could go on recounting the extremely serious allegations made by the AHRC regarding the law and order situation and law enforcement regime in Sri Lanka. The allegations, even if exaggerated (which they are patently not), would not bring credit for a practising democracy. There are, therefore, several subjects, apart from the overriding issue of a resumption of peace negotiations between the government and the LTTE, that President Kumaratunga and her administration need to address urgently and effectively. A healthy and truly flourishing democracy, with the hopes and aspirations of all the communities living within its territory satisfactorily taken care of, would be not only a credit for Sri Lanka but for the South Asia region as a whole where this particular form of government could have performed better than it has.

Notes

1. Even earlier, more than a year before the parliamentary elections were held, President Chandrika Bandaranaike Kumaratunga told the Colombo-based diplomatic community on 31 March, 2003, "For my part of head of state, I give the people of Sri Lanka, including those who belong to and support the LTTE, the assurance that whoever may be the government of the day, the process of seeking a peaceful resolution to our conflict will proceed without a pause...I have on numerous occasions, too numerous now to recount, stated and emphasised that I remain firmly committed to the furtherance of the peace process, which I began in 1994 and continued with, in spite of hindrances and obstacles placed in my way...the expression 'peace process' means no more than a process of seeking to achieve a peaceful resolution to the armed conflict, which has prevailed for more than two decades, by negotiations. This process cannot be an end in itself. It is a means of achieving an objective. That objective is the achievement of a just and durable peace, which can only come about if the legitimate aspirations of all our communities are met."
2. Ram Manikkalingam, *Tigerism and Other Essays,* Ethnic Studies Group, Colombo, 1995, pp. 4 5.
3. The media reported on 1 April, 2002, that Muslim MPs, cutting across party affiliations, made a united appeal to the government to safeguard their political rights, safety and security in the eastern province in the face of increasing intimidation, harassment and violence by the LTTE. The reports said that the rebels were targeting the Muslims, who accounted for one-third of the population in the Trincomalee district and much more in the Batticaloa and Ampara districts for collecting its 'tax.' The Muslims, being mainly traders, were the main target for revenue collection by the LTTE. Since the beginning of the ceasefire, the reports said, the number of Muslims being abducted for tax collection was rising steadily. *The Hindu* correspondent Nirupama Subramanian quoted Sri Lanka Muslim Congress leader Rauff Hakeem saying the Muslims feared that harassment for 'tax'

would increase if the LTTE was permitted to move freely in the Muslim enclaves of the east, as envisaged under the ceasefire agreement. Tension in the region increased after 'provocative' remarks made by the local LTTE leader S Karikalan to the effect that the Muslims were armed against the Tamils and that their safety could only be granted if they publicly declared their allegiance to the rebel group. It was from around this time that the SLMC leader Hakeem began demanding the representation of the Muslims in government-LTTE negotiations and he continues to repeat the demand till date. While meeting the Norwegian peace envoy Eric Solheim on 14 September, 2004, he urged all the Muslim MPs to present a united front at peace talks, if and when these were resumed. "We are told that there is no likelihood of an immediate resumption of peace talks but the SLMC will be discussing with other Muslim parties in the event we are summoned for peace talks, " he said. While the LTTE made peace gestures earlier, offering to return cultivable land taken forcibly from Muslim farmers to the rightful owners and the process of repatriation of land actually followed suit, Hakeem reported that the situation was once again worsening in September, 2004. "One positive result of our previous talks with the LTTE was that we were able to persuade the LTTE to help Muslim farmers to cultivate their lands without harassment. However, that situation has lately been deteriorating to the extent of forcibly retaking of farming land. Especially incidents in the east have become disturbing. We hope that the LTTE resumes the dialogue soon so that these issues can be addressed, " he said. The LTTE reneging on its promise to leave Muslim farmers unmolested was yet another indication that it had little desire to allow communal relations to improve in the eastern province despite its posture of being a political entity and its apparent expectation that future talks should be based on its ISGA proposals.

4. P K Balachanddran, *India-Sri Lanka defence pact will threaten peace process: LTTE*, HindustanTimes.com, 25 October, 2004.
5. P K Balachanddran, *Increasing US influence Over Sri Lanka Worries LTTE*, HindustanTimes.com, 4 October, 2004.

6. Ranga Jayasuriya, "No LTTE military build-up—SLMM" *Sunday Observer*, 24 October, 2004. The report further said that the ceasefire monitors could not, however, visit three alleged LTTE installations built deep inside jungles. "After visiting all but these three places, we did not see any 'military' presence of the LTTE in the area, " the SLMM spokesman said. He said that the three places were alleged to have been located deep in jungles. "Some civilians speak of the existence of these three installations in the jungle. But given the distance between these installations and the security forces camps, we don't think that would have any impact on the security situation, " he said. Most of these places, he added, were small installations of a few bunkers and were actually checkpoints. "Some of them are new and some are old. But all of them are well within the LTTE-controlled areas, " the spokesman said. The only LTTE camp built in the government-controlled area was the Wan Ela (Manirasakulam) camp, which was ruled a ceasefire agreement violation by the monitors. The SLMM had earlier submitted two preliminary reports to the government on its probe into the alleged LTTE build-up around Trincomalee. Both the reports had reached the same conclusion as the present one, saying that the monitors did not find evidence of an LTTE military build-up in the area. However, intelligence reports had warned that the Tigers were building up bases around the harbour and getting closer to the military artillery range.
7. Interview taken in Colombo on 17 September, 2004.
8. Jehan Perera, *International community playing a corrective role*, www.peaceinsrilanka.org, *11* October, 2004.
9. K Ratnayake, *Sri Lankan election produces a hung parliament and further political instability*, www.wsws.org, 5 April, 2004.
10. In an extensive interview to the *Financial Times,* London, South Asia correspondent Edward Luce, dated 17 November, 2003, Kumaratunga explained her policy towards the UNF government following her taking over of three important portfolios and suspension of parliament. Denying that she was facing a constitutional difficulty in her cohabitation with the opposition-

run government, she said, "I wouldn't call it a constitutional difficulty. By my action I resolved the constitutional conflict. The constitution clearly stipulates that defence should be entirely under the president. If there are any doubts about it, there was a Supreme Court ruling the other day which is one of the reasons I took it (the defence ministry) over. It was not removing or sacking ministers...All (the) three ministers are still in the cabinet. On taking over defence, in fact, I was correcting a constitutional problem that was there, which is that defence is inalienable from the president according to our constitution. All (the) previous presidents have held the portfolio of defence. ...In fact, it was their (Wickramasinghe's) previous government that pushed the Tamil people to war after the massacre of 1983...I came into power in 1994 and stopped all that —within 24 hours we brought back the rule of law, respect for fundamental rights and appointed commissions and all kinds of things. ' You shouldn't have any fears', I told the prime minister. But they didn't like it and he kept insisting on having defence. And I did the very unusual and unconstitutional thing of giving it to him only because of two things: he told me he would continue the peace process I had begun. I was very happy with that because in Sri Lanka we have this horrible habit of going against the other party....anyway, (Wickramasinghe) said he needed the defence portfolio because it was more convenient... (he) said to me, 'Every important defence decision will be taken in consultation with you.' But he did not...I did not take the defence portfolio back to attack some LTTE camp or other things. I had to take over defence. Even according to the ceasefire agreement, there are certain limits the LTTE (is) meant to follow. But the defence minister and (the) prime minister allowed some gross things to happen....Six shipments of arms (for the LTTE) were allowed to be brought in. Some of them were 60-tonne ships carrying surface-to-surface missiles. In other words, they allowed the LTTE to do things that no sovereign state would even dream of permitting. So all I did was (to) try to balance it. The LTTE has now surrounded the chief naval base of the country in Trincomalee, which is also

the second largest port in the country. They have surrounded it with seventeen camps put up in total violation of the ceasefire agreement. And the government is doing nothing about it...But the army and (the) navy were getting very restless and kept telling me, 'Do something about it.' ...and then the prime minister started saying that we were trying to sabotage this peace process. Obviously, I know it's a tightrope walk to keep the ceasefire and dialogue going with the LTTE and at the same time not permitting them to do all the things they are doing at the moment. But I think if one was firm they would understand it. So all I did was (to take) over (the) defence portfolio and (give) instructions as soon as I took over not to allow (the) LTTE to do anything that would harm the ceasefire arrangement." In similar comments to *Time Asia* (22 March, 2004), she said that she seized the government because Wickramasinghe's peace negotiations were a "farce". She accused the prime minister of making "secret promises" to the LTTE that threatened to split the country between the Sinhalese south and the Tamil northeast. Complaining that Wickramasinghe excluded her from peace negotiations despite her requests to be kept informed, she derided him as "a liar...(who) has no backbone" and who was "incapable of thinking big." She also fumed about what she perceived as his disrespect for her. Wickramasinghe would call her "madam" to her face "but sit there in (the) cabinet with a smirk on his face as his ministers abused me (with) the most horrendous insults." The report quoted analyst Paikiasothy Saravanamuttu saying, "In her mind, her future and the future of her party and the country are all tied together. Hurt one in that context and you hurt them all." Wickramasinghe was quoted saying that the real problem was her ego. "The president has said before that politics and power in Sri Lanka is a Bandaranaike family preserve."
11. G H Peiris, "A Presidential Intervention," *South Asia Intelligence Review*, 18 November, 2003.
12. It was in mid-October, 2003, that the Supreme Court arrived at a decision on the proposed 18th and 19th amendments to the Sri Lankan constitution, rejecting both and thus debilitating the

Wickramasinghe government from its design to take away certain rights enshrined by the constitution in the highest court of the land. The 18th amendment, which sought to place the newly created constitutional council out of the fundamental rights jurisdiction of the Supreme Court, was ruled unconstitutional. Had it approved of the amendment, decisions of the constitutional council would have been immune from the Supreme Court's jurisdiction. But it was the rejection of the 19th amendment that appeared to have struck a heavy blow at the government, which was immediately seized upon by Kumaratunga to begin the process of easing out Wickramasinghe from power. The amendment, if approved by the Supreme Court, would have taken away the presidential power to dissolve parliament and call for a fresh general election one year after the last election. The amendment would also have empowered MPs with cross-voting rights so that they could vote according to their conscience without being unseated for defying party whip. It is important to remember that the government brought the 19th amendment expressly in order to ensure that political instability induced by a dissolution of parliament, holding of fresh polls and new configurations in the composition of the next parliament would not have seriously impacted on the peace process. Thus, the power struggle between the president and the prime minister was intertwined with the peace process in a negative sense, further exposing the fundamental weakness of the Sri Lankan state in dealing with the ethnic conflict.

13. Interview taken in Colombo on 15 September, 2004.
14. A statement by the Asian Human Rights Commission, AS36-2004, 28 September, 2004.
15. Human Rights Commission of Sri Lanka, *Report for the period (01.04.2001-31.03.2003)*, pp.19-20.
16. Asian Human Rights Commission, *Urgent Appeal: Sri Lanka: Threat to life; Protection needed for the torture victim*, 7, September, 2004.

1
Frozen Peace Melting?

By the summer of 2004, certain things were clear in Sri Lanka. The split in the military machine of the Tamil Tigers with "Col" Karuna's defection (3 March 2004) had weakened it significantly and Velupillai Prabhakaran would not rest and could in fact, ill afford to rest until the control over the Tamil-inhabited areas of the east was regained.

Thus, even towards the end of the year, the Tigers and the defectors were killing each other off though the obvious advantage of numerical superiority lay with the former. But, what was clear above all, was that neither the Sri Lankan government nor the Liberation Tigers of Tamil Eelam (LTTE) was in a position to seriously do anything to derail the peace process, stalled since 21 April 2003, as sometimes they were suspected of intending to do.

As the stalemate over the resumption of peace negotiations continued to persist, the Bush administration was finding it difficult to keep the "little speck" of an Indian Ocean island on its rather crowded radar. After all, "dozens of international crises" appeared on the US agenda on a daily basis, as an administration official, seemingly out of justifiable frustration, put it.[1]

The international community too was finding it increasingly difficult to keep earmarking a substantial amount of hard currency ready for Sri Lanka's succour for an indefinite period. "Right now, there are a lot of competing situations," as Norwegian Deputy Foreign Minister Vidar Helgesen said without much ado, and therefore Sri Lanka could not expect the international community to sit with the money till both the warring parties agreed to resume their dialogue.[2]

Analysts suspected that one reason for the face-off over the resumption of peace talks could well be the $ 4.5 billion aid promised to Sri Lanka at the Tokyo conference (announced on 10 June, 2003). In October, the Tigers were cautioning the international community about assumed Sri Lankan designs to lay hands on the till even before talks could be restarted.

Between June and October 2004, the mood in the country, after living through a nightmarish ethnic war of 21 years vintage and approximately 65,000 (as most estimates claimed) deaths and unaccounted destruction rendering vast stretches of the northeast desolate and adversely affecting Sri Lankan economy, had almost turned the full circle and was relapsing into despair at the infinite folly of the leaders.

Yet, on the positive side, well over two years had gone by without a fresh outbreak of fighting, an achievement in any context. A substantial extent of developmental work had been accomplished in the northeast, with both the government and the LTTE participating in the endeavours and the Tamil Tigers easily outshining the Sri Lankan bureaucracy and military in registering their proven capabilities; and investment (mostly in the south and, rather spectacularly, from the Tamil Diaspora) had been in evidence.

True, the truce had grown pockmarked with violations of the conditions of the Ceasefire Agreement (CFA) by both the sides, necessitating the Sri Lankan Monitoring Mission (SLMM) to issue warnings to both periodically. However, this unaccustomed blissful period of peace, which had followed a ceasefire brokered by Norway and initiated on 23 February, 2002, gave way to a deepening sense of uncertainty in the mid-2004 in the wake of a series of killings of renegade Tamil rebels in and around Colombo; the perpetrators having clearly been the Liberation Tigers of Tamil Eelam (LTTE), bumping off members of the renegade "Karuna" band of loyalists.

The split in the LTTE in March 2004 with regional Tiger commander V Muralitharan alias Karuna breaking away and thus suddenly posing a serious challenge to the Tamil rebel organisation in the eastern Sri Lanka, which had traditionally provided male and female fighters and funds for the Tiger war machine, had finally begun to take its toll on the peace process itself, widening the circle of uncertainty and being stalked by the threat of resumed fighting between Sri Lankan government forces and Tamil rebels.

The circumstances that had periodically lent oxygen to the ethnic war in the Indian Ocean island seemed to have returned. Karuna's revolt against the Tiger rebel leader Velupillai Prabhakaran and his success in breaking off with 5, 000-6, 000 fighters (4, 000, according to some observers) had obviously weakened the parent organisation significantly, and the latter would now desperately need time to recoup.

Diplomatic circles in Colombo sensed a reluctance on the part of the LTTE to resurrect the disrupted peace talks at this particular juncture. "The Tigers are now militarily weaker in the east after Karuna's split," a news portal quoted an unnamed Western diplomat analysing the situation in early August 2004. "They are not likely to come for talks until they re-establish total control over the area."[3]

A month later, talking to the author, head of the Peace Secretariat of the Sri Lankan government and former senior United Nations official Jayantha Dhanapala said, "...the LTTE is not willing to talk now until they fully regain the east. But how many people can they kill?"[4]

This was, however, not the official version of the stalemate over the resumption of peace negotiations. Officially, both the government and the LTTE maintained that differences over the agenda for the resumed talks had held up progress, though in early September 2004, talking to the Foreign Correspondents' Club of Sri Lanka, Kumaratunga said that the Karuna factor "has also caused a certain blockage in the LTTE coming to the negotiation table early."

The agenda for the resumed bout of the dialogue, the Tigers had proposed, should be the constitution of an Interim Self Governing Authority (ISGA) for the north and east (see Appendix), a proposal that had brought forth a spate of panicked and angry protests from the professional ethnic baiters, the Janatha Vimukthi Peramuna (JVP), presently a powerful segment of the Chandrika Kumaratunga-led government, the Janatha Hela Urumaya (JHU) which had set a stiff challenge to the JVP over championing the majoritarian agenda and Buddhist monks, the latter having successfully maintained their unenviable record of exacerbating, rather than mending, ethnic relations in the perpetually troubled island nation.

More significantly, however, the Sri Lanka Freedom Party (SLFP), one of the two major Sinhalese political parties and the main constituent of the ruling coalition, had set forth its determined and extensively argued opposition to the ISGA proposals, alleging that the concept of an ISGA was nothing but a clandestine manner of "preparing the legal ground for a separate state." (see Appendix) The deep-seated mistrust between the largely Sinhalese establishment of the south and the Tamil rebels of the north remained exactly as ingrained as before.

There was, however, an important difference. Despite a rising tension in the relationship over the recent developments, both sides were willing to exercise restraint in their behaviour. The course of the shadow boxing over the issue of the agenda was itself an evidence that neither contending party was willing to stake all in order to score a point over the other. On 29 July, 2004, Sri Lanka Cabinet spokesman and minister Mangala Samaraweera told a media briefing in Colombo, almost in a Shakespearean vein, that "In thunder, lightning or in rain we are ready for negotiations and we hope the LTTE shows a similar commitment. What is at stake is much larger than the recent incidents reported in the east and in Colombo. Even though we do not agree with the Interim Self Governing Authority on principle, the government has agreed to open discussions on the ISGA, along with the final solution. I think the LTTE must show some flexibility on their part for the sake of the peace process."

On its part, the LTTE also climbed down significantly. While it had earlier stuck to the position that negotiations could be taken up only after the government had conceded the demand for an ISGA, it later softened its stand by saying that an agenda with discussions on the ISGA would be acceptable to it. By mid-September, 2004, with eleven months gone since the presentation of the ISGA proposals and no sign of the government in Colombo ready to start a dialogue, LTTE political wing chief S P Thamilchelvan was spelling out in as bold terms as possible that the proposals were negotiable. " They are not rigid or final and should be discussed at the negotiating table, " he told the *Daily Mirror* (15 September, 2004). "We want an interim structure that would enable the benefits of the ceasefire to go to the people and to provide humanitarian assistance. We felt (that) the proposals given by the former government on an interim structure to address these issues did not have sufficient powers. Then, the government and the international community requested us to put forward our proposals. We consulted a lot of people and put forward these ISGA proposals as a basis on which peace talks could resume. The former government accepted the proposals as a basis for negotiations."

In a wider political and public relations exercise aimed at a choice southern audience, Thamilchelvan had earlier met a delegation of Buddhist clergy, Catholic priests, trade unionists and media at the Tigers' political headquarters in the Vanni region in northern Sri Lanka on 2 August, 2004. Thamilchelvan said that the ISGA proposals were to address "urgent humanitarian needs" of the people in the areas of resettlement, rehabilitation and reconstruction and it was very unfortunate that politicians were using this issue to mislead the people in the south.

He said that the upholding of the Ceasefire Agreement (CFA) and taking steps to restore normalcy in the war-devastated northeast region were the most important and urgent steps to be taken to remove the impediments in taking forward the peace process. The Tamil people, he also said, were very disappointed that they had not become beneficiaries of the peace dividends. Normalcy for them was restoring their rights to go back to their homes, and being engaged in their professions like agriculture and fishing in their natural habitats. These were yet to happen and would be feasible only when the northeast issue was settled to the full satisfaction of their interests and concerns.

Not surprisingly, this was a deliberate exaggeration of the ground realities. Nearly half of the internally displaced persons (IDPs) had returned to the northeast, and the refugees still living in the welfare centres had either chosen to stay back or were unable to return home. Various factors were holding them back, such as, the large number of uncleared mined areas (one reliable estimate held that at least another six years would be required to fully de-mine the northeast); but, most significantly, it was the oft-confusing borders between the high security zones (HSZs) which in many cases almost tended to intervene into each other, thus heightening the danger of a sudden flare-up, and therefore, acting as a strong deterrent to the IDPs.[5]

As the situation was clearly worsening with repeated killings of renegades by the LTTE in and around Colombo in the aftermath of Karuna's defection, the perception of a deterioration in law and order sharpened with the abortive assassination attempt on minister and the Eelam People's Democratic Party (EPDP) leader Douglas Devananda on 7 July 2004 (interestingly, but not uniquely in the Sri Lankan context, the intra-LTTE killings and even the latest attempt on Devananda's life were largely perceived by the Sinhalese community as matters pertaining exclusively to the Tamils, and life therefore went on smoothly in Colombo and elsewhere in the south in the midst of the gory and otherwise unsettling incidents; it was the expatriate community which appeared to be much more concerned than the majority community about the law and order situation).

Nevertheless, it was obvious to perceptive observers in the majority community as well as elsewhere that the problem was no longer confined to the interrupted peace talks; it was far wider than the stalling tactics being deployed by both the government and the Tigers. In essence, the problem for the government was how to tell the people of the country and the larger world in a convincing manner that the initiative to influence the course of events had not relapsed into the hands of the Tamil rebels as had happened at each critical juncture in the chequered history of the ethnic conflict. Was the LTTE not exploiting the prolonged stalemate at the talks to settle its own score with its enemies, including in Colombo where the seat of the government was? Dhanapala was clearly irked by a question as to why the impression had gained ground that as in the past, the initiative had once again passed into the hands of the LTTE. With nearly a year having passed since the presentation of the ISGA proposals, it was the government which appeared to be not ready and equipped to formulate its response; and in that sense, the initiative had clearly passed on to the Tigers. But the peace secretariat chief reasoned otherwise, "One must appreciate that the government has to bear in mind the interests of the state, such as, its security, integrity and sovereignty, as well as

Frozen Peace Melting?

the welfare of the people, " he said. "On the other hand, the LTTE is free from such constraints and is able to pursue its exclusivist agenda."[6]

Unfortunately, however, the impression that the government was lagging behind the LTTE in image-building capabilities and in propagating its views in acceptable terms to the Sinhalese people appeared to be justified in the beginning of August 2004 when both the sides went public to reiterate their willingness to pursue the peace course. On 29 July 2004, the government resiled from its earlier stance to refuse pointblank to discuss the ISGA proposals with Dhanapala saying that "the president is willing to discuss the ISGA, along with government proposals, to set up an interim authority."

It was obviously not a straight offer to talk, as it was laced with the condition that the government proposals for an interim council (see Appendix) should also be discussed, something which were quite categorically ruled out by the LTTE when the concept was first aired. Most of all, the impression prevailed that the government was shying away from a serious dialogue with the political and public opinion in the south. The *Daily Mirror* said in its editorial on 16 September, 2004, "What is more important for the president is to get round the other parties and groups who are opposed to negotiations with the LTTE. They have to be convinced that there won't be any prospects for a durable peace, without making the LTTE a party to any settlement of the national question. Even if war is avoided, one will not see an end to the killing and violence. These parties are understandably opposed to the LTTE's ISGA proposals. There is none, except the LTTE, who supports (the proposals). Even the LTTE now expresses a willingness to consider any modifications to them suggested by other parties. What most political parties want is an end to the present impasse by resumption of talks....it is necessary for the southern parties to agree on a basis on which to resume talks with the LTTE. What is emerging as the greatest obstacle to forging a southern consensus is the main party rivalry now sharpened by the debate over the government's failure to honour the promises given at the last election."

A unique feature of the situation in the summer of 2004, which to an extent distinguished it from the previous stalemates in the earlier peace processes, was the more intimate involvement of the international community with the fortunes of the island nation. The two warring Sri Lankan sides were no longer posturing and shadowboxing for gaining tactical advantages over each other in reassuring isolation. They were under closer and constant watch of outsiders, the chief among them of course being the monitors of the implementation of the Cease Fire Agreement, and the facilitators of the peace process, the Norwegians. It was apparently a common desire of both the sides not to alarm the international community excessively that was inducement enough to exercise restraint.

The correlation between any expression of anxiety and despair by the international community and quick steps by the Sri Lankan government and the LTTE to signal that all was far from being lost was amply displayed during the most of 2004. It was on 19 July that the Sri Lanka Monitoring Mission warned that the ceasefire was under threat as both the sides were beginning to violate the CFA. Head of the SLMM Trond Furuhovde said in an identical letter sent to both the sides that "The SLMM should not be held responsible due to problems that arise after both (the) parties breach the agreement."

Media reports said at the time that following the unambiguous warning, the government quickly decided to engage itself actively in attempts to revive the peace process and called upon the Norwegian government to send an official to "push forward" the process.

As a result, the deputy foreign minister of Norway Vidar Helgesen spent three days visiting Sri Lanka and talking to the two sides. At the end of his visit, he was uncomfortably objective in his assessment of the situation. While the two sides, he said, were committed to peace, there was no progress towards an early resumption of talks. He told the media in Colombo on 28 July 2004 that he was not optimistic about an early return to the negotiating table. "This position remains the same," he said, while the security situation in the east and the recent incidents in those areas were disturbing the peace process. "There is no more clarification on the resumption of peace talks. We underline the security situation in the east and the incidents hovering those areas are not helping to bridge the gap between the two parties on the resumption of early talks. But neither party has a desire to return to war." He also spoke frankly about an unfortunate delusion that appeared to have led the people to believe that peace was at hand.

"The Ceasefire Agreement is not the peace agreement, " he said. "It only means that war has been frozen. Today, the frozen war is melting at the edges. That is not a good thing. People are strongly in favour of peace but, not in favour of the peace process." Saying that the president had demonstrated a deep commitment towards pushing the peace process ahead, he said, "But the president alone cannot operate in this regard. The parties, both government and the opposition, should perform their role to achieve peace."

While the Norwegian diplomat did not spell it out, he clearly sought to convey that the virtual impunity with which the two sides had manoeuvred to keep stalling a resumption of the peace process had been facilitated by "an incredible complacency among the general public" as they appeared to believe that peace had already been established. Significantly, when he was asked about the next step that the Norwegians should adopt, Helgessen said that his country expected to consult the international community in respect of re-energising the peace process. This could have meant only one thing, application of pressure on both the combatants, to pave the way for fresh talks, so that the risk of upsetting the delicately balanced no-hostilities situation could be minimised.

Helgesen's widely reported and quite dramatic announcement that the frozen peace had begun to melt at the edges apparently had some effect (not entirely unforeseen given the average Sri Lankan's acute sensitivities and the sometimes edgy relationship between the Kumaratunga presidentship and the Norwegians) on the Sri Lankan government which accused Norway on 29 July 2004 of "exaggerating" the existing state of affairs.

Cabinet spokesman and Media Minister Mangala Samaraweera said the government believed that Helgessen had exaggerated the situation and expressed his "full" confidence that neither the government nor the LTTE would go back to war. "Even if there is an impasse, to say that this is a slant towards war is an exaggeration, " he said.

The Sri Lankan government could not agree with the Norwegian diplomat's comment that there was a greater threat now of the peace process failing. Challenging Helgesen's remark that "the patience of the international community is being tested", he said he believed on the contrary that the international community was appreciative of the president's commitment to the peace process. "The president is committed and dedicated to resuming the talks. It is now left to the LTTE to respond in a similar manner. We have differences on the ISGA but they can be sorted out in a systematic manner if we sit across a table, " he said.

The sequence of the events established with adequate force the fact that the pressure of the international community exerted on the two quarrelling sides had begun to bear fruits.

Interestingly, the LTTE also found it expedient to assert periodically that it was not under any pressure from the international community for suing for peace. Thus, after a meeting in the mid-August of 2004 with a European Union (EU) delegation which apparently gave it a piece of its mind about the spree of killings of renegades, continuing child recruitment into the rebel outfit and abductions, all of which had clearly pushed the country towards a fresh fear of renewed bloodbath, the Tigers felt obliged to assert a basis for independence of action. Addressing journalists on 16 August, Thamilchelvan said that the Tigers were "not pressurised in any way by the visits of international delegations." He explained to the EU delegation the LTTE leadership's stand that it was "ready to restart negotiation with the Sri Lankan government on the basis of the ISGA proposals, which (were) endorsed by the Tamil people at the general election."

Clearly pushing hard the political demand for an acceptance of the ISGA proposal by the government, he also said that it was (the) "moral responsibility of everybody, including the LTTE, that the Tamil people's wish expressed as an overwhelming electoral mandate should be respected and talks should recommence without any further delay."

Letting out a fascinating glimpse into the way the LTTE was thinking about the renegades, Thamilchelvan also "explained" the situation in the east where "paramilitary forces" were being nurtured and promoted by Colombo and the Eelam People's Democratic party (EPDP) and the renegades "are engaged in activities aimed at disrupting the peace process."

Significantly, this statement was preceded by just a few hours by the shooting down of the EPDP propaganda secretary "EROS Bala"

Balanadarajah Iyer in Colombo, apparently by the LTTE. Condemning the murder, the government said that the recent killings "suggest (the) involvement of the LTTE" and pointed out that the shooting down of EROS Bala was the "latest in a spate of brutal killings that continue to be perpetrated in Colombo and the Eastern Province." Those killed included journalists, academics and activists who were targeted as a consequence of their political affiliation.

The following report posted on the website Tamilnet, considered in Colombo to be a virtual mouthpiece of the LTTE, dated 2 October, 2004, illustrates the professional coolness with which the killing spree was being carried out, "Special forces of the Liberation Tigers' Jeyanathan Regiment Saturday morning attacked a group of heavily armed paramilitary cadre northwest of Batticaloa, killing two and wounding three around 6.30 a.m., LTTE sources in the east said. The group of ten men from the paramilitary led by renegade LTTE commander 'Karuna' were in a safe house in Omadiyamadu near the Polannaruwa-Batticaloa district border, the sources said. "We recovered an AK-47-2 assault rifle from them. Those who escaped ran towards a Sri Lanka army position near Omadiyamadu. The bodies of the two paramilitary cadre killed in the attack were brought to Vakarai later in the day. We have asked their parents to take the bodies. The dead paramilitary cadre were identified as Vicky and Niththy. Omadiyamadu is about 28 km west of Vakarai." The LTTE had been describing the renegade Tigers as paramilitary in order to drive home its contention that Karuna's men were being sheltered and helped by the army.

To return to the plain speaking done by the EU delegation to the LTTE, the nonchalance displayed by Thamilchelvan to the media over it did not obviously reflect the seriousness with which the EU had viewed the situation and conveyed in unambiguous terms its concerns to the Tigers. In what was correctly described as the strongest statement made by the international community till date, the EU conveyed its "concern and alarm" to the LTTE over the recent increase in the violation of human rights and said that adhering to "good governance, pluralism, human rights and democracy" were vital if the rebels were to obtain "recognition as a political player in Sri Lanka."

Condemning the political killings, child recruitment and abductions increasingly being committed "as a breach of fundamental human rights", the EU also told the LTTE that "there is no excuse for such violence, which can never resolve the internal differences in Sri Lanka." Referring to its External Affairs Commissioner Chris Patten's call in 2003 to the Tigers to establish their absolute commitment to the peace process, the EU emphasised that issues such as good governance, pluralism, human rights and democracy, which were the cornerstones for everlasting peace in Sri Lanka, were also important for the rebels to qualify for the recognition as a political player.[7]

Thus, 2004 continued to witness the charade that was being played by the two adversaries. Even though a public relations gesture like a meeting with the LTTE leader would be an anathema in the existing backdrop of the stalled negotiations, this was precisely the idea that Kumaratunga came up with.

In an interview, she offered to meet Prabhakaran if progress were to be made in the stalemated peace talks. She said that she was willing to meet him "not for the sake of just shaking hands but if negotiations begin and we are progressing, quite definitely at some point we have to meet." However, speaking from the strength of being the head of state and government, she also said in the course of the interview that "the only way to control the situation in the eastern Sri Lanka would be to send in troops. I have never balked at doing what is required of me as head of state in the national interest. Even at the risk of my life, I have had attempted to the best of my ability to execute responsibilities handed to me by the people…at two presidential elections…We will not hesitate if it appears to us after long reflection that it is required in the national interest."[8]

She pointed out that her government had offered to step in and restore law and order in the LTTE-held eastern Sri Lanka following "Col" Karuna's revolt on 2 March "but the rebels had refused." She also explained the delay in restarting the peace talks by noting that the "main concern" of the LTTE leadership was to "stabilise the eastern situation before they come to talks." "It appears, " she said, "that the LTTE present leadership's main concern is this… And our impression is that the agenda is not the main point."

Frozen Peace Melting? 13

What is it that effectively blocks the political leadership of Sri Lanka from reaching the goal every time a serious bid for peace is made ? At one time, the blame lay squarely at the door of the LTTE for deliberately sabotaging peace initiatives. Beginning with the Indo-Sri Lanka Agreement "to establish peace and normalcy in Sri Lanka" of 29 July 1987, the history of the quest for peace in the island nation makes dismal reading.

That celebrated and much-maligned accord, which caused considerable unhappiness and bloodshed in Sri Lanka and an unaffordable unpopularity for the Rajiv Gandhi government in India, sought to "preserve the unity, sovereignty and territorial integrity of Sri Lanka" and at the same time to provide an assured space to the minority Tamil aspirations for regional autonomy and preservation of the salient aspects of a widely perceived and accepted Tamil way of life in its natural habitat (this very concept remains completely unacceptable to the Sinhalese community). Interestingly, seventeen years later, the LTTE, while presenting its proposal "on behalf of the Tamil people for an agreement to establish an Interim Self Governing Authority for the northeast of the island of Sri Lanka, " on 31 October 2003, also vowed "to bring lasting peace to all persons of the island of Sri Lanka"

One way of looking at the various attempts to bring about peace in Sri Lanka and reach an agreement over the future of the northeast is to conclude that these initiatives were probably doomed to fail because both the sides tended to exploit them to advance their respective agendas. Could this be the truth behind the prolonged struggle between war and peace in the country?

Prof. Jayadeva Uyangoda, a perceptive academic, for example, wrote sometime after the Indo-Sri Lanka Accord, "Politically, the Jayewardene regime clearly sought through the accord to regain its authority over the political process and to re-establish the stability of the state, since an end to the violent ethnic war without a serious military or political setback to the state was essential to restore the already lost political equilibrium in society. The accord, nevertheless, was a calculated risk taken by a section of the UNP (United National Party, the ruling party of the period), a risk (that) emanated from not-so-distant possibility of the accord being rejected by the militant and politically assertive sections of both Sinhalese and Tamil societies. Today, one year after the accord came into force, its objectives seem to be either partially fulfilled or not fulfilled at all. The real question, however, is not whether this or that individual provision of the accord has been duly implemented or not, but whether or not the political developments that followed it have diminished the political crisis in Sri Lanka."[9]

Needless to say, the answer would have been in the negative. Uyangoda continued, "The political conflict in society is assuming increasingly violent and uncompromising proportions, highlighting the inability of the regime to present a viable project of social peace. And to complicate the nature of the present crisis, no other political or social force seem to be able to mobilise the subordinate classes on a programme of social and ethnic peace which is essential to resolve the present crisis within the framework of the democratic state."

Writing fourteen years later on the latest quest for peace in Sri Lanka, as the current ceasefire appeared to find its feet and the United National Front government led by Ranil Wickramasinghe and the LTTE were inching towards the signing of a formal ceasefire agreement, Uyangoda felt that neither side was likely to move immediately into discussing political or constitutional issues. "Their primary focus will be on de-escalation." He said. "After all, this is the so-called 'realist' approach to peace. This reveals a fascinating convergence of approaches between the government and the LTTE on 'peace.' They seem to have a shared understanding of peace; de-escalation of war. In theoretical jargon, we may describe this as 'negative peace.' Which means the absence of war. It is basically a conflict management, pragmatic approach that falls far short of 'positive peace,' meaning the eradication of conditions that produced and may reproduce the conflict. Positive peace entails more than negotiations between the two adversaries. It involves addressing the structural causes of the conflict, reforming the state and political structures, community reconciliation and peace building, democratisation, returning to normal politics, human rights, reintegration of communities and many more reconstructive measures. It seems that both the UNF government and the LTTE are not interested in any of these transformatory objectives. Against such a backdrop, the present round of 'peace talks' may not produce anything beyond de-escalation. *For both (the) sides, containment of war has become a politically desirable goal.* Facing a disastrous economic collapse with a negative growth rate, the UNF government finds itself unable to finance the high intensity war, which is the legacy of the previous People's Alliance government's mishandling of the ethnic conflict. For the LTTE, in the context of the global 'war' against terrorism, political engagement with the government for some time to come is a basic compulsion. So, there is every reason for the present ceasefire to be formalized and extended for an indefinite period. *But, prospects for a negotiated 'settlement' do not seem to be as strong.*"[10]

Did Uyangoda sound uncannily prophetic? For, more than two years after he wrote the article in an Indian newspaper and after six rounds of peace talks, Sri Lanka in the last quarter of 2004 appeared to have been stalled in its track once the CFA had come into existence and very little had been achieved beyond that purely preliminary step. Little wonder, then, that the Norwegian diplomat took pains to point out that a ceasefire was not peace, that it merely meant a temporary cessation of hostilities and nothing more. Achieving peace required a lot more hard work and on different planes, none of which had even been attempted by either side in the Sri Lankan conflict.

And if the Jayawardene government had attempted to exploit the situation arising out of the Indo-Sri Lanka Agreement of 1987 in order to advance its own political agenda, the scenario was no different during the two years of the latest ceasefire. The government of the day, first the Wickramasinghe regime and then the United People's Freedom Alliance (UPFA) government, while liberalising a number of restrictive measures prevalent in view of the periodical hostilities, aimed at creating a conducive atmosphere to facilitate a gradual progress towards negotiations, clearly sought simultaneously to present itself as the sincere face of Sri Lankan efforts for peace and to manoeuvre to protect the interests of the majority community from the "machinations" of the LTTE at the same time. Ranil Wickramasinghe, heading the just installed UNF government in December 2001, made this clear when, in answer to a question on what way his government's peace offer would be different from the previous regime's which had failed, said, "We have a vision and a plan and a set of people who can implement it. The previous government did not. We will certainly bring back peace and economic prosperity to the country. It will be a gradual process, but we have decided to grasp the nettle."[11]

On the other hand, meeting the diplomatic community based in Colombo on 31 March 2003, President Kumaratunga said, "I have on numerous occasions, too numerous now to recount, stated and emphasised that I remain firmly committed to the furtherance of the peace process, which I began in 1994 and continued with, in spite of hindrances and obstacles being placed in my way. The expression 'peace process' means no more than a process of seeking to achieve a peaceful resolution to the armed conflict, which has prevailed for more than two decades, by negotiations. This process cannot be an end in itself. It is a means of achieving an objective. That objective is the achievement of a just and durable peace, which can only come about if the legitimate aspirations of all our communities are met."

Was there a meeting ground for the two views? While rightly Kumaratunga claimed to have initiated the peace process immediately after she became prime minister in 1994, it was equally true that her regime also witnessed the country relapsing into war. Writing about those days, this author noted, "There is little doubt that Mrs Kumaratunga started her stewardship of the divided nation on the right note. The healing touch was omnipresent in her statements on the ethnic conflict and she was acutely aware of the enormous initial advantage she had obtained by being perceived by the Tamils as one Sinhalese leader who could be trusted.....Sometime in 1995, when all the hopes for peace were finally buried and the relations between the government and the Tamils of the north had reverted to outright discord, Mrs Kumaratunga snapped at a western journalist for asking her at a press conference why the Tamils no longer trusted her. Evidently riled, she asked harshly, 'How many Tamils have you spoken to? I am surprised that you are making this unfounded criticism. I am in touch with the Tamils throughout every day and they know that I help them the moment they come to me. As the president of the country, I am in constant touch with the Tamils and I know that they do not harbour any such feeling (of mistrust in her).'" It could only be a measure of the difficulties faced by Sri Lankan leaders in tackling the ethnic conflict, pulled as they traditionally were by mutually conflicting and exclusive sentiments that in contrast to the robust self-confidence expressed in 1995, Kumaratunga found it necessary to emphasise at the end of March 2003 that she was not divorced from the Tamils.

"For my part as Head of State, " she told the diplomats, "I give the people of Sri Lanka, including those who belong to and support the LTTE, the assurance that whoever may be the government of the day, the process of seeking a peaceful resolution to our conflict will proceed without a pause."[12]

While the Sinhalese leaders found it politically expedient, at the time of every peace initiative, to emphasise that they were not divorced from the Tamil community and were adequately sympathetic to their aspirations, as part of their desperate endeavours to withstand aggressive sectarian opposition from the Sinhalese community laced with allegations of tilting dangerously towards the "trap" laid by the rebels, the LTTE on its part sought to utilise every respite from war to reiterate its exclusive right to represent all the Tamils and, of course, its determination to wrest self-rule from a reluctant and hostile majority community.

Analysing the defeat of the People's Alliance led by Kumaratunga in the December 2001 general election, Uyangoda commented, "On the ethnic conflict (one of the three factors having contributed to the defeat, the other two being the economy and political reforms), the Kumaratunga administration's policy during the past two to three years has been quite erratic and inconsistent; interspersed with the rhetoric of peace and a policy of war. Kumaratunga's contradictory strategy could not fully use the assistance offered by the international community to resume negotiation with the LTTE. She allowed the Norwegian mediation effort to go waste while moving towards a Sinhalese hardline position on the ethnic question. When the election time rhetoric of insecure Sinhalese nationalism was allowed to define the state policy towards the minorities, Kumaratunga could only ensure the breaking-up of the multi-ethnic coalition that she herself forged in 1993-94 with vision and foresight. Her shift began during the parliamentary election campaign of October 2000."[13]

Getting back to the summer of 2004, Helgessen hit upon a cardinal truth about Sri Lanka when he complained that while Kumaratunga remained steadfast in her commitment to seek peace, she was not getting help from either her government or her party, a remark which drew a sharp rebuke from the cabinet spokesman.[14] As one ploughs through the painful history of Sri Lanka's failed search for peace, one gathers the impression, howsoever imperfect it may be, that the deeply and perpetually divided majority community is by its very nature incapable of offering a steady and dependable platform to build a momentum for peace. It is this impression that appears to work behind the apprehensions expressed periodically by the international community about the prospects of peace. The almost cynical tone with which the world at large spoke at the beginning of this chapter emanated from this particular understanding of the Sinhalese psyche, which rightly or wrongly has been formed outside the country.

Equally perpetually, the LTTE, ever watchful to catch the Sinhalese off-guard, has played up the obvious divisions within the ranks of the majority community over the ethnic issue, thereby betraying a tendency to exploit the developing situation for mere brownie points rather than to stick to an honest search for peace.

In the wake of the latest manifestation of this Sinhalese propensity, *Liberation Tigers*, a newspaper widely believed to be a mouthpiece of the LTTE, wrote editorially on 2 August 2004, "Confusing and conflicting views of President Chandrika Kumaratunga and the instability of her government together have placed the peace process and the conducive environment built over time at grave risk, " it said. The government, while lethargic in its peace initiatives and acting in bad faith when it came to respecting the ceasefire agreement, wanted to only merely portray a peace environment to the international community, "but for the Tamil people it is a firm 'no' whether it be peace, development, resettlement or rehabilitation." The Liberation Tigers did have a moral responsibility to take on board the Tamil psyche as it was today in the context of the people's fear and suspicion as to whether there were subtle moves on the government's side to defeat (the) Tamil national uprising by the "peace trap", having failed to achieve (the) same through military means. The editorial also lambasted the Janatha Vimukthi Peramuna, the government's main ally, accusing it of preparing its propaganda for war while opposing the ISGA proposals. "The chauvinistic forces working overnight are engaged in a vicious propaganda against the ISGA proposals submitted by the LTTE, " the newspaper said. "The JVP takes the lead in this and the Sinhalese media too does its part in the business of racial-hatred mongering. The political landscape thus looks convoluted. The Sinhalese electorate, mostly in the rural areas, is fed with this poisonous racial-hatred by the JVP." However, the newspaper warned the majority community, that this kind of behaviour did not augur well for the peace process and was not at all conducive for the resumption of negotiations. Time was fast running out. The LTTE was, however, prepared to wait patiently to negotiate and resolve the Tamil national question. But if the government had a hidden agenda to protract the peace process and restage a game of deception, the Tamil people were not prepared to bear it any more.

As happens in all such cases, the LTTE was evoking the mantra of the Tamil nationhood and claiming to be speaking on behalf of the Tamil people. It was quite another matter that the Tamil people, left to themselves, would have loved to carry on with their daily life bothering little about self-rule provided the government of the day had discharged its normal democratic duties and responsibilities for their well-being. Needless to say that this was where the south-based government had failed throughout the post-independence period, thus facilitating the emergence of Tamil extremism and later the dominance of the LTTE enforced over the Tamils of the northeast.

The only feasible course left to the government in Colombo was to try to reach out to the Tamils of the north and east directly, sidestepping the LTTE. The latter understandably was vigilant to a fault to prevent the government of the day from achieving anything remotely close to such an objective. It should, however, be noted that the LTTE was also facilitated in this task by the propensity of the majority community to throw a spanner in the works of any government or southern political party which would betray a desire to move closer than before to the people in the north and east. No government till today has been fully able to withstand this peer pressure and has indeed found it expedient to succumb to the comforts of a majoritarian support base in the interests of retaining or regaining power.

The gradual degeneration of the laudable initiative for peace launched by the Kumaratunga government in the mid-1990's in the face of the twin obstacles of Sinhalese opposition and LTTE chicanery is a telling illustration of this vicious cycle that helps perpetuate the ethnic conflict and its myriad consequences.

In the summer of 2004, while Sri Lanka remained far from achieving a lasting end to the ethnic conflict, it was equally true that certain significant developments had meanwhile taken place which would irretrievably, even if at times almost imperceptibly, change the inherent situation in the island nation.

The most important of these was the duration of the ceasefire, by then more than two years. While the CFA had been violated on many occasions with both sides guilty of committing these acts, it was important to note that no major violation had occurred which would have pushed the ceasefire to an irretrievable failure. It was clear, and both the government and the Tigers had reaffirmed this, that neither side was willing to stake its all and throw the CFA out of the window. Apparently, the people's aspirations all over the country for peace had gained a certain credence which the Sinhalese, Tamil and Muslim political parties and the LTTE were no longer in a position to play around with to satisfy their own sectarian interests.

It was particularly relevant to remember that successive governments had been formed based on electoral promises of ending the war and bringing peace to the country. Perhaps, the day would not be far off when it would be counter-productive to play around with the sentiments and aspirations of the people and instead, politicians and guerrillas would likewise be obliged to address the core issues of peace, development and prosperity with the seriousness they deserved.

Secondly, this period witnessed a major split in the ranks of the LTTE with the defection of V Muralitharan alias "Col" Karuna, which had overnight weakened the LTTE in its strategic base in the east, specifically in the Batticaloa district. With the depletion in its ranks to the extent of 5, 000-6, 000 (or, conservatively, 4000) fighters, the rebel war machine was rendered incapable of adventuring into a resumption of armed conflict with the always numerically and weapon-wise superior Sri Lankan armed forces. This factor also contributed to the continuation of the ceasefire even though there were at times serious threats to its durability.

Thirdly, both the government of the day and the Tigers felt more intensely than ever before the progressively declining interest of the international community in the Sri Lankan problem as new conflicts were springing up in different countries all the time demanding immediate attention, and more importantly, its resources either to finance armed interventions or help rebuild destroyed economies, apart of course from meeting challenges of natural calamities like earthquakes, floods and famines in the developing world. Above all, the global war on terrorism grabbed both attention and resources touching almost every nation.

It was, however, worth noting that while the commencement of the global war on terrorism affected the Sri Lankan ethnic conflict mainly in two ways, firstly by placing the LTTE in graver danger having been branded a terrorist group by the United States and various other countries and, secondly, by facilitating the Sri Lankan government's fight against the Tigers, it did not confer the same importance and urgency to the Sri Lankan situation as it did to the situations in West, Central and South Asia, in Indonesia and the Philippines and in the USA and other western countries with Muslim populations. As a matter of fact, unlike in most of these countries, Sri Lankan Muslims were not branded as potential terrorists for the simple reason that the terrorism in Sri Lanka was not related to the community at all but to a different community, the Tamils. This factor also contributed to a downsizing of the Sri Lankan conflict in the context of the anti-terrorism global campaign.

This is not to suggest that the global war on terrorism has failed to bring benefits to the Sri Lankan government. There is a highly interesting theory, which may yet turn out to be the correct reading of the developments around this time, as to what really persuaded the LTTE to suddenly sue for peace on 19 December, 2001 (its unilateral ceasefire took effect from 24 December).

The Tigers thought it better to call a halt to the hostilities because it found the rising number of casualties among its military leadership prohibitive. And how were these leaders being killed? To go by the theory, they were being ticked off with an unrelenting regularity by the Sri Lankan army's long range reconnaissance patrols (LRRPs) that were penetrating deep into the Wanni to carry out their deadly missions. But how were these eminently successful LRRPs raised? After all, the army did not possess such target-efficient special groups before. The answer is: the LRRPs were raised and trained by the US special forces, navy seals and other elite arms of the US army, their services loaned under the global war on terrorism. The US armed forces are known to have helped their Sri Lankan counterparts in many other vital ways, mainly through training and exercise. There is yet another immensely significant field where the US has extended considerable assistance to the Sri Lankan government though it is far less dramatic than the military help. While the European Union holds the view that withholding the $ 4.5 billion aid package, Colombo could be reasonably pressured to start talking to the Tigers, Washington has come forward to clear funds by announcing that Sri Lanka is eligible for the Millennium Account facility. The US move has since been followed by Japan and the Asian Development Bank by removing the "coercive aid factor" from Sri Lanka's obligation regarding the peace process. Thus, while the LTTE continues its campaign to strengthen the case for not releasing the promised Tokyo aid package, the Bush administration has ensured that Colombo does not suffer on account of non-availability of foreign funds.[15]

The surest sign of the US support for the Sri Lankan government was made available during the mid-September, 2004, Colombo visit by ambassador-at-large J Cofer Black, State Department coordinator for counter-terrorism. Black told a media audience, "There's no question where we stand, there will be no compromise, there will be no wavering. Our policy is determined by the objective that the LTTE must negotiate with the government in good faith, but not just negotiate—it has to in good faith (renounce terrorism) in word and in deed. This is our view and we actively promote it, with our allies and with our international contacts in international fora."

Earlier, he said, "I want to make this very clear, and I don't want any misunderstanding—the LTTE is presently on our list of foreign terrorist organisations, and they are going to remain there until they show by word and deed, that they are negotiating in good faith (have renounced terrorism in word and deed), producing concrete results....It is also my responsibility to identify those groups, when it's appropriate, to suggest and recommend that they be removed and this is not the case with the LTTE. They need, by word and deed to (renounce terrorism and) enter into good faith negotiations with the government, and until that happens, I personally and professionally am convinced that they are going to be on this list until that is done."

Asked to specify any special plan to fight terrorism in the Sri Lankan context, the US official said, "Our approach is to support the government. We have, certainly the government has, the will to resist terrorism, to engage in negotiations, good faith negotiations. We do have programmes to support the government so that it could be in a position to negotiate effectively." The obvious emphasis was on strengthening the negotiating position of the government, and this point was buttressed in an answer to another question.

"We have a very good relationship with the government. We provide the type of support that puts it in a good position to negotiate. The object is peace, the object is not war, and we think that we have a good programme in place with the government for these times. Were the times to change, the United States would have to reconsider the type of support it gives." Was he hinting at more overt military support to Sri Lanka in case the war broke out again? Asked if the US thought there was any link between the LTTE and al-Qaeda, he said, "Put it this way, I am very disturbed at the LTTE's history as a terrorist organisation. It has been a purveyor of training, knowledge, and equipment to a spectrum of terrorist groups, and we currently see many of these groups being mutually supporting. So you can play the game of one group connected to another to another, and I guess one could make connections, but I think that I would just rest on solid ground that the LTTE has been a disseminator of knowledge on how to conduct terrorist operations and has equipped other terrorist groups, which in and of itself is sufficient cause for alarm, and concern. The community of nations should attempt to constrain its activities, and do everything it can to bring them to the negotiating table."[16]

It was immediately clear that the LTTE had taken the US official's blunt message quite hard. Equally apparent was its desire not to criticise the Americans directly, for the consequences could not be beneficial; it, therefore, fell back upon the convenience of using its parliamentary lobby, the Tamil National Alliance, to issue a rejoinder.

Within a few hours of the US official's roundtable with the Sri Lankan media, TNA parliamentary group leader R Sampanthan said in a statement that the event had caused much concern to "wide sections of the Tamil people." It was most unfortunate that ambassador Black's "tirade" was exclusively against the LTTE and that it had assumed that the Tamil guerrilla group was the root cause of all evil that prevailed in Sri Lanka.

"The Tamil people do not agree with this assessment and there is a need to ensure that the interests of the Tamil people are not harmed," he said. More innocent Tamils had lacked protection through the decades since independence more than any other people in the country. The Sri Lankan state sought to subjugate the Tamils through racial pogroms and genocidal attacks because it could not keep the commitments made to the moderate Tamil political leadership. This was where violence commenced in post-independent Sri Lanka. The LTTE was the manifestation of the failure to accommodate the legitimate political aspirations of the Tamils and of the unleashing of state-sponsored terrorism against them.

The Tamils were deeply conscious of the immense sufferings they had experienced and were offended when statements by important functionaries did not reflect this reality. Ambassador Black's statements did not reflect the deep divisions within the government nor the lack of bipartisan approach and the deeply entrenched political rivalry between the main political parties, which were serious impediments to the furtherance of the peace process. The statements did not refer to the virulent campaigns being conducted against the peace process by extreme elements within the majority people including vehement opposition to Norway's faciliatory role. The burning of the Norwegian flag had become a regular event at such demonstrations.

After a brief narration of the civil war and the LTTE's submission of the ISGA proposals, Sampanthan said that statements which condemned one side and which did not objectively address the several causes that impeded the furtherance of the peace process only tended to encourage the forces determined to disrupt the peace process. "The Tamil people would like to convey that the failure to adopt an even handed approach could cause immense harm to the peace process and would appeal that a more balanced approach be adopted in the cause of peace, which ambassador Black asserts he is committed to uphold."

There was enough substance in Black's tough talk and in the TNA's response for the Sri Lankan state and the Sinhalese-Buddhist community to draw inspiration from, and this was exactly where a neutral observer's misgivings would lie. The American official was making it abundantly clear that the Sri Lankan government would be provided the necessary assistance to attain a position from where it could dictate to the LTTE the imperative of joining the negotiating table; in other words, the position of the government would be strengthened to an extent to the exact parallel of which that of the LTTE would be weakened and that thenceforward the bargaining position would be exclusively the state's. If even this outright support to the state would fail to tame the Tigers, Washington might consider other options; in other words, an open military support to crush the LTTE.

How else would one read the following comment, "Were the times to change, the United states would have to reconsider the type of support it gives (to the Sri Lankan government)." Whichever way one read the hard-hitting words, the only reaction would be that coming as these words did on top of the continuing reluctance on the part of the majority community to accept the concept of federalism and sharing of power with the minority communities, the deeply entrenched intolerance of pluralism, diversity and federalism would be further strengthened and the country would move away from the prospects of ethnic and cultural liberalism and political catholicism.

Was Taraki, a perceptive Tamil journalist who had often run foul of the administration and security forces for his professional independence, being alarmist when he analysed the future in the light of Black's comments in the following manner, "...given (the) US commitment to keep the LTTE on the list of foreign terrorist groups and in the absence of the 'coercive aid factor', there is nothing today to compel the Sinhalese polity to radically restructure the unitary Sri Lankan state. Sinhalese nationalists can now rest assured that they can totally trash and indefinitely postpone talks with the Tigers without having to fear any effective external coercion. Of course, some European Union countries and India appear to think that the US move to neutralise the 'coercive aid factor' would create conditions that can precipitate another war…Very obviously, the US strategic and political interests here are squarely behind the Sri Lankan state. By keeping the LTTE on the Foreign Terrorist Groups list and thereby insisting that it should give up violence as a means of achieving political ends in "word and deed", the US has created a singular advantage for the Sri Lankan government. This advantage totally obviates the need for restructuring the Sri Lankan state as a federation…the manner in which the US has formulated its stand on the LTTE is clearly designed to preserve the unitary Sinhalese Buddhist state. America, of course, has to …pay lip service to a negotiated settlement…In this context, the desire to crush the LTTE militarily would inexorably come to the fore in the Sinhalese polity."[17]

It was only in the fitness of things that Black's bluntly critical statement about the LTTE and his unhindered expression of US support for the Sri Lankan government failed to convince all the Sinhalese Buddhists that Washington was up to its job of defending democracy and freedom around the world. The print media carried quite a few indignant articles and letters criticising the US official of not having been sufficiently harsh on the LTTE.

A strong grievance was expressed to the effect that Black had failed to criticise the ISGA proposals and he was asked as to why he did not reciprocate US assistant secretary of state Christina Rocca's statement at a Congress hearing that the proposals were a blue print for the establishment of a separate state. One article listed the points that should have been cleared by the visiting official. "Yes, a 'statement' from the US covering these points would be more than useful to take the peace process forward. ...this was indeed the opportunity for the US to have made a categorical statement on the ISGA, " it said. "Most unfortunately for this country, the country does not come first with our two major political parties. The government changed in April and it has taken six months for (the) two leaders to meet and that too does not appear to have been productive and we proudly boast that we are a working democracy—many in the UNP are so completely opposed to the president personally that they let this hate get the better of their judgement...As for 'statements' from the international community, none of them has been effective in reining in the LTTE; some have in fact been counter-productive. They were by implication assisting the LTTE to slip out of the signed commitment they made at Oslo for a 'federal structure within a united Sri Lanka.' Yes, we could have peace tomorrow if we agree to the ISGA—is this the 'peace' that the US and other members of the donor community wish? No, there can never be 'peace' on such terms. There is only one language that the LTTE understands and that is force—not necessarily military force...(the international community) must read the Riot Act to the LTTE and call them to order."[18]

The absolute US position on the LTTE, as stated by Black, may be considered a relatively new entrant into the Sri Lankan conflict since all other positions emphasise, apart from the overriding importance of preserving the unity, territorial integrity and sovereignty of Sri Lanka, the necessity of ensuring that the aspirations of the Tamil people are satisfactorily addressed in any final settlement. This is the position of the Sri Lankan state as well.

The point was very well brought out in the address that Kumaratunga delivered at the inaugural meeting of the National Advisory Council for Peace and Reconciliation on 4 October, 2004, "We arrived at the view that our conflict was engendered by the inability of our nation at the moment of decolonisation, 56 years ago, to weld together the separate sets of aspirations of the three main communities living in Sri Lanka, into one collective national vision, in which each community could live freely and in dignity within its own separate identity, in order to comprise one whole harmonious and united whole—a strong, stable and united state."

"We recognised that we had to build a new, pluralist, multi-ethnic and multi-cultural state based on the cultural, religious and social identity of the majority Sinhalese people who constitute around 75 per cent of our population, as much as the two main smaller communities, the Tamils and the Muslims, and the tiny groups of (the) Malays and Burghers, who constitute the rest of the country. We believe that the solution lies in seeking alternatives to the concept of a monolithic, unitary state—to blend power with principle, to reconcile authority with freedom. We are looking at a form of power sharing with a high level of democratic participation in decision making, law making and governance by the regional authorities or the devolved units."

"We do not believe that the dismemberment of the Sri Lankan state, demanded by the LTTE through the employment of terrorist means, would in any way be a solution to the Tamil people's problems. We are seeking a compromise that would satisfy the aspirations of all the communities of peoples living within our state—a compromise that would be democratic and pluralistic. We believe that the state must resolve the contradictions that have arisen between the state and the nationalist consciousness of the Tamil community. We have to find means and procedures to accord expression of this consciousness and to give constitutional, legal and political authority."

And where does the LTTE fit into this scheme of things, as spelled out by the president? Immediately after hearing ambassador Black's definition of the LTTE, Kumaratunga's categorisation of the Tamil group might be a bit unsettling. She said in the same speech, "My government shall continue to engage the LTTE, who we recognise as the primary actor, in the process of negotiating an end to the conflict and attaining peace. My government's dialogue with the LTTE will be a separate and priority process."

The precise description of the Tamil militant or terrorist group by the Sri Lankan president as the primary actor in the peace process is a mark of the distinction that one perforce has to draw between the LTTE and today's front-rank terrorist outfits Black referred to like al-Qaeda or the Taleban or the Chechen rebels. This is principally because the Sri Lankan government remains obliged to pursue a peaceful solution, along with the military one when the war is resumed, because the Tigers can successfully play the Tamil nationalist card.

Their ability to do so is vital to their survival and just as determined as they are in retaining this credential, so is the inability of the government to make a significant dent in this somewhat adulterated claim. It is significant to note that even today, when the global war on terrorism is being waged and even nation-states like Iraq, Syria and Iran are being brought under its purview, Colombo is not insisting that not just the LTTE but all the other Tamil political parties and groups should be represented in negotiations.

Far from such a position, the president herself describes the LTTE as the primary actor in the peace process; this is by no means a mean achievement on the part of the LTTE. On their side, the only success that the largely Sinhalese governments in Colombo have notched up over the years, thanks to the colonisation programme launched in the early years of independence to settle the Sinhalese in the eastern province, is the invalidation of the LTTE's claim that the east forms an integral part of the traditional Tamil homeland. This assertion is no longer tenable demographically. As for the LTTE's continuing claim of representing the northern province, the presence of the eight MPs of the Eelam People's Democratic Party certainly is a counter-argument and, to go by the EPDP's stand, a free and fair election in the Jaffna Peninsula would have fetched it several more seats.

EPDP leader Douglas Devananda told the author, "One reason why the LTTE wants to get me killed is the portfolios that I look after, agricultural marketing development, cooperative development and Hindu affairs and (assisting in) education and vocational training. All of these require that I interact with the common people and with the Tamils in particular all the time. The LTTE has never liked my position and knows that unless this relationship is brought to an end, my popularity and that of my party would continue to rise among the Tamils in the northeast. In fact, the LTTE prompted the Tamil National Alliance MPs to call on the president and demand that I should be removed from these portfolios. The president obviously did not listen to them because she knows that I enjoy sufficient support among the Tamils to deserve those ministries."[19]

In his brief but intensive probe into the prospects of a resumption of peace talks, the author obtained the impression that nobody was expecting a breakthrough in the stalemate during the remainder of 2004. "Not in the next six months, " some respondents ventured.

Their pessimism appeared to be well-reasoned; President Kumaratunga must win over the Janatha Vimukthi Peramuna in order to present a united face of the ruling coalition, which looked a rather formidable task. The JVP had been sensing a growing clout not just with its unprecedented 39 seats in parliament but also with the strong Sinhalese-Buddhist opposition to the ISGA proposals and the government's inability to convince the community about the need to start peace talks largely on the LTTE's terms.

Besides, the JVP was apparently quite mindful of the growing competition for the affiliation of Sinhalese Buddhists from the Jathika Hela Urumaya where no quarter could be given. Even though the JVP kept assuring that it was not opposed to talks with the rebels, it was not being taken at its words. Political and diplomatic circles in Colombo felt that when the time to act would arrive, the JVP would find it tactically difficult not to be tempted by the prospects of winning over the Sinhalese-Buddhist affiliation overwhelmingly by voting against a move to start talks with the LTTE on the basis of the ISGA proposals. In an interesting distinction that a JVP minister in the Kumaratunga government made between the ISGA proposals and a prospective interim administration for the northeast, JVP politburo member and Sri Lanka's minister for culture and national heritage Vijitha Herath said, "Some amount of devolution of power and decentralisation of administration" could help resolve the ethnic conflict and that talks with the LTTE should, therefore, be centred on an interim administration.

Asked whether the JVP would accept the concept of devolution of power on the lines of the Union of Regions proposed by the Kumaratunga government in 2000, he pointed out that it was not only his party but also the LTTE which had rejected those devolution proposals at that time.

He argued that it was not a question of "more or less" devolution of power between the centre and the regions but that any "final solution" should be based on the principle of "equal rights for all on an equal basis", which obviously would do away with the very concept of a Tamil homeland for any region as propounded by the Tamil Tigers.

The JVP, according to him, also remained opposed to the introduction of federalism which believed that the unitary character must be preserved in order to preserve Sri Lanka's unity, territorial integrity and sovereignty.

Not surprisingly, to go by what this minister said, the JVP was also keen that India came forward to help preserve the unitary character of Sri Lanka because a fragmented Sri Lanka would be against her interest. A prospective Tamil Eelam, he felt, would rather be like an Israel in South Asia facilitating the foundation of a US base in the region. This, the JVP would emphasise, should never be allowed to happen.[20]

"What is the JVP's final decision on the ISGA (proposals)?" In answer to this question, another Sri Lankan minister and JVP leader K D Lal Kantha said, "The stand of the JVP (in this regard) is very clear. We have stated it clearly that if the talks started based on the ISGA (proposals), the whole country would fall into the LTTE's trap. Therefore, talks should be based on a final solution and there is no interruption for that (sic). The question we have is as to why the international community (does) not force the LTTE to start talks based on a final solution instead of these ISGA proposals. We believe that there should be pressure on the LTTE. The LTTE, other Tamil parties and Muslim parties should all come to one table and should find a final solution. We agree to create an interim administration that would lead to such a final solution."[21]

It was, however, possible to discern completely contrary undercurrents beneath the usual JVP bluster regarding the ISGA proposals. The outright rejection of the LTTE blueprint for a self-governing authority for the northeast and championing of the unitary character of the country were not an end by themselves; they only served to camouflage the once-Marxist and presently widely compromising party's need for securing its political standing among the majority community.

As it found increasingly to its dismay that staying in power demanded its pound of flesh, it clearly marked out opposition to the LTTE proposals and to all attempts at liberalisation as a politically fruitful proposition.

In the last few months of 2004, the party, therefore, launched a campaign ostensibly titled " Who are the true enemies of peace?" but which in reality tended to be an assault on the ceasefire and a virtual call to renew war. According to one account of the campaign, the JVP's propaganda secretary Wimal Weerawansa delivered a lecture at Colombo's Youth Council Centre in late-August, 2004, when he denounced the advocates of a resumption of peace talks as stooges of the LTTE and branded the previous Wickramasinghe government, which had signed the ceasefire agreement with the LTTE, as "green tigers" (green being the colour of the United National party, Wickramasinghe's party). He naturally did not spare the Norwegian facilitators either and preferred to describe them as "white tigers" while the lowly non-governmental organisations, all motivated peaceniks, were calling for resumption of negotiations because they were actually "crowing for dollars."[22]

While not specifically calling for a return to war, the account said that Weerawansa attacked the emphasis being put on peace, saying that this had resulted from succumbing to the LTTE's pressure tactics. Peace, he said, had to take a back seat while "defence of motherland" had to be placed ahead of all other demands. In a comment that could only be interpreted as a warning to the JVP's allies in the ruling coalition United People's Freedom Alliance, he declared that even the government's survival had to take a second place to the defence of the country.

"In all our endeavours, " he said, "the security of motherland has to stay at the pinnacle," emphasising that the masses had to be mobilised to defeat "this so-called peace process." Elaborating on what his colleague Herath had said earlier in Chennai, he denounced the ISGA proposals not because the LTTE plan was undemocratic and communal in character but because it would weaken the unitary state. Even though the LTTE at its highest level had renounced its demand for a Tamil homeland to be separated from Sri Lanka, Weerawansa said, " the ISGA is nothing less than a separate Tamil Eelam. Even on an empty stomach, we will defend the unitary state of our motherland."

Analysing the JVP's stand on the peace process, the account held that Weerawansa did not attack the search for peace on a class basis (as it should have, since it claimed to be a Marxist party) nor did it point to the fact that the ceasefire was intimately connected to an economic restructuring agenda that was leading to mounting unemployment and poverty (the JVP had contested the 2004 parliamentary election promising a 70 per cent wage rise, which had contributed significantly to its popularity with the voters and which was towards the end of the year visibly proving to be a major embarrassment for the party).

"The JVP's opposition to the 'peace process' is entirely reactionary," said the account, "based on the defence of Sinhalese Buddhist domination. Far from articulating the needs of ordinary working people, the JVP reflects the position of sections of the ruling elite—the military and state apparatus, the Buddhist hierarchy and more backward sections of industry—who are deeply concerned that their interests will be compromised in any power-sharing peace deal with the LTTE."

The JVP's impressive political clout owes considerably to its unexpected show in the 2004 parliamentary elections, upsetting the SLFP's calculation to ride to victory on its back. Instead, what the JVP accomplished was to eat deeply into the SLFP's vote bank of the majority community and thereby improving its standing immensely. The party is now apparently loath to abandon the magic formula half-way and is working steadily to continue to add to its adherents among the Sinhalese-Buddhist community. In this endeavour, it is its strident opposition to the peace process that is obviously being counted upon to continue to bring results. Its case against resumption of negotiations with the LTTE rests solidly on the thesis that the ceasefire agreement was signed precisely at the moment when the Sri Lankan security forces had pinned the rebels down. "By the year 2001, " Weerawansa said in his speech referred to earlier, "the LTTE was a weakened force due to the valiant military campaigns of the Sri Lankan army. It was under the ceasefire agreement signed by the United

National Front of (the former prime minister) Ranil Wickramasinghe that the LTTE was able to politically defeat the Sri Lankan state."

Analysts point out that this line of thinking being propounded by the JVP is clearly calculated to bolster the opposition within the security forces to the peace process. Both the previous Wickramasinghe government and the present Kumaratunga government have been acutely aware of the widespread unhappiness within the military about the ceasefire agreement and the peace process.

It is no secret that both officers and men feel that the LTTE has been exploiting the ceasefire agreement to its advantage; the JVP's cynical exploitation of this anti-peace process feeling is potentially an unknown missile since it is difficult to expect the party to compromise on this point if and when Kumaratunga makes a genuine attempt to seek a resumption of negotiations with the LTTE. As of now, no analyst would venture that the JVP would rather be attentive to the survival of the coalition government than plunge headlong into the game of exploiting the Sinhalese-Buddhist chauvinism.[23]

On the other hand, analysts feel, the JVP would be happy to continue to exploit the continuing impasse over peace talks in order to strengthen its vote bank without threatening the duration of the coalition government. Meanwhile, while it is not incumbent on the party to actually honour its commitment to leave the ruling coalition in case the government goes for fresh talks, it pays to keep up the heat on the senior coalition constituent, the SLFP, by threatening to quit and at the same time to encourage further Sinhalese-Buddhist chauvinism. This scenario is likely to continue until Kumaratunga decides to take the bull by the horn and force a positive turn towards a resumption of talks with the Tamil Tigers.

However, in doing so, Kumaratunga must take into account the fairly entrenched opinion within her own party that unless the JVP is checkmated, it would continue to make damaging inroads into the traditional vote bank of the SLFP. This, many of her party members feel, has already reached unacceptable proportions and cannot be afforded any more. The dilemma for the party leadership lies in the pros and cons of taking an initiative to start peace talks, for such an act could only lead to further erosion of the vote bank to the advantage of the JVP and other chauvinistic forces of the majority community.

Notes

1. US Principal Deputy Assistant Secretary for South Asian Affairs Donald A Camp quoted in *The Sunday Leader*, 1 August 2004, Volume 11, Issue 3, "Peace process: Talks or bust" by Amantha Perera.
2. *ibid.*
3. *www.channelnewsasia.com*, 8 August 2004.
4. Interview of J.Dhanapala, Secretary General, Secretariat for Coordinating the peace process in the Presidential Secretariat, World Trade Centre, Colombo, taken on 15 September, 2004.
5. Interview of former Secretary Bradman Weerakoon to various presidents and prime ministers of Sri Lanka in Colombo on 17 September, 2004, and interactions with serving and retired military personnel during 8-18 September, 2004, anonymity maintained on request.
6. Interview of J.Dhanapala, taken on 15 September 2004.
7. V.S.Sambandan, "E.U.concerned at 'human rights violations' by LTTE," *The Hindu*, New Delhi edition, 17 August 2004.
8. Ravi R.Prasad, *United Press International*, "Sri Lankan president cautions rebels," 16 August 2004.
9. Jayadeva Uyangoda, *The Indo-Lanka Accord of July 1987 and the State in Sri Lanka*, contributed to "Indo-Sri Lanka Agreement of July 1987" edited by Shelton U.Kodikara, a publication of the International Relations Programme, University of Colombo, 1989.
10. Jayadeva Uyangoda, "A limited peace agenda", *The Hindu*, New Delhi edition, 4 February 2002.
11. In an interview to Nirupama Subramanian of *The Hindu*, dated 22 December 2001.
12. Apratim Mukarji, *The War in Sri Lanka: Unending conflict?*, Har-Anand Publications Pvt. Ltd., New Delhi, 2000.
13. Jayadeva Uyangoda, "Managing uncertainty", *The Hindu*, New Delhi edition, 10 December 2001.
14. A case in point is the following anecdote narrated by Sathya in the "Troubled peace process: Time for a reality check," 9 August 2004, www.peaceinsrilanka.com: "...it now appears that

President Chandrika Kumaratunga is willing to show some flexibility in commencing negotiation on an interim authority as indicated by the press release, following her meeting with Norwegian Deputy Foreign Minister on July 27, where it was stated that her government was 'willing and is keen to commence negotiations on an Interim Authority within the framework of a united state.' The hawks in her ranks, however, managed to insert a lead story in the Daily News of August 4 with screaming headlines, 'UPFA says no to LTTE's ISGA proposals.' The story attributed this stance to President Kumaratunga and cited SLFP General Secretary Maitripala Sirisena as the source. As a case of confusion confounded or as confusion clarified, *the Daily News* the following day carried the following clarification that 'the government emphasises that these media reports attributed to the statement said to have been made by the president at the executive committee meeting of the Alliance government at the President's House recently are totally misleading the public. In fact, what was stated by the president at the meeting was that the government's stance on the resumption of peace talks with the LTTE remains unchanged.' So, what exactly is the stance of the government? This was clarified in the government's official website which comes directly under the Presidential Secretariat, where it was stated that ' the president maintains that the government of Sri Lanka is willing to discuss with the LTTE its proposals for an Interim Administration alongside the talks to reach a final solution acceptable to all communities.'

15. Taraki, "A second look at US assistance to Lanka against terrorism", *Daily Mirror*, 15 September, 2004.
16. Media roundtable with US ambassador-at-large J.Cofer Black, State Department coordinator for counterterrorism, www.dailynews.lk.
17. Taraki, "A second look at US assistance to Lanka against terrorism", Daily Mirror, 15 September, 2004.
18. K.Godage, "Ambassador Black's visit—a missed opportunity" *The Island*, 15 September, 2004.
19. Interview taken in Colombo on 14 September, 2004.

20. "JVP not against interim administration", Sri Lankan minister and JVP leader Vijitha Herath spoke to the media in Chennai, India, *The Hindu* (Delhi ed.), 7 September, 2004.
21. "JVP queries CWC stand on ISGA", *Daily Mirror*, Colombo, 13 September, 2004.
22. Wije Dias, "The JVP intensifies its campaign against Sri Lankan peace talks," 31 August, 2004, www.wsws.org.
23. A typical example of the JVP's ways of exploiting the sentiments of the Sinhalese-Buddhist community was the following incident, reported with evident approval by the Colombo-based media. On 12 September, 2004, the JVP MP for the Trincomalee District (in the eastern Sri Lanka) Jayantha Wijesekara protested when it was discovered that the national flag was missing at the opening ceremony of the newly constructed Trincomalee courts complex, insisted that the flag must be acquired before the ceremony was held and hoisted the flag himself. His act of defiance of the LTTE (it was obvious that the organizers did not want to antagonise the rebel force which always hovered nearby) was widely acclaimed by the Sinhalese-Buddhist community. Equally predictable was the editorial that *The Island* carried on 15 September, 2004, which read in part, "...today we have no hesitation in commending the fearless, commendable and patriotic act of a JVPer, JVP MP for the Trincomalee District Jayantha Wijesekara. His patriotic act of hoisting the national flag in defiance of the orders of the LTTE at the ceremonial opening of the new High Courts complex in Trincomalee on Friday is a brave and clear message to the terrorists that they cannot bulldoze their way through."

2
Karuna's Revolt

The revolt by Vinayagamoorthy Muralitharan, better known by his nom de guerre "Col." Karuna, the erstwhile supreme commander of the LTTE in the eastern region comprising the Batticaloa and Ampara districts, became public knowledge when the rebel warrior himself talked about it, alleging 'discrimination' by the Jaffna Tamils against the eastern Tamils within the organisation and announcing his defection as an act of protest on 3 March 2004 (2 March, according to some accounts).

Three days later, the LTTE expelled him from the organisation. Still later, in late July, it called (according to southern media reports) for his assassination and offered a reward of Sri Lankan Rs.22.5 million to any person who would bring Karuna's head. It also let it be known at the time that Tigers' families which would be able to attack safe houses for Karuna's followers would be rewarded SL Rs.50, 000 for each house destroyed.

Scores of Karuna's followers and perceived sympathisers were killed in Colombo and in the east. With Karuna striking back effectively, there was widespread apprehension in the country that the internal fighting of the LTTE would lead to a situation necessitating state intervention, ultimately jeopardising the ceasefire and further delaying any prospects of a resumption of peace talks.

These developments proved that the LTTE had been badly shaken up by what it perceived to be a betrayal by its longest serving commander (17 years) in the much valuable east, the region which had traditionally provided fighters for the LTTE war machine and funds for financing the war against the state. Karuna himself said a few days after his defection, "It is discrimination against us within our organisation. I don't feel our leader (Prabhakaran) has given regard to the lives of our (eastern) fighters. From the time of the Indian army, our fighters have been martyred in the Wanni battlefields. Even now, there are 600 fighters there. Parents don't like their children to be deployed during peace. What we wanted was that the eastern fighters should be sent back. When the leader asked for 1, 000 more people, it was unacceptable. Then, of more than 30 administrative positions in the LTTE not even one is held by someone from Batticaloa-Ampara region."[1]

How honest was he being in asserting that he was forced to defect after Prabhakaran had made the impossible demand of recruiting another 1, 000 fighters from the east when the ceasefire was holding and there was no fighting? One well-informed analyst answers by asking the obvious question, "What is the cause of this estrangement between Karuna and the LTTE hierarchy? After the ceasefire of 23 February 2002, the LTTE's central command began expanding its activities into the regions, notably in the east. Earlier, this was not possible due to the war. In times of conflict the regional chiefs had practically a free hand in running their affairs. This was particularly so in the case of Karuna whose seniority and military ability was great. The central divisions were not answerable to the regional command and reported back to their heads alone, who in turn reported to Prabhakaran. Thus, several acts were being done in the east in the name of the LTTE that Karuna had no control over and, in many instances, no knowledge of. The LTTE courts, police stations, income tax offices and, more importantly, the dreaded intelligence wing TOSIS (Tiger Organisation Security Intelligence Service) all functioned in the east without being subject to any regional control."[2]

The situation was clearly becoming intolerable for Karuna who had till then risen impressively in power and stature within the LTTE by dint of performing major tasks, such as, rescuing the guerrilla outfit including its leader in the Mullaitivu District six years ago when government forces were closing in on Puthukudiyiruppu, Prabhakaran's traditional headquarters. By fighting a series of defensive battles with

3, 600 fighters, Karuna was able to rescue the LTTE from a major disaster.

He had since risen steadily, was made the overall field commander of the counter-offensive, "Unceasing Waves", that the LTTE launched in order to regain the control of the area extending from Oddusuddan to Omanthai. The offensive was successful, and Karuna returned to the east in triumph, elevated to the rank of the special military commander of the Batticaloa and Ampara districts. He was allowed to enjoy considerable autonomy in running the outfit in the east and even allowed to develop a parallel administrative set-up in the two districts.

His star was still rising when peace talks began and he became part of the LTTE negotiating team, the other members being the political wing chief Thamilschelvan and the political adviser Anton Balasingham. In yet another fresh post of responsibility, he was made the co-chairman of a committee to supervise de-escalation of military activities. In the talks with the government, he was treated as a representative not only of the east but also of the military wing of the LTTE. This saga of the rising star continued till the central command of the LTTE began to expand its own tentacles in the east to such an extent that not only Karuna's autonomy but also his very leadership of the eastern region was gravely threatened, obliging him to take rearguard action to protect his turf.

Thus, in essence, Karuna's defection and the resultant developments were part of a turf war that broke out within the so-called monolithic organisation. Apart from the leadership's decision to cut Karuna down to size (his eventual fate could have been far more debilitating, since in the traditional LTTE style, Prabhakaran summoned him to the Wanni headquarters where he would have been required to answer a series of damning charges against him drawn up by the TOSIS and would probably have then been executed, but sensing such a possibility Karuna refused to answer the summons and instead broke away from the parent organisation), a continuing rivalry between Pottu Amman (uncle), the 'Beria' of the LTTE running the feared TOSIS, and Karuna Amman (the popular name by which V.Muralitharan goes) appears to have contributed to the gradual estrangement of the latter from the parent organisation.

Karuna's Revolt

There is little doubt that the northern leadership's haste in expanding fast into what was essentially Karuna's turf exacerbated the situation, forcing the regional commander to finally break off. Besides, the traditional grievance of eastern Tamils against the northern dominance found fresh ground for protest when even the expansion of the LTTE in the east was supervised by northerners. Clearly, Wanni did not care to nurture the eastern Tamil on his own native territory, and Karuna could hardly stomach such a calculated attempt to decimate his fiefdom. Karuna himself commented, "I am not even concerned that (concepts such as the traditional homelands) will be affected because the northern Wanni leaders think arrogantly that they are the educated lot, that they can do everything and that they can suppress other communities. That is not acceptable. So when a country or a solution comes, what are they going to do? Even then, our people (eastern Tamils) will be suppressed. From the beginning, there have been severe problems between the Jaffna man and the Batticaloa man. There was discrimination. We thought war would change things. Within the organisation all was well; they took care of us well till their work was done. But with (the) passage of time, we find discrimination within the organisation. How can we continue to accept that?"[3]

A major factor to help build up the tension between the Wanni leadership and Karuna was the scheme to expand the LTTE's infrastructure and fighting strength by recruiting 1,000 fighters in the summer of 2004. This insistence on laying hands on new recruits occurred at a time when the international outcry against the LTTE's continuing child abduction and recruitment spree had grown particularly forceful, rendering Karuna's job materially much more difficult than before.

The latter, already scheming to break away from the LTTE, turned all the more reluctant to execute Prabhakaran's order; this could strike one as highly ironical too, since it was Karuna who had over the years forced children in the eastern province to join the LTTE's fighting machine. He himself talked about this when he said, "We gave 75 per cent of the (fighting) strength."[4]

The LTTE had always depended heavily on forced child recruitment for augmenting its fighting strength, thus earning for Sri

Lanka the dubious distinction of being in the company of such countries as Afghanistan, Burundi, Somalia and Colombia.

Amnesty International expressed its concern over the LTTE practice in a statement on 15 February, 2002, saying that it had written to the Tigers leadership providing details of the names, dates of birth and addresses of thirteen children who were recruited at the time. The list of the children abducted, including some who were as young as 12 years old, gained substance because it carried their names; this was noteworthy as even aggrieved parents would not normally venture to provide such details to outsiders for fear of reprisal.

A BBC report of the time mentioned that the list carried the names of six children who belonged to the Vavuniya District; this was considered significant because till then all child soldiers used to be recruited from the eastern province.[5] Other media reports of the time said that up to 300 young people had been abducted and recruited into the LTTE in the first fifteen days of 2002. Interestingly, the reports suggested that such a largescale recruitment drive targeted at schools was necessitated by the Tigers preparing for creating an educated cadre who would be able to fill up responsible administrative posts in case the proposed ISGA for the north and east became a reality through peace negotiations with the government (also indicating that far from discounting the possibility of a political settlement at the resumption of talks, the LTTE would have filled up all such posts with its own cadre in order to maintain complete control over such a body).

As the menace of child abduction and recruitment continued with impunity, the United Nations Security Council found it necessary to name Sri Lanka as a country, where notable degrees of child abductions took place in a new resolution adopted on 30 January, 2003. The resolution said that the Secretary-General of the UN had been requested to report by 31 October, 2003, on the progress made by parties to armed conflict "that recruit or use child soldiers" in violation of their international obligations. "This progress report applies not only to (Afghanistan, Burundi, the Democratic republic of Congo, Liberia and Somalia) but also to countries not normally on the Security Council's agenda where child recruitment is widespread. The latter include Burma, Colombia, Northern Uganda and Sri

Lanka." The Security Council indicated that if it was found that sufficient progress had not been made in the interim period with respect to child recruitment; additional steps could be considered, implying that even arms embargoes might be clamped on guilty countries.

A 27 April, 2004, report of the Human Rights Watch (HRW) laid bare not only the still continuing child soldier recruitment by the rebels but also how the fight that had broken out between the LTTE and Karuna was impacting on the unfortunate child soldiers. The report said that LTTE forces defeated Karuna's group on 9 April when, as the United Nations Children's Fund found out, at least two female child soldiers were killed in the fighting. There were unconfirmed reports that many more child fighters were killed in that battle or after having surrendered.

Both the LTTE army and Karuna's forces of nearly 6, 000 fighters included many child soldiers; many of the latter surrendered to the LTTE after the battle. A total of 209 of these children were released after their families demanded that the LTTE hand them over. An estimated 800 child soldiers belonging to Karuna's forces returned home on their own. Thousands more child soldiers were believed to have remained with LTTE forces in the north of the country, the HRW report said.

"The release of hundreds of LTTE child soldiers to their families is good news, " said Brad Adams, executive director of the HRW's Asia division. "The issue now is whether the Tigers will permit these children to stay home or force their return to the front lines." Fears of re-recruitment of the children by the LTTE rose when it was found that rebel vans were roaming the streets of the Batticaloa and Ampara towns asking members of Karuna's forces including those child soldiers released recently to report for re-registration.

The panic of parents was so much that international agencies present in the region including the UNICEF and the Sri Lanka Monitoring Mission were approached for safe shelter for children who ran the risk of being re-abducted. The HRW urged the international agencies to try to prevent the LTTE from perpetrating any such mischief. The HRW Asia division chief Adams was quoted saying,

"Children need to be kept away from the ranks of fighters, and the Tamil Tigers especially. International agencies must have a presence in the villages where these children live if there is any hope of preventing the LTTE from returning these children to its forces." The HRW also urged the Sri Lankan government to discharge its normal duty of protecting the children and facilitate the latter's rehabilitation in civilian life and re-integration into society by first declaring an amnesty for the child soldiers who had returned home.

While a February 2003 public pledge by the LTTE to cease all child recruitment was being apparently flouted with characteristic impunity, the HRW found out after a gap of about two months, in June 2004, that "the Tamil Tigers are stealing children from their homes to put them on the firing line. Despite all their promises, they are demonstrating absolute disregard for the most vulnerable part of the population it claims to represent."6

The UNICEF and local human rights groups reported that the LTTE was forcibly abducting children from their homes and threatening death to resisting and protesting parents. The rebels were targeting small, rather than large, groups of children in order not to create unnecessary alarm and draw unwanted attention to their activities. They were visiting villages, knocking on the doors of families with children, threatening dire consequences in the event of defiance and abducting 8-9 children from every village. The abducted children were transported by motorised rickshaws to the nearby lagoon and then by boat to the LTTE camp at Vaharai, avoiding Sri Lankan army checkpoints. In yet another equally chilling manifestation of child recruitment, parents were receiving letters asking them to attend meetings to be addressed by LTTE area leaders in Batticaloa. The UNICEF report said that at one such meeting addressed by area leader Yatharthan on 21 and 22 June, 2004, parents were told that they would have to hand over their over-16 years old children for armed service at Thihiliwatai two days later and that they should not delude themselves about any protection by the UNICEF.

"Although some parents have organised themselves in order to resist the LTTE pressure, " the HRW quoted Tej Thapa, its South Asia researcher saying, "there is considerable fear of reprisal in small communities with little or no government presence. The Tamil Tigers' ruthless and unforgiving tactics have terrified parents, children and human rights workers, who have no recourse to real protection from the Sri Lankan government...The Tamil Tigers are blatantly violating their obligations under international law [7] and ignoring the efforts of (the) UNICEF to protect these children. Children are being used to fill the ranks of the Tigers, while their parents face harsh retribution if they try to prevent it."

The Karuna revolt had another fallout on the LTTE's child soldiers. After the revolt which was followed by Karuna releasing hundreds of rebel child soldiers and letting them return to their families, LTTE intelligence officers threatened village government functionaries against issuing national identity cards to the released boys and girls. As a result, the latter could not qualify for national and international protection and for facilities for reintegration into society. In a clear defence of the LTTE's acts of abductions and forced recruitment of child soldiers, Tamil National Alliance (TNA) member of parliament Joseph Pararajahsingham told this author, "Why doesn't the international community talk about the exploitation of child labour all over Sri Lanka? While these children are forced to go into extremely exploitative jobs due to the poverty of their families, the boys and girls who are recruited into the LTTE do so in order to fight for their rights. It is baseless to allege that very minor children are being forced into fighting by the Tigers."[8]

An equally disturbing consequence, which attracted larger international attention due to its wider appeal, was the sudden spurt in reprisal killings, with both the LTTE and Karuna's group going the whole hog in attempting to decimating each other and with the former appearing to be scoring bigger hits by dint of its superiority in numbers and resources. In July, 2004 alone over a dozen men, either LTTE operatives or Karuna's followers, were gunned down. According to the government, during the two-and-a-half years of the ceasefire, the Tigers had killed as many as 250 political opponents. In the most hyped killing, Kandiah Yogarasa alias "PLOTE Mohan" (41 years old; his nickname derived from his long association with the People's Liberation Organisation of Tamil Eelam, which he left in 1994), a prize anti-LTTE intelligence operative, who had proved to be of immense value to the Sri Lankan armed forces and the police in hunting down LTTE cadre (he was said to have been associated with the Long Range Reconnaissance Patrols or of the armed forces prior to the ceasefire; the LRRPs were credited with having eliminated a large number of LTTE leaders, a factor which was said to have contributed to the decision of the LTTE to sue for a truce), was gunned down in a grisly shootout in the heart of Colombo on 31 July.

Media reports said that PLOTE Mohan was killed with a 9 mm. pistol around 11.20 in the morning on a sidewalk on the normally busy Duplication Road, which was however virtually empty on the Poya (full moon) holiday. The murder took people by surprise since PLOTE Mohan was always on an alert for possible attempts to kill him; after all, he had lived for many years under the threat of assassination by the LTTE.

Reporting the assassination, *The Sunday Times* of Colombo wrote, "The victim, who was clad casually in a blue T-shirt and beige trousers, fell face down in a pool of blood while eight empty rounds were found in the vicinity. The driver of the three-wheeler in which PLOTE Mohan travelled said that he had come shopping to the House of Fashion. (He) said that he waited at the vehicle while PLOTE Mohan went upstairs but found the place closed because of the Poya holiday. Then he saw PLOTE Mohan coming down while talking on his mobile phone and he started the three-wheeler. PLOTE Mohan then motioned him to wait a while, when he heard the shots."

The death of PLOTE Mohan was clearly linked with Karuna's defection because there were earlier reports that the former had visited the breakaway rebel at the latter's Thoppigala base following his defection. A similar fate had befallen Kandiah Yogarasa, also a former PLOTE man and later an informant for the Sri Lankan army intelligence who visited Karuna at Thoppigala and was killed soon after. *The Sunday Times* report claimed that more than 25 persons had been killed in a three week period prior to PLOTE Mohan's murder.

Media reports at the time spoke of security forces claiming that a detailed plan by Prabhakaran to attack camps run by Karuna in order to annihilate them had been revealed. *The Daily Mirror* said in a 31st July 2004 datelined story the security forces had received intelligence that in the previous week, Prabhakaran released a list of 100 names of Karuna loyalists, mostly leaders of various ranks, who were marked to be killed within a month. For the purpose of carrying out the attacks, a contingent of 2, 000 cadre consisting of four battalions had been sent to the east from Wanni in the course of a few days prior to the reporting.

The despatch of the contingent had been preceded by a survey of the east by the LTTE's intelligence wing in order to detect the locations, numerical strengths and fighting capabilities of the Karuna camps. Ahead of the impending attacks, about 1, 000 of Karuna's fighters were said to have fled and were regrouping for organising counter-attacks.

Parallel to the armed onslaught, the LTTE also launched a political battle in order to discredit and weaken Karuna. It asked the parliamentarians belonging to the Tamil National Alliance, widely considered to be a proxy for the LTTE in the Sri Lankan parliament, and Tamil politicians based in the east at a meeting held in Killinochhi on 17 July, 2004, to start a campaign to counter the defector's list of grievances against the parent organisation. The LTTE political wing leader Thamilchelvan told the eight TNA MPs and other politicians that they should carry out a political campaign to ensure that the LTTE's position as the sole recognised representative of the Tamil community was in no way jeopardised (a clear indication that Karuna's move to form a Tamil political party in the region run by the LTTE as its own territory had jolted the latter; the formation of the new party, Tamil Eelam People's Liberation Tigers with headquarters on the Lake Road, Batticaloa town, was announced on 12 October, 2004). The Tamil people had given a mandate to the MPs to carry out the policies of the LTTE. It was, therefore, imperative that the MPs moved closer to the Tamils in the east in order to defeat Karuna's efforts to create a hiatus between the two sides. The people in the east were apparently concerned over Karuna's "disruptive" activities which had led to an unstable security situation. This concern of the eastern Tamils must be addressed by an assurance of the LTTE that they would be protected.

The MPs should also extend the campaign inside parliament and elsewhere in order to expose Karuna. Significantly, the meeting was also attended by an important LTTE military leader, Ramesh, who led the LTTE forces in the Batticaloa-Ampara region. It was around this time that a double murder inside the Batticaloa prison attracted wide attention, necessitating a visit by the Peace Secretariat Chief Jayantha Dhanapala, who was the pointman for President Kumaratunga in peace negotiations with the LTTE. In an expression of the government's rising concern over the consequences of the LTTE-Karuna tussle, Dhanapala visited the prison where on 17 July, 2004, a former LTTE cadre shot dead two Karuna loyalists and injured another. Dhanapala also met regional military commanders and police commando officials at a meeting to discuss the adversarial impact the continuing feud was having on the maintenance of the ceasefire. The police said that the murders in the prison had followed a meeting between the LTTE leader in the Batticaloa town Senadhirajah and the killer; Senadhirajah was later attacked and injured by Karuna loyalists (he died three days after the prison incident). The prison killings were thus seen as a reprisal by the LTTE.

Apart from the fallout of the LTTE-Karuna break-up on the security situation and the unfortunate heightening of child abductions and forced recruitment, the attacks and counter-attacks, as both sides continued their vicious armed conflict in the rebel-held east and the government-held areas including Colombo, exposed for the umpteenth time the woefully inadequate (in most cases) and complete absence (in some cases) of the writ of the government over stretches of Sri Lanka.

Consider the following: in mid-July 2004, the LTTE urged the government through the Norwegian facilitators to allow its cadre to carry firearms when they found themselves in the government-held areas (banned under the ceasefire agreement) on the grounds that they faced a serious threat to their lives and limbs from Karuna campfollowers. Reports said that the request was made to the Norwegian ambassador Hans Brattskar by the LTTE's eastern political wing leader Kausalyan in the presence of the rebel group's political wing chief Thamilchelvan at a meeting held in Killinochchi on 13 July 2004. At the meeting, the LTTE pointed out that its cadre were getting killed with a regularity by Karuna's men. The only way to protect themselves from such attacks was to be armed, since Karuna's cadre were being helped by the army in carrying out the attacks.

Earlier, in this chapter we have seen how helpless the parents felt in the east in protecting their children from being abducted by the LTTE and how even the international agencies were being openly defied and challenged by the Tigers. The complete failure of the government to extend its writ even to the areas liberated from the LTTE, not to speak of areas still held by the latter, spoke of the rather uncomfortable realities of the Sri Lankan situation.

Even if credence were given to the LTTE's allegation that Karuna was being actively backed by the army, it would be difficult to explain the spate of killings that the LTTE was able to carry out inside the very national capital boasting normally of one of the most elaborate security covers witnessed in South Asia. Since there was no question of government forces facilitating the LTTE onslaught on Karuna, the only feasible explanation could be that the government was simply unable to stop the Tigers from carrying out their murder spree if and when these were carried out.

Just as the LTTE spoke and acted in the name of the Tamil people, so did Karuna. In his first telephone interview after going into hiding in March 2004, he told the BBC Tamil service that he was at the time in the eastern Sri Lanka where the people supported him. It was at this interview that he announced his intention to form a political party and enter politics. He also denied any covert link with the Sri Lankan military to facilitate attacks on the LTTE.

Explaining the disturbing spurt in violence as the rebel outfit and Karuna went on killing each other's leaders and ranks, he alleged that the Tigers themselves were responsible for the violence. "It is the LTTE which is killing our supporters and they are to blame for other violent incidents also, " he said in the interview. Prabhakaran did not believe in a negotiated settlement and was gearing up to resume the war. Acknowledging that the LTTE was getting better of the fighting in which a large number of his leaders and men were being felled, Karuna said, "I retreated because I didn't want thousands of my supporters to die in the fighting."

Intelligence from various sources continued to confirm that the LTTE was arming itself taking advantage of the ceasefire. Minister for Hindu affairs Douglas Devananda, who had just survived a suicide bomber attack on 7 July in his office in Colombo (apart from the number of attempts on his life throughout his active opposition to the LTTE), said in Chennai, India, on 13 July, "Such gruesome bloodletting, even while pretending to pursue the peace process, only further confirms the widespread suspicion that the LTTE is using the ceasefire to strengthen its war machine and carry on its policy of silencing, through violence, all forms of democratic dissent."

Referring to Karuna's utterances made at the time, he said the suspicion was being confirmed that the LTTE was arming itself. Devananda also confirmed his active support to Karuna in helping him to enter mainstream politics by forming and registering a political party. Talking to the author in Colombo in mid-September, 2004, Devananda said, "The Karuna issue was one of the factors why the LTTE wanted to get me killed (The abortive assassination attempt made on 7 July, 2004). It is also important to bear in mind that the ordinary people in the east continue to support Karuna. He will definitely join mainstream politics one day; I am helping him to form a political party. It is, therefore, imperative for the LTTE that I am rendered unable to continue to help Karuna in his attempt to break out of the past and start a new life aimed at becoming a legitimate political leader of the Tamils."[9]

While the spotlight was kept on the fratricidal killings and child abductions and recruitment, there was a potentially more disturbing development in the east. On 9 August, 2004, the Sri Lankan government made an official complaint to the Sri Lankan Monitoring Mission (SLMM) alleging that thirteen camps of the LTTE had been recently established along the southern mouth of the Trincomalee harbour, where the Sri Lankan navy's northern headquarters was located and where an oil tank complex was being run by the Indian government-owned Indian Oil Corporation (IOC). The complaint held that this development had violated the ceasefire agreement.

The SLMM despatched investigating teams on 12 August to check the veracity of the complaint by first assessing the location of the camps. The issue of the location of the alleged camps was particularly vital as, if this were true, the LTTE was clearly in a position to seriously disrupt the functioning of the harbour and thus jeopardise the main supply point to the government-held Jaffna Peninsula. The government complaint was followed by unconfirmed media reports that the camps were being fortified and bunker lines had come up along the coast.

The camps were also located in the vicinity of a bay at Illankanthai which would allow LTTE boats to be docked deep inland, thus safe from the navy's prying eyes, and unload logistical supplies. The SLMM indicated that verifying the government complaint was no easy task as some of the alleged camps were located deep inside the jungles of the Trincomalee Bay. While the SLMM enquiry was yet to start, LTTE political wing head Thamilschelvan denied the government charge.

While the matter remained unsolved for the time being, it was recalled that the Tigers had eyed the Trincomalee harbour from time to time during the ceasefire period in apparent attempts to strengthen its position in the strategically vital area. For example, the army complained to the SLMM in June 2003 alleging that the LTTE had set up a new camp at Manirasakulam on the south-western side of the bay. The SLMM found out that the camp was situated within 600 metres of the government-controlled areas and was, therefore, in violation of the ceasefire agreement. Interestingly, as an account reported more than a year later, the LTTE simply ignored the SLMM instruction and the camp continued to exist.[10]

While many more such deliberate contraventions of the provisions of the ceasefire agreement by the LTTE and, at times, by government forces continue to be cited (the SLMM estimated that in the 32 months of the ceasefire, between the late-February 2002 and the mid-October 2004, the Tigers had violated the provisions of the ceasefire agreement 2,439 times and the government 111 times) the uncomfortable impression that emerges from these violations is that both the SLMM and the government have oftener than not failed to rein in the Tigers and that the latter, if and when it pleases them to do so, can at will go on a rampage to attain a particular target, be it in the Wanni or in the east or in the south and even in Colombo.

Their marauding capabilities apparently can be stretched right inside the Jaffna Peninsula as well, which is indeed surprising since it is the control of this peninsula that has over the years defined the fortunes of the combatants and one could probably reasonably expect government forces to be adequately on the alert to be able to exercise their authority within their domain and foil LTTE designs in time. But, as students of Sri Lankan history know, the inadequacies of the security forces are legion.

Consider the following 7 August, 2003, Human Rights Watch report entitled "Sri Lanka: Political Killings During the Ceasefire": "Political killings are on the rise again in Sri Lanka. According to local human rights groups and Tamil political parties, at least thirty-eight people have been killed or were abducted and remain missing in politically motivated attacks against opponents of the LTTE since Sri Lankan prime minister Ranil Wickramasinghe and LTTE leader Vellupillai Prabhakaran signed a ceasefire agreement in February, 2002."

"Hundreds of others have been threatened, assaulted and injured. Most of the victims were members of or former members of Tamil political groups opposed to the LTTE, including some senior officials. Among those killed were Tamils who had worked for the Sri Lankan security forces. The Eelam People's Democratic Party (EPDP) and Eelam People's Revolutionary Liberation Front (EPRLF) of the Varathan faction, at present the LTTE's two main political opponents, have together lost thirty-two members or supporters killed or missing since February, 2002. The People's Liberation Organisation of Tamil Eelam (PLOTE) has had at least fifteen members or former members killed or injured in the same time period. TELO (Varathan), a breakaway unit of the Tamil Eelam Liberation Organisation that worked with the elite police Special Task Force in eastern Sri Lanka, has reportedly had at least four members killed or missing."

"The ceasefire has given the LTTE free access to towns like Batticaloa, Jaffna and Trincomalee (the first under only a nominal army control where rebels prevailed but the latter two firmly controlled by security forces where the Tigers could afford to enter at the risk of capture or death during hostilities—the author) for the purpose of opening political offices. Although the pact prohibits LTTE cadre from carrying arms in these areas, the prohibition is not well enforced. According to critics, the LTTE's new political offices have become useful points from which to coordinate surveillance, recruitment and extortion and, when necessary, the assault, abduction and assassination of rivals.

Three incidents out of several mentioned in the report signify the reach of the Tigers in carrying out their annihilation programme. In the first one, P Alahathurai (35) of Mandur, a member of the Varathan faction of the EPRLF and chairman of the Porativu local council, left his party office for his sister's home on the evening of 16 December, 2002. At around 7.30 p.m., witnesses saw him being led away by two known LTTE affiliates.

Two days later, his body was discovered near a lagoon at Kannapattai bearing signs of torture with one hand and ear chopped off. The two men identified as abductors were Ramiah Rajendran (Rajan) and Mylvaganam Paramanathan; the former was known to be attached to the local Porativu intelligence office of the LTTE while the latter was attached to the LTTE's political office in Mandur. The post-mortem examination of Alahathurai's body was delayed because local physicians were afraid to handle the case. After the post-mortem report was made available and on the basis of evidence before him, the Batticaloa magistrate ordered the arrest of the two suspects but the police took no action. Even eight months later, when the HRW report was prepared, neither suspect had been arrested. Notably, the incident took place in a government-controlled area.

In the second incident, Kadiragamanathan Ragupathy (35) was killed by unidentified motorcyclists on the Galle Road in the Colombo suburb of Mount Lavinia late in the evening of 18 March, 2003. The murdered man was a former PLOTE member who, at the time of his death, was working for the Sri Lankan Directorate of Military Intelligence. He had earlier told the Military Intelligence of his suspicion that he was being followed. The day he was killed, people considered to be under threat from the LTTE in Colombo received a warning that Mylvaganam Sivakumar, head of the LTTE intelligence in Batticaloa, had left the eastern town for Colombo. Sivakumar was known to have returned to Batticaloa one day after Ragupathy's death. The *Island* newspaper reported that he was the prime suspect in the murder case. The third incident took place in the morning of 14 June, 2003, when a sniper shot and killed Thambirajah Subathiran (Robert), 46 years old, deputy leader of the EPRLF (V) as he was exercising in his third floor office at the party headquarters in Jaffna city. He was the senior-most Tamil political figure to be killed between the beginning of the ceasefire and the preparation of the HRW report. The gunman reportedly fired from the neighbouring Vembadi Girls College. According to witnesses, the Nallur area leader of the LTTE Easwaran had visited the girls' school the previous day but, as the report says, the police had not questioned him till the writing of the report.

What was common to the three incidents was that all of them had taken place in government-controlled areas where the lawful administration was functioning. In two of them, suspected assailants or their possible accomplices were identified and the law and order authority duly informed. In one case, an arrest order was issued. Yet, there was no evidence that the administration took any initiative in pursuing the alleged culprits. Obviously, the reach of the LTTE was widespread.

That such a conclusion would not be outlandish is borne out by the audacious suicide bomber attack on Devananda on 7 July, 2004 at Kollupitiya in the heart of Colombo. A woman blew herself up at the Kollupitiya police station after trying to enter Devananda's office, killing five people, in the first ever such attack in the capital since the ceasefire came into force.

Giving his version of the incident, Devananda told the author, "A few days back I received a letter from a girl who had accompanied Sathya Leela, the would-be assassin in her mission to kill me. This girl escaped death and is now in custody. In this letter she has made a complete confession of what transpired on the day and how the entire incident was the LTTE's doing. She has even named those of the LTTE who were personally involved (in the plot). I have handed the letter over to the authorities for necessary action and the Norwegians have been informed for the clear violation of the ceasefire agreement as also as a proof of the LTTE's involvement in the assassination attempt. The girl has begged my forgiveness and I am willing to forgive her. But she would not be able to live a normal life if she is let off from the jail because the LTTE will most definitely bump her off. The contents of the letter show that Sathya Leela had come to live in Colombo under the assumed name of Thiagaraja Jeyarani about a year back. She was employed as a maid in a Sinhalese family. One month before the actual assassination attempt, she and the letter-writer had visited me in my office on a day when I received petitions from the people, and as the sole police woman to physically check all women visitors was absent that day, it looked to the would-be assassin that the access to my ministerial office could be had with no security checks. Obviously, she had concluded that on her next visit (when the attempt on my life would be made), she would not be detected. However, when the two came on 7 July, there was the usual strict security check and the girl-assassin was asked to go through it. It was then that she blew herself up, killing four police personnel and herself and injuring some more."[11]

Executive director of the Centre for Alternative Policy, Paikiasothy Saravanamuttu, who believed that the attack on Devananda was probably carried out by the Tigers, told aljazeera.net that the act was meant as a message to the government. "This must be seen in the context of the situation in the east of the country where the LTTE says the government is fighting a proxy war against it. And, particularly, it must be seen in the context of the last few days during which an LTTE loyalist was assassinated in Batticaloa. The LTTE is warning the government, 'If you try to get at us, we can put Colombo under a state of siege.' It is a reminder of the past and a warning about the future. A warning that the government better start getting serious about the peace process and start talks about some kind of interim government in the north and the east."

Referring to the LTTE allegation that Karuna had been propped up by the government to weaken it and that the military was waging a covert war against it using Karuna's services, the analyst said that there was probably some truth in the charge,: "The government has denied any link to Karuna but it is unlikely that he would be able to mount these attacks without some financial and military support."

Whatever the outcome of Karuna's revolt turns out to be, its consequences were unpleasantly clear in the months following the event. The very ceasefire was threatened and the fear was expressed by all quarters that Sri Lanka was edging towards a re-enactment of the 21-year-old secessionist war. While the international community urged both the government and the LTTE to resume talking to each other, all sides appeared to feel that the Tigers would not rejoin peace talks until the threat posed by Karuna was comprehensively dealt with.

However, despite the obvious support that the Karuna camp continued to receive from sections of the security forces in countering the determined LTTE onslaught, it was curious to experience the seemingly unhurried government response to the Tigers' annihilation spree. And a very curious comment was made reportedly by a government spokesman, Harim Peiris, who discounted any threat to the peace process by the ongoing violence. He told *aljazeera.net*, "It is the LTTE going after a political opponent. It is that and absolutely nothing else. It is resorting to violence to kill an opponent; it is not reverting to hostilities."

This seeming nonchalance, however, was not borne out by the ground realities. For, Karuna's revolt also posed a severe administrative and tactical challenge for the government as it entered the public domain on the eve of the April 2004 parliamentary elections. The principal challenge was to deal with it in a manner that would in no way jolt the ceasefire (which, by the very act of challenging Prabhakaran's authority within the LTTE, was by itself capable of accomplishing) , which was essentially an administrative issue.

But the tactical or political dilemma thrown up before the government (which was till then the bipolar arrangement with the president and commander-in-chief of the armed forces and the prime minister belonging to two sworn rival political parties of the south) was what to do with the act of revolt itself; should the necessity arise, would it be prudent for the government to extend some sort of official recognition to the defector?

This was prickly, to say the least, because the LTTE had been quick to allege that the military was fighting a proxy war through Karuna. Any kind of recognition at that stage would only serve to tilt the balance against the ceasefire, with the blame for destabilisation attaching itself squarely with Colombo.

With the SLMM and the international community watching the developments minutely, the government was forced to ponder over all probabilities with abundant caution. Karuna was already making sounds indicating his desire to enter the political mainstream by forming a political party (in which endeavour, the EPDP leader and minister Devananda was openly an enthusiastic facilitator, strengthening the impression that the government could after all be supporting the renegade) and seeking to establish his bona fides as a political, rather than a terrorist, entity.

His words and acts at the time also served to pose a challenge to the LTTE's well-crafted plan to fully control the participation of the Tamil community in the coming elections, obliging the two rival southern parties (which were also sharing a very painful coexistence in the government) to think over the impact of any extension of support or recognition to Karuna on the Tamil community of the north and east in terms of its potential electoral support to them, which was also of immediate interest.

The situation was further complicated by Karuna's direct challenge to the LTTE game-plan to send a large number of "proxy" members to the parliament-to-be in order to be able to influence the formation of the next government. He ordered the LTTE-chosen candidates contesting from the east to cut off all links with the Wanni leadership. This particular act of defiance appeared at the time to have pushed the situation towards further uncertainty and to have heightened the government's dilemma.

The challenges before the government, however, sorted themselves out, letting the government and the two contending political parties out without any effort on their part. Karuna's defiance on the eve of the polls simply evaporated and, as it turned out later, the newly elected Tamil National Alliance members of parliament from the east dutifully bowed to the dictates of the LTTE and were in fact participating with considerable enthusiasm in the political campaign launched against Karuna in the east. One of the MPs, Joseph Pararajahsingham told the author, "The TNA MPs do not dance to the tune of the LTTE.

During the last general election, we contested on four issues: the LTTE should be accepted as the sole representative of the Tamil people; the Tamils have the right of self-determination; the merger of the northeast Province has to be recognised; and the Interim Self Governing Authority proposals are to be the basis for steps for implementation. One must remember that 95 per cent of the Tamils voted for the TNA candidates. The TNA works as a political party and we hold discussions (on issues) with the LTTE."

While the Karuna saga remains unfinished at the time of writing this book, the question must be answered at some point how and why it happened. That this was no ordinary development in the Sri Lankan context was acknowledged by no less a person than President Kumaratunga.

Answering a question at the Foreign Correspondents' Club in Colombo on 3 September, 2004, as to what was wrong in helping Karuna (asked in the context of media reports that he was being helped by sections of the military), she said, "What is right in it? Karuna is as much a terrorist as Prabhakaran. I don't believe in any form of terrorism. I believe that all problems can be solved through negotiations, democratically, and in a humane fashion. I don't believe in killing. I don't believe in child conscription. Both these people (Prabhakaran and Karuna) have been entirely culpable of all these activities. To support one terrorist against another is just continuing the vicious cycle. I do not believe in that."

This author's random search for an answer as to how the Karuna defection occurred led to a plethora of explanations, sometimes mutually contradictory, but also ultimately to a semblance of coherent logic. Several factors apparently helped Karuna to conclude that the sustained ceasefire, which had rekindled the desire of the people in the northeast to live a normal life with myriad manifestations, like students enthusiastically pursuing their studies without interruption by war and by the constant fear of conscription by the LTTE and traders, farmers and fishermen redoubling their efforts to raise their incomes, offered an ideal opportunity to break out of the LTTE where his prospects were suddenly being threatened.

It is not clear if Devananda and his EPDP were already in touch with Karuna, but the Devananda model appears to have moulded his

Karuna's Revolt 59

thinking to a large extent. The EPDP leader himself was ambivalent about the exact timing of his contact with Karuna but he confirmed that since the latter's coming out in the open, the two had been in contact. "My help to Karuna to join mainstream politics is one of the reasons why I remain a target of the LTTE, " he said. "I am sure that he will join mainstream politics and shun terrorism for ever."

Pararajahsingham did not share Devananda's perception about the Karuna factor, asserting that, " (it) has failed to serve Chandrika Kumaratunga's purpose." The failure was due to the obvious lack of support for Karuna's line of thinking among the people of the east, which sought to undermine the unity of the Tamils. "Once the people realised that Karuna's criticism of the LTTE leadership was nothing but a camouflage for achieving his own political ambitions, while at the same time his actions were serving to weaken the Tamil people's movement for wresting the right of self-determination in the northeast, they decided to ignore him. The result is there to see; whatever gains Kumaratunga had hoped for from Karuna's defection have not materialised."

Speaking at the Foreign Correspondents' Club in Colombo, the president reiterated that her government was in no way involved in the Karuna affair. On the other hand, she alleged, it was the previous United National Front government led by Prime Minister Ranil Wickramasinghe which was deeply involved. "It was the previous government that helped Karuna to come to Colombo, " she said. According to her, a UNP MP (belonging to the United National Party led by Wickramasinghe and identified by her as Mr Moulana) admitted that he brought Karuna to Colombo.

"He has been dealt with by the UNP...he has been sacked since. The MP, Moulana, was arrested and questioned during my previous government (my first one, this is my third) for having dealings with Karuna at a time when the war was going on and the prevention of Terrorism Act was in operation, " she said. "But Moulana was given nomination even after that, to contest from the UNP or he was brought in on the National List into parliament. So, please do not say that (my) government helped."

Asserting that her government could not do much more than giving general instructions to the security forces to avoid any dealings with Karuna, she said, "…very clear instructions have been given right down the line by the president and commander-in-chief, to the commanders of (the) army that this kind of thing cannot happen. But we do not know who the individual (who helped Karuna defect) is, no individual has admitted to it; it is only a suspicion. We don't even know if individuals have helped. It is only a suspicion because (the) LTTE kept saying it was done. But one must also not forget that this is the first time in its 20-year history that somebody in the LTTE has successfully been able to contest the authority of Prabhakaran and get away with his life. So, may be the LTTE also has to make up stories to defend its authoritarian, dictatorial, positions. I have no evidence, as minister of defence and commander-in-chief, if any individual in the armed forces did it. There was some suspicion, especially because the LTTE kept saying 'we have evidence.' I have asked the LTTE for that evidence but they have not given me any evidence. The Peace Secretariat also has asked if they have any evidence at all, even some kind of evidence, but they have not been able to come up with it, or they have not yet. So, it is only a suspicion, and in case it happened, as it can happen in organisations, we have given all necessary instructions. That is the action we can take."

Later, Dhanapala told the author, "The president has given clear instructions (to people serving in the government) not to show complicity with Karuna."

Sitting in his sprawling, ornate drawing room, under the gaze of his illustrious ancestors, TNA MP and general secretary, All Ceylon Tamil Congress, Gajen Ponnambalam narrated a riveting event that took place in his Queen's Road residence.

For two days in April, 2004, the TNA parliamentary group, except two who were publicly supporting Karuna, were closeted to finalise a statement on the Karuna episode, which would clearly be against the defector. When a consensus was at hand and the MPs were preparing to sign the agreed statement, one MP contacted the army area commander in his district in the east by a mobile phone.

The latter in turn appeared to have passed on a message to the army and police contingents which had accompanied the MPs on their journey to Colombo and were camping outside Ponnambalam's residence. The officers and men then trooped in, demanding that the

MPs would have to accompany them immediately back to the east as further delay in departure might be harmful to their safety.

The parliamentary group disagreed, insisting that no MP would leave before the statement was signed by all. The officers then said that they were not in a position to disobey their superior officer's order to return to the east without delay and that as the security of the MPs was their responsibility, the latter would also have to return along with them. Since this unforeseen development would jeopardise the finalisation of the intended statement, the group then decided to contact the defence secretary and the army commander in order to arrange for a longer stay of the MPs.

"Despite our repeated efforts, we could not contact either officer and it became obvious that a situation was being created to prevent us from going ahead with the finalisation of the statement which would be highly critical of Karuna, " said Ponnambalam. "It became obvious to us that the then army chief was acting in a manner which was prejudicial to the interests of the TNA parliamentary group and was aimed at preventing us from issuing the anti-Karuna statement. This was one incident which made us suspect the army's role in the Karuna affair."

If the circumstances which led to Karuna's break from the LTTE continue to remain unclear, so was his whereabouts in the months following his decision to withdraw from the confrontation with the parent body and retreat, perhaps to recoup and think over his prospects.

Speculations were rife in the country that he was being sheltered by the military in Colombo; most guesses, however, placed him in his hideout in the Thoppigala jungles. But, at least one man, Devananda, who maintained that he was in touch with Karuna, asserted that the latter had been spirited away abroad. One international aid agency suspected that the ubiquitous Americans had played a hand in whisking Karuna away to a safe haven outside Sri Lanka. But, sources in the present government who agreed to talk on the subject rejected the idea outright that Americans or any other foreigner had been involved in the affair.

Diplomatic circles in Colombo tended to feel that above all other relevant aspects of the Karuna defection and its consequences, one thing that stood out was the Sri Lankan government's failure to exploit the situation. "The government had got an opportunity to dictate terms to the LTTE when Karuna defected because they had clearly suffered a setback and were weakened, " they said. "Unfortunately, instead of doing so, the government has merely allowed time and space to the LTTE to try to beat Karuna down to submission." The foreign diplomats who talked to the author were particularly aghast at the virtual impunity with which the LTTE could carry on its elimination campaign against Karuna's followers as well as intelligence operatives in the employment of the military, more shockingly in Colombo.

"This was almost an abnegation of the responsibilities of the state," they said. Despite the indirect facility provided by the non-action of the government, the LTTE, however, continued to remain weakened, having lost around 6, 000 (4, 000, according to pro-LTTE sources) fighters. What was of more importance at the moment was the Sri Lankan army's capability to wrest the east from the LTTE, though the Jaffna Peninsula might ultimately fall back into the hands of the guerrillas in case of a resumption of war.[13]

It was difficult to visualise how a resumption of peace talks could be accommodated in the midst of the mayhem that had been let loose in the wake of Karuna's revolt. The LTTE continued to defy its own commitments, belittle the provisions of the ceasefire agreement and even ignore the frequent harsh pronouncements of the Bush administration. The impending signing of a far-reaching defence pact between India and Sri Lanka with an expected strengthening of the security apparatus also failed to discourage it from its singleminded determination to exterminate the Karuna threat.

Thus, in the first week of October, 2004, there was obviously no improvement in the human rights situation in Sri Lanka owing to the continuing and mutually destructive killing spree between the LTTE and the Karuna faction.

On 5 October, representatives of the International Commission of Jurists (ICJ), Human Rights Watch (HRW) and Amnesty International (AI) met Thamilchelvan who was then leading an LTTE delegation to western Europe, in Geneva. They urged the LTTE to stop the killings and child conscription, which was also going unabated, and to respect the universally accepted human rights in Sri Lanka.

Nicholas Howen, secretary general of the ICJ, called upon the LTTE to prove its commitment to the lives and human rights of the people of Sri Lanka, show its respect for the universally acclaimed humanitarian and human rights, and asked the guerrilla group to prove its sincerity by actively helping in the observation of the rights. The HRW director in Geneva Loubna Freih told the LTTE functionary that the group must take concrete steps towards a resumption of negotiations with the Sri Lankan government and pointed out that instead of working towards consolidating peace, the Tigers were actually escalating their acts of political killings and continuing with child conscription without caring for its public commitment to stop this practice.

The AI representative Peter Splinter said that the LTTE had been assassinating with impunity members of rival political parties, Karuna faction cadre and intelligence operatives of the Sri Lankan operatives, all in violation of the ceasefire agreement. These acts were clearly a hindrance for efforts to resume peace negotiations. It was in a similar vein that Norway's deputy foreign minister Vidar Helgesen, actively involved in the Sri Lankan peace process, also spoke to Thamilchelvan when he said that the killings would only serve to jeopardise the peace process. He emphasised that his government strongly condemned the killings which should be stopped immediately in an effective manner.

Being buffeted by the rising tide of international criticism and warnings, the LTTE took the only step it could, not at all to stop the killings as it was being urged but to expedite the pace and effectiveness of assassinations and attacks, so that the Karuna factor was dispensed with decisively. This was made apparent when the entire security setup in the east was changed and the military command was passed on to military leader Bhanu who was also heading the artillery units of the Tiger force. The new commander, who had replaced Ramesh, immediately inducted battle-proven cadre from the northern command, mainly from the Jeyanathan and Charles Anthony brigades, into the east.

Soon thereafter, the LTTE scored a major blow against Karuna by killing his brother and second-in-command of the renegade force, Vinayagamoorthi Sivasundari alias Reggie. The latter was killed on 22 September, 2004, during an ambush near Karadiyanaru, east of

Batticaloa. Lately, the sniper attacks, ambushes and outright assassinations by both the feuding groups had centred around the Batticaloa town.

It was later known that the LTTE had picked up Reggie precisely at a time when he had become a genuine threat to it; he had managed to penetrate into the LTTE territory along with about twenty-five cadre, who had thereafter split into smaller units. One of these cadre had acted as a mole of the LTTE who kept the latter informed about Reggie's whereabouts.

Karuna vowed to revenge his brother's murder. In a statement broadcast by the London-based anti-LTTE Tamil Broadcasting Corporation on 23 September, he said that the martyrdom of Reggie had not made the dissidents "submissive to the fascist forces" and that it would only add strength and give a forceful thrust to the resistance movement. Reggie's death would be a guiding force in the struggle against the "Wanni group" (Karuna's description of the LTTE).

On 25 September, 2004, the LTTE's Batticaloa and Ampara political unit issued a statement saying that Reggie was killed not on the morning of 23 September but two days earlier. Tamilnet website reported the statement which maintained that Reggie was ambushed and killed by a crack jungle warfare unit of the Jeyanathan brigade (which was raised by Karuna in his capacity as the special commander of Batticaloa and Ampara) and that weapons and documents showing his links with some army officers were recovered from the scene.

Karuna went on record on the manner in which his brother was dispensed with by the LTTE; his fight was clearly weakened and he had to fight back hard. This he did by attacking the LTTE camps in Panchchankerni, north of Batticaloa; the significance of this mortar attack lay in the fact that the camps were within the LTTE-held territory. Five LTTE cadre and a civilian were killed in the attack. He also directed an attack on an LTTE bus carrying cadre but the attempt failed.

Judging by the trend of incidents since Karuna's defection and the breakout of the murderous feud between the two groups continuing well into October, almost eight months since the major split in the Tigers war machine, it was difficult to envisage a lessening of tension and conscious facilitation of a resumption of talks.

Karuna's Revolt

Both the LTTE and Karuna's men appear to be well settled to go to any length to score over each other; since the two sides are not equal, the parent group is likely to win in the dangerous game, and only then it might consider taking the necessary steps to return to the negotiating table.

Unless external factors like international pressure and active military support to the Sri Lankan military contribute to the unveiling of a different scenario altogether upsetting the present military-guerrilla fighting equation and thereby depriving it of the cosy time and space arrangement it has been enjoying under the ceasefire agreement, the LTTE seems inclined to go ahead with its agenda.

As the infiltration by Reggie's men into its territory was discovered following the ambush in which the Karuna group's second-in-command was killed, the Tigers deployed well-tested cadre in areas through which such attempts could be made in order to prevent any recurrence. The LTTE's senior cadre and various departmental leaders were instructed to restrict their movements and public appearances and the cadre were told to be less conspicuous than they were while moving into government-held territory where Karuna's men could be lying in wait for them.

The LTTE also brought about a qualitative change in the composition of its preventive personnel; its intelligence wing operatives and members of the dreaded "pistol gangs" took over from political wing cadre. These changes were soon followed by successful attacks against not only Karuna's men but also adversaries like the Eelam People's Democratic Party and Eelam People's Revolutionary Liberation Front (V).

In a tactical move, the LTTE changed its earlier tack and denied any involvement in the killings, probably in an aftereffect of the fusillade of international criticism and warnings to behave better. Amantha Perera of *The Sunday Leader* recalled Thamilchelvan's words, "There is no need for the Liberation Tigers to eliminate anybody. It is true that political assassinations are taking place. But we are also aware of the background of those killings. Fall guys are selected by some elements who are very much interested in promoting war and disrupting the peace process. The killings have all the hallmarks of the LTTE and the guys selected for it definitely happen to be vocal opponents of the LTTE but these are machinations of serious political hierarchies to attain a position of making the Liberation Tigers defensive on their political stand, whether nationally or internationally."[14]

Thamilchelvan was apparently hinting at the involvement of the Sri Lankan army, along with what it refers to as para-military, meaning Karuna's men, army intelligence operatives and anti-LTTE groups like the EPDP and EPRLF (V), in the killings since the army is known to have been unhappy about the ceasefire agreement. This, however, does not explain why the LTTE has been losing its own cadre who are known to have been entrusted with the job of finishing off the Karuna challenge. Besides, prior to the change in tack, it was quite boastful of the speedy manner in which the challenger's men were being disposed of, taking little care at that time to hide its own involvement.

Notes

1. V.S.Sambandan, "Rajiv assassination the gravest mistake: Karuna," *The Hindu*, New Delhi edition, 13 March, 2004.
2. D.B.S.Jeyaraj, "Tiger vs. Tiger in eastern Sri Lanka", *The Hindu*, New Delhi edition, 15 March, 2004.
3. V.S. Smbandan, "Rajiv assassination the gravest mistake, karuna," *The Hindu*, New Delhi edition, 13 March, 2004.
4. Ibid.
5. Frances Harrison, *Amnesty concern over 'child Tigers'*, BBC, 15 February, 2002.
6. Human Rights Watch, *Sri Lanka: Tamil Tigers again abduct child soldiers*, 29 June, 2004, London.
7. The Optional Protocol to the convention on the rights of the child protects children in armed conflict, prohibits the direct use of any child under the age of 18 years in armed conflict and prohibits all use of children under 18 years of age by non-state armed groups, such as the LTTE; Sri Lanka became a signatory and party to the protocol which has been in force since February, 2002.
8. Interview conducted in Colombo on 8 September, 2004.
9. Interview conducted in Colombo on 14 September, 2004.
10. Amantha Perera, "A violent ceasefire," *South Asia Intelligence Review*, vol.3, no.6, 23 August, 2004. The LTTE's blatant flouting

of the SLMM directive also brought up a fresh point of clash between President Kumaratunga and the then Prime Minister Ranil Wickramasinghe, leading ultimately to the former taking over the defence ministry, along with two other ministries, and eventually to the surprise dissolution of the Sri Lankan parliament and fresh general elections in April, 2004.

The LTTE had over the years provided enough examples to establish its abiding interest in the strategic importance of the Trincomalee harbour, which was integral to its demand for a Tamil "eelam" or homeland and would normally qualify to be the capital of the northeast. One such instance was a "nationalist" Pongu Tamil or "Tamil upsurge" celebration in the area in late-March, 2002, the significance of which was lost neither on the Sri Lankan nor on the Indian government, for this event was soon after followed by the first-ever visit by the then Indian high commissioner Gopalkrishna Gandhi to the Trincomalee oil farm in the fifteen years that had elapsed since the Indo-Sri Lankan Agreement of July 1987 (" The work of restoring and operating the Trincomalee oil tank farm will be undertaken as a joint venture between India and Sri Lanka, " as laid down in the 29 July 1987 letter the then Indian prime minister Rajiv Gandhi wrote to the then Sri Lankan president J R Jayewardene as part of the exchange of letters between the two leaders as annexture to the main body of the Indo-Sri Lankan Agreement), still later to be followed by the appearance of the Indian oil Corporation on the scene. More significantly, the Indo-Sri Lanka Agreement also laid it down that "Trincomalee or any other ports in Sri Lanka will not be made available for military use by any country in a manner prejudicial to India's interests." High commissioner Gandhi's unprecedented visit to Trincomalee took place in the backdrop of repeated urgings by Sri Lanka to New Delhi to get involved in the area more to act as an insurance against any future deliberate act of upsetting the ceasefire. Till then, New Delhi's approach had been to assert its "legitimate strategic" interests in Trincomalee diplomatically rather than in any relatively more tangible way. Yet another major indicator of the LTTE's designs was available when the incident involving a Tigers flotilla of three boats occurred eight nautical miles off the eastern Trincomalee port in the last week of April, 2002. The Sri Lankan navy intercepted the flotilla which was transporting LTTE fighters and arms by sea but let it go after the Sri Lanka Monitoring Mission intervened. President Kumaratunga, who had consistently cautioned the Ranil Wickramasinghe government against being duped by the LTTE and demanded that all security-related matters should be referred to her, summoned a special meeting of the National Security Council to discuss the unprecedented incident and demanded an explanation from the security forces for the unexplained release of the detained flotilla. The security forces explained that after the flotilla was detained, the SLMM was contacted under the provisions of the CFA and that the flotilla was released after the SLMM decided on that course of action.

Kumaratunga pointed out that while the prevention of Terrorism Act was no longer applicable after the ceasefire came into force, the obvious smuggling of fighters and arms could have been dealt with under the normal criminal laws of the country. She also asked the defence ministry to provide a full report on the incident. Later in the year, after she had cancelled an appointment with Norwegian deputy foreign minister Vidar Helgesen, she told an interviewer, "They (the Norwegian embassy in Colombo) sought a last-minute meeting as they had to change their plans to suit (LTTE ideologue and spokesman) Anton Balasingham's schedule. No, it (the cancellation of the appointment) was not in protest. But I do not agree with the way the Norwegians handle the peace process.

"Obviously, they have gone beyond their mandate. Not only them. Some other countries too were of the view that there is no harm in creating a separate state in the northeast if it brings peace. They justify their stance by giving all sorts of reasons. But when war breaks out again next time, it will be between two countries. It would be frightening even to think about it."

Former director of the Centre for South and Southeast Asian Studies, University of Madras, Chennai, India, Dr V Suryanarayan provides a comprehensive analysis of the importance of Trincomalee and the seas around Sri Lanka to the military and political ambitions of the LTTE in "Sea Tigers—threat to Indian security" (*The Hindu*, New Delhi ed., 28 July, 2004): "Although the ceasefire had been in existence for two years, the situation in the seas surrounding the north and the east continues to be volatile. Even as the Norway-facilitated talks continued (until the LTTE unilaterally withdrew, accusing Colombo of perfidy), the two sides built up their strength."

"The matter came to a crisis when the Sri Lankan navy sank a Tiger ship, allegedly carrying arms, on 10 March, 2003. Predictably, conflicting statements followed. The SLMM failed to clarify the situation as it should have. The Norwegian monitors played it safe and did not issue a conclusive statement of facts."

"In the days following the events in March 2003, the Tigers began to articulate their 'rights' in the seas. Prabhakaran has asked for a de facto naval status to the Sea Tigers. What is more, in its proposals for interim self-government, the LTTE has demanded control over marine resources and the right of access and exploitation over them. In case Colombo accepts these proposals, two-thirds of Sri Lanka's coastline will come under Tiger control. As far as the Palk Bay is concerned, the Sea Tigers dominate the entire coastline except the outer islands in the Jaffna Peninsula and the Mannar Island, which continue to be under the control of the Sri Lankan navy".

11. Interview of Douglas Devananda.
12. Interview of TNA MP Joseph Pararajahsingham, taken in Colombo on 8 September, 2004.
13. Interviews conducted on different dates in September, 2004, with foreign diplomats posted in Colombo.
14. *South Asia Intelligence Review*, October, 2004.

3
Is LTTE a Liberation Movement?

On 26 November, 2001, LTTE leader Velupillai Prabhakaran in his annual "Heroes' Day" radio address (which was noted with considerable seriousness by all sections of Sri Lankan society ritually every year) urged the democratic west to reconsider its act of labelling the Tamil Tigers as a terrorist organisation.

Terrorism should be redefined, he argued, in order to exclude groups like the LTTE from the terrorist list as they used violence for "a concrete political objective." He was not a terrorist, he asserted, as he represented a "people's movement." "We are fighting and sacrificing our lives for the love of a noble cause, that is, human freedom. We are freedom fighters, " he added.[1]

His argument was in the context of a ban and restrictions imposed by some governments on the LTTE; these were India and Sri Lanka (the latter also maintained an official relationship with the Tamil Tigers simultaneously as required by the compulsion to seek a political solution to the country's ethnic conflict), the United States (which designated the Tigers as a terrorist group for the first time in 1997 and had since maintained that status), the United Kingdom and Australia.[2]

The inadequacy of the international policing action against the LTTE was well brought out by a US Republican Congressmen, James A Leach, who was also the chairman of the Congressional sub-committee on East Asia and the Pacific. Speaking on 11 October, 2004, Leach urged an early resumption of negotiations between the

Sri Lankan government and the rebels and called upon the international community to consider additional steps to put pressure on the LTTE to abandon its tactics of terror and prove that its days of violence were over.

"It is remarkable, for example, " he pointed out, "that only four countries—the US, Britain, Australia, and India—have declared the LTTE to be sponsors of terrorism, frozen their assets and prohibited financial transactions with the Tigers. It is well reported that alongside a finely tuned propaganda campaign, the LTTE also runs a sophisticated international fund raising campaign."

Leach further said, " The majority of financial support comes from the Tamil diaspora in countries where there is no ban on transactions with the Tigers, including Switzerland, Canada and the Scandinavian countries. It is my understanding that the LTTE's overseas financing includes investments in real estate, restaurants, stocks, and money market funds. Even film, food festivals and cultural events may contribute to insurgent income."

Quoting the US Department of State, Leach said, "(It) also reports that expatriate Tamil communities in Europe have been tied to narcotics smuggling, another potential source of funding. In this context, surely the stark record of LTTE terrorism demands a firmer response from our friends and allies abroad."

Coming back to Prabhakaran's speech, the LTTE leader said that it had become all the more necessary to distinguish between "real terrorists" and freedom fighters in the context of the global war on terrorism. "Western democratic nations should provide a clear and comprehensive definition between freedom struggles based on the right to self-determination and blind terrorist acts based on fanaticism," he said. Arguing that the U S led global alliance against terrorism included the Sri Lanka state that "practises state terror against the minority Tamils", he urged that the international community should identify and punish such states. The basic "political" aspirations of the Tamil people were "neither separatism nor terrorism, " he said a few months prior to the offer of a ceasefire proposal that led finally to a ceasefire agreement between the Sri Lankan state and the LTTE. [3]

Prabhakaran's argument in favour of identifying the LTTE not as a terrorist outfit but as a liberation movement was neither unique nor unexpected. The launching of the global war on terrorism had clearly placed the Tamil Tigers in a particularly disadvantageous position as they were already branded as such by a string of powerful nations, leading to a significantly debilitating impact on their organisational strength, especially in respect of collecting funds and buying arms and ammunition as well as carrying out propaganda campaigns in those countries.

Thus, November, 2001, was clearly a time to attempt to break out of the restrictive net that had been imposed on the LTTE in the international arena.

The question crucial to Prabhakaran's argument is whether the LTTE is a terrorist organisation or a liberation movement. This brings us to the question of defining terrorism. A P Schmid and A J Jongman's *Political Terrorism* (New Brunswick, NJ; Transaction Books, 1988) provides as many as 109 definitions of the term "terrorism." In a much simpler manner, we will discuss here two definitions available, a social science definition and a minimum legal definition.

According to the first definition, terrorism is an anxiety-inspiring method of repeated violent action, employed by (semi) clandestine individual, group or state actors, for idiosyncratic, criminal or political reasons, whereby—in contrast to assassination—the direct targets of violence are not the main targets. The immediate human victims of violence are generally chosen randomly (targets of opportunity) or selectively (representative or symbolic targets) from a target population, and serve as message generators. Threat and violence based communication processes between terrorist (organisation), (imperiled) victims, and main targets are used to manipulate the main target (audience (s)), turning it into a target of terror, a target of demands, or a target of attention, depending on whether intimidation, coercion or propaganda is primarily sought. As for the proposed legal definition, terrorist acts should be considered as "peacetime equivalents of war crimes" (deliberate attacks on civilians; hostage-taking; killing of prisoners).[4]

It should, however, be noted that Prabhakaran's argument in favour of distinguishing liberation movements from pure terrorism is shared by various terrorist-liberation groups such as the Palestine Liberation

Organisation, Al-Fatah—Revolutionary Council, the Popular Front for the Liberation of Palestine, the Democratic Front for the Liberation of Palestine, the Irish Republican Army, the Basque Liberation Movement ETA, the Kosovo Liberation Army and the PKK or the Kurdistan Workers' Party.

On the other hand, attracting a definition of "Degenerate Guerrillas", the LTTE is also described as one of "the most dangerous terrorist groups in today's world. According to a report published in April 1997 by the US Department of State, 200 of the 311 deaths caused by 'international terrorism' in 1996 were attributable to the LTTE, and 76 of the 296 attacks counted by the US government last year were the work of the PKK."[5]

Seven years later, ever since March, 2004 till the second half of the year, the LTTE continued to indulge in a series of terrorist acts reaffirming its dependence on terrorism as a major tool for achieving its objectives. As in previous years, this went on parallel to its political moves like wooing the Sinhalese public opinion and the international community.

Among the many terrorist acts committed during this period was the shooting down of Somasunderam Varnakulasingam, a senior member of the Eelam People's Democratic Party on 23 September, 2004. Two "pistol" men of the LTTE (members of an assassination speciality group) visited Varnakulasingam's house around 2.30 in the afternoon, shot him in cold blood at a close range and escaped. The deceased was survived by his wife, also injured in the shooting, and three children.

It was around this time that the EPDP, which had continued to wage its long-standing fight against the LTTE despite constant onslaught, reported that Tamil migrants living in Germany had begun to experience the "fascist" actions of the LTTE. "Moderate intellectuals and those who favour democracy, " the EPDP said, "have come forward to enlighten fellow Tamils of the unethical attitudes of the LTTE. Some even advise them through leaflets and posters. The LTTE, having come to know of these actions against (its fascist) activities, (has) started to counter the protest. They threaten with death the people they find working against the LTTE, call them traitors and try to isolate them from other Tamils. The LTTE made use of the clash between the police and the workers during the last May Day rally and informed the police of some anti-LTTE activists as the people involved in the clash. Some of the persons arrested were released later after the German police held investigations."[6]

Though the LTTE earned some international notoriety in 1990 and 1995 by using chlorine gas against police and military installations in Sri Lanka, Prabhakaran might derive satisfaction from the fact that theoretically speaking, this act was not considered a terrorist act. Commenting on this distinction, David Claridge writes, "However, these attacks were part of a guerrilla war. The LTTE has never used weapons of mass destruction (such as chlorine gas) in terror attacks against civilians, despite massive conventional explosions in civilian areas. This strongly suggests (that) the group has, for some reason, rejected the use of chemical weapons as a part of its terrorist campaign." ("Exploding the Myths of Superterrorism", in Max Taylor and John Horgan ed. *The Future of Terrorism*, p.139)

The social science definition makes it clear that liberation movements such as the LTTE cannot lay claim to being purely political by virtue of seeking a political aim, the creation of a homeland for the Sri Lankan Tamils. The very fact that they employ terrorism in order to achieve their aim condemns them to be regarded as a terrorist group even if their ultimate aim is political. It would be interesting at this juncture to compare today's separatist and liberation movements which are essentially branded as terrorist movements with earlier liberation movements, such as, those in the northern (such as Algeria and western Sahara, the latter still continuing), western (such as the Congo), eastern (such as Kenya) and southern Africa (such as South Africa and Zimbabwe) and in Asia (such as, Indonesia, Vietnam, Cambodia and Burma), all of which used violent means to attain their goals, but an extensive examination of the question would require a separate space to be able to do justice.

Sri Lankan academic K M de Silva is, however, emphatic that the LTTE is seldom equalled as a terrorist organisation. He says, "Separatist groups which indulge in acts of calculated violence are often accused of being terrorist organisations. Few separatist groups operating in south and Southeast Asia have deserved this epithet more than (the) LTTE. Such separatist groups generally have a terrorist section operating in association with it or as a peripheral unit. With the LTTE, terrorism is part of its core, and has been so from its inception. How much of this terrorism derives from the political culture of internecine warfare, and of fratricidal violence, in which the LTTE has had to operate, and how much is due to the nature of its leadership and of its leader, Vellupillai Prabhakaran, are matters for debate. There is no doubt, however, that the latter's—the leader's—personal attributes have much to do with it. A recent *New York Times* issue (29 May, 1995) put it fairly when it stated that: '...He has shown a bloodthirstiness, in dealing with opponents, that has been compared with some of the cruellest figures in recent Asian history, including Pol Pot of Cambodia. Prabhakaran, who is 40, leads a movement whose deeds, in scale, pale alongside the genocide committed by Pol Pot's Khmer Rouge of the 1970s...but what they lack in scope, they make up in brutality...(He) has established a rule of terror in the city of Jaffna. According to scores of accounts from defectors and others who have escaped the Tiger tyranny, many of his own lieutenants have been murdered; Tamils who have criticised him, even mildly or in jest have been picked up, tortured, and executed; others have been held for years in dungeons, half-starved, hauled out periodically for a battering by their guards.'"[7]

Does the use of violence automatically categorise a liberation movement as a terrorist group? Louise Richardson makes an interesting and very plausible distinction between political and terrorist violence in "Terrorists as Transnational Actors" (Max Taylor and John Horgan ed. *The Future of Terrorism*), "...I see terrorism as politically motivated violence directed against non-combatant or symbolic targets which is designed to communicate a message to a broader audience. The critical feature of terrorism is the deliberate targetting of innocents in an effort to convey a message to another party. This is thus essentially different from the most proximate form of political violence, the irregular warfare of the guerrilla."

Richardson's definition appears to be closer to the Sri Lankan situation than any other definition available. The LTTE uses both purely terrorist attacks on civilians (mainly to spread panic and disorder and to disrupt normal life, sometimes also to harm the economy) and conventional militarist assaults (which are also on occasions a mixture of conventional and guerrilla warfare and terrorist acts such as suicide bombing; sometimes during fighting, suicide bombers are deployed to put army tanks and armoured vehicles out of commission) against the security forces in order either to retain or regain territory over which it wants to run a de facto government. These acts of violence are followed by essentially political moves, such as, the manipulation of the 2 April 2004 parliamentary elections to send a group of subservient members to the new parliament and thus create a niche for itself in national politics in the heart of the Sinhalese south (this was, however, not the first instance of such political manoeuvring. A group of Tamil MPs belonging to the Eelam Revolutionary Organisation of Students , led by Balakumar, was reputed to have played a crucial role in rescuing the then President Ranasinghe Premadasa from facing an impeachment move in parliament) or the frequent reiteration of its declared goal of shunning war and continuing the peace dialogue with the government.

While there are innumerable instances of the use of these seemingly contradictory methods by the Tigers in their search for the "Tamil Eelam", two from the 1987 vintage, when they were fighting the Indian Peace Keeping Force (IPKF), would suffice to highlight the behavioural pattern of this terrorist group. The first act was of pure terrorism when on 13 September 1987 they carried out a massacre of their chief rival militant groups in Batticaloa, killing 70 of them in one fell swoop and sending the survivors running helter- skelter into IPKF and Sri Lankan army camps in the east. This was soon followed by a sustained high-pitched propaganda of how the IPKF was acting on behalf of the Sri Lankan government and against the interests of the Tamils. The LTTE was apparently building a case for branding the Indians as agents of Colombo and anti-Tamil and thus seek to render them eventually ineffective in restoring full normalcy in the north and east.

The second move was the fast-unto-death by the LTTE political leader for Jaffna Amirthalingam Dhileepan[5], an Eelam fanatic and a highly capable organiser. The fast was undertaken near the

Is LTTE a Liberation Movement?

Kandaswamy temple at Nallur, Jaffna, where long after his death the occasion was turned into the most significant annual event in the LTTE calender, i.e., the Heroes' Week. The purely political nature of this Gandhian pressure tactic was underlined by the five demands that were declared, including one calling for an immediate end to the Sinhalese colonisation of Tamil-majority areas. The IPKF, however, decided not to attach any importance to Dhileepan's hunger strike, thus falling squarely into the clever trap that the Tigers had laid for it. As Dhileepan's condition worsened (he eventually died and thus became one of the most potent LTTE icons), the LTTE orchestrated popular anti-Indian campaigns which, as was intended, developed soon into violent and provocative demonstrations. By clever manipulations and manoeuvres, helped by the repeated failure of the Indians to read the writing on the wall, the comfortable and, at times, happy relationship that had grown between the IPKF and the civilian population was converted into one of mistrust, suspicion and, finally, outright hatred and hostility.

The sagacity of the LTTE in building the multi-pronged pressure on the IPKF soon began to pay dividends, one of which was the acceptance of the plan for a provisional provincial council for the north and east. [8]

This heady mix of a bloody massacre and a literal Gandhian fast-unto-death that the LTTE presented in the above instance clearly marks it out as a unique terrorist organisation, for seldom do such groups use non-violence as a means of achieving goals. But then, Dhileepan was no Mohandas Karamchand Gandhi either, for he was an active LTTE fighter and had lost parts of his intestines and liver in gunshot injuries caused in a battle with the Sri Lankan army at Vadamaratchchi. His hunger strike was, therefore, purely a means to arouse public sentiment and inform the people about the unacceptability of the IPKF and of the necessity to oppose it actively; in short, the LTTE used it as a weapon to agitate against the Indians in an effective manner and in no way signified a regular recourse to non-violence as part of its political weaponry.

If the above displays, the LTTE's dexterity in adopting different and, at times, mutually exclusive, methods to advance its cause, one feature that appears to distinguish it is its time-tested military prowess.

Apart from the fact that it has worsted Sri Lankan security forces in conventional battles many times over, sometimes inflicting crashing defeats, one salient aspect of its military record is its ability to take on forces which are infinitely superior in numbers, firepower and logistical support. Besides, government forces regularly receive training from major national armies, navies and air forces. Apart from the initial training that certain Tamils received in West Asia and in a much larger fashion, later in India, the Tamil Tigers and other Tamil militants in Sri Lanka have had scarce opportunities to equip themselves in a degree that would be comparable to what government forces possess.[9]

How does then one explain the impressive military prowess, including meticulous planning of attacks and retreats and an ability to dent the fighting morale of security forces, that the LTTE, an otherwise ruthless terrorist organisation which should normally carefully avoid confronting national forces, has exhibited on a number of occasions, especially when it is run by a dictator? A striking example of the Tigers' military acumen and capabilities was available in the crushing defeat they inflicted on the Sri Lankan army in Mullaitivu on 18 July, 1996, killing a massive number of 1, 200 soldiers, destroying completely one of the most fortified army bases and making off with prize weaponry and ammunition. The morale of the government nosedived and it took an unusually long time for it to acknowledge the devastating extent of defeat.

In understanding this unique fighting ability of the Tigers, one has to take into account certain extraneous factors that usually accompany Sri Lankan forces and LTTE battles. Aerial bombings by the air force cause a civilian exodus, apart of course from destruction of civilian properties. At the time of every battle, the LTTE propaganda machine starts working overtime to project the obvious sufferings of innocent civilians, placing both the government and security forces under an immediate obligation to take corrective measures to ensure that international outcry is neutralised.

A classic instance of this successful exercise was the circumstances that led to the Indian intervention in 1987 after security forces launched what the then Sri Lankan president Jayewardene declared would be "a fight to the finish. Either they win or we win." This was

"Operation Liberation", launched on 26 May, 1987, a full-scale assault on the Vadamaratchchi sector of the Jaffna Peninsula in which 8, 000 men of the army, air force and navy participated, preceded by leaflets dropped by the air force asking the civilian population to move into temples and schools for safety. Unluckily for both the sides, there was little safety in those places of worship as temples, churches and school buildings were hit killing scores of civilians sheltering there. Rohan Gunaratna says in *Indian Intervention in Sri Lanka: The Role of India's Intelligence Agencies* that recounting the time, President Jayewardene told him, "I told the generals to raze Jaffna to the ground, to burn the town and then to rebuild it. The Indian parliament did not meet in February, May and June. This was the best time. Otherwise, it would have been a headache also for Rajiv Gandhi (then prime minister of India). But Lalith Athulathmudali (the tough national security minister who was personally involved in the planning of the operation) wanted to hit the soft targets (periphery of the town such as the Vadamaratchchi sector) first."

However, in less than twenty-four hours, Indian intervention began to manifest itself, and the offensive was suddenly halted precisely at the point when government forces were sensing victory (within a week the entire Vadamaratchchi region had come under government control, forcing the LTTE to tacitly admit its defeat). Athulathmudali explained that the government decided to end the operation after New Delhi conveyed through diplomatic and private channels its determination of not allowing the fall of Jaffna and its intention "to arm the LTTE with surface-to-air missiles." The minister also informed the Sri Lankan cabinet on 12 August, 1987, that the Indian high commissioner in Colombo J N Dixit had told him not to touch Jaffna "lest India will intervene."

Just as the military offensive in which the LTTE was nearly defeated was called off, the Tigers fell back on their terrorist proclivity and organised a massacre of thirty-three Sinhalese, including thirty Buddhist monks, after a bus was stopped in Ampara District in the east on 1 June 1987.

In this particular instance, while government forces clearly got the better of the LTTE in a straight battle mainly by dint of superior strength, swiftness and a wider span of attack than anticipated by the rebels, the latter turned the table through the Indian intervention and sought to avenge its setback by staging the massacre of innocent civilians, a purely terrorist attack. Suffice it to say that no national force can match such a freedom of choice that can be availed of by non-state players.

The exploitation of the civilian population as a human shield or the natural human nature for an exodus for safety (a recurrent feature in the Sri Lankan war) which would eventually force government forces either to withhold fire to facilitate an escape bid for the Tigers or to suffer the rather weighty blame of violation of human rights is yet another weapon in the hands of the LTTE which is naturally unavailable to the other side.

The following news report filed by the author for *The Hindustan Times,* New Delhi (5 December, 1994) illustrates the point. "Intensified aerial bombings of Tamil rebels-held Jaffna Peninsula since the battle at Pooneryn by Sri Lankan air force supersonic jets have been wreaking havoc among the civilian population. Reports available with government circles and non-governmental organisations say that while air force jets bombed Jaffna city almost every day during the battle at Pooneryn and Nagaventhurai during 11-14 November, the sorties have been continuing since then. Though the defence ministry claims that only 'well-defined' rebel targets are being struck, the reports say that it is mostly civilians who are getting killed and maimed. Perhaps the most glaring example of the misdirection of air force bombings is what has happened to government agent K Manikawasagar and the katcheri (district headquarters). A supersonic jet hit the katcheri twice, first at 8.25 a.m. and then a few minutes later, on 12 November. Almost the entire upper floor has caved in, most of the furniture destroyed, and thousands of documents displaced and lost. The air force, according to reports available here, bombed a church on 13 November and an orphanage on 14 November. While the children ran out in time, a lady teacher was caught and injured in the attack. One leg was amputated. What apparently surprises the people in Jaffna is Colombo's inability to realise that aerial bombing can only kill more civilians while LTTE cadre mostly escape unhurt."

In another report entitled "Offensive in Jaffna leaves many homeless" (23 October, 1994), the author wrote, "More than 9, 000 families had to flee their homes and take shelter in school buildings, temples and churches and forty-two civilians died and eighty-three were seriously injured during the recent offensive by the Sri Lankan security forces against Tamil rebels in the Jaffna district. According to a Sri Lankan government report, the offensive, code-named Operation Yal Devi which was launched during 28 September-4 October, ostensibly to cripple the LTTE-run ferry service across the prohibited Jaffna lagoon, caused unprecedented misery to the civilian population in the Jaffna Peninsula and district in the war-ravaged north Sri Lanka. The report said that the widespread aerial bombings and shellings during the offensive caused so much panic that the entire population of the Pallai assistant government agent (AGA) division and more than half of that of the Chavakachcheri AGA division were evacuated. It was an exodus from the entire area of Operation Yal Devi, the report commented. Describing the travails of the evacuees, the report said the tragedy was that the displaced families, which had little time to leave their homes, were also subjected to severe attacks by helicopters while fleeing to relative safety. Citing one instance, it said that a young mother and her two infants, trekking to safety, were blown up in a rocket attack by an air force helicopter. There were instances when entire families were wiped out in aerial attacks. While the estimate of the displacement of 9, 000 families is preliminary, the actual number, expected to be much higher, is being ascertained, according to government circles. ...transportation of cooked meals to the various welfare centres opened in school buildings, temples and churches proved to be extremely difficult as the vehicles engaged for the purpose were regularly attacked by Sri Lankan air force planes and helicopters. The report explained that in view of the long hours and days the evacuees at times had spent without a meal, it was not possible to postpone transportation of meals until the curfew was over. The report mentioned that one welfare centre housing 849 families was attacked repeatedly and had to be shifted to nearby school buildings."

The government and the security forces always provided a standard explanation of why each military offensive almost compulsively brought untold miseries upon the civilian population (namely, that the "fascist" Tigers forced the people to act as a human shield), which eventually served to strengthen the Tigers' claim that theirs was a people's movement and that they were the true representatives of the Tamil people. If a campaign against the Tamil Tigers must mean that Tamil civilians would suffer as well in the process, so the LTTE argument ran, then in the eyes of the government the two were clearly identified as the same.

From this followed the logic that it was the Tamil people and not just the LTTE who were determined to fight for a separate homeland. A typical expression of this convoluted logic was the following statement issued by the then London secretariat of the LTTE on 22 October 1994, urging the Cyprus meeting of the Commonwealth Heads of government to recognise the right to self-determination of the Tamil people of Sri Lanka. "We believe that such recognition will pave the way for the resolution of the conflict which has taken an increasingly heavy toll in human lives and suffering during the past ten years and more," the statement said. "The Liberation Tigers have repeatedly made their position clear. If the government of Sri Lanka persists in its determination to subjugate the Tamil people, the Tamils will have no alternative but to continue to fight to restore their own sovereign state."

This chapter began with Prabhakaran's claim that he is not a terrorist, that he is a freedom fighter and that he represents a people's movement. This claim lies at the core of the LTTE's political approach to the task of persuading the world to recognise it as a political and liberation movement and as the sole legitimate representative of the Tamils in Sri Lanka. The problem for the LTTE is that in the beginning of its campaign against the Sri Lankan state, both the government and the international community appeared to have shared, even if only partially, a related impression but, as the group gained notoriety as one of the most ruthless terrorist organisations in the world, few people cared to cling to that perception. On the contrary, both the country and the world at large became increasingly conscious of the systematic campaign of annihilation with which the LTTE went on liquidating other, (at that time) far more representative Tamil organisations in order to secure its monopolistic position as a mouthpiece of the Tamils of the north and east.

Is LTTE a Liberation Movement?

The necessity to retain this monopoly over the right to represent the Tamils remains as valid today as before, and this was why "Col" Karuna's revolt, which clearly sought to undermine this position, rattled the LTTE so much. The impressively effective manner in which the annihilation campaign continued led analysts to feel that the revolt had in the end helped the LTTE to further consolidate its grip over the civilian population in its areas of influence. As an analyst sees in an interesting angle, "At a more tangible plane, the revolt has enabled Prabhakaran to strengthen his grip on the Tamil segment of Sri Lanka's population, and to control its politics more firmly than ever before by converting its political leaders, barring a very few exceptions, into a group of lackeys that has no voice or will of its own." Moreover, the period between Karuna's revolt and the 2 April 2004, general election allowed the Tigers to get as many as 22 Tamil National Alliance candidates, all beholden to uphold the LTTE agenda, elected to the new parliament, thereby considerably strengthening the terrorists' political bargaining power vis-à-vis the southern political parties and by a much wider constitutional platform. Nevertheless, one must deal with the legitimacy of the LTTE to represent the Tamils in order to understand the ethnic conflict in all its manifestations.[10]

Does the LTTE represent the Tamils or not? As one studies the conflict, one is aware of the fact that it is the LTTE and no other group which has succeeded in forcing the government and the majority community to consider the Tamils' grievances with seriousness, if not with the required sense of responsibility. There is a dramatic difference between the attitude of the late President Jeyawardene and that of the current President Kumaratunga, and among the larger Sinhalese community today than a decade or two ago. The late President Premadasa and his party United National Party used to boast that their policies had helped prevent the ethnic issue from becoming a problem in the south, which Kumaratunga and her Sri Lanka Freedom Party failed to preserve allowing the conflict to spill over into the south. This was in essence mindless politicking rather than a sober reflection on the most serious conflict the country had experienced. To Kumaratunga's credit went the fact that she had the guts to go and reach out to the Tamils during her first presidency. It was quite another matter that the LTTE sensed the inherent danger in her move and moved quickly and successfully to turn the tide against her government by systematically sabotaging all efforts at reconciliation and that the terrorist group was helped enormously in this endeavour by the ingrained anti-Tamil sentiments in the south. Kumaratunga today, having survived an assassination attempt, appears to have retreated significantly from the pioneering zeal of her first years in power, thus once again strengthening the bargaining power of the LTTE which has consistently portrayed her as being basically anti-Tamil.

To the question how representative of the Tamils the LTTE is, analyst Saravanamuttu says that the majority of Sri Lanka's ethnic Tamils think that the LTTE is their best bet of getting a good deal at the negotiating table. It is difficult to get at the truth as far as the Tamils living in the north and the east are concerned, but talking to ethnic Tamils living in the south and to Indian origin Tamils, one gets the distinct feeling that opinion on the issue is divided. Quite a few people would say that it is the LTTE which has earned for the community at least a grudging degree of attention from the government and the majority community. Reading the history of the ethnic Tamils' long struggle to gain equality and autonomy, one cannot escape the impression that had the south shown respect to the Federal Party and its commendable commitment to legality and constitutional propriety, the Sri Lankan history would have taken a different course altogether and probably Tamil militancy and terrorism would not have surfaced after all. "Sri Lankans need to look back and ponder if they want to look beyond," says M R Narayan Swamy in *Tigers of Lanka: From Boys to Guerrillas* (p.336). "If the Federal Party had been treated with some respect and its minimum demands accepted, there would have been no TULF (Tamil United Liberation Front). If the government had at least come to minimum terms with the TULF, in 1977 or even later, there would have been no raison d'etre for the LTTE and other groups, no anti-Tamil riots, no Indian interference, no (Indo-Sri Lanka) accord, no breach of accord. If Colombo, even much later, had not shortsightedly plotted to sabotage the EPRLF (Eelam People's Revolutionary Liberation Front)-led NEPG (Northeast Provincial Government), the latter would have been seen as some alternative to Eelam (homeland). The NEPG's collapse indirectly justified the LTTE's propaganda that the Sinhalese political leadership could never be trusted."

Compared to other terrorist groups, the LTTE displays certain characteristics not normally possessed elsewhere. Irrespective of its defiance of the criticism and outright hostility of the international community, it continues to enjoy a position from which it can dictate the timing of the next round of a peace initiative, most of the time also taking the credit for initiating such a peace process, as it does in respect of the latest ceasefire and the various rounds of talks with the government. This implies that its long list of blood-curdling deeds of assassinations, suicide bombings and massacres of the innocent has not really rendered it a pariah in the international polity. Far from it, each time the Tigers seek a pause in the ethnic conflict and proposes and generally declares a unilateral ceasefire, they are appreciated by the people of Sri Lanka and the international community and the government of the day is perforce obliged to reciprocate the peace gesture and resume the thread of peace negotiations left from the earlier aborted initiative.

This periodic return to the peace initiative is, therefore, yet another weapon in the LTTE's arsenal which is put into effective use whenever circumstances advise a lull in battlefield combat, usually to facilitate a vitally needed refurbishing of the fighting machine in terms of both fighters and arms and ammunition. Besides, each ceasefire brings a sorely needed respite for the civilian population in the war zone which, therefore, warmly welcomes such a move. The government of the day also seeks to gain from such a situation by liberalising the restrictions on civil life imposed by the exigencies of war and hopes to earn the goodwill of the beleaguered Tamils, but it does not end up making any lasting gain because the LTTE is vigilant enough to foil any such outcome. The Tigers achieve this objective by campaigning constantly during a ceasefire about the various perfidies allegedly committed by security forces and claiming that despite such provocations, the LTTE remains steadfast in its determination to safeguard the truce. Every period of ceasefire in Sri Lanka is replete with instances of the use of this clever and usually effective tactic. A typical example, set in the current ceasefire, illustrates the point: "We created the conditions for peace talks by unilaterally declaring a ceasefire in December 2001, " LTTE political wing chief S P Tamilchelvan said on 14 August, 2004, at a press briefing in Killinochchi. "Solution to the Tamil problem should be based on the basis of the aspirations of the Tamils because they are the ones who have faced discrimination, oppression and war for many years. It cannot be based on what the Sinhalese people want. It cannot be based on what the Sinhalese government wants. This is why the political pacts (the) Tamils made in the past with Sinhalese leaders came to naught. This is why it would be constructive to discuss the Interim Self Governing Authority (ISGA) proposals endorsed by the Tamil people than to discuss a proposal put forward by the Sinhalese government. The Tamil question has remained unresolved for more than fifty years because the governments in Colombo acted according to the Sinhalese people's political interest. No proposal put forward by the Sinhalese side has met any of the basic demands and the aspirations of the Tamils. In this context, we consider the counter-proposals by the government of Sri Lanka as a pretext to block us from coming to the negotiating table. The ISGA proposals (have) the Tamil people's full support and mandate. Therefore, talks based on the ISGA are the only possible way to address the Tamil question. The ISGA proposals we have submitted were drafted with the widest participation of the Tamil people and the proposals have received an overwhelming mandate of the Tamil people in the north-east. The international community is very well aware about this reality."

Tamilchelvan's statement is a classic instance of a clever mix of truths, half-truths and unvarnished lies. When he speaks of the traditional Sinhalese apathy and hostility towards the Tamils' quest for a legitimate share of say in running the northeast, he is obviously speaking the truth. But he turns Goebblesian when he coolly asserts that the ISGA proposals were drafted with the full participation of the civilian population in the northeast. We have seen how the Tamils live in the iron grip of the LTTE not only in the rebels-held territories but also in the government-controlled areas and that independent-minded Tamils are seldom protected from the Tigers by the government machinery. Besides, the all-too-frequent references to the "Sinhalese" government, instead of the Sri Lankan government, are a rather obvious attempt to establish that the national government is merely a representative of the majority community and, therefore, not of the minority communities. This is apparently a simplistic attempt to distance the government in Colombo from the Tamil community, but this is so patently untrue that it hardly deserves a refutation. Kumaratunga won her landslide victory with a 62 per cent of the valid votes cast in her favour in 1994 mainly on the strength of an overwhelming support from the Tamils. Besides, the Muslims, Malays and Burghers are also minority communities in Sri Lanka and they are traditionally enthusiastic supporters of the government of the day in Colombo.

It is apparent from the above account of the behavioural pattern of the LTTE that it would be inadequate to categorise it as a purely terrorist group and therefore condemnable; this will hold true as long as the Tigers are in a position to take into their hands peace initiatives and to compel the government to respond (this by no means implies that the government is less keen to pursue peace rather than war but the point to remember is that it continues to suffer from limited choices) and as long as the people of the country and the international community would continue to desire that the LTTE participates in meaningful negotiations with the government for a political settlement of the ethnic question. As was being witnessed in the third quarter of 2004, the LTTE was careful to draw a line between provoking the government and the international community by violating the ceasefire provisions while strengthening its military and political positions and reiterating its abiding interest in maintaining the ceasefire and working towards a resumption of the stalled negotiations. Its strategy was geared to the goal of maintaining and strengthening its deliberately cultivated dual personality, terrorist-militarist and political, and it would be loath to let go of this finely crafted duality of identity to tackle the infinitely superior government and the majority community. Credit must be due to the Devil, for the LTTE is a minority group in every sense of the word in the Sri Lankan context and has yet been able to confuse and mystify and, sometimes, even better the adversarial majority.

This comfortable niche founded on the dual identity of a terrorist organisation and a liberation movement was, however, facing a major and, perhaps insurmountable, challenge engendered by the global war on terrorism. Posed principally by the US government, the test that the Liberation Tigers were being called upon to face lies in its ability to convince the international community of the genuineness of its democratic protestations. Time and again, representatives of the Bush administration were insisting that the rebels must establish their democratic credentials before they could rightfully claim to be the political face of the Tamil community in the northeast. Speaking on this issue, US deputy secretary of state Richard L Armitage said, "…the United States government is encouraged by the vision of the LTTE as a genuine political entity. But for that to happen, we believe (that) the LTTE must publicly and unequivocally renounce terrorism and prove that its days of violence are over. The US will never accept the tactics of terror, regardless of any legitimate Tamil aspirations. But if the LTTE can move beyond the terror tactics of the past and make a convincing case through its conduct and its actions that it is committed to a political solution and to peace, the United States will certainly consider removing the LTTE from the list of Foreign Terrorist Organisations as well as any other terrorism-related designations."[11]

It would appear that in the intervening twenty months since Armitage's speech, the US attitude towards the LTTE had hardened significantly. The media roundtable that the US Department of state coordinator for counterterrorism J Cofer Black held in Colombo on 9 September 2004 (discussed in some details elsewhere in this book) provided a wide glance at the trend of US thinking on the nature of the LTTE. When asked by the media if the US planned to use methods other than persuasion to force the LTTE to mend its terrorist ways, Black said quite bluntly, "The object is peace, the object is not war, and we think that we have a good programme in place with the (Sri Lankan) government for these times. Were *the times to change, the United States would have to reconsider the type of support it gives* " (emphasis added), implying that tougher measures against the LTTE and a direct military support to the government could not be ruled out if the Tigers continued to be recalcitrant.

The LTTE was apparently alarmed by Black's message and, as noted elsewhere, responded through the Tamil National Alliance.

Is LTTE a Liberation Movement?

"Most unfortunately," the TNA group leader in parliament R Sampanthan said on 13 September, 2004, "ambassador Black's tirade is only against the LTTE and assumes that the LTTE is the root cause of all evil that prevails in Sri Lanka. The Tamil people do not agree with this assessment and there is a need to ensure that the interests of the Tamil people are not harmed."

What the Americans and the Indians have been emphasising for some time is that the qualification of a perceived popular support does not automatically preclude the LTTE from the label of a terrorist organisation and earn for it the sobriquet of a liberation movement. As has been amply demonstrated in this book and in innumerable publications and fora, International opinion is now rallied against the Tigers' defiance of democratic norms and extensive application of terror tactics to score over their political opponents who also represent segments of Tamil opinion. This image of the LTTE is entrenched irredeemably in the mind of the international community and no amount of camouflage, subterfuge and organised communal support would help dent it.

It is difficult to reconcile the Tigers' conscious pursuit of terrorism at this juncture when they are also intent on pushing hard the image of an evolving political entity, a claim without which they know it would be difficult to engage the Sri Lankan government in a serious dialogue on a political settlement of the ethnic conflict. How does one identify the perpetrators of a series of political assassinations and wanton acts of terrorism killing hundreds of civilians and non-combatants with the proponents of federalism in a unitary state seeking to provide genuine autonomy to fulfil the aspirations of a millions-strong gifted community of individuals? The two do not just gel.

This is why perceptive commentators across the world have been urging the LTTE to reform from within drastically to rightfully claim the identity and status of a fully legitimate political entity. By choosing to enter the political arena with the presentation of the ISGA proposals, the rebel group is no longer in a position to turn its back on this singular requirement. The proposals imply that the Tigers wish to be accepted as a democratic political entity which, in reality, they are not; the interregnum available before negotiations can be resumed, therefore, provides an opportunity to rectify this lacuna in its identity and functioning.

Will the LTTE rise to the occasion? There is absolutely no indication presently available that suggests even remotely such a possibility; on the contrary, the merciless pursuit of the renegade "Col." Karuna and his men and of the EPDP and other ethnic opponents shows with chilling precision that the rebel leader Prabhakaran has not moved one iota from his decades-old persona of a cruel fascist. If this is the correct reading, it would be difficult to expect the international community to support even a heavily watered-down version of the ISGA proposals nor would it be reasonable to expect the Sri Lankan government to enter a serious dialogue with the LTTE.

Yet, this is exactly what the Liberation Tigers appear to expect to happen, and hence their equally determined pursuit of a campaign to mould both the national and international opinion in favour of parleys devoted to the ISGA proposals.

To be realistic, neither Colombo nor the international community appears to suffer from any doubt about the right of the LTTE to claim its pre-eminent position in any dialogue concerning the ethnic issue. Every player, right from Sri Lankan president Kumaratunga to Norwegian facilitators to American officials, acknowledges this uncomfortable fact. Similarly, there is recognition all around that the LTTE will dominate any future interim administrative setup that may be agreed upon in respect of the northeast. All that the national government and the international community desire is that the LTTE accepts in principle the right of the Sinhalese and the Muslims to live and prosper in the northeast; in effect, there is absolutely no escape for the LTTE but to abandon its original intention to establish an exclusive Tamil region in the province. While the fact that the Tamils constitute two-thirds of the population in the merged northeast is well-accepted, there is equal keenness to ensure that the LTTE also accepts the reality of the substantial presence of the other two communities in the eastern province. By the same logic, the rebels are also obliged to accept the presence of representatives of these two communities in the interim regional government, if and when this is established, and their guaranteed peaceful existence in the region to be administered by that body.

As one analyst sees it, the Tamils constitute over two-thirds of the proposed ISGA territory and are entitled to have an absolute majority in the body (which is also conceded in the Wickramasinghe government proposals), but it will help if the Muslims and the Sinhalese are *overrepresented* in proportion to their numbers (as suggested in the government proposals). Further, there should be appropriate geographical distribution. For the system to work, the Tamil members should be acceptable to the LTTE, the Muslim members to the Sri Lanka Muslim Congress (this is conceded by the government but the LTTE nearly refers to appointment by "the Muslim community in the northeast") and there should be United National Front-People's Alliance concurrence on the Sinhalese members (this is not conceded by either the central government or the LTTE). It might be possible to negotiate a consensus on this basis.[12]

Pinning the LTTE down to the status of a terrorist organisation and without taking note of its claim to be a liberation movement giving voice to the aspirations of Sri Lanka's Tamil community does not, however, quite explain why the rebel group continues to be the main adversary of the Sri Lankan state; yet, it is important to understand this seeming illogicality. Research shows that it is very often the grievances of minorities concerning their perceived lack of political and civil rights which trigger violence. There is thus a consequential relationship between the two and this could be the premise on which one may propose to examine the standing of the LTTE in relation to the legitimate state (Feliks Gross, "Political Violence and Terror in 19th and 20th Century Russia and Eastern Europe" in vol.8 of *A Report to the National Commission on the Causes and Prevention of Violence*, James A Kirkham, Sheldon G Levy and William J Crotty (eds), (Washington DC: US government Printing Office 1969) (pp. 421-476).[13]

If one can juxtapose the Sri Lankan situation with those in the United States and in Britain since the late 19th century or in continental European democracies since the end of the Second World War, the failure of the same system of democracy that helped channel the frustrations of the minorities into constitutional politics and, therefore, away from terrorism but has failed in the Sri Lankan case due to various political, social and economic factors and disproportionately influenced by history becomes discernible.

Paul Wilkinson tells us that the overwhelming majority of ethnic grievances in western democracies cited above were able to find effective channels of protest, lobbying, and influence through the medium of constitutional politics or through the channels of both parliamentary pressure and extra-parliamentary protests, demonstrations, marches and rallies. This phenomenon is well illustrated by the struggle for the African-Americans' civil rights in the United States. In retrospect, it is astonishing that the black civil rights movement was so peaceful, especially when one considers the severity of discrimination and oppression of the African-American population in the segregationist areas of the south. This is not to deny that some militant activists opted for a strategy of violence, but they were very few in number and had only the most marginal influence on mainstream politics.

If one agrees with Wilkinson's analysis, one has to concede that the Sri Lankan Tamils proved to be far less forbearing than the African-Americans in pursuing the peaceful method of seeking justice from a discriminating state and that either the Federal Party gave up its pursuit of a non-violent protest movement too soon or the Tamil community proved to be intolerant of non-violence and in favour of violence as a means to extract concessions from the majority community. Wilkinson, however, draws a different conclusion from the success of non-violence in the African-American context. He says one obvious reason for the predominantly peaceful nature of the majority of civil rights movements in democracies has been that the penalties for violence, or any involvement in any activities deemed to be aimed at subverting or overthrowing the government, have been very severe. Thus, prudence rather than idealist views of civic duty may have been the predominant constraint against more violent dissent.

It is pertinent at this point to note that Mahatma Gandhi, who revolutionised the concept of social and political change including transfer of power through non-violence, always emphasised the importance of the prudence, alongside the ideology, of using non-violence as a means to confront the authority because the latter was infinitely more powerful than the protester and non-state violence would lead invariably to ruthless and overpowering state violence.

Is LTTE a Liberation Movement?

His advice to *satyagrahis* (practitioners of non-violent protest movements) was to strictly avoid violence even in the face of police brutality but always with prudence rather than mindless defiance.[14]

But, as Wilkinson notes, a more pertinent factor (in the Sri Lankan context) that helped avoid major conflagrations in western democracies tackling minority grievances was the introduction of enlightened political and socio-economic reforms and ameliorative measures by successive governments. Attention to much needed reforms to adapt to changing popular needs should be a central concern in the daily business of governments, not simply seen as a device for heading off potential civil conflict and violence, but because it is the central duty of democratic governments and political parties to serve the needs of the people. There is overwhelming historical evidence that effective, and preferably, timely, programmes of political and socio-economic reform are the best antidote against the rise of anti-democratic mass movements of the extreme left or the extreme right.

Directly in the Sri Lankan context is what Wilkinson follows with. It is salutary realism for us to recognise, he says, that to date there is no wholly successful example of a peace process leading to the comprehensive and effective transformation of a terrorist organisation into a democratic party. There have been *partial* successes, however. For example, in the 1970's and the early 1980's the political wing of ETA did respond very positively to the Spanish government's initiative of 'social reinsertion', which meant that almost all of them were able to secure their liberty on the clear understanding that they would abandon terrorist violence and participate in purely non-violent democratic politics. This partial achievement is highly encouraging, but we should bear in mind that the hardliners of ETA-military refused this pathway out of terrorism and continued stubbornly in their campaign of terrorism. It was not until 1998, after it caused outrage by kidnapping and murdering a young councillor, that ETA's hardliners were at last willing to declare a ceasefire, but it appears that they used it to regroup and in December, 1999 they renounced their ceasefire and resumed violence.[15]

While Wilkinson's analysis of the behaviour pattern of terrorist organisations, which also claim to be liberation movements at times, should find a sympathetic chord in the minds of Sri Lankans, he nevertheless lists certain tentative conclusions concerning the prerequisites for an effective peace process compatible with democratic principles and values, which hold eminent relevance for Sri Lanka.

These are: 1. There must be a sufficient political will among both parties to a conflict, both to initiate and sustain a peace process; 2. The role of individual leaders in mobilising and guiding their population/community/movement through the peace process is crucial; 3. In many cases, though not invariably, external mediators or brokers for peace may be invaluable to the process, and this may mean a key role for the United Nations, for a regional organisation, or for a major power such as the United States, capable of bringing not only enormous influence but also the substantial economic resources which may be crucial in rehabilitation and recovery following severe conflict; 4. Patience and a spirit of compromise together with the courage to take risks for peace are essential qualities for the leaders and negotiation on both sides is required if they are going to avoid being blown off course by inevitable crises and setbacks during what is likely to be a very protracted and highly complex process; and, 5. A key requirement is for at least a minimal degree of bipartisan consensus in favour of the peace process among the major political parties in the legislature.[16]

Observers of the Sri Lankan situation would easily recognise almost all the prerequisites that Wilkinson lists as either already present or desired or seemingly unattainable. For example, it is clearly the lack of political will on the part of the Sri Lankan state that hampers, rather than facilitates, the peace process though lately, since the current peace process began over two years ago, the government displays a certain degree of political will to attempt to continue with the peace process; as for the LTTE, the question hardly rises because it is a dictatorial organisation with the command emanating from a single source, its leader Prabhakaran. The second prerequisite is almost totally missing in the Sri Lankan scenario. The third prerequisite is not only present but has been instrumental in the maintenance of the ceasefire and in continued efforts to bring the two sides back to negotiations. The fourth prerequisite remains highly desired and present only nominally in Sri Lanka; otherwise, neither the ceasefire agreement nor the few rounds of peace talks would have been possible. After all, as already widely commented upon, the failure to resume talks has not yet meant a collapse of the ceasefire and return to fighting. Clearly, both the state and the rebels have displayed a certain sense of responsibility and forbearance which is commendable. As for the fifth prerequisite, this is the most vitally needed precondition that the Sri Lankan government looks forward to; unless and until, all the UPFA constituents and particularly the JVP parliamentary group, decide to fall in line with Kumaratunga's oft declared desire to re-enter the dialogue process, there would apparently be no progress.

Notes

1. Prabhakaran gave a detailed interview, "How I became a freedom fighter", to a Tamil literary magazine published from Jaffna., *Velicham* (April, 1994), in which he made his case for being considered a freedom fighter. "It is through books that I learnt of the heroic exploits of Alexander and Napoleon, " he said. "It is through my habit of reading that I developed a deep attachment to the Indian freedom struggle and (to) martyrs like Subhash Chandra Bose, Bhagat Singh and Bal Gangadhar Tilak. It was the reading of such books that laid the foundation for my life as a revolutionary. The Indian freedom struggle stirred the depths of my being and roused in me a feeling of indignation against foreign oppression and domination. The racial riots which erupted in Sri Lanka in 1958 and the agonies that the Tamils had to endure as a result were the factors that impelled me to militancy. The 2. 3. 4. 5. 39 6.reports that appeared in the dailies unleashed a hurricane of fury in me. When I read the novels of Tamil Nadu writers like Kausiyan (Paminip Pavai), Sandilyan (Kadat Pura) and Kalki (Ponniyin Selvan), I learned how our forefathers had established and ruled over great, flourishing empires...Why shouldn't we take up arms to fight those who have enslaved us: this was the idea that these novels implanted in my mind."

2. The US government describes the LTTE as a terrorist organisation that has relied on a guerrilla strategy including the

use of terrorist tactics. *Patterns of Global Terrorism, 2003*, US Department of State, June 2004 states: "The Tigers have integrated a battlefield insurgent strategy with a terrorist programme that targets not only key personnel in the countryside but also senior Sri Lankan political and military leaders in Colombo and other urban centres. The Tigers are most notorious for their cadre of suicide bombers, the Black Tigers. Political assassinations and bombings are commonplace. Exact strength is unknown, but the LTTE is estimated to have 8, 000 to 10, 000 armed combatants in Sri Lanka, with a core of trained fighters of approximately 3, 000 to 6, 000. The LTTE also has a significant overseas support structure for fundraising, weapons procurement, and propaganda activities. The Tigers control most of the northern and eastern coastal areas of Sri Lanka but have conducted operations throughout the island. Headquartered in northern Sri Lanka, LTTE leader Velupillai Prabhakaran has established an extensive network of checkpoints and informants to keep track of any outsiders who enter the group's area of control.

The LTTE's overt organisations support Tamil separatism by lobbying foreign governments and the United Nations. The LTTE also uses its international contacts to procure weapons, communications, and any other equipment and supplies it needs. The LTTE exploits large Tamil communities in North America, Europe, and Asia to obtain funds and supplies for its fighters in Sri Lanka." The report names the following as "known front organisations" of the LTTE: World Tamil Association, World Tamil Movement, Federation of Associations of Canadian Tamils, The Ellalan Force, and The Sangillan Force.

3. Nirupama Subramanian, 'Prabhakaran Asks West to Redefine Terrorism," *The Hindu*, New Delhi ed., 28 November, 2001.

4. Alex.P.Schmid, *The definition of Terrorism. A Study in Compliance with CTL/9/91/2207 for the UN Crime Prevention and Criminal Justice Branch* (Leiden: COMT, January 1993), quoted in A.P.Schmid, "Terrorism and the Use of Weapons of Mass Destruction: From Where the Risk?" in *The Future of Terrorism,*

edited by Max Taylor and John Horgan, Frank Cass Publishers, UK, 2001, reprint, pp.128-9. Incidentally, Schmid's article contains a table showing "Selected high fatality >100 Incidents 1973-1998" listing "1987: Car bomb in bus station in Sri Lanka 113", referring to the 21 April, 1987, incident at Colombo's main bus terminal at the business district of Pettah, when a powerful bomb left in an autorickshaw exploded during the evening rush hour killing 113 and injuring nearly 300 people (p.107).
5. EPDP News (English), 25 September, 2004.
6. Quoted in Xavier Raufer, *New World Disorder, New Terrorisms,: New Threats for Europe and the Western World* (*The Future of Terrorism*), p.37.
7. K.M.de Silva, *Reaping the Whirlwind: Ethnic Conflict, Politics in Sri Lanka*, Penguin Books India (P) Ltd., pp.323-4.
8. Apratim Mukarji, *The War in Sri Lanka: Unending Conflict?*, Har-Anand Publications Pvt.Ltd., New Delhi, 2000, pp.95-6.
9. Indian intelligence and security analyst B Raman writes, "The influence of the PLO, its Al Fatah, the PFLP and other terrorist organisations of west Asia on the LTTE's modus operandi could be seen in the following characteristics: its use of suicide terrorism, its networking with the Sri Lankan Tamil diaspora in different countries through a web of non-governmental organisations not overtly connected with the LTTE, but secretly working under its direction and control; and its business interests centred around its shipping fleet used overtly for legitimate commercial purposes, but covertly for narcotics and gun-running and other clandestine purposes. The fleet provides it with an important source of revenue and with the clandestine means for keeping its arsenal replenished. Initially, it built up its network of contacts with the clandestine world of arms and ammunition with the help of its west Asian friends, most of them based in the Lebanon. Subsequently, it benefitted from its contacts in Myanmar, Thailand, Cambodia, Singapore, and Malaysia." *The LTTE: Its Metamorphosis*, Paper no. 448, 29 April, 2002, South Asia Analysis Group, www.saag, org.

10. G.H.Peiris, "A Mutiny Disintegrates," *South Asia Intelligence Review*, April, 2004.
11. *Sri Lanka: Prospects for Peace*, remarks by US Deputy Secretary of State Richard L. Armitage to the Centre for Strategic and International Studies, Washington DC, 14 February 2003.
12. Devanesan Nesiah, *The Proposed Interim Self Governing Authority*, Polity, vol.1, no.5, January-February, 2004.
13. Quoted in Paul Wilkinson, "Politics, Diplomacy and Peace Processes: Pathways out of Terrorism?", in *The Future of Terrorism*, pp.66-82.
14. "This became Gandhi's target, " writes Louis Fischer in *The Life of Mahatma Gandhi*, Jonathan Cape, London, 1951, p.93. "To be strong not with the strength of the brute but with the strength of the spark of God. Satyagraha, Gandhi said, is 'the vindication of truth not by infliction of suffering on the opponent but on one's self.' That requires self-control. The weapons of the satyagrahi are within him....Satyagraha is the exact opposite of the policy of an-eye-for-an-eye-for-an-eye-for-an-eye which ends in making everybody blind. You cannot inject new ideas into a man's head by chopping it off; neither will you infuse a new spirit into his heart by piercing it with a dagger. Acts of violence create bitterness in the survivors, and brutality in the destroyers; satyagraha aims to exult both sides." One of the best portrayals of the non-violent resistance movement technique gifted by Gandhi and practised so successfully decades later by the African-Americans in the United States was provided by the one-time enemy of Gandhi and the then prime minister of South Africa General Smuts. "I must frankly admit, " he said, 'that his activities at that time (leading the Indians' resistance movement against the Asiatic Registration Act which sought to restrict Indians to specific provinces, thus turning them into virtual ghettos) were very trying to me...Gandhi...showed a new technique...His method was deliberately to break the law and to organise his followers into a mass movement...In both provinces (of South Africa) a wild and disconcerting commotion was created, large numbers of Indians had to be imprisoned for lawless behaviour

and Gandhi himself received—what no doubt he desired—a period of rest and quiet in jail. For him everything went according to plan. For me—the defender of law and order—there was the usual trying situation, the odium of carrying out a law which had not strong public support, and finally the discomfiture when the law was repealed." Fischer adds, "Part of Gandhi's effectiveness lay in evoking the best Gandhian impulses of his adversary. The purity of Gandhi's methods made it difficult for Smuts to oppose him. Victory came to Gandhi not when Smuts had no more strength to fight him but when he had no more heart to fight him."(p.135-6)
15. Quoted in Paul Wilkinson, "Politics, Diplomacy and Peace Process: Pathways out of Terrorism" in *The Future of Terrorism*.
16. *Ibid*, p.78-9.

4
Sri Lanka and India

As one steps into the reception hall of the Indian high commission on the Galle Road, Colombo, one is greeted by a quotation of Mahatma Gandhi from 1939 which at the first glance appears to be a rather curious choice, "It is, at least it should be, impossible for India and Ceylon to quarrel."

One is struck by two competing reactions on deciphering the quotation, the appropriateness of the quotation in the Indo-Sri Lankan context and, on a broader canvas, its very inappropriateness in describing any bilateral relations. When one talks about the relations between two countries which is later chosen to be a quotation, one normally does not emphasise negative aspects; in this quotation, attention is firmly on the propensity of the two neighbouring countries to fall out with each other, peppered with a gentle admonition ideally not to indulge in it.

It was somewhat in an extension of this curious relationship, popularly described as a love-hate relationship, that in the summer of 2004, Sri Lanka wondered aloud about two imponderables, the likely duration of the stalemate in the peace process and India's probable attitude towards the latest turn in the endemic ethnic conflict.

"What is India's attitude?" An Indian visiting the country would be asked, and the enquirer could be anybody from the prime minister to the man-in-the-street. Everybody, it would seem, was genuinely interested to find out how India's mind was working: would there be an indefinite continuation of the strict hands-off policy, pursued ever since the 21 May, 1991, assassination of Rajiv Gandhi? Or, would there be a new look at the realities of the day and, perhaps, a reassessment of the Indian policy towards Sri Lanka? After all, India could not continue to shrug Sri Lanka off as it had been wont to do during the last thirteen years or so. Its interests were so intimately interlinked with those of its tiny neighbour.

The stage at which segments of Sri Lankan society, including all the politically significant communities, would begin to rethink about an Indian role in finding a way out of the latest tricky situation was reached in a graduated fashion, as had been the case earlier. One catalyst to push into focus the desirability of India's involvement in favour of all the mutually competing sides was a perceived unsatisfactory manner in which the problem was being dealt with at the Sri Lankan level.

The following comments, made by the ideologue of the Tamil Tigers and the chief peace negotiator of the Wickramasinghe government respectively, provide a clue as to the intrinsic worth of that exercise.

Anton Balasingham: "We are aiming at a political solution, a final solution when the LTTE can enter into a democratic, political framework. That is the objective of the peace process itself. There's no...you shouldn't have any doubt about it."

G L Peiris: " I think the very fact that the LTTE is here taking part in a media briefing, such as this, indicates more convincingly than any words could do, that they are engaged in a transformation into...into a political organisation. They are getting to grips with political realities, political tensions, political complexities and the best example of that is what is happening in this very room today."

This rather fetching display of over-enthusiasm and possible indiscretion by Prof. Peiris, the head of the Sri Lankan government delegation, took place during the media briefing that followed the conclusion of the second session of the peace talks with the LTTE at Nakhorn Pathom, Thailand, on 3 December, 2002, exposing the considerable gap that existed between the two negotiating sides on the understanding of the dynamics of the unravelling negotiation process.

The LTTE was participating in the talks not out of its quest for avenues to enter the political mainstream but to wrest whatever benefits it could get out of the process for furthering its objectives, the chief of which was to earn regional autonomy for its area of influence in the north and east. (Prabhakaran had for the first time said in his annual rebel radio broadcast in 2002, that the LTTE was ready to drop its long-standing demand for independence and that it would settle for provincial autonomy and self-rule in Tamil-dominated areas of the north and east). The Tigers were not at all attending the talks to learn from a better-qualified side about the democratic process but to assess the prospects for the concessions they were after and, if feasible, to obtain them while retaining the opportunity to use arms whenever required. Thus, the unsought-for certificate from the good professor was misplaced and rather indiscreet, if nothing else.

The very fact that the sixth peace effort, as the government describes the current peace process, begun with the LTTE declaring a ceasefire unilaterally, as had happened several times before, signified the terrorist group's determination that it was time for a period of peace in order to recover from certain disabilities (for example, in less than a month after its declaration of ceasefire, the Tamil National Alliance, loudly sympathetic to the Tigers' cause, demanded of the Norwegian peace delegation that "the ban on the LTTE in Sri Lanka should be lifted immediately to facilitate the commencement of peace negotiations") and correct some imbalances that had crept into its war against the state.

It was clearly looking at a fresh peace process as an interregnum and not as a way forward to a permanent peace, as it had been its wont on earlier occasions. It is also important to note that it was the LTTE which took the initiative to suspend the talks on 21 April 2003 while reiterating its commitment to peace which, translated into non-political language, meant little since the choice to resume fighting had not been abandoned. From a reading of the history of the ethnic conflict, nobody could accuse the Tigers of raising false hopes that the time for a true end to the war and beginning of a lasting peace had already arrived. Yet, Prof. Peiris's words tend to give precisely the impression that the government had been unduly impressed by the LTTE's gesture.

While both the government and the LTTE share the responsibility for the stalemate in the negotiations, the virtual irrelevance of the facilitator Norway (the irrelevance was not of choice but the result of certain circumstances) in tackling the tricky situation has been increasingly underlined. The facilitator's outburst in July, 2004, that clearly irritated president Kumaratunga drawing a sharp rebuttal from her, also indicated the growing helplessness of Norway in finding a way out of the impasse ("The Norwegians have no fresh ideas, " said Peace Secretariat chief Jayantha Dhanapala to the author in September, 2004, commenting on the then ongoing Sri Lanka visit by Eric Solheim). It was in this sudden vacuum of ideas and actions that the perennial issue of India's possible role in solving the intractable ethnic problem was revisited.

Thus, in the summer and autumn of 2004, as the LTTE and its breakaway faction fought a vicious battle of attrition all over the country heightening fears of a renewal of hostilities with security forces, there were already murmurs and louder noises being made in Sri Lanka about the propriety of involving India in the island nation's latest woe. As always, advocates for and against such involvement multiplied by the day, reinforcing the unfortunate but persistent impression that Sri Lankans would always get into such debates without getting down to the job of setting their own house in order and solving the ethnic conflict by themselves.

It is important to remember that true to the tradition, efforts to get India involved ran throughout the latest peace process, beginning with the LTTE suggesting on 8 January 2002, that India should be a venue for talks. A few days earlier, the newly elected Sri Lankan prime minister Ranil Wickramasinghe (who, for good reasons, usually claimed to enjoy excellent personal rapport with Indian leaders) said, while explaining the importance of apprising India of the development in his country, that "India is a country that can have an influence on the events in Sri Lanka. It has been involved directly or indirectly in events in Sri Lanka since the time of the Indo-Sri Lanka Accord, and there is a lot that India could do."[1]

This was followed up by the LTTE a few days later when it argued that the two sides (India and the Tigers) must bury the past and move ahead by forging an understanding based on what it intriguingly described as "mutual interest". A Tamil newspaper quoted an unnamed LTTE leader saying, "If the US and Russia can cooperate with each other, so can India and the LTTE."

The chief of the terrorist group's intelligence wing and one of the prime convicts in the Rajiv Gandhi assassination case Pottu Amman was quoted in the same news story saying, " It is not events or incidents but an absence of mutual understanding that is the main reason for the differences between the LTTE and India." In what could only be described as the height of impertinence, he added, "Let us forget the bitterness of the past. Both sides have done good and bad."[2]

Prabhakaran himself joined the chorus when he said in his first ever press conference in twelve years , held in Killinochchi town on 10 April 2002, "India's participation is crucial for the peace process. We do not want to alienate India. Without the support and sympathy of the people and government of India, this problem cannot be solved."

Thus, in a span of a little over three months, both the Sri Lankan prime minister and the LTTE leader spoke in the same vein about the justifiability of their suggestion for Indian participation in the Sri Lankan peace process. India, of course, reacted absolutely predictably. In less than twenty-four hours after the argument of Prabhakaran, who was held responsible for the horrible death of a former Indian premier Rajiv Gandhi, the incumbent Prime Minister Atal Behari Vajpayee dismissed the notion outright. "We are not going to be part of any negotiations or interfere in any talks between the Sri Lanka government and the LTTE, " he said, adding that the ban on the Sri Lankan terrorist group would continue. "In front of us, " he said, "there is only one proposal and that is for providing medical treatment to (Anton) Balasingham in the country."

This Indian position on the issue continued to be maintained since then, with a reaffirmation on 15 October, 2003, when India's foreign minister Yashwant Sinha said, "Third parties who facilitate conflict resolution should avoid mediating or offering guidance." There was a further confirmation of India's continuing policy of strict neutrality on 29 April 2004, when the Sri Lankan foreign minister Lakshman Kadirgamar was visiting New Delhi.

"The foreign minister of Sri Lanka apprised the Indian side of (the) recent developments in Sri Lanka, including on the peace process," said the external affairs ministry of the Indian government. "The government of India expressed the hope for an early resumption of the peace process and for a negotiated settlement acceptable to all sections of Sri Lankan society within the framework of a united Sri Lanka and consistent with democracy, pluralism and respect for individual rights." The statement ended with the punch-line, " India believes that an enduring solution has to emerge purely through internal political processes, " emphasising the irrelevance and ultimate folly of any country other than Sri Lanka to try to solve the problem.

Earlier, in December, 2003, this was what India said with reference to the Interim Self Governing Authority proposals mooted by the LTTE and over which a duel with the Sri Lankan government had ensued, echoing Colombo's stand in the matter, "Any interim arrangement should be an integral part of the final settlement. India would welcome a resolution of the current impasse in the peace process and an early resumption of negotiations."

Following was a representative sample of the myriad pressures that India periodically faced from various segments of Sri Lankan society in uneasy times. The leader of the truncated Sri Lanka Muslim Congress (SLMC) Rauff Hakeem, who visited New Delhi in early August 2004 argued that while his party would very much like India to take an active part in the Sri Lankan peace process, it would rather caution against forcing it to take on such a role.

"Certainly, we would very much wish India to play an active role, but this is a matter for India and India alone (to decide). She has her own domestic compulsions, " he told a New Delhi newspaper in an interview on 3 August, 2004. "India has always shown goodwill towards Sri Lanka. She has had a specific interest in our problem, but unfortunately, because of bitter experiences of the past, she would be quite reluctant (to take an active role) and we understand that. What is comforting is that despite changes in the administration in Delhi, the policy towards the ethnic crisis and its resolution remains almost the same." Hakeem held discussions with both the Indian minister for external affairs K Natwar Singh and the national security adviser J N Dixit. "As an important stakeholder in the peace process, Natwar Singh was keen to know from us more about the current stalemate in the peace process in Sri Lanka and about the various means to overcome the stalemate, " he said. Spelling out the SLMC's approach to India, he said, "Muslims in the northeast are in a difficult situation, particularly because of the India-sponsored merger of the northern and eastern districts (provinces) to form a united northeastern province. The merger had made the Muslims politically weak. But now, we are politically organised and are a vibrant force, which has repeatedly got the mandate of the people."

Why was it then that the SLMC was now suggesting an Indian role in Sri Lanka? Hakeem provided an interesting explanation: India had, in the intervening years, changed its attitude to the Muslims and was now showing a readiness to accommodate their interests. "India is obviously inclined to amend it (its earlier stand) and find a reasonable modus vivendi for resolving issues relating to an autonomous arrangement that we are seeking in the northeast to ensure that we (the Muslims) have self-rule along with shared rule in a federal arrangement, " said Hakeem.[3]

While the SLMC made explicit its reason for seeing India getting involved in the peace process just as did both the Sri Lankan government and the LTTE, each sparring side hoping to strengthen its respective bargaining position through an assumed Indian support, a completely unexpected development took place during the political vacuum created by the stalemate in the peace process.

Public opinion in the southern Sri Lanka, generally representing the hard-line Sinhalese majoritarian approach, began to speak out publicly in support of an Indian role. This was remarkable even in the light of the fact that the concept was not being aired for the first time; both hardline political parties, the Janatha Vimukthi Peramuna (JVP) and the Jathika Hela Urumaya (JHU), notorious in not so distant a past for carrying out virulent anti-India campaigns, and sections of the intelligentsia in the south had been talking about the desirability of an Indian role for quite some time.

In the late summer of 2004, the majority community in Sri Lanka tended to look upon itself as a victim of an unsympathetic and outright hostile attitude seemingly ingrained in the western mind; in its perception, this predominantly partisan mindset had been well-reflected throughout the peace process in the attitude and behavioural pattern of the facilitator Norway and other western-dominated international agencies and organisations.

Various manifestations of this strong wall of resentment against Norway occurred during the period, beginning with foreign minister Lakshman Kadirgamar declaring on 15 November 2002, that Norway was no longer acting impartially. A rather serious development took place in the following December when the JVP wrote to President Kumaratunga protesting against an import of equipment for the clandestine LTTE-run Voice of Tiger radio consigned, strangely enough, to the Norwegian ambassador in Sri Lanka Jon Westborg, prompting the question, "Why was the equipment imported in the name of the ambassador?" This was seen as a blatant display of the Norwegian sympathy and covert support for the LTTE. This public airing of the consignment, however, forced the Wickramasinghe government to come out with the explanation that it had granted a broadcast licence to the LTTE peace secretariat to run an FM radio station and also arranged for the import of the broadcasting equipment. President Kumaratunga, grabbing at what she perceived to be yet another instance of the opposition-run government playing into the hands of the Tigers, wrote to the Norwegian prime minister on the issue criticising the involvement of the ambassador in the deal. She also asked the Sri Lankan prime minister for a report on the issue.

Wickramasinghe, not liking the attitude of the president, wrote back to caution her, "Be cautious to ensure continued Norwegian facilitation." In yet another curious twist, the Norwegian prime minister committed what could only be construed at the least as an act of indiscretion and at the worst as an interference in Sri Lankan affairs by replying to Kumaratunga in the following manner, "The government of Sri Lanka has already answered your concerns."

As a matter of fact, the charge that the Norwegians were interfering in Sri Lankan affairs and thus going far beyond their given task of monitoring the ceasefire recurred throughout this period of Sinhalese chagrin. A typical example was the following; K T Rajasingham wrote on 17 November 2002 in www.asiantribune.com: " In the president's opinion, the Norwegian government appears to be stepping beyond its original role. Already, President Kumaratunga expressed her concern (at) what she sees as the Norwegian government's increasing interference in internal matters when Norway's ambassador Jon Westborg met her last week to brief her on the second session of the peace talks in Thailand. We already had earlier one viceroy—J.N.Dixit, the former Indian high commissioner in Colombo, who negotiated with Prabhakaran face to face initially for an interim provincial council for the north and east, after the signing of the Indo-Sri Lanka Agreement in July, 1987. Recently we were told of the existence of the viceroy no.2 by Mangala Samaraweera, chief opposition whip.

"When objecting to a comment, attributed to Westborg, to the effect that the recent Colombo High Court verdict, sentencing Prabhakaran to a 200-year jail term, could have 'torpedoed' the peace process, Samaraweera said at a press conference that the ambassador should 'stop behaving as if he is the viceroy of Sri Lanka.'"

On 16 May, 2003, the Sinhalese sense of outrage found a strong expression in an open letter that the Alliance of Expatriate Organisations for Peace in Sri Lanka, an umbrella organisation for expatriate Sinhalese, lambasted the Norwegian facilitators alleging that the latter were continuing their attempts to establish de facto institutions like a clandestine navy by the Tigers within Sri Lanka. This was unacceptable, the organisation said, pointing out that the primary responsibility of the SLMM was to monitor compliance with the ceasefire agreement between the Sri Lankan government and the LTTE and to bring any violation to the notice of the two parties.

"We reiterate that (the) Norwegian facilitators and the SLMM are not trusted by a majority of Sri Lankans who cherish democracy," the organisation asserted. "We do not believe (that) you have sufficient empathy with South Asian culture to play a meaningful role in putting to end terrorism in this part of the world. Based on your unsuccessful mediation in the Israeli-Palestinian conflict, we have no confidence at all in your ability to contribute positively to achieving (a) stable, long lasting peace in Sri Lanka. We also condemn your mission's attempts to mislead the public by trying to contradict criticism of biased actions, or at times, inaction by your mission. Your report on the LTTE's attack on the Chinese fishermen is a good example of your bias towards terrorists."

A much sober yet hard-hitting criticism of the SLMM was made later by the minister of public security, law and order and acting defence minister Ratnasiri Wickremanayake who said on 26 August 2004,

"As the government, what we expect from the mediators is to enquire into complaints made by both parties and communicate their opinion to the public rather than limiting themselves to the four corners of their room."

The period also afforded a glimpse of the frustratingly twisted Sri Lankan mindset about India. Certain sections of the print media published tantalising details of the purportedly dark deals that the powerful northern neighbour was forcing down the hapless Sri Lankan throat. The bete noire of the media in particular was the "invasion" of the fuel distribution system by the Indian Oil Corporation whose local arm, the Lanka Indian Oil Company (LIOC), was already a visible presence in the country with petrol stations displaying its logo all over the capital and outside; also drawing uncharitable attention were a software deal on the point of being awarded to a Hyderabad (India)-based company to install a high-technology information system at the National Water Supply and Drainage Board and India's Sethusamudram navigational channel dredging project for the eastern sea coast, which was projected as one to irretrievably harm various Sri Lankan interests.

The Sri Lankan cabinet discussed the Indian project and set up a high-level inter-ministerial committee headed by the foreign ministry to study the implications of the project for Sri Lanka and draw up the plan for an appropriate response to the Indian move.

The cabinet spokesperson Mangala Samaraweera said on 16 September, 2004 that the Sri Lankan government was seriously concerned about the Sethusamudram ship canal project. "Therefore, the cabinet has decided to appoint the committee which will act as a forum to assess the impact and make recommendations on proceeding with this issue with the relevant Indian agencies as soon as possible, " he said.

The committee comprised the environmental and natural resources ministry, ports and aviation ministry, fisheries and aquatic resources ministry, defence ministry and science and technology ministry.

Samaraweera was quoted in media reports saying that while the proposed Indian project envisaged the creation of a canal through excavating and dredging in the Adams Bridge and parts of the Palk Strait and linking it with the Gulf of Mannar, it would involve the digging of a 44.9 nautical mile channel between India and Sri Lanka.

"The project is aimed at reducing the present 400 nautical mile naval route around Sri Lanka to reach the east coast of India due to the non-availability of a continued navigable route, " he said, claiming that the project would have a serious impact on the Sri Lankan ports as it aimed to change the existing international shipping route. "There will be adverse effects on international traffic now using the Colombo port and also on the envisaged ports in Galle and Hambantota, " he said.

The negative environmental impact in the process of extensive dredging including sea erosion and adverse effects on marine environment and the livelihood of fishermen were among the other "serious" concerns that had been identified.

To go by Samaraweera, the Indian project would even have a certain amount of pressure on Sri Lanka's security in the northeastern territorial waters. *The Hindu* (New Delhi ed. 20 September, 2004) lent support to the Sri Lankan opposition to the Indian move, saying that "Another important task is for the government of India to brief the government of Sri Lanka in a friendly way on the Sethusamudram Ship Canal project to rule out any kind of bilateral problem. New Delhi must also keep in perspective the 1982 United Nations Convention on the Law of the Sea, which both Sri Lanka and India ratified and acceded to in the mid-1990's."

The case for Sri Lanka's unhappiness and concern rested mainly on the argument that it had been taken by surprise at the sudden Indian move to go ahead with the project. Accordingly, the media played up the latest Indian act of malevolence. It, however, soon transpired that the very impression that New Delhi had been going ahead with a project of multinational dimensions without bothering to keep the would-be affected parties informed was faulty.

P K Balachanddran reported in *Hindustan Times.com* (14 October, 2004) that "Contrary to the impression in certain quarters in Sri Lanka, India did not keep Sri Lanka in the dark over its plan to cut a shipping canal in the sea between the two countries, a well-placed official source in New Delhi told Hindustan Times."

Reacting to official and media criticism in the island that India had sprung a surprise on its neighbour by taking a decision to launch the Sethusamudram project, the source said that Sri Lanka was briefed at a very senior level immediately after the Indian cabinet took the decision to go ahead with the project, he wrote.

Even though it was well within India's sovereign rights to cut a canal in its own territorial waters, the Sri Lankan foreign office was briefed in view of the friendly and good neighbourly relations between the two countries, Balachanddran quoted the source saying.

On the complaint, widely aired in the Sri Lankan media, that Sri Lanka was not consulted before the Indian cabinet took the decision, the source said that the question of consulting Sri Lanka simply did not arise because the canal was to be well within Indian waters. Moreover, the aim of the project was to facilitate shipping between the western and eastern coasts of India and this was to be done with no hindrance to any activity on the Sri Lankan side, the official was quoted saying.

The image that a third country citizen would derive of India in the Sri Lankan context from unnecessarily alarmist media reports was one of a wily, unscrupulous grab-all combined with the portrait of a powerful giant regional power unmindful of the woes of its infinitesimally tiny and helpless neighbour, exploited throughout history.

By no means, a flattering picture; in other words, the ugly Indian. It was perhaps on the strength of various facts and circumstances that Mahatma Gandhi made his wry comment, which was later judged by the Indian diplomatic establishment as encapsulating India-Sri Lanka relations and immortalised in the plaque in the premises of the Indian high commission in Colombo.

A characteristic sample of the highly critical campaign that these sections of the print media carried on in the summer of 2004 was the following, "Ceylon Petroleum Corporation (CPC) has sought the attorney general's advice in restraining the Lanka Indian Oil Company (LIOC) from taking over franchise dealer outlets around the island. The CPC claims (that) the LIOC is adopting unethical practices in luring franchise dealers into (its) network."

Speaking to *The Sunday Leader,* power and energy minister Susil Premajayanth said (that) at the time of privatisation the Indian companies were given 102 filling stations but now they had bought 140. "This is because they go after the franchise dealers. In another couple of months, they might increase the number even to 200. They earn money from here and also take over more filling stations. We want to put an end to this and we have referred this matter to the attorney general.'" (The issue of 12 September, 2004) The news report apparently showed the Indian company as a scheming Shylock extracting the last ounce of profit from whatever it was allowed to touch.

The truth, as in most such cases, was otherwise; the LIOC had won the contract through a perfectly legal tender system and had since expanded its business strictly in conformity with the provisions of the agreement.

While the newspaper report made the Indian company look like a fly-by-night operator, it was a company owned and operated by the Indian government; it was taking over franchise dealerships because the existing dealers found its offer lucrative and it was fully within the provisions of the agreement. It was buying land to set up filling stations because the agreement would allow it to open filling stations after the cut-off date of 31 December, 2006.

In short, the company was acting as a legitimate and professionally run business entity strictly within the law of the country but clearly the debilitating factor was its Indian origin. The report even carried allegations purportedly made by CPC officials to the effect that the Indian company was winning the game (of doing business in Sri Lanka) by using underhand tactics.

The travails that the LIOC was going through at the time, however, reflected much more than the proverbial Sri Lankan suspicions about Indian motives and objectives. Rightly or wrongly, the author found during his visit to Sri Lanka in September, 2004, that Indian business interests and deals were identified in the popular perception with a wanton aggressiveness and a desire to grab all. He also heard about a particular case where even unskilled labour was imported to construct a major project in Colombo, clearly a highly

Sri Lanka and India

visible act which would be unlikely to be accepted in good grace by the local population. In diplomatic circles in Colombo, he came across tales which would appear to be uncomplimentary to the acumen of Indian diplomats. As a matter of fact, media comments appeared at times to be as uncharitable and unfriendly towards a particular high commissioner as was experienced only during the height of anti-Indian feelings in 1987 and seldom since then.

As the stalemate over the peace process was prolonged, the desire for an active participation of India in smoothing out the uneasy situation became increasingly manifest. At least one former diplomat thought out a particularly bold way of reining in India, by suggesting that the two countries should adapt the India-USSR Peace, Friendship and Cooperation Treaty of 1971.

Speaking to an Indian newspaper, the former ambassador and Peace Secretariat official Kalyananda Godage said that Sri Lanka and India should revisit the 1990 Sri Lankan and Indian proposals for a comprehensive treaty of peace, friendship and cooperation, aimed at accomodating a whole range of issues of concern to the two countries and build on them to take into account the current needs and realities on both the sides of the Palk Strait.

The new treaty should include a clause to the effect that if there was a perceived threat to the unity, sovereignty and territorial integrity of either country, the other contracting party would render all possible assistance to counter it. The basis of this exercise should be the Indian "counter-draft" handed over to the Sri Lankan government in Colombo on 12 January, 1990 (the Indian document was in response to a Sri Lankan draft, prepared by the Premadasa government which was campaigning against Indian interference at the time, aiming at preventing Indian interference in Sri Lanka's internal affairs including the ethnic conflict. In yet another irony of history, the very Indian response to that draft was being advertised in 2004 as justifying Indian interference in helping sort out the ethnic conflict).

Godage emphasised the appropriateness of Article 2 of the Indian draft for the prevailing circumstances. The provisions under this article were related to non-use of ports for military purposes to the prejudice of the national interest of either contracting party; deportation of nationals who activated or advocated separatism or secessionism with respect to the other country; maintenance of peace and tranquility in the Palk Strait; non-use of the countries' respective territories for hostile activities against either of them; and the stoppage of the illegal movement of people and arms and contraband across the Palk Strait by strengthening all arrangements and by mutual cooperation.

In his view, Article 5 of the "counter draft" assumed immediate relevance as it provided for economic and technical and scientific cooperation. The new treaty, he believed, should stress this aspect of cooperation as well in conjunction with the recent improvement in Indo-Sri Lankan trade and economic ties in the aftermath of the Free Trade Agreement.[4]

Godage returned to his theme, extending it further, by writing to *The Island* (15 September, 2004) in the following manner, "Statements or pledges such as supporting Sri Lanka strongly, ring hollow unless something tangible is done. At the risk of seeming to be presumptuous may I suggest that India as the regional power take the initiative along with the US, Norway and the European Union and summon a peace conference to which the main political parties in Sri Lanka and the LTTE should be requested to attend, recall the agreement at Oslo—a federal structure within a united Sri Lanka which the LTTE signed up for. The conference could examine the LTTE's Interim Self Governing Authority proposals; the previous government's counter proposals and the proposals of the present government. And the proposals of the Muslim community in the east and, not the least, a referendum must be held under international supervision to determine the status of the eastern province; this is a democratic right of the people of the eastern province and must be respected by the international community. A real peace would then emerge if India and the international community have the political will to ensure an end to this conflict which has taken 60, 000 lives and could take another 60 or more thousand lives if left to the adversaries to resolve."

While the majority of Sri Lankans, belonging to the majority Sinhalese and the minority Tamil and Muslim communities, the author spoke to felt that India should change its mind and play a direct role in finding a universally acceptable solution to the ethnic problem, an exercise in which the international community should play a supportive and facilitatory role, only a few of them could articulate specific ideas for doing so. One section of Sinhalese opinion would go to the extent of suggesting that India was morally obliged to put its neck out in order to redeem its honour lost during the 1980's while Tamil guerrillas were nurtured on Indian soil. They would of course prefer to ignore Premadasa's role in arming the LTTE on Sri Lankan soil and the loss of over 1, 100 Indian servicemen while fighting a purely civil war. Commenting on such thought processes, one perceptive Sri Lankan observer commented, "They want India to fight Sri Lanka's dirty war. But they should acknowledge that India had done so once and paid a very heavy price indeed. Why should India stick out its neck again for a job which may turn out to be as thankless as before?"

Indian naval chief of staff admiral Arun Prakash visited Sri Lanka precisely at a time, September 2004, when the cry for India was threatening to develop into a wail. His words and actions were, therefore, closely scrutinised in an intensive search for the way India's mind was working.

The Interim Self Governing Authority (ISGA) proposals of the LTTE had generated considerable anxiety in the Sinhalese mind, suspicious as it was by habit of any idea emanating from the Tamil Tigers, and the Indian admiral's visit was, therefore, an opportunity to try to get a glimpse of India's thinking about the primacy of the need to preserve Sri Lankan sovereignty over the long northern and eastern sea coasts which, in case of a total acceptance of the LTTE proposals, would be under the Tigers' control.

It was significant that the newly appointed Sri Lankan navy chief and chief of defence staff vice-admiral Daya Sandagiri described the Indian navy chief's visit as "a source of inspiration." During the visit, Sandagiri said, the Indian navy chief had also agreed to provide military support, including training, to the Sri Lankan navy. Within a month of the admiral's visit, the Indian and Sri Lankan governments finalised the draft of the proposed Indo-Sri Lanka defence agreement. The latter said that some of the fields that would be included in the agreement were military training, exchange of military intelligence and information and maritime surveillance to prevent illegal activities affecting both the countries. It also informed that the draft pact had been ready and kept on hold for more than a year. The Sri Lankan defence ministry said that the pact would also facilitate joint military exercises.

The Indian admiral's assessment of his five-day visit, as narrated by him to Indian correspondents based in Colombo, could only have served to reassure the Sri Lankan government that it had succeeded in convincing the important neighbour about the correctness of its own estimate.

Admiral Prakash said that India was "solidly behind" Sri Lanka's integrity and sovereignty and that it was India's stated policy that "it would like to underwrite the integrity" of Sri Lanka. Explaining the reason for his visit, he said, "I felt (that) the situation warranted us to come (on) a first hand assessment" of the Sri Lankan situation.[5]

On the all-important presumed threat to the Trincomalee harbour by the Liberation Tigers, the Indian admiral gave a rather diplomatic answer. Pointing out that the Indian interest in the harbour was basically about the Indian Oil's acquisition of the oil tank farm, he said that the strategic significance of the Trincomalee port and harbour was "more important to the Sri Lankan navy."

Adding he had been told that "the LTTE has also focussed on this as a part of their overall plan", he said, "there is some concern that it should not fall into the wrong hands. It seems to me that at the moment, the LTTE is closely bearing down on Trincomalee." He could not have been more explicit in agreeing with Colombo that the LTTE's activities in the Trincomalee area required a close watch.

He was equally forthcoming on the question of the Sea Tigers. Asked if the Tigers naval force could be deemed to be a third navy in the region, he said, "The LTTE is a proscribed, terrorist organisation. There is no question of a naval wing or anything like that. We don't recognise entities of that nature." How effective was the Sea Tigers? "Like any fanatical and suicidal organisation," he said, "they have the potential to cause a certain amount of damage."

The Indian navy chief was even charitable towards the Sri Lankan navy on one of the few perennial fields of conflict between the two countries. Saying that the intrusion of Indian fishermen into Sri Lankan waters was "a very vexed issue", he remarked he was "fairly certain" that the island's navy "does not inflict violence on our fishermen." Quite rightly, he added that the situation "is not muddled by the presence of the LTTE. At this moment, we are not sure who is creating the mischief." Spelling out India's desire to find a workable way out of the otherwise intractable problem, Prakash said that one of the key areas of his visit "has been to come to a very clear understanding with the Sri Lankan navy as to the rules on the ground." Pointing out that the question of Tamil Nadu fishermen being arrested in Sri Lankan waters was a very emotive issue in the Indian state, he said, "If we sit down and talk to each other, get some ground rules going, we should be able to resolve it."

He was equally optimistic about resolving the Sri Lankan concern over the Sethusamudram ship canal project; noting that the project would facilitate India's coastal shipping considerably, he said, "I think (that) there is enough traffic for all of us. We can come to an understanding." Besides, the Indian project would only ease the movement of smaller ships and larger ships would continue to go around Sri Lanka. Incidentally, the Sri Lankan concern over the project was not at all raised during his visit, he said.

However, what drew immediate attention was Sandagiri's declaration that the Sri Lankan navy was the country's only navy that could use the territorial waters and no other force could claim that it shared this authority.

His other comment which caught attention was that the Trincomalee harbour continued to be under heavy threat from the surrounding LTTE camps. "We cannot say that the Trincomalee harbour is not under threat, " he told the media on 15 September, 2004. "We have to remember that it came under attack in the 1990's." The forces, however, were ready to face any eventuality. Pointing out that the eastern harbour was a strategic point in the overall defence of the country, he remarked, "We are well prepared to meet any enemy attack." Opinion in Sri Lanka differed on the extent of actual threat to Trincomalee and the author heard dissenters asserting that the navy chief was being unduly alarmist.

Still, vexing questions perturbed the Sinhalese: fairly representative of the collective Sinhalese psyche trying to unravel the LTTE's perceived game-plan was the following critique of the ISGA proposals by the Sri Lanka Freedom Party, the main constituent of the ruling UPFA government.

Clause 18 of the ISGA proposals sub-titled "Marine and off-shore resources" appeared to have truly raised the hackles of the majority community, which read, "The ISGA shall have control over the marine and off-shore resources of adjacent seas and power to regulate access thereto."

The SLFP commented, "This is a very significant provision highly dangerous to the sovereignty of the state. If control over the marine and off-shore resources of the adjacent seas passes to the ISGA, the territorial integrity and sovereignty of the state of Sri Lanka will be very considerably compromised. There will be a grave threat to international shipping lanes that pass the east coast of Sri Lanka, and needless to say, to the security interests of India. The power to 'regulate access' means that the Sri Lankan navy will no longer be able to regulate access to the adjacent seas and will therefore not be able to perform its duty to protect the territorial integrity of the state. It must be remembered that the coastline of the seas adjacent to the north east go all the way down to Hambantota in the east and Mannar or below in the west. The northeast coastline comprises almost 2/3rds of the coastline of Sri Lanka."

This particular LTTE proposal managed to disturb the Sinhalese mind to such an extent that the newly appointed navy chief was obliged to emphasise that there was only one navy in the country (implying that despite its clandestine efforts, the LTTE would not succeed in getting its Sea Tigers the recognition of a national navy and that in Sri Lanka the navy meant only the Sri Lankan navy and no other force).

It was this very proposal that in the Sinhalese mind appeared to justify beyond a shadow of doubt the logic of the demand for India's immediate involvement in Sri Lankan affairs ensuring that the ISGA proposals could never become a reality in their entirety. For, even if the government of the day succumbed to the "wiles" of the Tigers, as the Wickramasinghe government was apparently getting in to a position to do, India should take stock of the situation and put its foot down firmly to say no. In other words, the ISGA proposals in general and this provision in particular should act as an adequate warning to the Indian government which should initiate appropriate measures to safeguard Indian security and other interests.

Interestingly, commenting on the same provision of the ISGA proposals, a leading Sri Lankan analyst Dr Devanesan Nesiah, director of the well-regarded Marga Institute, showed far less alarm. Acknowledging that the proposal was meant to establish the ISGA's control over marine and off-shore resources, he remarked, "This should be negotiated with the central government with a view to reaching a compromise that would take account of both equity and environmental considerations."[6]

The majority view in Colombo in the months following the presentation of the Tigers' blueprint for an interim administration in the northeast, irrespective of ethnic affiliations, appeared to be overwhelmingly against any acceptance of the ISGA proposals in original form and against certain provisions (such as Clause 18) even with modifications. For example, Clause 3 "Elections" was opposed by the SLFP because while dealing with elections, "it is also an extremely important indication of the LTTE's ultimate objective. It says that if after five years of the agreement coming into force no final settlement has been reached and implemented, then an independent election commission appointed by the ISGA shall conduct a free and fair election. This is the clause that conceals the power or right to secede. The LTTE can say after five years—'no agreement has been reached, we will hold an election', and then declare a separate state having explained to the world why, as the preamble indicates, they were driven to take that ultimate step. The fault for not reaching a final settlement, acceptable to the LTTE, will be attributable solely to the government of Sri Lanka."

The SLFP document is significant in comprehending the Sinhalese mindset about the LTTE as it is fairly representative of the genre. The ISGA proposals in the preamble say that the history of relations between the Tamil people and the Sinhalese people has been a process of broken promises and unilateral abrogation by successive governments of Sri Lanka of pacts and agreements entered into between the government of Sri Lanka and the elected representatives of the Tamil people.

While this assertion is clearly borne out by the history of the country since independence in 1948, the SLFP prefers to look at it in a predictable light altogether, "This is an important part of the case for ultimate separation." Similarly the LTTE position that successive governments have perpetrated persecution, discrimination, state violence, and state orchestrated violence against the Tamil people gets the following response, "The implication is that LTTE terrorism is justified as being in self-defence."

That such thinking, apparently devoid of any intellectual responsibility with which the LTTE allegation should have been dealt with since it constituted the core of the Tamil community's litany of grievances against the Sinhalese, could still survive on a large scale in a country after more than two decades of desperate fighting must otherwise rank as a wonderment.

It is important at this juncture to note that sane Sinhalese voices were also being heard at the same time as there were sections in the majority community who were questioning openly the correctness of the traditional approach to the Tamil question. "The Sinhalese are not prepared to accept that the minorities are to be treated with equality, " said Uyangoda by way of explaining the continuing resistance of the community to accept the fact that the twenty-one years of armed conflict, 65, 000 deaths and destruction and non-development of vast stretches of the country had wrought some fundamental changes in the sociological, economic and political environments of the country.

As an example of the traditionally skewed view that the majority community took of the Tamils, he referred to what he called the conditionality approach to the LTTE. "The conditionality approach seeks reforms only in the LTTE, " he pointed out. "It has not yet seen the need for changes in the Sinhalese polity or the state as a whole. It also assumes that the changes in the north should occur and be demonstrated rapidly, in accordance with a timetable as set out by the external actors."

Interestingly, the conditionality approach was echoed by Dhanapala, the seniormost bureaucrat in charge of the peace process on behalf of the government, "There has to be a change of heart in the LTTE. Countries like India are in a good position to exert pressure on the LTTE in this regard, without necessarily having to recognise the organization, " he argued bringing India as well into a wholly domestic situation.[7]

The voice of sanity, though infinitesimal in the context of the majority community, was nevertheless persistent, steadily questioning why the Sinhalese must remain confined to their traditional mindset which had clearly failed to equip them for a better handling of the ethnic issue. A parallel issue was the question of reacting to the concept of federalism in a country which had known the concept of centrism as integral to the wider concept of Sri Lanka as a Sinhalese, Buddhist country.

"There is an increasing curiosity in the Sinhalese community about the concept of federalism, " said Loganathan Ketheeswaran, a former functionary of the Eelam People's Revolutionary Liberation Front and presently an analyst with the Centre for Policy Alternative, Colombo. "The concept, following the Oslo Declaration (2-5 December, 2002, when the Sri Lankan government and the LTTE agreed to explore federal models with a view to find a solution to the ethnic strife within a united Sri Lanka with the LTTE retaining the right to self-determination and secession as a last resort), has come into the public domain. Our centre conducted a poll among the people in the south and, not surprisingly, the majority of the respondents said that they did not know about federalism."

"The question as to why the federal concept has not been propagated in the intervening years can be answered in several ways. From the perspective of the LTTE and the Tamil people, various betrayals perpetrated by the Sinhalese acted against popularising the concept. But, the duplicity displayed by the LTTE has not also helped selling the idea of federalism. The ISGA proposals have further served to crystallise the resistance to the concept, since these almost make out a case of a parallel state. The question, therefore, that confronts you is: how do you integrate the concept with the ingrained Sinhalese perceptions? Meanwhile, the reluctance of the LTTE to address the core issues is complicating matters."[8]

Chairman of the Colombo-based Civil Society Forum Dr Kumar Rupasinghe, who led a delegation from the south to the northern headquarters of the LTTE in August, 2004 and who was among the few notable Sinhalese social activists propagating the concept, was, however, optimistic about the prospects of its eventual acceptance by the majority community. "The federal concept is suitable for our country," he said. Hence, the government should commence peace talks on the basis of the ISGA.

He argued that as it was, the government and the LTTE had progressed considerably towards a broad consensus on many related issues; a recent examination of the ISGA proposals and those of the government presented to the country in 1995, 1997 and August 2000 revealed that agreement had been achieved with the LTTE in as much as 70 per cent of the cases; there were grey areas in about 10 per cent of the issues and that serious differences existed only in about 20 per cent of them.

"So, negotiations are all about resolving these 20 per cent of what are seemingly intractable issues," he said. Quoting the LTTE political wing chief Thamilchelvan, Rupasinghe said the LTTE believed that the Sinhalese people had failed to understand correctly the federal concept. This was mainly because political leaders in the south were not consistent with their political stand. The southern political leaders had been in the habit of saying one thing in the morning and a completely different thing in the evening. Thanks to newspaper reports, the identity of the victim of Thamilchelvan's satire, the president, was not lost on the Sinhalese and the quotation was cited with abandon in Colombo and elsewhere in the country for days together.

But Thamilchelvan's satire should also make one pause and take stock of the disquieting situation in the country over one of the central issues around which the ethnic conflict revolved. An astonishing degree of a lack of trust between the leaderships of the two communities underlined the difficulties that any attempt at reconciliation would encounter.

Tamil National Alliance MP Joseph Pararajahsingham was hardly indulging in a falsehood when he told the author, "The Tamils are suspicious of Kumaratunga's duplicity, more so after the manner in which she sabotaged the peace process by taking over three portfolios including defence from the Wickramasinghe government and then dissolving parliament. They are no longer in a position to believe her. There is now complete mistrust between the two sides."

If this indeed were true, how did one expect the government and the LTTE to put their heads together in order to get going with negotiations? Uyangoda brought out this serious shortcoming in the context of the situation prevailing before the 2004 general election, "...the general sentiment among the Tamil people appears to be one of disappointment over the inability demonstrated so far by the Sinhalese leadership to offer a serious and constructive response to the LTTE proposals. As I have noticed in a recent visit to the north, they even feel slighted. In political conversations with (the) Tamil people, one can see a sense of deep disappointment and even the possibility of being let down once again by the Sinhalese political leadership."

"They feel that the memorandum of understanding has not been adequately implemented and that demilitarisation of the civilian life in Jaffna has been conveniently forgotten by the government. This mood of disappointment was of course heightened by the political uncertainty that suddenly erupted in Colombo just a few days after the LTTE unveiled its proposals."

"The government does not seem to communicate with the Tamil people at all. They don't get positive political messages from the south. They get only negative signals." Significantly, what Uyangoda commented about the political setup in the south at the time, the Kumaratunga presidency and the Wickramasinghe premiership ("The president and the prime minister as well as the UNF government's chief negotiator need to realise that any further delay in exploring constructive engagement with the LTTE around the ISGA proposals would undermine the confidence of the Tamil people on the peace process as well as the capacity of the Sinhalese political leadership to do serious politics with the north") would hold true about the situation later in the year with both the presidency and the premiership with the United People's Freedom Alliance (UPFA).

Despite the coherence achieved in the governance of the country with the irritant of the UNF prime ministership and cohabitation removed, the homogeneous Kumaratunga government failed to show any progress towards formulating a cogent political response to the issue of resumption of negotiations. True, the government time and again reiterated its determination to resume talks on the basis of the

ISGA proposals, but once more a key ingredient in the task of facilitating a dialogue with the LTTE, the necessity to educate about and win over the Sinhalese community to the concept of federalism (which would be an inherent and essential part of any political arrangement that could be eventually worked out in a meaningful effort to eradicate the ethnic conflict) was missing. Whatever efforts were being made towards that direction in the south in the second half of 2004 were in the realm of individual and non-governmental organisational initiatives and certainly not by the government.

The following instances of such enterprise would also serve to bring out the virtual absence of a meeting ground between those who were advocating federalism and those stiffly opposing the very notion of it. A newspaper report in August, 2004, said international experts had held that the key to the crisis in Sri Lanka lay in a solution based on a federal structure.[9]

Addressing a seminar organised by the Centre for Policy Alternatives in Wadduwa visualising several possible scenarios for the national problem and the future of Sri Lanka, Bob Rae, chairman of the Forum of Federation (a Canada-based international network on federalism) and a former prime minister of Ontario, who had just returned after visiting the war-ravaged north and holding a meeting with Thamilchelvan, said that the federal solution presented itself as an unavoidable choice for Sri Lanka to make.

Both Prof. David Cameron, the vice dean at the University of Toronto, who had accompanied Rae, and the latter stressed the need to establish a separate administrative mechanism for the northeast until a final solution to the ethnic conflict was worked out; they also emphasised the need to grant urgent humanitarian assistance to the civilian population in the war zone.

The report said the experts were of the view that the reality that had not struck the majority in the south was that within Sri Lanka, there existed two states. One was the government of Sri Lanka, a democratically elected body recognised internationally. And the other was the de facto LTTE state controlled by the Tamil Tigers. The de facto state was dictatorial with no democratic mechanism and lacking respect for human rights. But the de facto state had its own judicial, economic and educational systems; a de facto army and police, etc. The government, by signing the memorandum of understanding and the ceasefire agreement with the rebels, had accepted the existence of the de facto state.

One possible scenario, the experts felt, was that Sri Lanka would slide back to war and the government forces would ultimately win it but defeating the LTTE militarily would not end the ethnic crisis because there were genuine aspirations of the Tamil people which needed to be addressed. To accomplish this task, the government would have to start negotiations with Tamil representatives and ensure that their grievances were addressed. In the other scenario, if the LTTE won the war, they would have to talk to the government again to make arrangements for a power-sharing mechanism since a self-declared LTTE state would not gain international recognition.

One of the participants at the seminar, peace activist and academic Rohan Edirisinha said that while the ISGA proposals were clear on the issue of self-rule, they were apparently silent on the issue of shared rule, an equally important concept in a federal structure. Power should go down to regional levels from the central government and it was also important to share power within a region.

Similarly, in making possible a federal system of governance, it was necessary that the rights and aspirations of regional minorities as in the northeast, the Muslims and the Sinhalese, would also have to be taken into consideration.

The other instance was yet another seminar which dealt specifically with the question of secession in a federal constitution. Here, a leading Sinhalese constitutional lawyer H L de Silva preferred to describe a federal solution to the ethnic conflict as a snake that a drowning man would clutch to save himself. "One wonders whether for Sri Lanka, federalism is that beguiling serpent which by its fatal sting will bring about the death of the republic." The eminent lawyer was giving expression to the quintessential apprehension in the Sinhalese mind, no doubt born more of ignorance than anything else (though, certainly not in his case) and reared in the comfort of a unitary system of government always overwhelmingly dominated by his own community, about federalism.[10]

The report quoted de Silva saying, "It would appear from reports in the media that at the peace talks held in Oslo, the government of Sri Lanka has agreed to the adoption of a federal system of government as a solution to the problem, though even the broad outlines of this have not been disclosed. This has been done without prior consultation with other political parties and without an adequate consideration of all the dangers that a federal government entails in the context of a highly volatile atmosphere of deep-seated ethnic conflict. There is a strong body of opinion that is opposed to the adoption of a federal framework as being unsuitable in the context of Sri Lanka and entertain credible fears that it would lead to the exacerbation of the problem and an inevitable secession."

It is for more academic reasons than otherwise that we record here a reaction to de Silva's opposition to federalism in the Sri Lankan context. The report quoted an eminent Tamil scholar Dr K Vigneswaran, adviser to the EPDP, saying that he was depressed by the Sinhalese lawyer's views. "The 1972 constitution simply forgot the Tamils and it led to the 'Vaddukoddai Resolution' (which declared that the establishment of a separate sovereign state in the northeast was the only viable course left open to the Tamils to realise their political and fundamental rights)."

Vigneswaran also refuted Dayan Jayatilleka of the University of Colombo who had contented that secessionism had always been an inherent part of the Federal Party's political project, by pointing out that the founder leader of the Federal party S J V Chelvanayagam had campaigned against secessionism when C.Suntheralingam urged the Tamils to vote for a separate Tamil state in the by-election to the Muttur electorate in 1961. He said that Sri Lanka would not have had to face the present crisis if the Sinhalese polity had cooperated in finding an acceptable solution to the Tamil question in the 1950's or at least in the 1960's. "The LTTE should not be an excuse to sweep the problems of the Tamils under the carpet, " he said.

Bob Rae, also speaking at this second seminar, said, "The current conflict in Sri Lanka, it would appear to this observer, really turns on two questions. The first is the extent to which Sri Lanka itself conforms positively to the criteria set out (in the Canadian supreme court's ruling on Quebec's right to secession consequent to the 1995 referendum to the effect that a state whose government represents the whole of the people or peoples within its territory, on a basis of equality and without discrimination, and respects the principles of self-determination in its internal arrangements, is entitled to maintain its territorial integrity under international law, and to have that territorial integrity recognised by other states). The second is the legitimacy of the tactics and methods by which self-government is pursued."

The seminar reflected a growing opinion in the Sinhalese community opposed to federalism (since that would give rise to an ethno-federal system leading to disintegration along Sri Lanka's ethnic fault line) but in favour of maximum regional autonomy to be made possible by enhancing by sufficient safeguards and additional powers the 13th amendment to the Sri Lankan constitution under which provincial councils were established in 1987 following the India-Sri Lanka Accord.

Jayatilleka, speaking out the Sinhalese point of view, felt that Sri Lanka could learn from two examples, Yugoslavia and the USSR, which "fell apart along ethnic fault lines" as well as from the fact that newly introduced market economies and the compulsions of democratic electoral politics precipitated the disintegration of ethno-federal states. The Tamilnet website noted that the Tamils were not enamoured of the concept of maximum regional autonomy because it glossed over the fundamental issues at stake in the ethnic conflict.

Jayatilleka also felt that the unification of Germany by Bismarck could be an inspiration for solving Sri Lanka's ethnic problem. Arguing that an interim administration would not be an interim administration (a purely temporary arrangement until a final solution) if it were tagged on to a powerful army (as was the case with the LTTE demanding an Interim Self Governing Authority with its fighting force intact), he hinted that defeating the Liberation Tigers militarily could be a desirable pre-condition for establishing a federal system in Sri Lanka. He pointed out that Germany became a federal state after Chancellor Otto von Bismarck crushed all the regional military forces in that country in the 19th century. He further pointed out that "it took 650, 000 casualties to consolidate the American Federation—to crush the parallel military machine of the southern states of the US in the American Civil war."

The extensive reference to the arguments for and against federalism in the Sri Lankan context suggests rather strongly that it would be an uphill task for the Sri Lankan government to try to sell the concept of federalism to the Sinhalese community.

There is little doubt that the task has been made infinitely more difficult by the failure of the Sri Lankan leadership to address itself to the all-important urgency of formulating a positive political response to the LTTE in order to revive negotiations.

President Kumaratunga's September invitation to all the political parties in the south to participate in the peace process by joining the proposed National Advisory Council for Peace and Reconciliation, which was thoughtfully kept open in order to persuade late comers, appeared to have fallen far short of the kind of initiative that would have been workable.

The Sri Lankan media went to town reporting the leader of the opposition in parliament Ranil Wickramasinghe's polite decline of the presidential invitation to co-chair the proposed advisory body along with her Prime Minister Mahinda Rajapakse, but when asked about it the former prime minister laughed derisively and told the author, who was somewhat surprised to hear him say, "But she did not offer me anything of the kind. There was no offer to co-chair such a body and, therefore, there was no question of my declining it. She certainly asked for our cooperation in parliament in case an agreement was in sight (with the LTTE) and I of course said that we would extend all cooperation in parliament once the government had sewed up a pact with the LTTE. So, where is the problem?"[11]

Throughout 2004, as the stalemate over the question of resumption of peace talks continued and threatened at times to degenerate into unpredictable uncertainties, sending the international donor community into fresh throes of anxiety, two factors which were clearly responsible for such an unhappy state of affairs stood out in sharp focus: a solidly entrenched hiatus between the Sinhalese and Tamil perceptions over the very fundamentals of the history of the last fifty years or so (such as, the history of the deprivations of the

Tamils under the Sinhalese-majority rule. But was there really such a bleak history as was being made out by Tamil terrorists? the Sinhalese would always want to know, and even in 2004); and the lack of a consensus among the majority community on two planes, (a) the need to make a truly cooperative effort to sit down and talk to the LTTE, and (b) the imperative of going for federalism as the only feasible panacea for curing the ills of the Sri Lankan state.

Where do all these leave room for India to play a healing role? Or, does the majority community in Sri Lanka expect India to play a completely different role, one that takes adequate care of the "nuisance" that the LTTE has grown into and thus help preserve the traditional unitary form of the Sri Lankan state? Listening to some of the best Sinhalese minds like H L de Silva and Dayan Jayatilleka, one might be tempted to think that that could well be the case.

Without venturing into hypothetical situations and keeping in view the experiences of the earlier Indian misadventure, the contours of an Indian response to the potentially grave Sri Lankan ethnic issue could be discerned, which incidentally would not appear to be significantly different from the present Indian policy.

Despite its relative successes in projecting itself as a people's movement by developing a de facto Tamil state in the original "Tamil homeland" now shrunk considerably, the LTTE remains primarily a terrorist group under international law and will continue to be so as long as it refuses to abandon terrorism as a tool to achieve its objectives and as long as it does not reform itself by evolving into a democratic institution wedded to constitutionalism with all its implications, including observing respect for human rights and equal political, economic and social rights for all the communities living in Sri Lanka and living within the northeast.

Notes

1. Nirupama Subramanian, "Peace process will move forward, says Sri Lankan PM", *The Hindu*, New Delhi edition, 22 December, 2001.
2. Nirupama Subramanian, "Let's bury the past, LTTE tells India", *The Hindu*, New Delhi edition, 4 February, 2002.

3. Meenakshi Iyer, "Don't force India into active role in Lanka peace bid: Muslim Congress," *Hindustan Times*, New Delhi ed., 6 August, 2004.
4. P.K.Balachanddran, "Plea for India-Lanka treaty on lines of 1971 Indo-Soviet pact/Colombo Diary," *Hindustan Times.com*, 2 August, 2004. Balachanddran adds, "The Premadasa government's draft had aimed at preserving Sri Lanka's complete independence and sovereignty in internal matters and the ethnic issue was seen as an internal matter. However, 2004 is not 1990. Much water has flowed down the Palk Strait since 1990. Those who violently and vigorously demonstrated against Indian intervention between 1987 and 1990, are today pleading with India to intervene, on the grounds that only India has a genuine interest in keeping Sri Lanka united and free from separatism and terrorism. In 1987-90, these forces did not want Indian help for striking a deal with the minority Tamils and in tackling the LTTE. But today these very forces want India to come to do what it was prevented from doing so decisively a decade-and-a-half ago." He quotes Godage to argue that the objections of these forces do not hold water in the changed domestic, regional and global context. "Jean Bodin's concept of a sacrosanct sovereignty is not valid any more. Sovereignty is observed more in the breach now, " Godage said.
5. V S Sambandan, "India solidly behind Sri Lanka's integrity", *The Hindu*, New Delhi ed., 17 September, 2004.
6. Polity, vol.1 no.5, January-February, 2004, Colombo.
7. Interviews of Prof. Jayadeva Uyangoda of the University of Colombo and Jayantha Dhanapala, secretary-general, Secretariat for Coordinating the Peace Process, government of Sri Lanka, World Trade Centre, Colombo, on 13 and 15 September, 2004, respectively.
8. Interview taken in Colombo on 15 September, 2004.
9. Rashomi Silva, "Case for federalism", *Sunday Observer*, Colombo, 29 August, 2004.
10. "Federalism is a beguiling serpent," www.tamilnet.com, 28 July, 2004.
11. Interview taken in Colombo on 17 September, 2004.

5
Colombo Continues to Miss Out

It is a measure of the persistent inadequacies of the Sri Lankan leadership that even after more than two decades of civil war, it is not yet in a position to persuade the people to accept that the national coastline, so vital for survival and prosperity in the island nation, is well cared for and that Tamil guerrillas cannot rule unilaterally over any stretch of it.

Towards the end of 2004, as the stalemate over the stalled peace negotiations continued through an uneasy period of uncertainty, threatening at times to develop into a sudden flare-up of hostilities, the sense of apprehension and anxiety in the Sinhalese mind was intensified with what was widely perceived to be an ultimate LTTE design, to wrest control over two-thirds of the coastline through Clause 18 of the ISGA proposals, sub-titled "Marine and offshore resources." (discussed in some detail in chapter four).

The apprehension about the perceived scheme was so widespread and so liberally aired that the newly appointed naval chief was obliged to declare, almost theatrically, in September 2004 that the jurisdiction of the Sri Lankan coastline rested solely with the national navy and with no other force. However, the sense of Sinhalese outrageousness was already heightened with the periodic LTTE reiteration that the ISGA proposals alone could constitute the basis for a resumption of dialogue, and the matter was not helped at all by the Kumaratunga government's characteristic flip-flop over it, first rejecting the demand outright and then conceding it in instalments, the very process having been perceived in some quarters to be a proof of capitulation to the wily Tigers.

As discussed in the previous chapter, all through this period an undercurrent of a desire to see the Indian navy play a role in helping Sri Lanka preserve its sovereignty and territorial integrity was discernible. The emphasis naturally was on the possible adversarial effects a manifestation of the ISGA proposals would have on India's security concerns, which would then by the sheer weight of logic justify an Indian role in the Sri Lankan waters.

In his discussions with Sri Lankan bureaucrats, retired and serving military personnel and academics, the author sometimes found himself facing questions, such as, what would be the Indian navy's policy if it had intelligence of an LTTE ship smuggling in arms and ammunition when the ship was in the high seas or in the Indian or Sri Lankan waters? Would it intervene and arrest the ship if it was still in the high seas or had crossed into the Indian territorial waters and pass on the intelligence to the Sri Lankan navy if it had entered the Sri Lankan waters and assist the latter in apprehending it? What would be its policy if, in the third scenario, fighting broke out with Sea Tigers? Would it be neutral or join in the fighting to help the Sri Lankan navy?

While it was beyond the capacity of the author to provide any substantive answers to such questions, what was noticeable was the depth of the Sri Lankan anxiety over probable LTTE designs behind that particular ISGA clause.

While it would be churlish to dismiss such misgivings about a hypothetical scenario (since the long history of LTTE manipulations of various situations is easy to recall), one must also appreciate the intensive shortcomings that the successive Sri Lankan governments suffered from in dealing with the phenomenon of the LTTE. Yet, even recent history tells us that the situation would have been less worrisome if Colombo had displayed better foresight and less paranoia about India's assumed hidden agenda (this point particularly comes to mind as the clamour for Indian intervention in support of Colombo grows louder). On 7 July, 1991, barely forty-five days after the benumbing assassination of former Indian prime minister Rajiv Gandhi in which the LTTE was involved, the Indian government suggested to Colombo joint patrolling of the eastern Sri Lankan coast by the two navies, aimed at effectively choking off and largely depriving the Tamil Tigers of military supplies. And how did the Sri Lankan government react?

President Premadasa, whose singlehanded contribution to the mess created by the enforced departure of the Indian Peace Keeping Force a little over a year ago was impressive, to say the least, rejected the Indian offer categorically and instantaneously. His officials were aghast at the sheer illogicality of the rejection but there were few souls, and certainly not a single one in the Presidential Secretariat at the Galle Face Green, in those days who would have dared to reason with him. But this act of pure peevishness merely served to underline the propensity of Sri Lankan leadership to crave for and spurn Indian assistance simultaneously, at times injudiciously carried away by political and sectarian considerations. Clearly, the personal idiosyncrasies of the camouflaged autocrat prevailed upon an impassive analysis of the country's security concerns. It was difficult for India to appreciate that this particular Sri Lankan leader lost sight of the simple truth that the LTTE was a military force and should, therefore, be sought to be weakened militarily and one effective and necessary means of achieving this would be by cutting off its supplies of military hardware. Had Sri Lanka accepted the Indian offer all those years ago, the Sri Lankan navy would have been in a far better position to tackle the Sea Tigers and it would not have been necessary for the country to feel intensely threatened about its coastline in 2004.

Had the Sri Lankan president been less malevolently disposed towards India and approved of the proposal at the time, it could be safely presumed that much of the subsequent strengthening of the guerrillas' military prowess could have been checked. An example of the effectiveness of the Indian navy in this respect was soon available when the rebel ship carrying a huge load of weapons and with rebel leader Kittu (returning from the UK after the British government did not extend his visa) aboard was waylaid and brought to the Madras (renamed Chennai) Port where the crew blew it up. The loss of the weapons and of Kittu was a major blow to the LTTE whose fighting ability was considerably undermined at the time.

It was again true to the peculiarly sensitive Indo-Sri Lankan relations that years later and what could only be regarded as an ironical twist of events that Sri Lanka found it expedient to make a similar offer to India. The latter reacted in a mature fashion, taking due consideration of the pros and cons of the proposal, and agreed to collaborate. Ever since then, co-operation between the two navies, though not on the scale of intensive patrolling that India had suggested, had continued, bringing in more benefits to Sri Lanka than to India for obvious reasons, and the rebels had certainly found arms smuggling more troublesome than before. Premadasa's contemptuous rejection of the Indian proposal of 1991 was even more ill-advised as Sri Lanka was by then fully aware of the supreme folly of having forced the repatriation of the IPKF from its soil; around this time, state minister for defence Ranjan Wijeratne, no friend of India but an honest politician, had publicly announced, "The IPKF had virtually finished them (the LTTE) off. They were gasping for breath in the jungles. It was we who provided that oxygen to them."

The LTTE was not only back in the northeastern province but had also established a semi-homeland in its sprawling territory. It had decimated not only the rival Tamil parties and groups but had also killed nearly 700 policemen and taken over police stations over a wide area in the northeast. Sri Lankan security forces had proved to be incapable of taking up the rebels' challenge effectively and the mess that Colombo had created was beginning to stink. We can listen to Wijeratne with more profit. "The LTTE went through thirteen months of discussions (with the government), " he told a public meeting at a southern town on 1 July, 1990. " We accepted (their) intentions as honest. But what happened? They attacked and captured the police stations in the east. They slaughtered the captives."

Elsewhere, he sought to explain how the security forces were worsted by the rebels. "The police and the security forces were taken unawares and they were not ready or prepared to fight. This was because till then the LTTE was not an adversary of the government but an adversary of the IPKF. If they were our adversaries, would we have accommodated them in five-star hotels paying millions of rupees and given them protection and aircraft?" The Sri Lankan state's inability to evaluate correctly the contribution of the IPKF towards its well-being must rank among the most scandalous follies recorded in history.

Fortunately, the state appears to have mended its ways to some extent since then and, at the very least, relations with India are handled with sophistication rather than through prejudice-induced myopia and knee-jerk reactions. The relations have indeed travelled to such a length that the top leadership of both the main Sinhalese political parties today enjoy personal rapport with that of the Indian ruling and opposition parties and the medium of frequent consultations and briefings between the two countries, as and when required, is continued with unflappable regularity. This process has also been facilitated by the desire of the international community that New Delhi is kept fully informed of all relevant developments by Colombo.

As far as the Sri Lankan state is concerned, it clearly has transcended the traditional misgivings about assumed Indian intentions and appears to be well assured that come what may, India would never betray Sri Lankan sovereignty, territorial integrity and unity. At the same time, India's abiding interest in a final settlement of the ethnic question ensuring full protection of the Tamil community's aspirations is well taken note of.

On its part, India takes full cognisance of the tremendous stride made by the two prime leaders of the country, Kumaratunga and Wickramasinghe, in providing ample evidence of their personal liberalism towards the Tamils, though the perception prevails that this does not always percolate to the political parties led by them. Note is also taken of the highly complex demands of parliamentary democracy that tend to play havoc with party policies, especially in the context of the ethnic conflict; and it is realised that the situation is further complicated by the rather erratic compulsions of coalition politics.

Still, particular note has been taken of Kumaratunga's rendering of a state apology to the nation over the anti-Tamil riots that occurred during 25 July-3 August, 1983, describing them as the most shameful crimes ever perpetrated in Sri Lanka, in which more than 1, 000 people were killed and about 18, 000 Tamil properties were destroyed.

On the occasion of the 21st anniversary of the July 1983 anti-Tamil pogrom, which changed the face of Sri Lanka for ever, Kumaratunga offering state apology said on 25 July 2004, "As we know all nations have great achievements, which they are proud of; they also have moments in their history, which they need to be ashamed of. Only very few nations seem to have had the courage or the right leadership to accept the blame for their moments of shame. At least now I believe that we as a nation and especially the Sri Lankan state should come of age, look the truth in the face and make a national apology, first to all the victims of that day in Black July and then beyond them to the entire nation. Perhaps it is the responsibility of the state and the government to engage in that exercise first and foremost, and then all of us as the nation. Every citizen in this country should collectively accept the blame and make that apology to all of you here who are the representatives or the direct victims of that violence and through you to all the other tens of thousands who suffered by those incidents. I would like to assign to myself the necessary task on behalf of the state of Sri Lanka, the government and on behalf of all of us, all the citizens of Sri Lanka to extend that apology. It is late but I think it is still not too late. Maybe if all of us can collectively put behind us all the little pettiness that has bound us in shackles, free ourselves from those many and numerous hatreds, jealousies that make of us little men and women, then I am sure we could move forward towards working, living as one nation in harmony, in a search for that very necessary unity within the diversity that is Sri Lanka, the diverse ethnic communities, the diverse religious communities, and various other social groups that live together in this country. We cannot forget, we cannot blind ourselves to the mistakes we have made; we will have to accept collective guilt for the wrongs, and then move forward. When I say collective guilt I mean first the state of Sri Lanka for the horrors they perpetrated upon one section of our peoples, 21 years ago, and at other lesser moments, but I also mean all the others on the other side of the divide who have also used young children as suicide bombers, and killed hundreds of people and caused much suffering to other people. I hope on this day, and I know that all of you here would hope and pray with me, that all those who call themselves leaders, amongst the Sinhalese, the Tamils, the Muslims, the Hindus and everybody else, would be able to reach at least for a brief moment that level of greatness that is required of us mere humans, those of us who pretend to be leaders to reach that greatness in order that we resolve this problem for our peoples. We are willing to do that; I hope all the others are also ready to do that. I am sure the government will receive the support from all the citizens of this country, irrespective of who they are, or to what community they belong, in this enterprise which is the most difficult, the most challenging and the most dangerous any government of this country has undertaken."

This apology, read together with the report of the Presidential Truth Commission on Ethnic Violence (1981-84) chaired by a former chief justice S Sharvananda, which corroborated the well-publicised course of events during the anti-Tamil pogrom, served to persuade the international community that Sri Lanka at long last was on the right road to a healing of its wounds. However, those who knew Sri Lankan affairs adequately felt that the president had also attempted to score a point or two against her political rivals through the apology and that, in that sense, it was more of a political one-upmanship than a genuine apology tendered to the Tamil community. The reactions of the latter were, however, an eye-opener for those who thought that Kumaratunga was an honest liberal, a humanist and the kind of leader the country badly needed.

Predictably enough, the reaction of the LTTE was not complimentary; the relations between the two had been bruised enough ever since her military misadventure and, thereafter, what the Tigers perceived to be an undisguised act of sabotage, first by fighting at every step with the Wickramasinghe government during the peace talks (which was no doubt facilitated by the latter's often clumsy attempts to bypass and markedly ignore the president) and then withdrawing three key ministries including defence, which led to the collapse of the dialogue process, and finally the dissolution of parliament and calling for fresh parliamentary elections.

True enough, the talks were far from being revived towards the end of 2004. Commenting on the apology tendered by the president, an LTTE functionary S Elilan, who was the district political head of the guerrilla organisation, said, "We regard Kumaratunga's public apology for the 1983 pogrom as a deceptive attempt, driven by political expediency rather than principles...It is politically convenient for Kumaratunga to blame the United National Party which was in power during that period. Has she forgotten that her father was in power when the first communal riot broke out in Sri Lanka in 1958? Why has she failed to apologise for all ethnic riots and massacres of Tamils by government forces during her regime and when her father and mother ruled the country? Crimes were committed against Tamils under the chauvinistic politics of (the) Sinhalese leadership of both (the) parties."

Sarath Kumara, writing in www.wsws.org on 6 August, 2004, was full of bitter sarcasm, "When the Sri Lankan ruling elite starts to speak about honesty, it is always laced with a heavy dose of hypocrisy. That is certainly the case with President Kumaratunga's recent public 'apology' to the country's Tamil minority for the 1983 communal pogrom, which cost hundreds of lives, turned tens of thousands into refugees and marked the start of the country's devastating civil war. The 'apology' was accompanied by nominal compensation to some of the victims. Just 72.3 million (Sri Lankan) rupees (US$ 702, 000) will be paid to 937 people or an average of 77, 000 (SL) rupees (US $ 750) for the injuries and destruction they suffered. Leaving aside the cost in lives, the loss of property alone in 1983 has been estimated to run into billions of rupees. Kumaratunga's sweeping declaration that 'every citizen' was to blame (for the riots) is to consciously obscure the role played by the ruling elite in Colombo not only for the pogrom itself but their deliberate resort to anti-Tamil chauvinism over the preceding decades and since. Ever since independence in 1948, the ruling class has responded to mass opposition and every challenge to its rule by fomenting communal divisions. Between 1958 and 1983, there were seven major anti-Tamil riots. While the president now offers an empty apology for the events of 1983, her Sri Lanka Freedom Party (SLFP) was responsible for institutionalising the anti-Tamil discrimination in the 1960s and 1970s that paved the way for the pogrom and the war. Along with the UNP, she and the SLFP ruthlessly prosecuted the (racist) war against the LTTE to ensure the predominance of the Sinhalese elite over their Tamil counterparts. 'Every citizen' was not to blame for the tragic events. It is open secret that this violence was instigated and organised by the then UNP government of President J R Jayewardene...the pogrom was no accident or aberration. The Sri Lankan ruling class can no more meet the basic needs and aspirations of working people today than in 1983. And it will just as readily resort to the communal violence to preserve its rule."

It is no idle and irresponsible speculation to say that anti-Tamil pogroms can still occur in Sri Lanka; the following is an unfortunate confirmation of this grim reality.

On 25 October 2000, twenty-seven Tamil youths, all LTTE suspects, were done to death at the Bindunuwewa Rehabilitation Centre, Bandarawela. According to the survivors, this was what happened that morning. On the morning of the 25th when the detainees got up, they saw a large number of civilians surrounding the camp and a number of police officers standing by. The mob, consisting of both men and women, started to pelt stones and came in and attacked the Tamil detainees with knives, matchets, clubs, iron rods etc.

The detainees were attacked when they were in the halls of residence. The halls were set on fire by the mob and two or three inmates were thrown into the fire. Many were clubbed to death. The police officers did nothing to stop the crowd. When some of the detainees tried to run for safety, one of them was shot down by the police. One survivor was apparently shot in his hand as two fingers were found missing. When some detainees sought shelter in a police truck, the mob attacked them there with two police officers watching closely and doing absolutely nothing.

Investigating the incidents, the Human Rights Commission of Sri Lanka, later said, "From all the information that we received in the course of our enquiry it is clear that the police officers, approximately 60 in number, have been guilty of grave dereliction of duty in not taking any effective action to prevent the acts of violence that resulted in the deaths of 27 inmates and injury to several other inmates of the Bindunuwewa camp. There are various estimates of the crowd that entered the camp that morning, ranging from a few hundred to several thousands. From what we could gather from the evidence available to us, we felt that the large estimates of 2, 000-3, 000 exaggerated the size of the crowd. These estimates must be received with caution as they appear to be calculated to mitigate the inaction of the police. In any event, the crowd that collected had not possessed any firearms and were armed only with knives, poles and implements. The police, on the other hand, were fully armed and could have easily brought the crowd under control and dispersed it. At least some of the persons who were leading the crowd could have been arrested. The inmates of the Bindunuwewa Rehabilitation Centre were all young persons sent to the centre on a rehabilitation order of the defence secretary. They included both suspects arrested under the Prevention of Terrorism Act as well (as) persons who had surrendered voluntarily to escape the LTTE. Some of them were as young as 11-14 years. The policy of sending all these persons to one centre and treating them alike is inadvisable and needs to be re-examined. The location of centres of this type would also need careful consideration. In some cases, where inmates cannot get back to their homes on account of the LTTE, the release after they complete their term of rehabilitation poses problems which need to be satisfactorily resolved. The commission proposes to examine all these problems and make recommendations for dealing with them. One of the disturbing conclusions emerging from the Bindunuwewa incidents is that *our society is still not free from racial violence and that it can express itself in very brutal forms.* (emphasis added) The Bindunuwewa tragedy needs to be enquired into fully and all the underlying causes that led to the atrocity uncovered. The disturbances and unrest within the centre, the unusual speed with which a group mounted a poster campaign, the violence in the plantation areas that followed the incidents which included the killing of two detainees from the plantation areas, the inaction of the police and the participation of local people regardless of the numbers involved, all point in different directions and open different lines of investigation. No doubt, investigations have to be pursued on all these lines and everyone responsible for the incidents of the 25th and who has any complicity in them need to be brought to justice speedily. At the same time, it would be necessary to strengthen all the initiatives that have been taken in the recent past to promote ethnic harmony and reconciliation and involve the local communities more effectively in those efforts. On our return to Colombo and learning of the disturbing developments in the plantation areas, we contacted the secretary of the ministry of national integration and ethnic affairs and stressed the need for immediate action, such as, the formation of peace committees at the local level with the support of religious leaders and civil society organisations. There is also need for launching a medium and long-term programme of national integration and ethnic harmony drawing lessons from the Bindunuwewa case."[1]

From the above account of the Bindunuwewa atrocity, the chilling similarities with the July 1983 anti-Tamil riots strike one immediately. The Human Rights Commission of Sri Lanka itself noted this, "Of the (human rights) violations that occurred in 2000 by far the worst was the massacre of the youths detained in the rehabilitation camp in Bindunuwewa. It recalled the atrocity committed in 1983 when Tamil prisoners were killed by fellow prisoners but the brutality of the Bindunuwewa killings had certain features which were even worse. The victims were all very young, some of them children. Apart from the human tragedy and the shock and trauma for the survivors and surviving relations, the massacre was a serious setback for the country's efforts to improve the human rights situation. One redeeming feature has been the prompt action taken by the state. The investigations by an independent police team sent from Colombo, the arrest of the officers who at the least had to be charged with grave negligence and inaction and the appointment of a presidential commission which will enquire into all aspects of the incident set a welcome precedent for future action." Read together with Kumaratunga's state apology for the 1983 riots, the promptitude displayed by the government in unearthing what lay behind the Bindunuwewa incidents indicated that the Sri Lankan state had moved away from the days of blind Sinhalese chauvinism of the Jayewardene-Bandaranaike variety.

This image of the Sri Lankan state was reinforced when Kumaratunga told the media at the United Nations headquarters in New York, "We remain committed to the concept that we do not like war. We are determined to do our maximum to persuade our adversaries, the LTTE, to engage in the process of negotiations in order that we can together formulate a satisfactory and lasting solution to the conflict."[2]

It was, therefore, somewhat uncomfortable to encounter a completely negative attitude towards her and her government's liberalism among the political and intellectual elite of Colombo; this was certainly very pronounced and rather aggressively expressed by members of the Tamil community who appeared to be inordinately disenchanted with her words and actions.

Without going into personalities, however, the real depth of the Sri Lankan state's quest for a truly liberal ethnic policy could be gauged by the fact that even a solemn occasion like offering the state apology to the Tamils was turned unmistakably into yet another occasion to berate Kumaratunga's bete noire, Ranil Wickramasinghe.

While analysts trace the seemingly pathological rivalry between the two leaders to a traditional competition between the two main Sinhalese political parties, the UNP and the SLFP, apparently handed down through generations of leadership, the phenomenon deserves analysis as it definitely impinges on the ability of the government of the day to carry on any meaningful and sustained dialogue with the militants in the ranks of the Tamil minority community.

Sooner or later, the government finds it strategically and politically expedient to switch over from a liberal stance to a posture of toughness. This transition is frequently accelerated by LTTE manoeuvres which senses the arrival of an opportune moment to exploit to its advantage any cleavage appearing in the ranks of the majority community. The LTTE's apparently well-considered withdrawal from peace talks following a forceful presidential intervention in the functioning of the UNF government, preceded by a series of acts of brinkmanship by both Kumaratunga and Wickramasinghe, was the latest example of such exploitation of an inherent shortcoming in the Sinhalese polity.

The eventual failure of the Sinhalese leadership to present a united front while bargaining with the LTTE continues to be the bugbear of Sri Lankan history. While that history is replete with carcasses of Sinhalese bids to outsmart the Tigers through political moves, in an incisive analysis of the situation in the beginning of 2004, Uyangoda wrote, "Unlike the war, peace talks have brought the state reform agenda to the centre of ruling class imperatives. It is in this backdrop that entering the next phase of talks as well as negotiating a compromise with the LTTE requires the political unity of the two power blocks. Ruling class political unity is fundamental to any breakthrough in future peace negotiations with the LTTE."[3]

This brings us to a disquieting feature of the Sri Lankan situation present throughout 2004. Why is it that while both the major Sinhalese political parties continue to be committed to the concept of federalism, there is no sustained campaign, both at the levels of the parties and the government, to educate the majority community about it? The concept of federalism, as an analyst told the author, is out in the open in the south; the media regularly carry articles, news reports and letters on the subject and seminars and workshops are being organised to propagate the concept.

The effort, however, does not go deeper, and there is no intensive campaign as such, mainly because of a lack of state and political initiative. It is noteworthy that the LTTE has taken the initiative in popularising the idea of federalism in the south through a sustained campaign, by organising trips to the north by select groups of the Sinhalese, especially including segments assumed to be fiercely opposed to federalism such as Buddhist monks. TNA MPs have been instructed to mount a campaign on federalism right in the den of the lion, so to speak, by organising public discussions in the south (there was considerable hesitation on the part of the MPs to do as bidden, and in September 2004, they told the author that the time for such a bold and unconventional approach was yet to come). It is also important to remember that the south has been obliged to turn its attention to the concept of federalism principally because the LTTE has thrown into its lap the ISGA proposals, creating a widespread fear psychosis and automatic rejection syndrome, but nevertheless making the majority community study the proposals before rejecting them.

If one may adopt Uyangoda's categorisation, the LTTE has presented a post-federal vision of the future Sri Lankan state through the prism of the ISGA proposals, but the Sinhalese polity remains bogged down within the traditional pre-federal framework, which thus becomes yet another defining challenge to the laggard Sinhalese leadership.

Whatever post-federal framework is being attempted in the south remains confined to what is euphemistically called the "Colombo elite", like most other intellectual activities, implying thereby that discussions and debates somehow steer clear of the people at large. An instance of this limitation was available when the author met members of a truly elitist group, The Citizens Movement for Good Governance (CIMOGG) in Colombo.

Consisting of mostly retired senior bureaucrats, technocrats and social activists, the group apparently is interested in helping to stop the drift in the affairs of the nation and find a way out which, it believes, it already has. "Our commitment is to promote every aspect of good governance, based on democracy and the rule of law, " it says calling for the establishment of a new political order in the country. The new order will make small village communities and the nation itself more self-reliant; this is one answer to the negative aspects of globalisation, which pose new challenges to the weaker nations. The real problem in Sri Lanka is identified as the growing dissatisfaction with the present political system and the electoral process, as evident in the fact that over five per cent of the total votes cast in the 2001 general election was spoilt, which increased to over seven per cent in the local elections in some districts that followed. The votes were obviously spoilt deliberately as ballot papers carried rude remarks, indicating the extent of frustration amongst voters who participated while three million others who did not vote at all.

Calling the electoral process a lawless one with money and muscle playing an increasingly decisive role, the group says that the situation is compounded by the absence of good governance due to the all-powerful executive presidency, lack of transparency and accountability at all levels of government and political authority monopolised by a small, highly privileged class not accountable to the people. After much consultation and discussion at various levels of society and in many parts of the country, the CIMOGG has come up with the following solution: the new political order will be based on the concepts of accountability, subsidiarity and the trusteeship of power. Accountability will be ensured by such means as the forum where representatives will answer to the people, voters will have the right to recall representatives, the referendum and the right of petition. The proposed political structure will be based on the following principles: transparency and accountability of elected representatives; peace, security, equality, and harmony among all sections of the people under the rule of law; devolution of power to smaller units; the cheapest possible free and fair elections; and maintenance of the integrity and security of the state and of its territorial waters and ocean resources. The proposed structure will consist of peoples councils, divisional councils, territorial assemblies, a national assembly, a second chamber to be called the consultative assembly, and a supreme council. The CIMOGG explains that its plan for a new political order draws inspiration from Switzerland where participatory democracy is truly practised.

But how does the CIMOGG propose to deal with the immediate over-riding problem, the ethnic conflict, without dealing with which no major reformatory initiative can hope to gain legitimacy? Commenting on the preamble to the ISGA proposals submitted by the LTTE, it says that it agrees with the insurgent group on the importance of achieving lasting peace but believes that Norway as the facilitator of peace talks should be assisted by other countries.

More significantly, however, it says it recognises that "groups of Sri Lankans" have been responsible for acts of violence and terrorism against each other, which is on record (implying thereby that the Tamils may not have any special grievances in this respect since they are equally guilty of acts of violence and terrorism against the Sinhalese). As a matter of fact, the CIMOGG response to the ISGA proposals devotes considerable space to establish that the principal Tamil grievances are shared by the Sinhalese as well since the fountainhead of all the problems in the country is the existing political system. "The existing political structure has marginalised not only the people of the north and the people of the east but also the people in the rest of the country" as proven by the Janatha Vimukthi Peramuna rebellions. The distinction made by the CIMOGG between the people of the north and the people of the east is similarly no accident; by this formulation, it apparently wishes to demolish the LTTE case for a Tamil homeland comprising the currently conjoined north and east. Countering the

LTTE proposals which aim to get in place an interim autonomous body to administer the northeast monopolised by its nominees, the Colombo group suggests the formation of an all-inclusive negotiating council of Sri Lankan representatives of the national polity, to be chosen from the present MPs and the LTTE.

In what may appear to some as the true purpose of the CIMOGG exercise, the group says that it cannot, however, accept the position that the LTTE is the sole representative of the Tamil people unless and until democratic elections have been held based on "accurate and updated" electoral lists to establish this position. The CIMOGG also disputes that the LTTE enjoys effective control and jurisdiction over the majority of the north and the east either through physical presence or under the terms of the ceasefire agreement or under accepted norms of international law.

This is followed by something of a coup de grace: the CIMOGG does not accept the assertion that subsequent to the Vaddukoddai Resolution of 1976 ("Whereas throughout the centuries from the dawn of history, the Sinhalese and Tamil nations have divided between them the possession of Ceylon, the Sinhalese inhabiting the interior parts of the country in its southern and western parts from the river Walawe to that of Chilaw and the Tamils possessing the northern and eastern districts...'the Tamil United Liberation Front' resolves that Tamil Eelam shall consist of the northern and eastern provinces 'of Sri Lanka'), the Tamil people mandated their elected representatives to establish an independent, secular state because the 1977 election results proved: that more voters opposed the TULF in the eastern province than those who supported the party in the northern province (thereby implying that the east did not wish to be merged with the northern province into a single political unit) and even after taking the two provinces together, as much as 53 per cent of the voters opposed the TULF, thereby establishing that the separatist party did not obtain a mandate to set up a separate state. Thus, apparently satisfied that all the fundamental aspects of the case for a Tamil homeland have been adequately taken care of, the CIMOGG proceeds to suggest that while an all-inclusive negotiating council should embark on the negotiation process, an international advisory group, subdivided into Norway and Pakistan or Bangladesh in one group, India all by itself in another and Japan, the US, the EU and the Commonwealth in the third, should facilitate the process. The process will be further assisted by a non-political advisory group and a technical advisory group.

A purely private initiative such as the CIMOGG has been quoted at such length in order to illustrate the principal tragedy that besets this beautiful but unfortunate country. The psychological divide between the north and the south is shocking, to state the obvious. The CIMOGG is not even prepared to acknowledge the fact of the political, social and economic discriminations that the Tamils have gone through though it goes through the motion of taking note of them. But, cleverly enough, it soon seeks to equate the Tamils' grievances with those of the Sinhalese. It is astonishing that the history of independent Sri Lanka can be glossed over to such an extreme extent, but the CIMOGG probably exemplifies a new sophistication achieved by the majority community (though the group is said to count among its illustrious members representatives of other communities as well) in its continuing quest for denying the Tamils any right to feel aggrieved.

The author was somewhat surprised at the enthusiasm with which a distinguished member of the CIMOGG sought to establish the "archaeological" evidence of Sri Lanka having been an exclusively Sinhalese-ruled country throughout history. The gentleman also urged a quick settlement of the ethnic issue because, as he saw it, the LTTE was taking full advantage of the continuing impasse and "systematically destroying the archaeological evidences of Sinhalese rule strewn all over the northern province." The only way to stop this "vandalism", he felt, was to establish full government control over the province in the quickest possible way. When asked about the relevance of digging into distant history while searching for a solution to the ethnic conflict, the gentleman replied that this was necessary as it was the Tamils who first dragged history into the issue by claiming about a "fabled" Tamil kingdom. Besides, one always learned from history.

Listening to him the author recalled his own description of the Sri Lankans' morbid obsession with history, " There are few countries, other than Sri Lanka, where history has been turned into an unshakable burden, an albatross that must hang around the collective neck of the nation, binding it to an eternal curse of reliving history in order to perpetuate myths in a vicious circle. The obsession of the Sinhalese and Tamils with their mutually exclusive versions of Sri Lankan history strikes a foreigner for its intensity through newspapers, seminars, lectures; in fact, almost at every intellectual exercise. Through these obsessions the two quarrelling communities try continuously to outwit each other, proving more to themselves than to others the impeccability of their respective positions. In the process, even archaeology, which is scientific enough to banish myths, has turned out to be the handmaiden of the manipulated history...History and archaeology have got inextricably mixed with ethnic nationalism in Sri Lanka because both are perceived to be instrumental in establishing the two communities' historical bona fides, beginning with an enquiry into their mutually disputed antiquities."[4]

There was, however, a whiff of fresh air when a leading archaeologist urged an unbiased, scientific and multi-disciplinary approach to the Sri Lankan history in view of the considerable damage done to the national fabric by unscientific studies and incorrect or biased reading of the past. Prof. Sudharshan Seneviratne of the University of Peradeniya said that history and archaeology in Sri Lanka had been badly politicised, and that politicisation of this sort had contributed to the Sinhalese-Tamil conflict.[5]

He held that both the Sinhalese and the Tamils had been responsible for this state of affairs as both had distorted history to serve narrow and competitive political ends. Regretting that little or no effort had yet been attempted to stem the root, he said while delivering the G C Mendis memorial lecture in Colombo in early October, 2004, that "a new breed of charlatans and political animals in these disciplines are responsible for the emergence of a historical and anti-historical bias in schools, at seats of higher education, and in the country as a whole."

Archaeologist Seneviratne was, however, almost a lone voice advocating treatment of history as a scientific means of learning the past, a very thin strain of thought initiated by G C Mendis who first called for a methodology to distinguish historical persons from supernatural or mythical beings, historical stories from legends and historical facts from religious beliefs. Foreigners are usually shocked beyond belief when told by well-meaning Sinhalese-Buddhists that the Lord Buddha visited Sri Lanka thrice in his lifetime, usually flying down from India. Encounters with such esoteric obsessions illustrate a fundamental lacuna in the Sri Lankan polity, that the majority community without whose consent no constitutional and administrative structural changes can be brought about has just not been prepared to be able to appreciate the nature of these changes. This is clearly a singular failure of the Sinhalese leadership, both in government and opposition. Once it was determined that a military solution to the ethnic conflict was not forthcoming (or, was such a determination ever made?), it became imperative for the leadership to initiate an educative process for the Sinhalese to learn and appreciate the nuances of federalism. Unfortunately, little spadework has been done in this respect; and even the elite class remains prone to examine the question of dealing with Tamil aspirations in a badly convoluted manner, thus failing to rise to the occasion.

A group of social scientists have argued that the Tamil liberation movement in the north (with its primary focus on ethno-linguistic difference) and the Janatha Vimukthi Peramuna uprisings in the south (with their primary focus on class disparity) reflect an inadequate post-colonial national vision and strategy. As a result, political discrimination in governance, a lack of equitable development policies, and a failure to preserve and respect local and cultural knowledge have become endemic. While the conflict in the northeast has a major ethnic component, the war is not reducible to ethnicity; it is just not the Tamils vs the Sinhalese, not that simplistic at all. "Poverty, inequality and intra-ethnic divisions played a part in fuelling the conflicts in the north and south alike. A just and sustainable peace will require understanding the complexity of Sri Lanka's two post-colonial conflicts as well as transcending competitive ethnic politics," the group says.[6]

Looking at today's Sri Lanka, one realises how immeasurably tough a job it would be to implement the recommendations of the group to achieve sustainable peace. Appearing to travel the same track that the CIMOGG travels but differing fundamentally in the underlying philosophy, the group of social scientists suggests that the proposed vision for Sri Lanka should be based on and builds from an acknowledgement and appreciation of the island's historic, largely pacific and multi-cultural past with due recognition of its more violent and divided present.

And how would that be worked out? One example is: acknowledgement of Sri Lanka's mixed cultural geography and ancient multiculturalism entails recognition that a majority group in a region is bound to respect and protect those who are in the minority in that particular region. The toughness of the task is apparent when this requirement is juxtaposed against the Bundunuwewa incidents, which happened a mere four years ago. When the author posed this particular recommendation before representatives of the Sinhalese community, some of the latter responded by pointing out that the Tamils had repeatedly failed to protect the Sinhalese and Muslims in the northeast. While advancing this argument, they did not consider it relevant to note that Tamil perpetrators of atrocities against the minorities in Tamil-dominated areas were regimented LTTE cadre and not the civilian population and preferred to equate the Tigers with the Tamil community as a whole.

The second recommendation that the group makes appears to be even more challenging to the Sinhalese, unprepared and possibly unwilling as they are to re-educate themselves, since no example is being set by their leadership. For example, an elitist group like the CIMOGG is likely to reject the very formulation that the group makes, namely, that while all communities suffered during the two decades of violence, the people of the north and east bore the brunt of the violence, displacement and destruction. We have seen the CIMOGG's effort to equate the sufferings of the northeast with those of the south.

It may be mentioned here in passing that when the author sought to gauge the attitude of the majority community to the enduring ceasefire (in the context of the known Tamil reaction of a sense of relief and gratitude), analysts often responded by noting a qualitative difference between the two categories: they said that the Sinhalese' experience of the war could in no way be equated with that of the Tamils who lived in the war zone and as a result suffered extensively. Those who lived in the south through the war years never suffered losses in any comparable degree, such as, losing homes destroyed in fighting and being forced to flee for safety elsewhere (there were Tamil families which became internally displaced persons as many as six or seven times within the two decades of the civil war). Therefore, the Sinhalese and others living in the south and west would be happy in a general way that the ceasefire had lasted but because they had few memories of personal losses (such as, losing family members who lost their lives while serving in the police and security forces and participating in the war), they would not be truly internally concerned, except by such vital factors as rising costs of living due to the war.

The social scientists' group also calls for a recognition (again a tough proposition for the largely uninitiated majority community) of the strength of ethno-national consciousness developed during the war years, the need for power sharing under a federal system and equally, the need to balance the claims of diverse groups. Striking at the core of Sri Lanka's myriad problems, the group recommends that power sharing should reflect the country's multi-ethnic, multi-religious and multi-lingual society and mixed cultural geography. A political tradition of inter-ethnic consultation has to be evolved.

"A political culture and social acceptance of diversity and inclusiveness is needed at all levels—from the centre to the periphery. Whereas there should be no politically motivated colonisation, whether by the centre or by the region, no territory should be regarded as ethnically exclusive. The concept of traditional habitations is legitimate (e.g. for cultural purposes), but there should be no concept of a mono-ethnic homeland. Every citizen of Sri Lanka should be free to live and work in any part of the island, " the group recommends.

This particular recommendation brings to mind an unexpected experience that the author had while visiting Sri Lanka during the extended ceasefire. Viewed from his perspective of the early 1990's, he felt that the over-two years of no fighting must have been seized upon by the Sinhalese intellengtsia, especially the media, to not only visit the northeast periodically but also to cover events and developments in the region regularly through the services of correspondents posted there (nobody except foreign correspondents and international aid workers could travel to the north during the first, second and third eelam wars). Surprisingly, no Colombo-based English newspaper covered the northeast directly, except by making sporadic attempts. Rather strikingly, there was no regular coverage of the living conditions of the people in the war-ravaged region; there was just no way one would know what was going on in the northeast except isolated reports on the LTTE's factional fights and briefings by the military, the Peace Secretariat or the various ministries or international aid organisations.

The failure of the Sinhalese community to respond to the vitally altered situation in the country, the ceasefire that has held for over two years and, by all accounts, is expected to hold on, is also sharply etched in the world of Sinhalese cinema. Has cinema, features and documentaries, moved to the northeast to chronicle the joys and pains, the hopes and aspirations, of the people who have lived with twenty-one years of a civil war?

Discussing the Sinhalese cinema's response to the single enormous change in the country, the doyen of the genre Lester James Peiris told the author, "In terms of the ceasefire, one would have thought that the Sinhalese cinema would have gone northward and confronted the situation directly. I am sorry to say that nothing of the sort has happened. We are behaving as if nothing of substance has changed or occurred in the country that we should sit up, take notice and portray it in our medium. The sole exception I can think of is the TV semi-documentaries that Ashoka Handagama has made, depicting the Muslim and Tamil situations. In these films, the viewer sees people recounting their experiences of the war; and, quite predictably, most of the stories are about the dispossessed and the disappeared. Besides, Sinhalese film makers and theatre artistes and producers got together and went to the University of Jaffna and showed their works with English sub-titles. By all accounts, the screenings were highly successful, and a kind of dialogue between the Sinhalese artistes and the Tamils ensued. If I remember correctly, two or three Sinhalese plays were staged with a good deal of enthusiasm. But what we have found is that we cannot confront the ethnic problem head on, and the job has been made difficult by the fact that parables and fables have not emerged from the civil war."[7]

This lack of initiative to bring the previously estranged but presently united northern and southern regions, even including the areas still under LTTE control, during the protracted ceasefire points to the second major shortcoming in the Sri Lankan polity, the first being the absence of a public awareness campaign aimed at the majority community to prepare its members for a post-federal scenario. It certainly does not speak well for the well-being of the polity that none of the major institutionalised stakeholders like the government, the media or the academic world came forward to initiate familiarisation and peer-group exchange programmes in order to encourage and increase people-to-people contacts, more for the benefits of the people living in the south than for the other side (as it is, the people in the northeast have been travelling to the south throughout the two decades of fighting either to find berths within or outside the country or simply to obtain necessities of life before returning to the deprivations of living in the war zone).

It is significant that the LTTE has taken advantage of this lack of southern initiative and launched an apparently well-planned campaign to introduce southerners to the life in the rebels-held territory. In the south, several well-meaning social activists have come forward and are organising friendship tours of the north but, since these are basically isolated initiatives often suffering from a dearth of funds and volunteers, the impact appears to be minimal. More shockingly, there is resistance by segments of Sinhalese society to participate in such sponsored tours of the war zone.

More than two years of "negative peace", as an analyst described the ceasefire, provided an unprecedented opportunity to the Sri Lankan state to reach out to the people in the war zone and to bring out the southern people out of their comforting but eventually self-defeating seclusion and help them get close to and understand the situation in the northeast at first hand. The consequences of such initiatives could only have been beneficial for the state, provided it remained steadfast in its determination to pursue peace and a final settlement of the ethnic conflict to the satisfaction of all.

Far from such affirmative actions, both the Sri Lankan polity and the majority community have allowed the considerable time and space to pass by. What is even more disconcerting is the fairly widespread lack of consciousness in the Sinhalese community of its failure to grab the unique opportunity and take a move forward to heal the debilitating ethnic divide. Unfortunately, this is true of civil society as well except for a few bravehearts who regularly commute between the north and the south with batches of well-intentioned individuals eager to build bridges across the ethnic chasm. These honest efforts must, however, fall woefully short of the vast requirements of the moment.

What the country needs now, says another group of social scientists, is a highly diversified and broad-based peace movement with links and leverages in all communities. Strategic alliances should be formed to engage with all political actors and for building up a critical mass of agents of change within the civil society. Insiders representing all stakeholders should form networks of close cooperation with outsiders from transnational civil society to make the international support of the peace process as multi-partial and proactive as possible. The citizens of the country have to be prepared for reconstituting Sri Lanka as a multinational federal state.[8]

Clearly, the task of educating and training Sri Lankan society to think in terms of federalism would be an enormous task, if it is ever taken up. As often noted earlier, there is as yet no concerted move in that direction and certainly not one in which the state would occupy the widest space. The job is rendered many times difficult by the absence of a tradition of a peace movement, apart from the fact that even during the last two years of the ceasefire, no peace movement has emerged on the scene. The isolated attempts being made are still too brief in their scope and cannot add up to the beginning of a meaningful peace movement.

But, perhaps the rudiments of a nationwide peace movement are being formed. Even if these are numerically insignificant, ideas are surely being generated in minds across the divide, and though all the three principal actors, the state, the political parties, and the media have failed miserably to rise to the occasion, it is at least no longer impossible to dream of a diversified yet united society with various communities pursuing the goals of a normal life.

The majority community thus finds itself facing several major challenges which are inter-linked and have to be tackled simultaneously. There are analysts who believe that the process of transforming Sinhalese society in order to equip it to deal with the post-federal scenario would not, however, take off until the political leadership of the community is reconciled. Uyangoda writes, "Already the gulf between the Sinhalese and Tamil polities in the vision for a future Sri Lankan state has become starkly clear. While the LTTE has presented a post-federal vision through its ISGA proposals, the Sinhalese polity remains within a pre-federal framework. The challenge for the Sinhalese political leaders is to bridge this gulf between the majoritarian pre-federalism and the minoritarian post-federalism. It is not an easy task. It requires a radical intellectual turn around as well as a new political self-understanding on the part of the Sinhalese ruling elites. Such a qualitative shift can only rest on a new political unity among the Sinhalese ruling strata."[9]

As we have seen elsewhere in this book, western democracies which handled minority community grievances successfully channeled the protest movements, such as the anti-segregationist African-American civil rights movement, towards a settlement through the media of corrective constitutional, social, political and economic measures and also through the presentation of the state as a tough disciplinarian whose diktats could be ignored only at great punitive risk.

Paul Wilkinson's words need to recalled when he says in 'Politics, Diplomacy and Peace Processes; Pathways out of terrorism" (in "*The Future of Terrorism*" ed. Max Taylor and John Horgan, Frank Cass, London, p.67), that "One obvious reason for the predominantly peaceful nature of the majority of civil rights movements in democracies has been that penalties for violence, or any involvement in any activities deemed to be aimed at subverting or overthrowing the government, have been very severe."

Judged against this fairly common trait in democracies dealing with political movements which have the potential to turn into violent armed struggles, Sri Lanka in 2004 appeared to be a terribly bad loser. While the wanton killing spree being indulged in by the LTTE and the Karuna group spread wide across the island spoke of a demoralisingly ineffective law and order machinery, one incident that happened in Vavuniya in late-October, 2004, simply defied credulity.

The Tamilnet website reported on 23 October that the inauguration of an all Ceylon women's netball championship being held in Vavuniya was delayed in the morning because some local groups objected to the hoisting of the national flag and the singing of the national anthem. The function was allowed to proceed only after the organisers agreed not to hoist the national flag and to cancel the singing of the national anthem.

The event could only be considered extraordinary for the following reasons: Vavuniya had been under government control since 1991; the sports meet was organised by the Sri Lanka Inter Netball Association; and was attended by the Wanni region military commander Maj.Gen. B Kulatunge, senior police commissioner Mahinda Baddewela, LTTE Wanni District head of sports Thamilmaran, government officials, students and Vavuniya residents. Both the national flag, also known as the Lion Flag, and the national anthem had been resented by the Tamils as symbols of Sinhalese chauvinism. The Sri Lankan state thus stood exposed for its incapacity to protect its very symbols as it was seen yielding easily to the obvious machinations of the LTTE. This latest instance of the crumbling of the authority of the state occurred well within government territory and in the presence of senior army, police and civilian officials.

The history of the Sinhalese-Tamil relations since the late 1950's shows an uneven political and administrative response to situations which were initially peaceful and constitutional protest movements, turned gradually into aggressive and violent movements and finally yielded place to armed guerrilla operations. The Sri Lankan state either chose to ignore or react disproportionately to the first stirrings of the Tamil uprising when the legality and constitutionality of staging protests against the state were strictly adhered to. Observers of Sri Lanka were left to lament in later years this singular lack of sound judgement on the part of the Sinhalese leadership, for it became obvious in the following years that the Tamils were not being cowered by state terror and were in fact beginning to see terror as their weapon as well.

This was what a left Tamil intellectual, Ram Manikkalingam, preferred to call Tigerism. Writing in 1992, he showed how the politics of Tamil nationalism, which began as a reaction to Sinhalese nationalism, had come to acquire its own internal dynamics and this independent dynamics was impelled by the growing dominance of a vicious and extreme form of Tamil nationalism espoused by the Tigers. The emergence of this nationalism could be traced to the dilemmas of a national movement. A nationalist movement would use a dual approach to oppose a dominant power by invoking the violation of democratic norms, such as individual liberties and freedoms, in the status quo, while it would seek to mobilise a community on the basis of ties of ethnic solidarity.

However, in a dynamic movement ethnic ties would not always hold together and differences of opinion would surface, giving rise to tension between internal democracy and the need for a unified struggle. This contradiction could be solved in various ways, such as through dialogue and non-violent confrontation to violent coercion. In the case of Tamil nationalism, Manikkalingam noted, the Tigers set out to eliminate all opposing parties, organisations and individuals and unity was asserted at the expense of internal democracy. "The Tigers, thus, represent an extreme aberration of the emphasis on ethnonational solidarity at the expense of democracy...The Tiger emphasis on a monolithic unity is a consequence of their attempt to invent a new Tamil identity, where the basis of political programmes and alliances are of an ethnically essentialist character, " he argued.[10]

If one could go by Manikkalingam's hypothesis of the birth and growth of Tamil nationalism or Tigerism, one would arrive at the conclusion that the Sri Lankan state or, specifically, the Sinhalese leadership, paved the way for the transformation of Tamil nationalism from an essentially pluralistic and liberal background to Tigerism which would prove to be as chauvinistic, rigid and narrow-minded as its Sinhalese counterpart.

Manikkalingam has many contemporaries who reciprocate his understanding that the success of the LTTE lies in its ability to usurp the identity of Tamil nationalism which, to begin with, had nothing to do with extremism and armed insurrection. As we have seen earlier in this volume, the LTTE is continuing to struggle to maintain its stranglehold over the Tamil identity through its claim that it is the only representative of the Sri Lankan Tamils. Its hold on the usurped title of the sole envoy of the Tamils constitutes the core of its political and military strength and it is naturally loath to let this slip out of hand. Hence, the violent reaction to "Col." Karuna's defection.

By failing to exploit the situation created by Karuna's "betrayal", the Sri Lankan state thus missed yet another cue to rally back in the fight to preserve the unity and territorial integrity of the country. Had Colombo successfully played up the Karuna card, the Tamil community would have had one narrow breathing space to look beyond the LTTE. By choosing to close that option and by continuing to allow the Tigers to finish the job of annihilating Karuna, the state had merely further facilitated the supremacy of the Liberation Tigers over the Tamil community.

Notes

1. Human Rights Commission of Sri Lanka, Colombo, *Annual Report (01.01.2000-31.03.2001)*.
2. Media conference held on 22 September, 2004.
3. Jayadeva Uyangoda, *Peace Watch*, Polity, vol.1, no.5, January-February, 2004.
4. Apratim Mukarji, *The War in Sri Lanka: Unending Conflict?* (2000), Har-Anand Publications Pvt.Ltd., New Delhi.
5. P.K.Balachanddran, "Call to Stop Politicising Sri Lankan History," *HindustanTimes.com*, 11 October, 2004.
6. Darini Rajasingham-Senanayake, Fara Haniffa and Devanesan Nesiah, *A Vision for Sustainable Peace in Sri Lanka*, Polity, vol.1, no.5, January-February, 2004.
7. Interview taken in Colombo on 13 September, 2004.
8. Tyrol Ferdinands, Kumar Rupasinghe, Paikiasothy Saravanamuttu, Jayadeva Uyangoda and Norbert Ropers, *Sri Lanka's Peace Process: Towards Phase II*, Polity.
9. Jayadeva Uyangoda, *Peace Watch*, Polity, vol. 1, no. 5, January-February, 2004.
10. Ram Manikkalingam, *Tigerism and other essays*, Ethnic Studies Group, Colombo, 1995.

6
Somebodys vs Nobodys

A wit in Colombo said that Sinhalese politics had always been about nobodys trying to be somebodys and somebodys hating nobodys for that very reason and ensuring that the status quo was maintained but politics was also about changing fortunes and one day nobodys would actually succeed in becoming somebodys, leaving the original somebodys thoroughly scandalised, and the rivalry between the original and pariah aristocrats would continue for ever. "Though it may be considered simplistic, the fact is that Sinhalese politics has always been about the Senanayakes vs the Bandaranaikes," observed one of the most experienced Sri Lankan bureaucrats, Bradman Weerakoon.

The personality clash between President Kumaratunga and leader of the opposition in parliament and former Prime Minister Ranil Wickramasinghe, which dominated Sinhalese politics throughout 2001-2004 as it indeed did the earlier decade as well, was an extension of this time-honoured battle for supremacy between the two political traditions, the United National Party (UNP), led by the Senanayake father-son duo and John Kotelawala and the Sri Lanka Freedom Party (SLFP) led by the Bandaranaike husband-wife duo.

While both the batches of leaders found their followers among their own social class, the anglicised and traditional landed aristocracy, the Bandaranaikes held the Senanayakes in contempt as they lacked the former's legacy of Kandyan aristocracy, the very epitome of Sinhalese aristocracy. In the beginning of the long heritage of political rivalry, therefore, the Bandaranaikes started as the original somebodys and successfully projected the Senanayakes as the first set of nobodys.

This tradition of contempt, which apparently ceased to be one-sided before long and became mutual, has come down the line till today, when Kumaratunga and Wickramasinghe are continuing to treat each other with their inherited sense of superiority for self and contempt for the other party.

It would appear from the unflattering history of intermittent bickerings between the two main Sinhalese political parties that the power struggle between the UNP and SLFP leaderships or the rivalry between the two ruling families and the two ruling individuals of today in Colombo has come to enjoy precedence over national issues, such as, dealing with the LTTE and finding a permanent solution to the ethnic conflict.

This was in stark evidence all through the period of Kumaratunga's rise to power since the mid-1990's, with Wickramasinghe and her upstaging each other at every opportunity with an apparent lack of concern for the country. Chronicling the cataclysmic events of another summer four years ago, when at one point an eventual takeover of the Jaffna Peninsula by the Tamil Tigers appeared to be inevitable, the author wrote, "...the foremost lesson that Sri Lanka, one hopes, has already drawn (since every single external power has emphasised it), is the imperative of forging unity among the political parties and groups representing the Sinhalese, Tamil and Muslim communities over an acceptable devolution package."

" The world must witness, sooner than later, a concrete instance of the willingness of the Sri Lankan political parties to join hands in this endeavour. If, on the other hand, the age-old bickerings and the game of one-upmanship continue, pushing the acceptance of a devolution package to a further prolonged period of uncertainty, the country would lose the sympathy and understanding of the larger world it still enjoys....Will the Sinhalese parties agree to the unit of devolution, the true bone of contention which has bedevilled a political solution all these years? Will the majority community accept at last the Tamils' demand for a contiguous autonomous region as a Tamil-majority province? Will the Tamil-majority parts of the eastern province be merged permanently with the northern province?...One main reason why the devolution package of 3 August, 1995, never took off was the LTTE's manoeuvres; the rest was of course firstly the UNP's determined opposition and, secondly, President Kumaratunga's deliberate mishandling of the opposition."[1]

It does credit to no party involved that four years later, all the issues mentioned above continue to remain unsolved. Devolution of power is the essence of federalism, and the very concept of it remains totally unacceptable to the majority community even if individuals and groups, including the very top political leadership, are publicly aligned with it. It is clear that neither the Kumaratunga-led Sri Lanka Freedom Party nor the Wickramasinghe-led United National party is in a position to go to polls over the issue of federalism.

Nor is there any sign of prospects for better working relations between the two top leaders. Since the summer of 2000, the relations between the two main Sinhalese parties have revolved around constant personality clashes and narrow partisan interests. In the December, 2001, parliamentary elections, the People's alliance of Kumaratunga lost out to Wickramasinghe's United National Party and the latter became prime minister.

Since then began the sad saga of uneasy relations between the presidentship of Kumaratunga and the government of Wickramasinghe; it was perhaps inevitable that the rivalry and competition between the two entities would revolve around the issue of the peace process the preliminaries of which were launched soon thereafter.

A little over a year later, in February, 2002, the Wickramasinghe government and the LTTE signed a permanent ceasefire agreement which continues to be in force today but which also witnessed a flare-up in the already constrained relations between the president and the prime minister.

All through the period of the government-Tigers peace talks, Kumaratunga continued to be stringently critical of the "concessions" that Wickramasinghe was willingly handing over to the LTTE, and by May, 2003, she was threatening to sack the government if she felt that too many concessions had been granted to the rebels.

Right in the early days, when Prime Minister Ranil Wickramasinghe advocated de-proscription of the LTTE, a banned outfit in Sri Lanka, the former foreign minister in the Kumaratunga government and the main campaigner in those days for a world-wide ban of the LTTE as a terrorist organisation, Lakshman Kadirgamar advised the government not to act in haste. "The question of deproscription should be considered with deep circumspection and caution, " he advised.

The president wanted the government to use a possible lifting of the ban on the LTTE as a leverage to wrest certain guarantees which would be vital for maintaining peace. Her spokesman Harim Peiris said at the time, "Is the LTTE committed to not carrying out killings of civilians, assassinations and suicide attacks on economic targets? Would there be a memorandum of understanding with the LTTE on these issues? These are some of the issues for which there are no answers, but they have to be taken as part of the process."

An outright opposition to the dawning of the peace process was not possible, even if the rival-led government eventually succeeded in cornering the glory of bringing peace. The president was, therefore, always careful not to create an impression that she was a spoil sport; her spokesman made this clear when he said, "We would place no obstacle to the peace process. We remain fully committed to it. But the peace process should be correct in order to be successful."

This would be a major point of disagreement between the two centres of power, with both the president and her men and the prime minister making out their mutually contrary positions in an increasingly stronger language. When Kadirgamar urged caution, Wickramasinghe maintained that the ban on the LTTE should not be allowed to become an impediment to peace talks, arguing that while the international community recognised the Tigers as a terrorist organisation, it also wanted Sri Lanka to hold a dialogue with it.

In a typical instance of the developments those days, Kumaratunga sent a firm message to the government on 29 October, 2002, saying that the proposed joint mechanism with the Liberation Tigers for overseeing development work in the northeast should be rooted in law and should conform to the norms of constitutional governance.

The proposed joint task force, she said, should be "rooted in the law. Constitutional principles of governance applicable to the rest of the country should be part of this, " as government spokesman and chief government negotiator Prof. G L Peiris represented her view to the media. By raising the objection, she was implying that the government, which was a constitutional body, could not participate with an extra-constitutional body like the LTTE in any activity on an equal footing.

The president was also pressing at the time for "core issues" to be taken up in the negotiations as early as possible. She felt that discussion on these issues should not be delayed indefinitely as transitional mechanisms like the proposed joint task force could be used by the negotiating parties to evade political accountability and a human rights framework. As mentioned earlier, in most of her objections about and criticisms of the peace talks, she took care to let it be known that she did not wish to jeopardise the talks in any manner.

Partly driven by her instinctive desire not to allow the UNP grab the full credit for any eventual peace deal with the Tigers and also to introduce a legitimate broad-basing of the talks, so crucial to establish peace in the country, Kumaratunga proposed a national commission for ethnic reconciliation and sustainable peace that would include, apart from the government and the LTTE, all the parties and groups represented in parliament and major non-governmental organisations.

"A clear action plan must be formulated, " she said in an address declaring her intent to pursue the re-democratisation and re-humanisation of Sri Lanka, " with the purpose of bringing (the) military conflict to an end and finding a durable solution to the causes of the conflict."

Regretting the anti Tamil riots that broke out two decades ago giving rise to the ethnic conflict, she said, "The clear failure of the Sri Lanka state to protect its Tamil citizens in July, 1983, is a watershed event in ethnic relations. It was a failure which I deeply regret." She described the riots as "a true tragedy of epic proportion."

The cold war between the president and the government over the conduct of peace talks continued, not always in the form of acrimony but sometimes disguised in diplomatic manoeuvres. Thus, Kumaratunga was quick to welcome the outcome of the peace support mission in Oslo on 25 November, 2002, at which the donor countries demanded that the LTTE renounce terror and that human rights and democratic values be included for negotiation in the peace process.

Her spokesman Harim Peiris told the media, "The appeal by the US to the LTTE to give up violence and its armed struggle and the reference in the Oslo Declaration to human rights and democracy shows that the president's concerns have been taken into consideration." It was quite another matter that the LTTE did not commit itself to a straightforward renunciation of violence if the talks failed; all it conceded at the time was that it would try to avoid conflict in future.

After ensuring that the Oslo Declaration would rather add to her credit than to that of the prime minister, Kumaratunga emphasised that she continued to be concerned over the LTTE's conduct during the peace process which was not at all being faithful to the spirit of the ceasefire as the rebel outfit was seeking to expand its "illegal kangaroo courts" and "police stations", thus seriously eroding the state's judicial power and sovereignty.

As an example, her spokesman referred to the LTTE-organised protests against the Eelam People's Democratic Party, which was the only opposition to the Tigers in the Jaffna Peninsula, an act which clearly went against the chief Tigers negotiator Anton Balasingham's claim in Thailand that there would be no fetters on political activities in the northeast. Thus, as the government continued to parley with the LTTE, the president quietly stepped in to protect the EPDP by instructing the police and the navy to provide protection to the party cadre and office in Delft Island.

Kumaratunga was also insisting at the time that decommissioning of weapons by the Tigers should begin as the talks went on. There should first be a renunciation of weapons and then its implementation on the ground. "It is the president's clear stance that decommissioning should take place, and this is a good time to make a beginning, " said her spokesman. Besides, the president was still keen, even as the talks were continuing for some time, that her nominee should be accommodated as an observer in the negotiations. This was necessary as the regular briefings after each round of talks by a senior minister were proving to be inadequate. She was thereby implying that she was not being told the entire truth about the talks.

As the battle of wits continued between the president, the government and the LTTE over the contents of peace talks, the norms of behaviour appropriate to the occasion and the implementation of the provisions of the ceasefire agreement, the difference of perception between the president and the government became clearer day by day.

In hindsight, it is interesting to see that when the president was digging out various misdemeanours on the part of the Tigers and acts of omission and commission on the part of the government, the latter was preoccupied with defending the peace process and thus necessarily appearing to protect the interests of the LTTE.

Reacting to Velupillai Prabhakaran's 26 November 2002, annual address over the clandestine rebel radio, the cabinet spokesman, chief government negotiator and constitutional affairs minister G L Peiris said, "We find much of the substance (of Prabhakaran's address) helpful and encouraging. They are now shifting away from the demand for a separate state to a solution within the country."

Curiously, Peiris took it upon himself to defend Prabhakaran in respect of his threat, made during the course of the speech, to revive the campaign for independence if the demand for self-rule based on "internal self-determination" was rejected by the government. Arguing that the speech was markedly different from the previous ones, he said that the secessionist option was merely related to a "hypothetical situation" in the case of a breakdown of talks. In any case, there was little prospect of talks failing because the government was ready to offer substantial devolution of power to the Tamils.

The positions of the government and the LTTE were not antithetical to each other; "There are and there will remain differences, but the purpose is to narrow them down." "Of course, we don't agree with all of it, " he added, "there may be some deficiencies." Such statements could only exacerbate the president's anxiety to take care of the interests of the Sri Lankan state from the hands of a government which probably did not know what it was talking about.

To be fair to the Wickramasinghe government, however, it was taking steps at this time to dismantle any LTTE court that may have come up in the government-controlled territory; it was to these rebel courts and police stations that the president had earlier referred and ordered their dismantlement.

The sporadic presidential acts to rein in the government which appeared to be rushing into a "peace trap", to use a favourite Sinhalese phrase describing the peace process, came to be crystallised into a policy statement by her party, Sri Lanka Freedom Party, demanding a larger role for her in the negotiations. At the same time, the SLFP made it clear that it was against granting an interim administration for the northeast, which would apparently be dominated by LTTE nominees, before a final solution could be agreed upon.

In a subtle touch of the traditional rivalry with the United National Party led by Wickramasinghe, the SLFP said that it supported a negotiated settlement of the ethnic conflict and would not sabotage the peace process in the "destructive" way that the UNP did to its own peace initiative. However, it listed conditions that must be met if the UNP wanted its cooperation. Chief among these was the demand that the president played a larger role in the peace process by recognising that she was the head of state, head of the executive and of the government, head of the cabinet, commander-in-chief of the armed forces and the leader of the SLFP and of the People's alliance.

The SLFP response came at a time when Wickramasinghe, preoccupied with pushing the peace process down the throat of a hostile Sinhalese community, had appealed to the polity to move away from confrontational politics in the interests of building a pluralistic society.

It was, therefore, in the fitness of things that the SLFP asked the government to practise what it preached by adopting a united approach to the peace process. "As the LTTE has pronounced time and again, for a sustainable solution to be found to the ethnic problem it is essential that there should be agreement between the two main parties and at least consultation with other parties, " the party said in a statement. It also suggested that a standing committee should be set up under the joint leadership of the president and the prime minister to guide the peace process.

Do all these sound a bit ironical in today's context when Kumaratunga, who had continued to be the president, was found using the same argument to persuade the UNP to come forward and share responsibility for the peace process? Three years ago, it was the

UNP and its leader Wickramasinghe appealing for the SLFP's and the president's cooperation and the latter were demanding a larger role in the peace process in exchange for cooperation.

The sequence of events leading to the signing of the ceasefire agreement indicated that the government did not want the president to start opposing before the act was sealed; the agreement had to be a fait accompli.

Accordingly, Prabhakaran signed a copy of the agreement, handed over by the Norwegian ambassador, on 20 February 2002, in Killinochchi. The following day the agreement was shown to the president. Then, on 22 February 2002, Wickramasinghe signed the agreement in Vavuniya, the northern town. Two days later, the Sri Lanka Monitoring Mission arrived to begin monitoring the observance of the ceasefire agreement.

Three days later, on 27 February 2002, the president wrote to the prime minister with the following observations: that the ceasefire agreement had been submitted to her at the eleventh hour; the legality of the document was in question because article 4.1 of the agreement required only the signatures of the prime minister and the LTTE leader and not of the president; certain articles of the agreement could impinge on national security; the agreement should not be made an end in itself and the government should ensure that substantive issues were raised and settled at the talks; the implication of Art. 1.2 "offensive naval operations" needed to be clarified; Art.1.3 appeared to disallow the Sri Lankan navy from engaging LTTE boats even if they were suspected of carrying arms; the government should give clear instructions to the navy as to its powers and duties regarding illegal arms shipment by the rebels; and despite the ceasefire, the LTTE was continuing to violate its own assurances given to the United Nations on child recruitment.

As the tussle between the president and the prime minister continued with the tension mounting following the presidential letter, the chief LTTE negotiator Anton Balasingham chose to describe Kumaratunga's objections to the manner in which the government was conducting the peace process as "irresponsible, injurious and ill-advised."

Balasingham said that the president's so-called concern was untenable and fallacious as the demarcation of territories between the government and the LTTE reflected the ground realities and, without taking them into account, the ceasefire agreement could not have been achieved.

The LTTE then went to the extent of demanding, as was already being demanded by elements in the ruling United National Front, that unless the president was removed, she would wreck the peace process. Sources well-informed about the LTTE's thinking said that the rebels were concerned over the continuance in power of president Chandrika kumaratunga and the perceived inactivity of prime minister Ranil Wickramasinghe in taking meaningful action to remove her from office.

The rebels chose to link any progress in the peace process with the removal of Kumaratunga from office, saying that she was posing a perpetual threat to the process and that the Wickramasinghe government should lose no further time in getting rid of her. Unless the end of the road was in sight for co-habitation (the system of the president and the prime minister belonging to different political parties but running the same government) they felt, there could not be meaningful progress for the peace process.

Behind all this bluster was the knowledge that under the Sri Lankan constitution, the president was all powerful and that it was Kumaratunga and not Wickramasinghe who could actually move to unseat the other. The only constitutional way the president could be removed from office was by impeaching her and finding her guilty of misdemeanour in office.

That would not be easy as her objections to the ceasefire agreement and the manner in which the peace process was being handled found strong resonance in the popular Sinhalese opinion; it was also no secret that the armed forces had been unhappy about the ceasefire agreement on the grounds that it was the rebels who were cornering all the advantages and privileges of the cessation of hostilities.

The denouement came on 4 November 2003, when Wickramasinghe was visiting the US; the president took over the ministries of defence, interior and mass communications (state media) on the grounds that the security of the country was being threatened and that the policies were not being adequately reflected in the government-controlled media. For a few months more, the government hobbled on but the peace process came to be abruptly halted as the government felt that without the key ministries in hand, continuing the talks had become impossible.

The two leaders are thus saddled with a baggage of history which they are condemned to carry as part of their leadership heritage unless they pause to reflect on the enormous opportunity, history has thrust upon them to make a clean break from the sordid past of hypocrisy, narrow partisanship and self-defeatism practised by them and their predecessors.

This has become imperative as the quarrelling Sinhalese leaders cannot escape addressing the stiffest political challenge posed by the LTTE so far, through the ISGA proposals. The majority leadership must find an acceptable response to the Tamil Tigers' fait accompli and by all indications, this would not be possible until there is unity in the leadership.

Analysing their mutual bickerings earlier this year, Dr Jayadeva Uyangoda wrote, "...both leaders appear to practise the worst aspects of the legacy of the J R Jayewardene school of politics, manipulation and deceit. Both Kumaratunga and Wickramasinghe appear to think that manipulation and deceit make them smart and sophisticated politicians."[2]

The pity was that nearly at the end of the year, the two leaders continued to try to outmanoeuvre each other, pushing the prospects of an understanding further back.

On 3 October, 2004, Kumaratunga wrote back to Wickremasinghe regretting the UNP's decision to boycott the inaugural meeting of the National Advisory Council on Peace and Reconciliation which was expected to be a truly representative body of all political parties and groups elected to parliament and now stood bereft of its raison d'etre since the main opposition party had decided to shun it.

"I am rather perplexed at the reasons you provide for this unfortunate decision and sincerely hope you will reconsider this for the following reasons, " Kumaratunga wrote. She argued that the UNP should reverse its decision and cooperate with the advisory body because: firstly, discussions with the LTTE would not be exclusively on the interim authority but on a "wider agenda" though they could be so initially (which would thus take care of the main complaint of the UNP); and, secondly, the present government was firmly pledged to resumption of negotiations with the LTTE which were broken off when the latter walked off from talks being held with the UNF government.

While Wickramasinghe wanted the present government to start discussions with the LTTE on the ISGA and UNF government proposals, it was pertinent to note that the LTTE had unequivocally rejected the latter proposals many times over. "It is thus crystal clear that you are advising me to resume negotiations with the LTTE on a basis, part of which, as you are fully aware, has totally been rejected by the LTTE, " Kumaratunga argued with a fair amount of logic.

She clarified that she was not seeking a consensus of the parliamentary parties in the advisory body "as a precondition either to begin talks with the LTTE" or to make the body responsible for decisions concerning the talks (which would, therefore, answer the UNP's unspoken reason for steering clear of the advisory body) and followed up by making "honest and workable" suggestions. The advisory body would be a consultative forum for the government enabling it to keep the country informed and to be abreast of the views of the people through their representatives in parliament. "We do not in any way wish to use this process of consultation through the (advisory body) to run away from the government's total responsibility of seeking means of resolving the conflict of the northeast."

In her parting shot, Kumaratunga said, "The country is aware that I have during the past ten years made numerous efforts to find ways to bring the country's two major political parties, the UNP and the PA (People's Alliance), to work together in the national interest—especially with regard to the ethnic conflict—and that these efforts failed to come to fruition due to the consistent rejection of each of my proposals by the UNP."[3]

Wickramasinghe on his part announced, with a lot of apparent magnanimity, on 10 October 2004, that he was giving carte blanche to revive the stalled peace talks with the LTTE. "We have given you and your government carte blanche to proceed with the engagement with the LTTE in talks, " he said in a letter to the president. But behind this ostensible gesture of reasonableness lay a totally expected twist in an honest representation of the relations between the two eternally feuding leaders, which took nobody by surprise.

It was on 9 September, 2004, that Kumaratunga and Wickremasinghe met at President's House to discuss the government's invitation to the latter to co-chair the proposed advisory body and to support the efforts to resume negotiations with the Tamil Tigers. On 12 September, Sri Lankan newspapers reported that the leader of the opposition had declined the offer though he had promised his MPs' support in parliament to any decision that the president would succeed in arriving at with the LTTE. The reason for not agreeing to associate with the consultation process, according to the reports, was that not being part of the decision-making authority but being part of the advisory body, Wickramasinghe would not have full control over the process but would, nevertheless, be held accountable for its actions and decisions. This might affect his credibility and would restrict his ability to negotiate with the LTTE once he was back in power as his credibility would have been harmed by his association with the advisory body. "Chandrika's peace trap and Ranil's googly" was how one newspaper headlined its analysis of the latest spat between the two top Sinhalese leaders.

This was, however, followed by the UNP's announcement on 16 September of its unreserved support to the government as it considered the resumption of peace negotiations a national endeavour. In a typical caveat, UNP spokesman and the chief peace negotiator of the Wickramasinghe government. Prof. G L Peiris, thereafter, added, "But before we extend our support, the government should make its stance clear regarding the basis for the resumption of the talks. The Janatha Vimukthi Peramuna, which is the main coalition partner of the United People's Freedom Alliance (UPFA), has been strongly opposing the ISGA proposals as a basis for talks and this is the main stumbling block."

A second caveat put forward was that once this inner contradiction was resolved (a very unlikely possibility given the inner politics of the coalition government and the JVP's clear stand against the ISGA proposals), the UNP would support the interim structure that was agreed on and announced through the Tokyo Declaration. "It is on that basis that the international community agreed to give their financial and other support to Sri Lanka, " Peiris said. "Today we also see another build-up where the Ceylon Workers' Congress, the new entrant to the UPFA government, calling on the president to restart talks with the LTTE even without the support of the JVP...however, the JVP has said that all partners in the UPFA coalition must conform to the agreement of the alliance." The UNP would throw in its lot once the government sorted out its differences. "Otherwise, it would be a futile exercise on the part of the government to call on the opposition to express their views on restarting talks." Thus, there was no change in the position of the UNP with regard to responding to the president's call for cooperation in the matter.

Daily Mirror commented on the same day, " But it is discernible that the avowal of support (in parliament) is perfunctory, clearly devoid of the sincerity or seriousness that the present situation demands. This statement smacks of an indifferent attitude to the president's suggestion made with a view to getting the opposition also actively involved in the peace process at a time when the whole country wants these two parties to act unitedly on this issue. Will the president's appeal to place the country's interests before party interests—an appeal repeated ad nauseum by politicians while assiduously boosting the latter—have any effect, in this context?"

Kumaratunga was obviously not in a position to honour the UNP's caveat and was perforce obliged to go ahead with the exercise of convening the advisory body, knowing fully well that irrespective of the validity of the two caveats, the UNP would not have responded affirmatively to her invitation to join the consultation process. Thus, Wickramasinghe's letter to Kumaratunga and Peiris' statement meant little and the "carte blanche" part of the UNP response amounted to nothing because the government needed not the UNP's permission but its cooperation in going ahead with peace negotiations. But the UNP obviously had no intention of doing so.

But a day later, what truly surprised the author was Wickramasinghe's flat denial that he had been offered the cochairpersonship of the advisory body. "The offer to make me the co-chair was not made, " he said. "It was mere newspaper speculation; that was why I or my party did not bother to contradict it. She sought our support in parliament and I said we would give you full support provided you first come to a decision with the LTTE. But can she first carry her government with her?"[4]

While saying this, the former prime minister made a typical gesture of enjoying the turn of events by slightly swaying his head to and fro.

Unfortunately for Sri Lanka, the endemic personality-based political rivalry between the two main Sinhalese parties appears to have acted negatively in helping them resolve the country's principal conflict. For example, looking at today's enormous mess created mainly by a continuous overdose of Sinhalese Buddhist chauvinism, which also went for Sinhalese nationalism and came into being mainly as a tool to outplay either party (epitomised in the Bandaranaike-led SLFP's decisive victory in the 1956 general election), it would be difficult to realise that Sri Lanka's first prime minister D S Senanayake (1947-52) presented an image of a staunch believer in the pluralism of the polity as a source of strength, not of weakness, and identified the establishment of a sense of Sri Lankan nationalism through a resolute subordination of ethnic and religious identities as one of the principal and most urgent concerns of any transfer of power in a political settlement.

To quote Dr K M de Silva, the essence of Senanayake's policies was contained in Clause 8 of the Ministers' draft constitution of 1944, prepared under his leadership and drafted by his constitutional adviser Sir Ivor Jennings (then vice-chancellor of the University of Ceylon) and a constitutional expert. Under that clause, legislation which sought to prohibit or restrict the free exercise of any religion, to make persons of any community or religion liable to disabilities or restrictions to which persons of other communities or religions were not liable, or to confer on persons of any community or religion any privileges or advantages which were not conferred on persons of other communities or religions, or to alter the constitution of any religious body except with the approval of the governing authority of that religious body...would require a special two-thirds majority in the lower house of the legislature. It is noteworthy that in the aftermath of independence, debate in Sri Lanka revolved, apart from two other subjects, around the emerging conflict between supporters of the primacy of Buddhism and the Sinhalese in the polity,; the other two being the dominion status and membership of the Commonwealth and a defence pact with the UK which was seen to be pushing the country into the Anglo-American block in the emerging Cold War scenario.

It is also necessary to note that while only the leftists were vocal in the debates over the latter two subjects, there was a much wider popular support base in the debate over the primacy of Buddhism, indicating the nature of things to come. As de Silva shows, the debate over religion vs secularism remained restrained mainly because of its mature handling by Senanayake. This became apparent during the following two prime ministerships, that of his son Dudley Senanayake (1952-55) and of Sir John Kotelawala (1953-56), who yielded ground gradually to Sinhalese-Buddhist chauvinists in the hope of appeasing them and in turn get re-elected to office for a second term. Political opportunism had won over from D S Senanayake's principled stand on religion and secularism and Sri Lanka was beginning a dangerous journey to unknown destinations.[5]

Very quickly thereafter, in the course of a few months during 1954-55, all the familiar facets of Sinhalese-Buddhist chauvinism came on the surface challenging the principles of pluralism and secularism, and Sinhalese nationalism began to claim its supremacy in the country. The 1956 elections came, and S W R D Bandaranaike exploited the emerging Sinhalese-Buddhist chauvinism to the hilt. De Silva writes, "His decisive victory was a significant turning point in Sri Lanka's history, for it represented the rejection of the concept of a Sri Lankan nationalism based on an acceptance of pluralism as an essential feature of a democratic political system, and its substitution by a more democratic and populist nationalism which was fundamentally divisive in its impact on the country, because of its unmistakably Sinhalese and Buddhist orientation."

This was also the year of the 2, 500th birth anniversary of Lord Buddha, and the resurgent Sinhalese-Buddhist chauvinism exploited this platform to make the movement totally oriented towards the

Sinhalese language, and the phenomenon of linguistic nationalism hit the island nation, so long cocooned in the warmth of a foreign language that had nurtured the ruling class since the preceding century, with the force of an unexpected gale. The unique force was reinforced in its gathering strength by a simultaneous evocation of Sri Lanka's past, which was perceived to be all Sinhalese and Buddhism and very idyllic in which there was no room for any other dispensation.

"All the major Sri Lankan political parties of Bandaranaike's day were baffled by this novel phenomenon of linguistic nationalism, " writes de Silva. "Yet, the imperatives of their calling compelled each in turn to define their attitude to it. Most of them eventually succumbed to the blandishments of linguistic nationalism. None understood the perils involved. They may have been less complacent if they had turned to the history of Europe where this phenomenon had appeared in the mid-19th century and had such a destructive impact on the politics of central Europe... In Sri Lanka, (linguistic nationalism) has contributed greatly to disturbing the civil peace since the mid-1950's."

The consequences of this transformation of nationalism for the processes of state-building in Sri Lanka were: firstly, the concept of a multi-ethnic polity ceased to be politically viable any longer; and secondly, the validity of this change derived from the majority status of the Sinhalese-Buddhist community in the total population.

Disputes and clashes began to appear at this juncture as the Tamil community in particular and the Sinhalese christians as well refused to accept the contention that Sinhalese nationalism and Sri Lankan nationalism were synonymous. While the following decade witnessed rising tension between the majority Sinhalese community and the minority Tamil and Christian communities mainly over the phenomenon of linguistic nationalism, which was forcing the Sinhalese language down the throat of the people, the period right up to the 1970's also saw the strengthening and establishment of Sinhalese-Buddhist chauvinism as the decisive factor in Sri Lankan politics.

The influence of the latter grew so much that even leftists, including the true-blue Marxists, found it increasingly expedient to succumb to its charm as the compulsions of parliamentary democracy continued to mould their policy of siding with the Bandaranaikes-led Sri Lanka Freedom Party. Describing those days, de Silva writes, "Indeed, the two Bandaranaikes (S W R D and Mrs Sirimavo) between them had established a new equilibrium of political forces within the country, and their own supporters and their associates (such as the Marxist Left) as well as their opponents (such as the UNP) had to accommodate themselves to this political reality in the 1960's and 1970's at least."

"The primary feature of this new balance of forces had been the acceptance of the predominance of the Sinhalese and Buddhists within the Sri Lanka polity, and as a corollary of this, a sharp decline in the status of the ethnic and religious minorities. Neither the UNP nor the Marxist Left (was) entirely happy with the latter situation, but political prudence required them to refrain from any public repudiation of at least the first part of this arrangement. This was especially difficult for the UNP since it was the alternative government for much of the 1970's and aspiring to power."

"Repudiation of both these conditions came during their long term in office, from 1977 to 1994, but by this time they were confronted by a sharp radicalisation of Tamil political activity in the north of the island and a burgeoning separatist movement."

It is, however, possible to differ with K M de Silva in his narration of the early years of independent Sri Lanka in terms of the relations between the majority and minority communities. For example, some commentators believe that D S Senanayake was not entirely above Sinhalese chauvinism either; otherwise, why did he go after Tamils of Indian origin and disenfranchised nearly a million of them by bringing legislation, the Citizenship Act of December, 1948, and the Parliamentary Elections Amendment Act of 1949, reducing the representation of the minority communities to less than 20 per cent of the total number of seats in parliament?

"What these Acts did was to make non-citizens of the Tamil plantation labour who formed about 10 per cent of the national population or about a third of the minority population, and deprive them of their votes. What was surprising, however, was that almost all of the Tamil elite representing the Ceylon Tamils through both

Mr Senanayake's United National Party and the Tamil Congress, either voted for the bills or were not serious about opposing them. The Sinhalese elite discovered very early that they could easily call the bluff of the Tamil elite, especially the Colombo Tamil", wrote *The Broken Palmyra*.[6]

To go by this seminal work on the travails of the Tamil community in Sri Lanka, what almost certainly motivated Prime Minister Senanayake was "his alarm over the strength in parliament of the working class-based parties of the left, which comprised 20 out of a total of 95 seats in parliament." The UNP had obtained only 41 seats, seven short of a simple majority. With their strength, the left members could in future even manage a berth in a coalition government. "It was thus natural for the UNP to think of perpetuating its political and class dominance by knocking out a large section of the working class which was the most easily isolated." In the very next elections in 1952, the UNP's strength rose to a comfortable 54 seats. The passing of the discriminatory acts left its mark on Sri Lankan history. Leader of the leftist Lanka Sama Samaj Party Dr N M Perera said, "I thought racialism of this type died with Houston Chamberlain and Adolph Hitler. I do not believe that any one claiming to be a statesman would ask us to accede to a bill of this nature...We cannot proceed as if we were God's chosen race quite apart from the rest of the world; that we and we alone have the right to be citizens of this country."

Thus, while Senanayake's secular credentials were under a cloud, he was also guilty of being cynical and playing ethnic Tamil interests against those of the Indian or plantation Tamils and succeeded in getting parliamentary support from ethnic Tamil MPs to facilitate the passing of the legislation. But clearly the seeds of Sri Lanka's future nemesis lay in this act of Senanayake though only one man, S J V Chelvanayakam could discern the writing on the wall at the time. After he had resigned from the Tamil Congress in protest against the party's stand on the Indian Tamil question in 1948, Chelvanayakam predicted, " Today it is the Indian Tamils. Tomorrow it will be the Ceylon Tamils who will be axed."

Were the seeds of the future discord which would engulf the country one day into a seemingly interminable bloody conflict, laying vast tracts of the land waste, thousands of its citizens killed and maimed and thousands more driven out, planted in those two Acts of parliament? Colombo had certainly perpetrated its first folly; in the years to come, the follies would multiply tearing the country apart. And in all this, tragically, the rival UNP and the SLFP could only calculate their own electoral gains lending scant regard for consequences for the country.

It was the political career of Solomon West Ridgeway Dias Bandaranaike, father of President Kumaratunga, a born Christian and a typical South Asian product of British colonialism, which chronicles with a chilling faithfulness the transition of Ceylon (and, in later years, Sri Lanka) from a largely innocuous feudal rural society into a virulent pro-Sinhalese, pro-Buddhist and anti-minority country, racked by communal and insurrectionist violence. He quit the UNP in 1951 and formed the Sri Lanka Freedom Party (SLFP); in less than five years, riding the newly roused communal passions of the majority community, he would romp home to form the first SLFP-led coalition government. The electoral politics (beating the rival in the hustings by any means) of the majority community would thus continue to give shape to the ethnic divide that would lead one day to the ethnic conflict.

The first major indication of a rapidly growing ethnic divide was available in the violent anti-government campaign that erupted in the Sinhalese-Buddhist region following Prime Minister Sir John Kotelawala's announcement in Jaffna in 1955 that his government would accord an equal constitutional status to the Sinhala and Tamil languages. To the government's dismay, a diabolic twist was given to its announcement by spreading a rumour that the actual plan was to force the Sinhalese majority to study Tamil (is it not immensely ironical that a suggestion was being made in the late-2004 by sections of the Sinhalese community that members of the two communities should learn each other's languages?). This was the opportunity that SWRD Bandaranaike, an eminent product of Anglo-Asian liberalism till then, was apparently lying in wait for. As the ruling UNP stood sharply divided over the issue, he took up the leadership of all pro-Sinhala language groups and demanded that the majority language be declared the sole official language and Tamil could be allowed only "reasonable use" in government work (one grievance that Tamils today harbour is that despite the parity restored between the two languages, Tamil is not being given due recognition in government work which requires that every document, circular, etc., is translated into the language as well and that this is not being done as thoroughly as it should be).

Sir John, the other true-blue anglicised liberal, then did a breathtaking volte face, as his support base in the ruling party slipped dangerously, declaring that he was equally in favour of making Sinhala the sole official language. To him, this outright betrayal of the hopes and aspirations of the Tamils was the only political ploy in hand to checkmate the SLFP's Bandaranaike. His capitulation before the threat from Bandaranaike was a graphic illustration of how the Sinhalese electoral politics was getting inextricably mixed with the Sinhalese-Tamil relations.

His next act, calling for fresh parliamentary elections, was naturally based on his optimism that he had outmanoeuvred his opponents. In reality, the 1956 elections pushed the country inexorably towards further blunder and chaos. The language issue continued to dominate the election campaign with Bandaranaike sounding even more chauvinistic and declaring that within the first 24 hours of his election victory as the next Prime Minister Sinhala would be made the sole official language; as he sensed that the majority community was now fully roused on the communal line, he conveniently dropped his earlier call for allowing Tamil "reasonable use" in government work.

The next step that he took, the enactment of the popularly called "Sinhala Only Act" sealed the fate of Sri Lanka, exposing the essentially communal politics (tagged necessarily to the urgency of outwitting the rival party) that the ruling SLFP and the opposition UNP exploited shamelessly, without pondering over the inevitable consequences. The worst folly of them all had been committed, and the country continues to pay a terrible price after forty-eight years of independence and twenty-one years of armed conflict later.

All histories of modern Sri Lanka record at this stage the few sane voices from the Sinhalese community who clearly foresaw the seeds of the future Armageddon being planted. LSSP member of parliament and a giant of Sri Lankan politics Colvin R de Silva, participating in the debate over the "Sinhala Only" bill, uttered words which later became immortal and were destined to be remembered with a sense of de'ja` vu, "Two torn little bleeding states may yet arise out of one little state (if the bill is passed)...One language, two countries; two languages, one country." Another LSSP member Leslie Goonawardene prophesied that if the Tamils felt that a "grave and irreparable" injustice was being meted out to them, "there is a possibility of their deciding even to break away from the rest of the country." It is remarkable with today's hindsight to realise that these two Sinhalese leftists and one Tamil liberal could clearly foresee the extreme possible repercussions of the legislative steps that Sri Lanka's first prime minister and himself a liberal initiated which culminated in a few years' time into what another prime minister, again an avowed liberal to begin with but later turned by opportunism into an ethnic chauvinist, completed.

Sinhalese foolhardiness goaded constantly by the Sinhalese-Buddhist chauvinism did not, however, remain confined to the legislative arena. As the "Sinhala Only" bill was introduced in parliament on 5 June, 1956, Chelvanayakam led about 300 Federal Party members in a peaceful sit-in demonstration on the Galle Face Green opposite Parliament House (later the presidential secretariat). As the Tamils demonstrated peacefully, a mob of Sinhalese-Buddhist monks and others, which had reached parliament to express solidarity with the bill, pounced upon and thrashed, kicked and spat upon them as the police watched disinterestedly.

Appalled by the naked display of communal passion and the partisan role of the government, Chelvanayakam, who had been spared personal humiliation, called the demonstration off. The passion let loose by the opportunistic majoritarian politics, however, quickly went out of control; anti-Tamil riots spread all over the country; and while the law and order machinery began to hit back, the tally at the end of the mayhem was 150 killed, most of them Tamils and women and children to boot. Tamil-owned business establishments were, of course, a special target of the raging Sinhalese mobs. The face of Sri Lanka was now changed for ever; it had clearly ceased to be a tolerant society, poisoned by the deadly virus of communalism. The moment also marked the demise of Tamil liberalism reared in a fusion of the best European tradition and the Indian freedom movement, and the rise of radicalism, symbolised by the fall of Chelvanayakam and the rise of Appapillai Amirthalingam.

A little over two months later on 19 August 1956, the Federal Party, badly shaken by the confrontation with the Sinhalese-Buddhist communalism, held a national convention in Trincomalee and adopted a resolution, demanding that the country's unitary constitution be replaced with a federal one, that the Tamil and Sinhala languages should be at par, that the highly discriminatory citizenship laws should be repealed forthwith, and that the deliberate colonisation of Tamil-inhabited areas by the repatriation of Sinhalese families should be immediately stopped. It is worth noting that 44 years later, the Sinhalese are yet to accept the concept of federalism despite the presentation of the devolution package by the government of the day in the mid-1990's. As for the colonisation of the eastern province that the Federal Party took strong objection to all those years ago, it is a fait accompli today and constitutes the bulk of the logic of the majority community in refusing to concede the province as part of any assumed Tamil "homeland."

If the sit-in demonstration on the Galle Face Green had ended in a fiasco, the Federal Party was threatening to organise a civil disobedience movement throughout the northeast if the demands made out in Trincomalee were not honoured. The Trincomalee convention itself was preceded by a long march by thousands of visibly indignant Tamils led by MPs who walked from Kankasenthurai in the north and Tirukkovil in the south. It was becoming increasingly obvious that the accumulated grievances of the Tamils, who were so long battling growing incidences of racial discrimination silently and individually, had at last found a powerful means of expression through an organised people's movement.

Newer forms of protests against the Sinhalese-Buddhist chauvinism were coming to the fore as time passed. The following independence day, 4 February 1957, was marked by Tamils in many areas as a day of mourning and would continue to be observed thus for almost ten years. However, the perceptible toughening of the Tamil opinion appeared to have alerted Bandaranaike to the dangers ahead and may have prompted him to think of granting a sop to the roused Tamils.

As a result, he negotiated the Bandaranaike-Chelvanayakam Pact of 29 July, 1957, providing for autonomous regional councils in Tamil-dominated areas; if implemented in sincerity, this could have proved to be a stepping stone to a limited devolution of power in the future. The promised privilege of regional councils was, however, granted on a compromise that the Tamils made on their demand for a parity between the Sinhala and Tamil languages. The UNP, which had been relegated to the wilderness of opposition, sensed the Bandaranaike-Chelvanayakam Pact as the opportunity it had been waiting for to catch the government off-guard and improve its electoral prospects.

Sinhalese leaders, thereafter, went around rousing anti-Tamil passions as part of the UNP's wreck-the-pact campaign, and the star campaigner proved to be the future President Junius Richard Jayewardene who led a landmark march from Colombo to Kandy opposing the pact. As communal passions raged, the government not only dithered over implementing the controversial pact but also sought to pamper the majority community by bringing about a law seeking to prefix the Sinhala letter "Sri" in motor vehicle number plates. The aroused Tamils served notice of their vehement opposition to the move, described by them as further communalisation of Sri Lankan society. They blackened all "Sri"s in the number plates of government buses plying in Jaffna.

This in turn enraged Buddhist monks further, sending them protesting against government inaction outside Bandaranaike's residence. The latter, surrendering once more to the inherently dangerous politics of majoritarianism, soon announced the abrogation of the Bandaranaike-Chelvanayakam Pact much to the joy of the victorious Buddhist monks and to the universal dismay of the Tamils who felt that they had been freshly betrayed by the Sinhalese leadership.

Meanwhile, with the inevitability of a classic Greek tragedy, the much graver anti-Tamil riots of 1958 had broken out in a spree of loot, arson and killings. For the first time, with Tamil retaliation in the north, the Sinhalese also became refugees. The process of the sucking of the country into the vortex of a debilitating ethnic strife was clearly intensifying. Tamil refugees in Colombo had to be repatriated to Jaffna and Trincomalee by ship from the southern port. There were many who asked if the two communities had reached the point of no return. Fate then caught up with the main Sinhalese player in the tragedy, Bandaranaike, who was assassinated (the first political assassination in the island nation, to be followed by many more and continuing in 2004) by a Buddhist monk on 25 September, 1959, after he had made a half-hearted attempt to propitiate the dark Tamil mood by getting a bill allowing "reasonable use" of Tamil in government work adopted by parliament.

Bandaranaike's assassination was followed by a dissolution of parliament. Fresh elections were held in July 1960, in which rank communal passions dominated the scene in Sinhalese-majority areas. The elections also threw up the world's first woman Prime Minister, Mrs Sirimavo Bandaranaike, SWRD's widow and President Kumaratunga's mother. These elections also witnessed the leftist LSSP abandoning its pro-Tamil image and going the whole hog in embracing Sinhalese chauvinism. Apparently, the overriding electoral compulsions were playing havoc with the surviving ideological scruples of the sole Sinhalese-dominated party which had remained a bridge between the two drifting communities.

Recalling the history of the first few years of independent Sri Lanka until the rise of Sinhalese-Buddhist chauvinism is instructive in several ways, the principal of them being the realisation that nearly fifty years later, the Sinhalese polity is being called upon to restore the lost validity of multi-ethnic pluralism and Sri Lankan nationalism to the country. This is enormously educative because the vehicle through which this message has been conveyed is the Tamil insurgency and the instrument through which the act of restoration of the lost ideals and principles could be attempted is federalism.

Fortunately, the country is not entirely mired in the mindset that made the transition from the age of D S Senanayake to that of S W R D Bandaranaike possible and both the concepts of multi-ethnic pluralism and federalism are being debated and certain advancement has been made with regard to federalism, though the draft constitution remains confined to paper.

The majority community is still far from accepting either or both the concepts though accepting the first concept would facilitate embracing the second concept, a logical and therefore, much easier step.

The primary responsibility of educating the majority community to the extent where the acceptance of the concept of federalism becomes possible, however, rests with the Sinhalese political leadership, and that is precisely where the danger of a failure lurks. It is more than ironical that while both the leaders, Kumaratunga and Wickramasinghe, have publicly accepted the justifiability of federalism in the Sri Lankan context, they may yet fail to complete the task of persuading the majority community to go along with them in embracing the concept because they are unable to cooperate with each other.

As the former prime minister made clear in his conversation with the author, Kumaratunga should find it beyond her capacity to persuade the JVP to fall in line and support dialogue with the LTTE. "The internal politics of the ruling alliance prevents any such possibility," he said, drawing apparent satisfaction from the stalemate reached between the president and the JVP over the matter.

As in the electoral rivalry between the UNP and the SLFP, so in the tussle between the SLFP and the JVP it is electoral politics and not the ethnic conflict that continues to determine the behavioural pattern of the players. The JVP has already made dangerous inroads into the SLFP's traditional vote bank, the Sinhalese-Buddhist constituency in the countryside. The party has been assiduously pursuing policies to grab more space in the constituency, and the principal policy in this enterprise is a very stiff opposition to a resumption of negotiations with the LTTE, especially over the ISGA proposals. It is to counter this pressure from the JVP that sections of the SLFP are turning increasingly hostile to the idea of fresh talks with the Tigers.

The UNP's response to the president's peace move will hence continue to be partly based on the evolution of the SLFP-JVP equation in parliamentary politics. Only if Kumaratunga succeeds in weaning the JVP away from the easy lure of electoral gain by sticking stubbornly to oppose a dialogue with the LTTE, the UNP would be forced to rethink its own recalcitrance in refusing cooperation with the government. Otherwise, it is fine with Wickramasinghe to play the role of a satisfied spoilsport in the revised scenario; a year ago, it was he who desperately wished cooperation from across the traditional party divide. The bitter history of the contemptuous relations between the two ruling parties intervened then; it continues to put a wedge between the two today.

Notes

1. Apratim Mukarji, *The War in Sri Lanka: Unending Conflict?*, Har-Anand Publications Pvt. Ltd., New Delhi, 2000, pp.146-7.
2. Jayadeva Uyangoda, *Peace Watch,* Polity, vol.1, no.5, January-February, 2004, Colombo.
3. *President regrets UNP decision to boycott Advisory Council on Peace* (3 October, 2004-10.00 GMT), Current Affairs Sri Lanka, www.priu.gov.lk, the official website of the government of Sri Lanka.
4. Interview taken at the UNP headquarters in Colombo on 17 September, 2004.
5. K M de Silva, *Ethnic Conflict: Ethnic Politics in Sri Lanka—Reaping the Whirlwind*, Penguin Books, 1998, pp.22-23.
6. Rajan Hoole, Daya Daya Somasundaram, and K Sritharan, *The Broken Palmyra: The Tamil Crisis in Sri Lanka—An Inside Account*, University of Jaffna, Jaffna, Sri Lanka, published by The Sri Lanka Studies Institute, 112, Harvard Avenue, Suit 66, Claremont, CA 91711.

Epilogue:
Tsunami and Dialogue

Six months into 2005, even the gigantic task of rebuilding the tsunami-wrecked parts of Sri Lanka appeared to have lost its urgency as a brave president battled on with her southern Marxist allies, determined to involve the Tamil rebels in a joint mechanism to undertake reconstruction work. While the JVP withdrew from the coalition government reducing the UPFA to a minority in parliament on 16 June, the LTTE sensed a further weakening of Colombo's authority.

One pro-LTTE newspaper wrote, "The political turmoil which engulfed Sri Lanka this week was utterly predictable, following as it does, a depressingly familiar pattern that has characterised ethnic relations in Sri Lanka since independence. Today's bone of contention is, of course, the proposed joint mechanism between the Liberation Tigers and the Sri Lanka government for sharing tsunami-related aid. But the Post-Tsunami Operation Management Structure (P-TOMS, also known as the Tsunami Relief Council) is merely a device around which a much deeper dispute, that of the status of the Tamil people in the Sinhalese-dominated country, has once again emerged. We emphasise people, because the rhetoric of pluralism as commonly deployed in Sri Lanka marginalises the notion of a Tamil collective identity…"[1]

The tsunami had devastated vast areas of Sri Lanka on 26 December 2004, killing outright over 30,000 people and displacing approximately 500,000 people, destroying more than a quarter of a million dwellings in seaside villages and towns in the south, the north and the east. The presidential secretariat said in a statement on 6

Epilogue: Tsunami and Dialogue

January 2005 that the human cost of the disaster was unparalleled, definitely in Sri Lanka, and every effort had to be made (already significant work by non-governmental organisations, government agencies, and the Liberation Tigers of Tamil Eelam had commenced, though without the benefits of an overall plan and strategy, and was progressing—the author) to alleviate the situation on an urgent basis. Notwithstanding the calamity caused by the tsunami disaster, it was important that the rest of the economic, social, and development activity enunciated by the recent UPFA budget, was not derailed in the process.

However, the government also responded on the same day to a rather predictable offshoot of the disaster. It said it was unfortunate that the LTTE and its "agents" were carrying on a campaign to the effect that rebels-held areas were not receiving disaster aid from the government. "The people in the affected areas in Jaffna, Killinochchi and Mullaitivu (districts) have in fact, been receiving more government assistance than those affected in the south," it said. "The government is perturbed at the conflicting statements of Thamilchelvan to the international media, that LTTE areas are not getting assistance from the government."

The campaign by the Tamil rebels soon developed into a well-mounted demand that the government permit the LTTE to play a worthwhile role in ensuring an "equitable" distribution of aid to be received from international donors. While the president responded positively and started working out a mechanism for the purpose, the rebels' demand was well-received by the international donor community which felt that a joint body comprising the government and the LTTE engaged in the tsunami-affected areas of the north and the east in reconstruction work would encourage understanding and cooperation between the two old adversaries.

Why did the LTTE turn hostile so early in the post-tsunami period when cooperation with the government should have been its obvious priority in order to fetch relief to thousands of Tamils living in the affected areas in the quickest time possible ? According to a credible report, the swiftness and spontaneity with which the Sri Lankan armed forces threw themselves into rescuing the people caught in the vicious tsunami and the rapid relief work that they began to render almost as soon as the disaster struck the north-eastern coast appeared to have alarmed the rebels who felt threatened by the unexpected development.[2]

The report said that to those whose memories of the armed forces were associated with the massacres and disappearances of 1990 and before, the tidal wave brought new revelations. The story was the same everywhere along the government-controlled seaboard along the east. It was spontaneous, uncoordinated, and not part of conventional military training.

When the disaster struck on 26 December, the army had its camps along the Vadamaratchchi coast, and itself suffered much loss. Yet, many people (later) testified to the courage and unselfishness shown by the army in helping and rescuing people. A fisherman from Katkovalam, east of Point Pedro, who was himself rescued by the army, testified that the army helped all those it could and was uniformly kind to everyone. As with many soldiers, this man was hurt when (he was) thrown against barbed wire fencing along the coast by the force of the wave.

Along the seaboard of the Trincomalee town and north of it, the navy was the only body at hand to help the civilians (mostly Tamils and Muslims). Around the 8th Mile Post (Kuchchaveli Road), in the wake of the turbulence the navy asked the civilians to run inland to the Agampodai Hill, and later in the afternoon brought food and water for them.

Similar reports came from coastal areas close to the Batticaloa town, Kallady, Amirthakali, and Navalady. Testimonials were of the army going into the water, pulling out people, and getting them to safety. "Strangely, what the media largely ignored was not lost on the Batticaloa people (living) abroad. A Batticaloa (resident) said that he (later) received telephone calls from several of his friends in Australia and New Zealand, asking him to convey their gratitude to the army brigadier in Batticaloa for the good work done by his men," the report said.

Describing the attitude that the LTTE took at this juncture, the report said that even more remarkable was its behaviour. In all these areas where the LTTE had been unremarkable in the immediate aftermath of the disaster, it began to assert itself subsequently, trying to take over the refugee camps, and demanding that all relief materials and work should be controlled by its cadre. It followed up by launching a virulent campaign against the armed forces, bringing up false charges.

Among these were that the army had burnt a refugee camp in Kudathanai, Vadamaratchchy, had supplied bad rice to the refugees, and was obstructing relief. While the army cleared the road from Vadamaratchchy to Point Pedro making it reusable for traffic, the LTTE claimed that the work was actually done by the Sea Tigers and the people.

The government, however, pointed out that the peace secretariats of the two sides had "always maintained regular dialogue on matters of mutual interest" and that since 26 December 2004 "coordination of post-tsunami relief and reconstruction have been the main topics of dialogue." It also informed that after receiving the president's letter inviting them to participate in humanitarian work, the rebels agreed to discuss the matter while the two peace secretariats began to explore ways and means of achieving this objective.

It also said that at the LTTE's request, the rehabilitation ministry purchased and despatched a fleet of pick-up trucks, tractors, generators, and water pumps to the affected areas in the north-east. Steps were also being taken to rent heavier machinery and equipment to be used for debris clearance and reconstruction in the region where these were in short supply.

Around this time, the government also took the opportunity to emphasise that there was no question of practising discrimination in relief distribution between the government-held and LTTE-controlled areas in the north-east. Foreign minister Lakshman Kadirgamar told *The Hindu* (26 January 2005) the government was acutely aware that the funds coming into the country were "other people's funds." The government was, therefore, determined to ensure equitable distribution of funds. As for the LTTE-controlled areas, a common effort would be necessary to ensure that funds were properly and effectively deployed. The funds would come to the government and it would, therefore, be its duty to ensure that there was equitable distribution.

Equally, it would be the LTTE's duty to cooperate (with the government) in an equitable distribution of funds and in the implementation of reconstruction projects in the areas controlled by it. "I have reason to believe," he added, "that the LTTE is also fully aware of the implications of the tsunami in this respect."

Kadirgamar also revealed how the government's mind was already working on the scope of further cooperation between the two adversaries even though the contours of such a relationship were not even in the horizon. "I think the best way of putting it is to say that this is a kind of a cruel blessing in disguise," he said. "Disaster has forced upon us an acute awareness of the imperative of working together in a development scenario. The concept of working together in a development scenario is something we have been talking about for decades but (the) tsunami has forced (it) within a week." As for any likelihood of resumption of peace negotiations at that juncture, the minister noted that the question was not "a matter for consideration at this point of time," and that attempts to resume talks were "definitely" on hold.

However, five months later, participating in a hearing before the US House International Relations Subcommittee for Asia and the Pacific, the US Assistant Secretary for South Asia Christina B.Rocca said on 14 June 2005, "...The cease-fire of 2002 is holding, although violence is ongoing and the peace process has stalled. This is due in part to divisions within the Sri Lankan government and the absence of trust between the government and the LTTE, which continues to use assassinations and suicide bombers, underscoring their character as an organisation wedded to terrorism and justifying their designation as a Foreign Terrorist Organisation. Recovery from last December's tsunami preempted the peace process as the primary concern of both (the) parties for the past several months. With Norwegian assistance, the parties have been negotiating an agreement to regulate the distribution of tsunami reconstruction aid. This agreement, a Joint Mechanism, is an opportunity to build trust between the parties and is, therefore, an important contribution to the peace process should it come to fruition."

President Kumaratunga expressed this sentiment rather forcefully on the day the JVP announced its withdrawal from her government

Epilogue: Tsunami and Dialogue

in protest against her determination to implement the proposed joint mechanism. "It is unfortunate ," she told the nation in a televised address, "that some sections of the media continue to project this proposed joint administrative arrangement as a 'monster.' On the contrary, this is one of the best openings in the path to reach a negotiated settlement to a 21-year-old conflict."

She also took head-on some of the principal objections raised by those who felt that the proposed body would eventually pave the way to a stronger demand for a "Tamil Eelam" (Tamil homeland). She asked the JVP to explain why the LTTE should not be absorbed into the democratic mainstream "if we were to progress as a nation." Pointing out a fundamental change in the rebel group's policy, she noted that the LTTE, which at one point in time did not recognise the government or even other communities such as the Muslims, had for the first time agreed to work with them.

Asking what was wrong in working with such an organisation in order to help the tsunami-affected people, she said that Sri Lanka should follow a path to achieve rapid economic development. The ethnic conflict and the tsunami had delayed achieving this objective. Several friendly overseas nations and peoples came forward to assist the country. They had shown faith in the management structures and stability and were confident (that) the funds pledged would be properly utilised. "Therefore, this administrative arrangement is a significant milestone in our path towards peace and prosperity," she argued.

Similarly, countering the most frequently voiced criticism of the government for seeking to collaborate with a terrorist organisation, Kumaratunga asked if the JVP, a Marxist organisation, was friendly only towards the Sinhalese, and in that case if the Sri Lankan state should allow the Tamils and Muslims to starve. "The people affected by the tsunami in the north and east are our citizens too (and) they should be rescued," she added.

Since the question why the government was keen to involve the LTTE and not other Tamil groups was being raised all over south Sri Lanka, she said that although the rebels did not represent the entire Tamil population, it did represent a certain section of the Tamils and should, therefore, be engaged in the reconstruction work. "We know that a certain percentage of the Tamil population will vote for the

LTTE if there were to be an election tomorrow," she argued. "Therefore, their representation is essential."

She had dwelt at length on this point in her 14 June response to the JVP general secretary Tilvin Silva, emphasising that the Tsunami Relief Council did not accord any recognition to the LTTE as the only representative of the Tamils. It only admitted the LTTE as a party which should play a role since it was "the only armed group" which waged war (against the Sri Lankan state) and controlled "certain areas affected by the tsunami catastrophe. This position will not imply that the LTTE is the only representative of the Tamil people." She also pointed out that the council, a purely administrative mechanism to rehabilitate the affected areas in the northern and eastern coastal belt, would only be functioning up to two kilometres inland from the beach.

Not only the president herself but also the chief officer in her Peace Secretariat, Jayantha Dhanapala, sought repeatedly to persuade the Sinhalese Buddhist community to accept that the government was in no way endangering the integrity of the republic by involving the rebels in the distribution of aid for reconstruction. "...for the specific of a crash programme to rebuild the tsunami disaster zone in the six districts of the north and east the Post-tsunami Operation Management Structure (P-TOMS) is considered vital," he said. "We engage the cooperation of the LTTE to implement that task. It also has a long-term benefit of inducting a rebel group with a notorious terrorist record in a democratic process working with other parties and the government to the benefit of the people of all ethnic communities in the north and east."[3]

Asked if he could guarantee the LTTE's eventual commitment to a political settlement of the ethnic conflict and return to peace talks if the P-TOMS was implemented, Dhanapala said he could only hope that the rebels would make the transition from their terrorist past to being a political party capable of working in the democratic mainstream as other rebel groups had done in so many countries, including in Sri Lanka.

An almost similar scenario prevailed in the post-tsunami period in Indonesia, the Asian country most wrecked by the December 26,

2004 upheaval, where identical issues surfaced. The rebellion-hit Aceh province was the hardest hit part of the country, and the government soon faced the question of partnering the Free Aceh Movement (GAM) in reconstruction work. However, unlike in Sri Lanka, peace talks were resumed in Indonesia within a month after the tsunami.

This was apparently a surprise though it was soon learned that efforts were already continuing in the pre-tsunami period to resume talks. However, the very fact that peace talks were taking place at all in the backdrop of the massive destruction of life and property in the rebellious province was clearly a significant breakthrough. Importantly, however, and very unlike what was happening at around the same time in Sri Lanka, it was the tsunami tragedy that clearly accelerated the resumption of peace talks between the Indonesian government and the GAM in Helsinki.

Just as the international donor community has kept persuading the two Sri Lankan adversaries to seek cooperation and an eventual return to peace talks, so did the tsunami donor community urge Jakarta and the GAM (the majority of its leaders was based in Sweden) to accord the highest priority to emergency relief work for the people of Aceh. While relief materials and aid were pouring into the tsunami-hit areas, all the sides concerned could see the logic behind cooperation: Aceh could only be rebuilt successfully if the decades-old conflict was resolved. Both the government and the GAM acknowledged the significance of the new circumstances thrown up by the tsunami and agreed that peace negotiations should begin.

There was, however, an important difference between the situations in the two countries. The brutality of the Indonesian army in suppressing the Aceh rebels had led to such an outcry that General Wiranto of the army was ultimately forced to offer a public apology for his men's collective guilt. Even one day before the tsunami struck Aceh, it was under the repressive emergency law and was a closed territory run for all practical purposes by the army. The devastation, however, forced the government to open the province up as foreign medical aid, food, and shelter had to be rushed in and the national and international media allowed to report on the devastation. Shocked by the extent of destruction of life and property, international attention was immediately riveted upon the province, and its quick rescue, reconstruction, and rehabilitation became an international concern. The Indonesian army had little choice but to give in to the diametrically changed circumstances.

It is noteworthy that the rebel leadership displayed at this juncture both political courage and diplomatic skills by agreeing to participate in the Helsinki talks proposed by the facilitator CMI, a non-government organisation, headed by a former Finnish president Martti Ahtissari. Similarly, the Indonesian government showed its prudence when the GAM sought to include various issues into the talks, such as, a discussion on self-government for the province and the future of the rebel group as a mainstream political party.

Disruptive tendencies, however, developed soon thereafter, and as in Sri Lanka, the hardliners in the Indonesian ruling party and government began to oppose any compromise with the rebels, while the Acehnese on their part displayed a reinforced sense of mistrust in the intentions of the government in Jakarta. As several analyses put it, the cycle of violence in Aceh had created a deep distrust among many Acehnese towards initiatives taken by the government. Rebuilding trust and goodwill was, therefore, vital before they could again be involved in a peace process. War weariness was widespread among the Acehnese, which meant that the main thrust of a peace agenda should include a process of transformation from violence to peace.

In late May 2005, however, the situation had deteriorated so much due to renewed fighting that the GAM demanded a United Nations intervention to investigate human rights violations by the Indonesian army. The Australian Broadcasting Corporation reported on 21 May that the orders from the top military leadership were simple and "brutally expressed"; the army Commander-in-chief Endriartono Sutarto had been touring the province, telling his troops that every GAM rebel who would offer resistance must be exterminated.

Jakarta of course reacted fiercely to the GAM demand for a UN intervention. The spokesman for the foreign ministry Dr Marty Natalagawa told the ABC that the events in Aceh were purely internal developments, "affairs of Indonesia." "We see in our own neighbourhood, the Philippines, with the southern Philippines, about the MILF and the like. Do we hear similar calls for that type of intervention by the UN ? We have similar separatist tendencies in some European countries...in the UK with the IRA, in Spain with the Basque. Do we have calls for the UN to get involved ? These are sovereign rights of certain countries to exercise. Our country has been threatened, been torn asunder, by a group of terrorists who represent no one but themselves, who derive their authority from the barrel of the gun."

The swift petering out of the very sensibly initiated peace effort in Indonesia resulted in the inevitable. Six months after the tsunami left 130,000 Acehnese dead out of the total tally of 220,000 killed in eleven countries, 37,000 were still missing but presumed dead, and skeletons were still being dug out. But even more poignantly, reconstruction and rehabilitation were a long way behind the expectations of the Acehnese who were promised seven billion dollars worth of aid. As one newspaper report pointed out, in the town of Krueng Raya where almost every building was wrecked and throughout the province, the reconstruction process was painfully slow. The town, once a densely populated place, had been reduced to desolation, still carpeted with debris, and "there is ... an overwhelming sense of nothingness, of a void where a thriving community once stood...only a handful of new houses has sprung up." The people were desperate to build permanent homes but, due to the non-availability of adequate building materials, they had been forced to live in pathetic shacks.[4]

The massive human tragedy and devastation wrought by the deadly tsunami in both Indonesia and Sri Lanka thus gave way eventually to the intractability of the long-established state-rebels conflict in the two Asian countries. It was, however, truer in Sri Lanka than in Indonesia that apart from being called upon to tackle the unpredictability of the response of the rebels, Colombo was also required to adjust to a new status, that of a minority government following the 16 June withdrawal of the JVP from power-sharing. A saving grace was the decision of the UNP not to jump into the traditional game of engineering an immediate collapse of the government.

Going over the objections raised by those who opposed the government move to bring in the LTTE as a partner in reconstruction work, it appeared that though considerable emphasis was being placed on the wisdom of allowing the rebels a perceived equal footing with the legitimate regime in Colombo, the basic question was related to permitting them to handle part of the massive $ 3 billion aid promised by donor countries for reconstruction purposes (on 16 May at the Sri Lanka Development Forum held in Kandy).

It could also be seen that the suspicion of the opponents about the ultimate fate of the huge aid basket emanated principally from the conditionality attached by the donor countries (except India) that the aid would be released only on the establishment of a joint government-LTTE mechanism to administer reconstruction efforts. The opponents appeared not to have reconciled themselves to a reported earmarking of "as much as" (as a prominent commentator put it) sixty per cent of the pledged aid to reconstruction in the northeast.[5]

Though the opponents acknowledged the apparent logic of earmarking the lion's share of the promised aid to the northeast since nearly seventy percent of the people killed by the tsunami and sixty-two percent of the dwellings destroyed belonged to the region, they also preferred to emphasise the terrorist nature of the LTTE and its propensity to exploit every available opportunity to reinforce its "ultimate" objective of seceding from the country.

The opponents also claimed that fifty percent of the tsunami-affected people in the northeast were Muslims, the very community which had been systematically "brutalised" by the LTTE and asked how the government could expect the rebels to be suddenly sympathetic to them.

This particular argument found a powerful backing when the Sri Lanka Muslim Congress (SLMC) said on 18 June that the Muslims entertained "a variety of concerns" regarding the proposed joint mechanism and that if these were not addressed and the joint mechanism suitably amended, the party would not be able to extend support to the move. The Muslims' chief concern was that they were not involved in the formulation of the mechanism and that they were apprehensive about the eventual effectiveness of their representatives

Epilogue: Tsunami and Dialogue

in the proposed mechanism. Media reports quoted SLMC leader Rauf Hakeem saying that "Not to involve elected Muslim representatives (in the formulation of the proposed mechanism) is a serious flaw" though the community was required to be "an active party in the process and (to) sign the document." The Muslims had fears about the ability of their representatives to decide upon reconstruction projects which would correctly address the problems facing them, he added, in the context of the proposal (not yet officially disclosed) for a three-tier structure with an equal representation of the government, the LTTE, and the Muslims at the apex level and with a ten-member regional body comprising five LTTE nominees, three Muslim party nominees, and two Sinhalese (government).

The Muslims' demand to be included in the process of setting up the P-TOMS received a boost when Kumaratunga conferred with the representatives (all senior clergymen belonging to all the three eastern districts) of the Eastern Muslim Council on 21 June and discussed in detail the structure the government was aiming to put in place. The priests demanded that the community should be a signatory to the proposed body and that its representatives should be allowed to participate in the reconstruction of the tsunami-affected areas. The president assured them that the rights and security of the community would be safeguarded and respected and that it would be given its rightful share in the reconstruction implementation body. She also informed that the Norwegian deputy foreign minister Vidar Helgesen, visiting Sri Lanka at the time, had been requested to convey the concerns and aspirations of the Muslims to the LTTE at his meeting scheduled the following day. With the sudden signing of the aid deal on 24 June, however, the Muslims felt that irrespective of the president's assurance, their concerns had not been really addressed. Kumaratunga conferred once more with the Muslims parliamentarians, including ministers and deputy ministers in her government, on 27 June, listened to their suggestions for improvement in the already agreed arrangement, and assured their consideration and possible implementation.

Predictably enough, the tussle over the desirability of the proposed joint mechanism gave rise to a fresh bout of exhibitions of Sinhalese-Buddhist and Tamil sentiments in the south and north-east respectively.

Colombo continued to witness massive demonstrations organised mostly by the JVP where the strongest Sinhalese-Buddhist chauvinist sentiments were given a free rein. Typically, slogans such as "The country needs a government to defeat separatism, not to nourish it" and "We will agitate the president for her resignation" were raised.

In the north-east, where the LTTE had been organising protest rallies in support of the joint mechanism proposal, slogans and speeches dwelt at length on the spectre of a resurgent Sinhalese-Buddhist chauvinism and how this development was once again pushing the country back into the throes of renewed hostility. Typical of this was the declaration made on 19 June to the effect that "We, the Tamil people, declare that we will defeat Sinhalese-Buddhist chauvinism and regain our traditional homeland from the occupation of armed forces. We will exercise our right to self-determination in our land with our own strength." Speaking on the occasion a Catholic priest said, "Even now (the) Sinhalese political leadership is not prepared to provide a simple structure that could facilitate the rehabilitation and reconstruction of (the) tsunami-destroyed coastal areas in the north-east province."[6]

While much of this sabre-rattling by both the communities was essentially politicking, there was increasing indication following the pullout by the JVP from the government that Kumaratunga was being called upon to tackle an accelerated crisis. The shrill campaigns in the south and north-east could only encourage further ethnic divisiveness, which Sri Lanka could well have been spared as the immediate task of setting up the multi-community P-TOMS and then the long-elusive task of achieving a consensus on the ISGA proposals remained. While the UNP's assurance to the president to continue to support the joint mechanism proposal was considered a positive development, it was also noted that the main opposition party soon thereafter confabulated with the Tamil National Alliance, a transparent LTTE-promoted parliamentary group, on the same issue. Interestingly, the TNA was not satisfied with a similarly positive response of the UNP but suggested that the latter made its policy public, which UNP leader Ranil Wickramasinghe agreed to do.

Kumaratunga and her party would also be called upon increasingly to deal with a political development which had serious electoral ramifications. The JVP's extreme measure of withdrawing from the government coupled with an intensified campaign against the proposed joint mechanism was aimed principally to further woo the Sinhalese-Buddhist electorate; and there was considerable optimism that the party's popularity should rise handsomely along with an anticipated increase in chauvinistic feelings. This should be considerably worrying for the SLFP, the president's party, which continued to depend chiefly on the support of the Sinhalese-Buddhist community and which had already paid a high price by conceding the JVP's rising popularity among the community during the last parliamentary election.

The only way to counter this could be by continuing to persuade the JVP to rejoin the government on a future date, now that there was strong indication that the regime would not collapse following its relegation to the status of a minority government in the 225-seat parliament. The SLFP would, therefore, maintain that the JVP's pullout did not automatically signify a complete and final break of the coalition and that the party's return to power-sharing, which was always politically gainful, should not be ruled out.

The JVP, however, had other ideas, among which was one of acquisition of sufficient electoral mileage to help achieve a still more effective role in government-formation than had been possible so far. In the post-withdrawal period, the party pursued this particular objective with determination. In a special statement made in parliament on 22 June, the JVP parliamentary group leader Wimal Weerawanse took care to "thank" a number of SLFP ministers in the Kumaratunga government for their "cooperation" and said that his party, on behalf of the "inspiration of millions of people" (sic), wished them success in defeating the "minority NGO clique" which had wriggled its way into the government (in order) to destroy it.

If the ministers' struggle to defeat the conspiracy of this minority clique "sustained by foreign aid of some NGOs" was successful, "maybe we will meet on one platform." If, however, the minority clique in the minority government moved to sign the joint mechanism, the JVP would have to reconsider its desire to defend the stability of the government and the provincial councils while acting as an independent group in the opposition. However, it had no intention of making the country unstable. It was also not prepared to abandon its responsibility for the masses who, with immense hope, voted for the UPFA "including us" in 2004.

A truly worrying development, however, took place in the east where the LTTE defector "Col." Karuna felt threatened by Kumaratunga's determination to bring in the LTTE as a partner in aid distribution for reconstruction work and decided to wreck the prospects to the extent he could. This became apparent as his faction started targeting LTTE-sponsored NGOs in the east, notably the Tamil Rehabilitation Organisation (TRO).

Equally interestingly, the JVP which had been extending support to Karuna in his fight with the LTTE, including his plan to set up a political party, appeared to have coordinated well in its decision to pull out of the government and in respect of its continuing anti-joint mechanism campaign. The Karuna group welcomed the JVP's withdrawal from the government as it felt that such a gesture capable of generating unforeseeable repercussions would strengthen its case for excluding the LTTE from the proposed joint mechanism.

Karuna's vehement opposition to the LTTE's inclusion in the P-TOMS was apparently based on his reading that such a development would immeasurably enhance the rebel group's position in the northeast and would concurrently act to diminish the space he was creating for himself with considerable sacrifice and risk. He knew that once the P-TOMS became a reality with the LTTE publicly perceived as functioning on an equal footing with the government in aid distribution and reconstruction work, his own position among the same target population would be seriously threatened and that the only way to prevent this possibility from actually happening was to strengthen the JVP in its opposition to the joint mechanism. Interestingly, pro-JVP Sinhalese newspapers and journals proved to be the best source of news about the Karuna faction during this period.

For the president, however, the continuing delay in the formation of the P-TOMS spelled increased challenges in various other spheres as well. Apart from the certainty that the promised massive reconstruction aid would not be released until the joint mechanism was in place, her chief unfulfilled task remained the continuing deadlock over the question of resumption of the peace dialogue (which meant, first, an understanding to be reached with the LTTE over the Interim Self Governing Authority, which had eluded the country and the government till the tsunami hit the Sri Lankan coastline).

Clearly, Kumaratunga was no longer in a position to handle both the seemingly unachievable tasks either simultaneously or serially. Since the tsunami aid issue had come to the forefront and must be dealt with first, she had little choice in preventing the outcome of the battle over the P-TOMS from influencing the result of the conflict over the ISGA.

Ironically but not surprisingly, the failure of the government to achieve a national consensus on the two issues held up billions of dollars worth of promised aid which, if forthcoming, would have gone a considerable way in shoring up a sagging economy. While the promised aid thus remained locked up, Sri Lanka also needed an easy flow of foreign funds to energise the principal sectors of economy. There had been little improvement in the economy, especially in the unemployment rate, since the last parliamentary election when the southern electorate in particular turned its face away from the Wickramasinghe government for its failure to generate jobs in a high-cost economy. The president only knew too well the eventual price that she would be called upon to pay if a consensus over both the P-TOMS and the ISGA remained elusive. It was noted that while the position regarding the P-TOMS was principally discussed at the 21 June meeting between the president and the visiting Norwegian deputy foreign minister, they also went over the existing status of the ceasefire and on the need to review its implementation in due course.

When Helgesen met Thamilchelvan in Killinochchi, where the LTTE was headquartered, on 22 June, the latter expectedly sounded as condemnatory of the president as prudent in continuation of the pressure tactic adopted to coerce the government into coming out with the joint mechanism document. "(The) message from Colombo (as conveyed by the Norwegian diplomat) contained the word 'very soon' in relation to the (proposed) joint mechanism," he told the media following the meeting. "We cannot rely on words. The joint mechanism requires signatures. And more importantly it has to be implemented in the spirit in which it is written. We see no sign of this happening soon. We gave a frank and detailed description of the situation on the ground to the Norwegian delegation and explained to them that the ceasefire agreement is under serious strain. We told the delegation that (the) Tamil people have lost faith in the peace process and the situation is explosive in Tamil (inhabited) areas." What was essential today, he said, was to salvage the peace process which was being threatened seriously by ceasefire violations, for the CFA was the key to the entire peace process and "if that is hijacked by scheming elements," then there was no useful purpose in the joint mechanism or any mechanism for that matter.[7]

The head of the LTTE's political wing said in relation to the Muslims' demand to be included in the formation of the P-TOMS (so that they could participate in decision-making in reconstruction projects in their habitats) that the LTTE was firmly committed to ensuring that the Muslims were represented in the post-tsunami reconstruction structures in consonance with the destruction they had suffered in the disaster.

Complaining that the LTTE was, however, unable to send any message to the Muslims "as we cannot fully rely on Kumaratunga's assurances on the aid deal", he added significantly that the rebels' commitment to ensure a fair and acceptable representation of Muslims in the joint mechanism remained firm "once the deal is signed. This has been our position from the very beginning." The Muslims, however, did not clearly trust the rebels any more and felt very strongly that the latter had a game-plan to neutralise their representatives in the tsunami aid distribution and reconstruction body and that this must be foiled.

On his part, the Norwegian diplomat characteristically sounded optimistic, noting that although the parties had not signed the joint mechanism yet, they were nevertheless "moving forward."

Four days later, however, the history of Sri Lanka took a dramatic turn with the signing of a memorandum of understanding (MoU) for establishing the P-TOMS to be in force for the next one year and with an option for extensions through consensus. Representatives of the government and the LTTE signed the document in Colombo and Killinochchi (as was the practice whenever the two sides were to put their signatures on any document). A very determined president had

Epilogue: Tsunami and Dialogue

clearly snatched the initiative from the loud and increasingly aggressive Sinhalese Buddhist nationalists (the JVP members threw the parliament into turmoil on 24 June, the day the MoU was signed forcing an adjournment; the party went to court challenging the aid deal; and in a possible act of one-upmanship, the National Bhikku Front urged the senior most Buddhist prelates to withdraw the blessings they had given Kumaratunga as the head of State and to declare her a non-Buddhist) and given a hard push to the dithering nation towards a definitive objective. At the same time she had forced the LTTE to face a challenge it had earlier failed to live up to; that of working in good faith together with the government for the welfare of the ethnically diverse people of the north-east. The rebel group would now be called upon to treat the Sinhalese and Muslim neighbours of the Tamils in the province on equitable terms; with political acumen it would also be in a position to convert the challenge into an opportunity to establish its bona fides as a true people's movement.

At the same time, to her credit the president took painstaking care to educate the country about the P-TOMS. Picking up each of the objections advanced by the opponents, the government said on 29 June that "...adequate safeguards against misuse and mismanagement of regional funds have been built into this arrangement, which has been designed to ensure complete transparency and accountability."

The opponents of the P-TOMS felt that it could lead to undermining of the security of the country with the LTTE constructing bases and controlling the entire 2 km stretch of land and pressuring the government to remove security forces camps and installations. The government said Clause 2 (f) of the aid deal specifically stated that the Ceasefire Agreement (CFA) would continue "in full force and effect" and "nothing in the MoU shall be construed to prejudice or alter its terms in any way." Article 1.12 of the CFA specifically provided for the exclusion of the High Security Zones (HSZ) from the ambit of the CFA while guaranteeing their security under the security forces. Therefore, the P-TOMS could not in any way affect the existence of the HSZs or military camps and installations.

The Trincomalee harbour was under the government's control and the LTTE enjoyed no access to these establishments. The

Trincomalee harbour, the Kankeshanthurai harbour, and the Palali military camps were not under the P-TOMS. The CFA specifically mentioned in Art. 1.12 under the section on "freedom of movement" that the government had the right to deny entry to specified military areas. Art.1.3 of the CFA recognised that the Sri Lankan armed forces would continue to perform their legitimate task of safeguarding the sovereignty and territorial integrity of the country.

The LTTE and the Sea Tigers would exercise control "only in areas they did under the CFA." They would not have a right to control any areas outside this, even if these were affected by the tsunami. "It should be noted that the powers vested in the P-TOMS is limited to tsunami relief, rehabilitation, and reconstruction," the government said.

The fear that the P-TOMS would enable the LTTE to rebuild their military bases within the 2 km area was completely unfounded. Overall project proposals based on "accepted needs assessment" for the reconstruction of civilian infrastructure damaged by tsunami could be handled by the P-TOMS; and no funds could be allocated for any military activity, reconstruction or otherwise from the donor funds that would be disbursed for the tsunami-related reconstruction work exclusively.

Explaining the working of the regional fund, which lay at the core of the arrangement, the government said that the purpose of the fund was to provide funds expeditiously to the six tsunami-affected districts in the north-east, Ampara, Batticaloa, Jaffna, Killinochchi, Mullaitivu, and Trincomalee "following proper approved procedures" to help speedy implementation of relief, rehabilitation and reconstruction programmes.

The regional fund consisted of unspecified (programme) and secretariat funds; the former would be composed of foreign funds exclusively while the latter would consist of both foreign and local funds. The former would be used to finance post-tsunami reconstruction programmes or projects in the affected districts, while the latter would be used to cover recurrent costs of the regional secretariat.

The regional fund would not operate differently from the manner in which all government ministries, departments, and institutions

Epilogue: Tsunami and Dialogue 205

functioned with regard to financial matters. All the existing laws and financial regulations would apply strictly to the administration of the regional fund which would operate under the authority of the Treasury. Similarly, adequate safeguards had been built into the joint mechanism to ensure that the projects and programmes to be financed were properly reviewed and approved by the regional committee and thereafter by the high-level committee, and then submitted to the finance ministry. It would be only thereafter that the Treasury would allocate and disburse the relevant funds for the approved projects. The moneys would actually be granted to the relevant government institutions authorised to implement the projects.

Since the opponents of the aid deal felt very strongly that the Tamil rebels would be particularly keen to exploit the foreign funds, the government clarified that all donor funds for tsunami relief, rehabilitation, and reconstruction would be maintained in a separate account of the central bank. The allocated programme funds for the six districts would be transferred to the regional fund from the Central Bank with the approval of the Treasury via a suitable ministry after the high-level committee had made the relevant request. It was important to note the procedures ensured that no donor funds could be transferred directly to the regional fund.

The regional fund itself would be held and administered by a custodian, appointed by the parties to the deal, who would sign contractual agreements with the relevant implementing agencies. Specified projects funds would be coordinated directly by the donor agencies and the Treasury, and these would be outside the purview of the regional fund. The custodian would be required to submit quarterly progress reports on projects financed by the regional fund to the Treasury and the P-TOMS. To ensure fool-proof accounting, he would commission globally accepted auditing and accounting procedures for preparing progress reports. The government apparently felt that this exhaustive explanation of the manner in which the P-TOMS would be operational should satisfy all those who had entertained various apprehensions and doubts about its implications.

Significantly, the president also lost no time in turning the attention of the nation, riveted so long on the seemingly impossible business of reaching a consensus on the joint mechanism, to the next task of resumption of the deadlocked peace talks. She described the P-TOMS as "a window of opportunity to recommence the stalled peace process." She said that Sri Lanka "will soon achieve a negotiated durable peace which will ensure the rights of all communities" and appealed "all concerned to put an end to divisive and confrontational politics."

With one stroke, Kumaratunga had redeemed her image of a secular liberal, which had taken many a battering through the last few years as her efforts to steer the country away from war and towards a negotiated peace were foiled time and again by an opportunistic political opposition and a deeply ingrained majoritarian chauvinism. Her achievement in roping in the LTTE in the administration of tsunami reconstruction aid in the face of a stiff and expanding opposition by the majority community forced three different entities to deal with a challenge from which they would not be able to get away easily; they were the southern political opposition parties, Sinhalese Buddhist chauvinists, and the Tamil rebels. How each of them would respond to the challenge would shape Sri Lankan politics of the coming days.

The Hindu wrote in its 25 June editorial, "President ... Kumaratunga has shown exemplary courage...As Sri Lanka's only truly non-chauvinist, non-majoritarian leader, (she) has had one overriding goal through two terms as president: to bring peace to her country. At times, this goal seemed to have slipped out of her grasp, as the LTTE and the opposition UNP played dangerous games with her plans for peace. Now, with a year to go before her second and final term comes to an end, (she) has taken the path that she believes is just and the way forward, not merely for post-tsunami reconstruction but also for a permanent peace."

The political challenge gathered further momentum from its timing; for the presidential election would be due in 2006 and speculation was rife in Colombo after the dramatic turn of events of 24 June that Kumaratunga could even go to the extent of dissolving parliament and order a fresh general election next year. Since such an initiative would rest solely with the president, the challenged entities could only consider their responses in terms of such an eventuality and could base their strategies more on speculation than on authoritative declarations and actions.

Epilogue: Tsunami and Dialogue

Meanwhile, a reality check was introduced by the publication of the Amnesty International (AI) report covering Sri Lankan events during 2004. Pointing out the long way that the government still had to travel to introduce an improved human rights situation in the country, the report noted that in November the government announced a reactivation of the death penalty in respect of rape and murder cases and narcotics dealings. Noting that this signalled the end of a 27-year-old moratorium on executions, the report pointed out that the reactivation of the death penalty occurred in response to the murders of a high Court judge and his police guard.[8]

Torture in police custody was widely reported and victims seeking redress faced threats and violence. "There were numerous reports of torture by police as well as some reports of death in police custody. Some of the torture victims seeking redress in the courts were reportedly put under pressure to withdraw their cases. Among them was Gerald Perera, a torture victim due to give evidence against seven police officers in the High Court, who was shot on 21 November (2004) and subsequently died," the AI report stated.

The AI noted that in August (2004) the National Police Commission announced that addressing torture by police would be its top priority and that it would be responsible for the disciplinary control of all police officers, revoking the previous authority of the Inspector General of Police (IGP) in disciplinary matters relating to officers below the rank of inspector. The National Human Rights Commission (NHRC) established a Torture Prevention and Monitoring Unit to investigate allegations and to carry out surprise checks on places of detention. However, in September (2004) the IGP issued a directive, based on the Attorney General's advice, stating that the NHRC must notify senior police officers before inspecting police barracks and other unauthorised places of detention. Besides, there was little progress towards holding security forces to account for past human rights violations. Religious minorities came under threat, with attacks on Christians and Muslims, as well as the tabling of a private member's bill aimed at curbing religious conversions.

Alarmingly enough, the human rights situation in the north-east deteriorated following a violent split within the LTTE in April and a dramatic increase in politically motivated killings (a reference to "Col." Karuna's defection and the resultant mayhem, which was continuing through 2005—the author). "The continued killings and intimidation created an atmosphere of fear among the civilian population in the east as well as putting the ceasefire under strain. A number of people were also killed in Colombo," the report noted.

The AI said that although the LTTE had released a large number of child soldiers during the "internal fighting", it continued to recruit children, including through abduction.

The UN Children's Fund reported the recruitment of 448 children as soldiers during the first six months of the year, while acknowledging that the actual figure could well be much higher. There were reports that a large number of child soldiers were deployed in the fighting between the LTTE and the Karuna faction in April (2004, as discussed in details earlier in this book) and some of them were killed.

If the AI report was disquieting enough, the Kumaratunga regime was also called upon at the time to deal with the continuing sluggishness in the economy, and, more importantly, with the failure of the country to attract investment despite the unprecedented boon of four consecutive years of peace. "Achieving a permanent peace is undoubtedly one of the important steps Sri Lanka can take towards improving its investment climate," said Peter Harrold, World Bank country director for Sri Lanka, as quoted in a joint study conducted on the country's economy by the Asian Development Bank and the World Bank.

Summarising the assessment made by the study, he said that if sustainable poverty reduction was to be achieved by Sri Lanka, it was required to raise the overall level of investment. The joint report presented the first comprehensive scientific analysis of the factors that were inhibiting investment, domestic and foreign, urban and rural. Based on an island-wide survey of more than 2,000 enterprises, the study highlighted the difficulties that small-scale rural entrepreneurs faced in starting and developing their units. It found that small businesses in rural areas were hampered by poor transport, limited access to the formal financial sector, and frequent outrages. Although the country owned a dense road network, as much as 90 percent of the roads were in poor condition because of a lack of maintenance.

Epilogue: Tsunami and Dialogue

This factor alone dramatically increased travel times and contributed to almost half of all agricultural produces rotting before they reached customers.

The helplessness of business firms operating in the northeast was reflected in the finding that to achieve sheer survival, these units had developed over the years what could be called coping strategies by reducing their inventories, production centres having been located in residences, and allocating larger outlays on ensuring security. An unsatisfactory power situation had obliged as many as 75 percent of urban manufacturing units to own generators (as compared to 27 percent in China). As a result, their production costs had gone up by as much as 300-400 percent reducing their productivity by half. Electricity and transport including the road network, therefore, needed urgent attention and investment.

While Sri Lanka had lost years when it should have dealt with and solved its myriad problems including the ethnic conflict, President Kumaratunga's bold step forward in launching the P-TOMS in June 2005 should open up the closed doors to peace, development, and progress. As she reiterated and as the world at large spontaneously acknowledged, the road henceforth should lead resolutely forward and not be blocked any further by fresh displays of human failings.

It was, however, important to keep in mind the untested status of the P-TOMS as a vehicle through which the first limited experiment of government-rebels cooperation was being launched. As a Western scholar remarked, the reconstruction process could now begin but it would not be easy. The reconstruction of war-ravaged areas had encountered serious problems in the pre-tsunami period; in particular a shortage of skilled artisans to rebuild as well as a lack of equipment plagued reconstruction at the time. This problem could actually deteriorate in the face of massive reconstruction efforts once the P-TOMS became operational. The joint mechanism being put in place should, therefore, ensure an efficient allocation of funds which ought to take care of both the shortages through a fair distribution of labour and equipment.[9]

In late June 2005, therefore, there was a sudden environment of measured optimism in Sri Lanka. The JVP had not succeeded in bringing down the government; on the contrary, it was being called upon to mend its mindset and join the new movement toward a possible peace just as the LTTE in the northeast could no longer enjoy the luxury of manipulating the vagaries of war and peace according to its strategic and tactical needs.

All of Sri Lanka, the north-east, the south and the west, could at last begin to hope for a new chapter in its largely bleak recent history. Those who remained staunchly unresponsive to the concept of federalism would also get an opportunity to experience the first stirrings of sharing responsibility for community welfare not only between Colombo and the provinces but also between the legitimate central government and the illegitimate but de facto rulers of a part of the country. Ethno-centric nationalism which verged on chauvinism on both the sides of the divide would also be required to grapple with reason and reality and change itself. Would the LTTE pass the test satisfactorily, convincing its fierce opponents in the south of its bona fides as a genuine people's movement or would it relapse into its terrorist mould and push the country into a renewal of hostilities? Having travelled an already testing distance, the Kumaratunga government should no longer be vulnerable to counter-productive forces. That much appeared to be certain. The international community could only be encouraged by the turn of events and facilitate the long-pending return of Sri Lanka to a renewed peace dialogue. Perhaps the dangerous interlude would come to an end and it would be opportune to talk and negotiate between the government and the rebels.

Notes

1. *Tamil Guardian*, online edition, 16 June 2005.
2. http://www.priu.gov.lk, 14 June 2005.
3. *University Teachers for Human Rights (Jaffna) Sri Lanka UTHR* (J) *Information Bulletin No. 37*, 'A Tale of Two Disasters and the Fickleness of Terror Politics', released 10 January 2005.
4. *The Independent, 19* June 2005.
5. G.H.Peiris, 'Tsunami Reconstruction and the Illusion of Peace' *South Asia Intelligence Review*, Vol.3, No.45, 23 May 2005.

6. www.tamilnet.com, 19 June 2005.
7. www.tamilnet.com, 22 June 2005.
8. Amnesty International, *Sri Lanka Covering Events from January-December 2004*.
9. Robert C.Oberst, professor of political science, Nebraska Wesleyan University, USA, quoted by www.tamilnet.com, 29 June 2005.

Postscript to Epilogue

Between June and August, 2005, Sri Lanka once again swung between hope and despair amidst rising fears that the ceasefire would finally disintegrate under the shattering impact of the 12 August assassination of Foreign Minister Lakshman Kadirgamar. The affable and remarkably successful diplomat was felled on the late evening by a sniper shooting from a neighbouring house. Did this signify that the new beginning towards dialogue and eventual peace, which appeared to be within reach, was after all premature? President Kumaratunga vowed two days later that she would redouble her efforts and the commitment of her government to implement the task of devolution of power "based on a democratic and pluralistic society, through dialogue with all the communities inhabiting our land". This reinforced optimism at this dark hour of national tragedy. In Colombo, secretary general of the Peace Secretariat, Jayantha Dhanapala said on 16 August that in the light of the assassination, there would have to be a serious review of …certain policies and procedures followed up to now in relation to the peace process. However, on 18th August, the LTTE political wing Chief S.P Thamilchelvan threatened that while "war is not an option…if war is thrust upon the Tamil people, we will have no option but to face it" This serves as a jerking reminder that peace and war remain equally indeterminable in today's Sri Lanka.

The two most important questions on the assassination of Kadirgamar, who had killed him and why he was killed, were answered within hours of the act. The inspector-general of Sri Lanka police Chandra Fernando told the media on 13 August that the evidence available and the weapons brought by the assassins (there were at least two, the police guessed) pointed to the involvement of the LTTE. "Looking at the weapons used and the style, it is definitely the work of the LTTE. There is no other group with weapons like this," he said. The sniper had struck from a toilet in a house next to Kadirgamar's private residence. The police had recovered a tripod used to mount a long-range rifle and found that a hole had been bored into the window through which the swimming pool in the minister's house could be observed. They also recovered four 7.62 mm spent cartridges from the scene of the assassination which had taken place at around 11 p.m. on 12 August after Kadirgamar had finished his swim. Also recovered from the neighbouring house was an unused 40 mm grenade launcher. Though the tripod of the killer rifle was found, the weapon itself was missing. The police also realised that the assassins had spent considerable time in observing Kadirgamar before striking him down as food including cheese, biscuits, and mixture packets were found left behind in the toilet. On 16 August, the neighbour, Lakshman Thalayasingam told the preliminary enquiry at the Colombo magistrate's court that he was unaware of the assassination until soldiers alerted him at around 1 a.m. on the 13 August morning. The toilet from where the assassins had shot Kadirgamar was rarely used, and there was no access to the upper floor of the house from the backyard.

But why should the LTTE kill Kadirgamar? Once again, not only the government in Colombo but also everyone who could shed any light on the question felt convinced that the Tamil rebels had the most compelling reason to ensure that the foreign minister did not continue to be a nuisance to them any more. President Kumaratunga said in her address to the nation on 14 August, "Initial indications of the investigations seem to reveal the responsibility of the LTTE in (the) brutal murder...The LTTE has denied involvement in the murder. Their denial contradicts the facts and our knowledge of their long-held desire and repeated attempts to murder both my Tamil Cabinet colleagues (the other minister being Douglas Devananda)...Kadirgamar was a Sri Lankan nationalist, who believed passionately in a united and democratic Sri Lanka...He envisioned a negotiated political settlement of the ethnic problem that combined devolution of power with pluralism and democracy...He constantly grieved the subjugation of the Tamil people to LTTE authoritarianism...During my first government, he was instrumental in having the LTTE recognised internationally for what they are, an armed terrorist group. Consequently, they were proscribed in the leading nations of the world. The USA, the UK, Australia followed India."

The international community too shared the belief that Kadirgamar had been done in by the rebels. "This senseless murder," said US Secretary of State Condoleezza Rice on 13 August, "was a vicious act of terror, which the United States strongly condemns. Those responsible must be brought to justice." Norway's minister of foreign affairs Jan Petersen described the assassination as "a gruesome deed, which is deeply tragic for Sri Lanka. Japan's prime minister Junichiro Koizumi said that he was "greatly shocked and saddened at the tragic news". Secretary-general of the United Nations Kofi Annan said that he was shocked and saddened and deplored in the strongest of terms "this criminal and senseless act" and hoped that the perpetrators would be found and brought to justice. China condemned the assassination as "an act of terror". The European Union said that the killing was a brutal and senseless terrorist act. India "unreservedly" condemned the assassination, the external affairs ministry saying that the killing had been a heinous act. Reflecting the popular perception, The *Hindu* of India wrote on 15 August, "There is not the slightest doubt that the (LTTE) planned and executed this fiendish crime. ...Kadirgamar was known to be at the top of the LTTE's hit list, just below President...Kumaratunga...The LTTE and also its agents and apologists...denounced this son of Jaffna Tamil parents as a 'traitor.'"

The LTTE was quite prompt in denying its involvement, though it was equally ready to underline that Kadirgamar, the Tamil was unacceptable to the rebels. "The collective Tamil thinking and judgment...of the man is that he is a traitor," said Thamilchelvan. "This does not necessarily mean (that) he (had) earned his death, because it is not just Mr Kadirgamar who did this. An eye-for-an-eye and a tooth-for-a-tooth (are) not the concern at the moment when we are strongly committed to the ceasefire agreement. We are seriously interested in the ceasefire agreement." Adding a twist to the question "whodunit ?", he said, " (Kadirgamar) had 24-hour security. So if in the end someone had been able to infiltrate into that set-up and meticulously carry out a killing, definitely there is an inside element in this matter."[1] The Sri Lankan government did not seem to attach importance to the LTTE's denial of involvement; and instead referred to similar denials about various other acts of terrorism (such as, the 21 May, 1991 assassination of former Indian prime minister Rajiv Gandhi in the Indian state of Tamil Nadu, and the 1 May, 1993 assassination of the then Sri Lankan president Ranasinghe Premadasa) where its culpability was exposed by investigation.

Apart from reaffirming its determination to continue with the ceasefire and seek resumption of negotiation, the government did take another significant step. The Sri Lankan foreign secretary H M G S Palihakkara, while addressing the diplomatic community in Colombo on 14 August, called for concerted international action that would be immediate and tangible against the LTTE. He said that while the government appreciated the "accurate" characterisation of the assassination as a " truly vicious terrorist act" by many distinguished international statesmen in their condolence messages, the evidence was incontrovertible that the act had been committed by the LTTE. The need of the hour was then to follow up on the recognition of the nature of the terrorist act by taking practical and effective measures as required by international law for the prevention and suppression of terrorism. These measures could include sanctions and internationally isolating responsible entities and individuals, and engaging in international law enforcement cooperation, against terrorist activities. Sri Lanka's ambassador in the United States Bernard A B Goonetilleke followed up with an elaboration of Colombo's stand, pointing out it was clear that the LTTE had agreed to the ceasefire in order to buy time after the international climate suddenly turned adversarial in the aftermath of the 11 September, 2001, terrorist attacks on U.S. soil.

Clearly sensing that its denial of involvement in Kadirgamar's assassination had cut no ice with the international community and that Colombo might yet succeed in turning the screw tighter around it with global backing, the LTTE was quick to accept the Norwegian invitation to "participate in a review of the implementation of the ceasefire agreement in order to find practical ways of ensuring full compliance by both (the) parties". Norway's foreign minister Jan Petersen and his deputy Vidar Helgesen met the LTTE's political adviser and chief peace negotiator Anton Balasingham in London on 17 August and handed over the facilitator's proposals in this regard.

Balasingham later said that the LTTE leader Prabhakaran had positively considered the Norwegian proposals and agreed to send a high-level delegation to participate in talks to be held in Oslo shortly, adding that discussions would also focus on the escalating violence in the north-east and related issues.[2]

By quickly agreeing to participate in talks with the government, the LTTE obviously desired to deflect international attention away from it in the aftermath of the assassination of Kadirgamar, for which it had become the solitary suspect. The implementation of the ceasefire agreement had proved to be highly contentious throughout its three-year existence, with both the sides alleging violations of its requirements by the other side and complaining of various shortcomings. It was on 4 August that President Kumaratunga had expressed her government's readiness to a 'review' (as distinct from a 'renegotiation') of the ceasefire agreement so that ancillary arrangements could be put in place to remedy the current gaps in the agreement and build confidence on the basis of mutual responsibility and reciprocity between the two parties. She also reiterated her commitment to reopen direct negotiations with the LTTE at the meeting with Helgesen. Kadirgamar, who was killed eight days later allegedly by the LTTE, was associated with Kumaratunga in the discussions.

Apart from trying to buy time once again in the face of the strong suspicion of its involvement in the murder, the LTTE had another compelling reason for agreeing to return to talks on the ceasefire agreement. The agreement had brought it many benefits which it was apparently loath to forego. While the Sri Lanka Monitoring Mission headed by Norway had reported as many as 2,903 ceasefire violations by the rebels and 131 violations by the government (as quoted by the Sri Lankan ambassador in the U.S.) and both the parties were demanding a proper implementation of the agreement, the LTTE had also successfully converted the provisions of the agreement into a 'weapon'.

Exploiting the ceasefire, the rebels set up a de facto administrative control in the north-east, forcing government officials posted in the region to implement their orders. A parallel administration to the official set-up had thus come up with the rebels collecting taxes and running their own police force. The ceasefire line had been converted into a virtual international boundary with the rebel outfit issuing "visas" to visitors for onward travel. The truce was also utilised to reinforce the rebel fighting force, as had always been the case; an additional 'achievement' was the setting up of an air wing. Diplomacy on a heightened scale was also deployed during the ceasefire in an attempt to persuade critics to turn soft. All the three years of ceasefire had been spent in a frenzied pace of diplomacy with senior rebel leaders touring Europe, while Prabhakaran continued to receive and talk to international visitors at his base in the Mullaitivu jungle, seeking to establish the identity of a leader of a "liberation" movement purportedly accepted by a wider world. The LTTE was also able during the ceasefire to place the government in a situation where it was obliged willy-nilly to provide every facility to make possible such visits to the jungle hide-out in order to honour the provisions of the ceasefire agreement; while technically the rebel group remained outlawed in four countries and Interpol "red corner" notices remained in effect against its leader.[3]

The period of the ceasefire also provided an opportunity for the LTTE to re-establish its presence in the entire north-east as the "sole" representative of the Tamils. This was achieved by setting up political offices all over the region administered by the government, as permitted by the ceasefire agreement; by forcing non-LTTE political parties and groups to withdraw from the area as they had to turn in their weapons under the ceasefire provisions; those who resisted and stayed back were soon to be liquidated by the LTTE. The culmination of this strategy was the successful hijacking of the March, 2004 parliamentary elections when the rebel group was able to ensure that its 'proxy' candidates of the Tamil National Alliance got through the hustings and became its collective propaganda team right in the heart of democratic Sri Lanka, the parliament.

This long list of military, administrative, and political advances achieved during the period of the ceasefire indicated a well-planned and efficiently executed campaign to exploit the peace interregnum to strengthen the LTTE's position as a challenger to the government. Some analysts felt that its goal was much more ambitious—it had planned from the very first day of the truce period to push the rebels' cause for an 'Eelam' (Tamil homeland separated from Sri Lanka) to be achieved obviously not through a negotiated political settlement (which would not permit secession) but through war. Each act of the LTTE since the very beginning of the ceasefire, such as, the forced recruitment of child soldiers through abductions; intermittent violence against Muslims; the determination with which the rebel outfit fought the government diplomatically and politically to force its role in controlling post-tsunami reconstruction finances, and the continuous campaign of murders to obliterate the challenges posed by "Col." Karuna and the pro-government Tamil political parties and groups not only in the north-east but also in the national capital, could only be interpreted as conscious stepping stones towards achieving a separate state and definitely not towards creating a federal Sri Lanka.

The assassination of the widely popular but very staunchly nationalist foreign minister, an ethnic Tamil of the Jaffna vintage, was also seen at the time as two important signals being sent out by the LTTE. One, that the rebel group would not care too hoots for international opinion but use terrorism as and when required to achieve specific goals, as it had done throughout its history. Second, that the act of assassinating the second most important member of the Kumaratunga government threw a challenge that Colombo would not be able to counter in a punitive manner because that would be risking a resumption of hostilities in the face of a nationwide peace constituency and a steady international clamour for taking up the interrupted thread of negotiations for a political settlement of the ethnic conflict.

Endnotes

1. Reuters interview of the political wing head of the Liberation Tigers of Tamil Eelam, S.P.Thamilchelvan,www.tamilnet.com,17 August 2005.
2. *LTTE agrees to participate in talks on Ceasefire Agreement,* www.tamilnet.com, *19* August 2005.
3. Nirupama Subramanian, "Requiem for a peace process," *The Hindu, 15* August 2005.

Appendix

URGENT PRESS RELEASE
LTTE Headquarters
Killinochchi
Tamil Elam
27 November 2004

'Tamil Tigers Will Launch Freedom Struggle If Peace Talks Are Further Delayed'—LTTE Leader

The leader of the Liberation Tigers of Tamil Eelam, Mr Velupillai the Spelling of Prabhakaran Used by the LTTE, in his annual statement marking Heroes' Day, cautioned the Sri Lanka government that his organisation would be compelled to launch the freedom struggle of the Tamil nation if peace talks were further delayed and the suffering of his people continued.

In an urgent appeal the LTTE leader called upon the government of Sri Lanka to resume the peace talks, without conditions, on the basis of the Interim Self Governing Authority as proposed by his organisation.

The following is the official translation of Mr Prabhakaran statement issued on 27 November 2004.

"Today we are faced with a critical and complex situation, unprecedented in the history of our liberation struggle. We are living in a political void, without war, without a stable peace, without the conditions of normalcy, without an interim or permanent solution to the ethnic conflict. Our liberation struggle will be seriously undermined if this political vacuum continues indefinitely.

"Three years have lapsed since we entered into a ceasefire agreement with the government of Sri Lanka, after three decades of protracted armed struggle. You are fully aware that during this period of ceasefire we have been making every endeavour, with sincerity and commitment, to seek a negotiated settlement to the Tamil national question through peaceful means. In various capitals of foreign nations, with Norway as facilitators, we engaged in peace talks with the government. The six sessions of negotiations held over the duration of six months, turned out to be futile and meaningless. Sub-committees that were set up for the de-escalation of the conflict, for the restoration of normalcy, for the rehabilitation and resettlement of the displaced and for the reconstruction of the war damaged infrastructure, became non-functional. In the meantime, the Sri Lanka government, having excluded our liberation organisation, participated in the donor conference held in Washington, thereby undermining our status as equal partners in the peace process. It was in these objective conditions that our organisation decided to express our displeasure and disappointment by temporarily suspending the talks. Our intention was not to terminate the talks and put an end to the peace process. During the period of suspension we urged the government of Mr Rani Wickramasinghe to formulate and submit a draft proposal for an interim administrative structure. We emphasised that the envisaged interim administrative mechanism should be invested with adequate authority to deal with the rehabilitation of the war affected people and to reconstruct the war devastated Tamil nation.

"We were not satisfied with the three successive draft proposals on an interim set-up submitted by Ranil's government. The draft frameworks lacked adequate administrative authority and they were unacceptable to us. Ultimately, we decided to formulate our own set of proposals. We discussed with our people at different levels and consulted political experts, legal specialists and constitutional scholars in the Tamil diaspora and finalised our proposals for an Interim Self Governing Authority. This is an original and pragmatic framework embodying necessary structures and mechanisms to address the urgent existential problems of our people. The proposed framework is invested with substantial authority to effectively and expeditiously undertake all tasks of resettlement, rehabilitation, reconstruction and development in the Tamil homeland. We submitted this proposal to establish an Interim Self Governing Authority to Ranil Wickramasinghe's government on the 1st November last year and also released it to the media for public debate.

"Some international governments welcomed our proposal, because it was the first time the Liberation Tigers had clearly and explicitly spelt out their political ideas in writing. Ranil Wickramasinghe's government did not reject our proposal for an Interim Self Governing Authority to deal with the rehabilitation of the war affected people and to reconstruct the war devastated Tamil nation. His government viewed our proposals as different from their drafts, yet it agreed to resume peace talks on that basis, whereas the Sri Lankan Freedom Party outrightly condemned our interim administrative framework as the foundation for a separate Tamil state. As the leader of the Sri Lanka Freedom Party and as President Chandrika Kumaratunga went a step further by taking punitive action that plunged the southern polity into a crisis. Ranil Wickramasinghe's regime was suddenly and seriously destabilised when President Kumaratunga took over three key ministries, including defence. Eventually, following the dissolution of Parliament by the president, Ranil's government collapsed.

"The ethnic contradiction between the Sinhala and Tamil nations became acute as a consequence of the general elections held at the beginning of the year. The elections paved the way for the hegemonic dominance of Sinhala-Buddhist chauvinistic forces in the southern political arena. The Janatha Vimukthi Peramuna (JVP), an anti-Tamil political party steeped in a muddled ideology of racism, religious fanaticism and orthodox communism, won a substantial number of seats and became the third largest Sinhala political organisation. President Chandrika has embraced this racist political party as the most important ally and partner in her coalition government. This government is constituted by an unholy alliance of incompatible parties articulating antagonistic and mutually contradictory views and policies on the Tamil national question.

"While the verdict of the general election helped to reinforce Sinhala-Buddhist hegemonism in the Sinhala south, Tamil nationalism arose as a unified collective force in the northeastern Tamil homeland. The political ideals of our liberation organisation received the overwhelming support of the Tamil people. Our organisation received the popular endorsement as the sole representative of our people. Our proposals to establish an Interim Self Governing Authority received a mandate from our people. The Tamil National Alliance gained a sweeping victory by winning twenty-two seats, thereby becoming the political voice and the democratic force representing our liberation organisation. As never before, this general election has polarised the Sinhala and Tamil ethnic formations into two distinct nations, as two separate peoples with divergent and mutually incompatible ideologies, consciousness and political goals.

"Though there was a change of government in southern Sri Lanka and chauvinistic forces were able to gain political power, we continued to observe ceasefire and wanted to promote the peace process. We informed the Freedom Alliance government of Chandrika Kumaratunga, through the Norwegian facilitators, that we were prepared to resume peace talks based on our proposal to set-up an Interim Self Governing Authority. It was at that time, confusion and policy differences emerged within the ruling coalition.

"Politically, the most powerful partner in the alliance, the JVP, vehemently opposed granting political rights or devolution of power to the Tamil people. It has severely criticised the Norwegian government, which plays the role of facilitator. It has also outrightly rejected our proposal for an Interim Self Governing Authority. The JVP has warned that it would break away from the ruling coalition if peace talks resumed on the basis of our proposal. The extremist, hard-line attitude of the JVP towards peace and ethnic reconciliation has become a major challenge to Chandrika Kumaratunga.

"The government of Kumaratunga is facing a multi-dimensional crisis. On one side, the international community is exerting pressure on the government to resolve the ethnic conflict through peaceful means. On the other, the donor countries continue to insist that granting of the pledged aid package is conditional upon progress in the peace talks. Furthermore, the economy of the country is sliding into an abyss. With these multiple problems, the government is compelled to engage the LTTE in peace negotiations. But the internal contradictions and the fundamental policy differences in the ruling alliance have become a stumbling block to the resumption of peace negotiations. There is no clear, coherent policy orientation, or a consensus approach within the political parties of the coalition government. Since she has aligned herself with political parties drenched in anti-Tamil racism, militarism and Sinhala-Buddhist hegemonism, the president cannot advance the peace process based on a coherent, consistent strategy and policy. This is the authentic political reality prevailing in southern Sri Lanka. This political reality of the lack of consensus is skilfully covered up and concealed to the international community.

"We submitted our proposals for an interim administration at the final stage of our negotiations with Ranil Wickramasinghe's government. The leadership of the United National Party continues to insist that peace talks can be resumed based on our set of proposals, but the Kumaratunga government is imposing a condition for the resumption of talks. The government says that any form of interim administration should be an integral part of a permanent settlement. While we are demanding an interim administrative set-up, the Kumaratunga government is insisting on talks for a permanent settlement to the ethnic conflict.

"There are important reasons as to why we are insisting on the formation of an interim administrative set-up as early as possible. As a consequence of a brutal and protracted war our people are facing urgent existential needs and immense humanitarian problems. Hundreds of thousands of displaced Tamils continue to languish in refugee camps in appalling conditions. In the meantime, the donor governments have pledged a massive aid package for the relief and rehabilitation of the war affected people. Therefore, it is of critical necessity that an interim administrative mechanism should be instituted with adequate powers to undertake the task of providing relief and rehabilitation to the suffering Tamil population and to reconstruct the war devastated Tamil homeland.

"Though we have entered into a ceasefire agreement and observed peace for three years and participated in the peace talks for six months, our people have not yet received any peace dividends. The intolerable burden of the day-to-day life problems is suffocating our people. Our people are desperately anticipating relief and resolutions to their urgent existential problems. For these reasons we want the immediate resumption of peace talks, based on our proposal, so that an interim administrative authority can be established as early as possible to address the grievances of our people. If some elements of our proposals are deemed problematic or controversial, these issues can be resolved through discussions at the negotiating table. Once the interim administrative authority is institutionalised and becomes functional we are prepared to engage in negotiations for a permanent settlement to the ethnic problem. That is our position. Our position is reasonable. We are advocating this position in relation to the actuality of the concrete conditions prevailing in the Tamil homeland. Nevertheless, President Kumaratunga is inviting us for talks on a permanent solution, advancing a position that even an interim administrative set-up should be worked out within the contours of a final settlement. We can point out different reasons as to why she gives primacy to talks on a permanent solution. One reason could be her strategy to satisfy extremist racist elements, particularly to placate, to satisfy extremist racist elements, particularly to placate the JVP, who are deadly opposed to our proposal for an interim administration. The second reason could be to impress upon the international community that she is genuinely committed to resolving the Tamil national question. The third reason could be to prolong the peace negotiations indefinitely by opting to talk on a most intractable and complex issue. We can come up with several other reasons. Whatever the real reason, we can clearly and confidently say one thing; it is apparent from the inconsistent and contradictory statements made by President Kumaratunga that her government is not going to offer the Tamil people either an interim administration or a permanent solution.

"I do not wish to elaborate here the bitter historical experience of political negotiations we have engaged in with the Sinhala political leadership for more than fifty years to resolve the ethnic problem of the Tamil nation. Over a long period of time, we had talks on linguistic rights, on equal rights, on regional autonomy, on federal self-rule and entered into pacts and agreements, which were later torn apart and abrogated. Our liberation organisation is not prepared to walk the path of treachery and deception once again.

"The Sinhala political organisations and their leadership, which are deeply buried in the mud of Sinhala-Buddhist chauvinism, will never be able to comprehend the political aspirations of the people of Tamil Eelam. None of the major Sinhala political parties are prepared to recognise the fundamentals underlying the Tamil national question. None of the Sinhala political organisations is prepared to accept the northeastern region as the historical homeland of the Tamil-speaking people, that the Tamils constitute themselves as a distinct nationality and that they are entitled to the right to self-determination, including the right to secede.

"The southern political movements do not have the maturity and magnanimity or the political sagacity to understand and accept the fundamentals of the Tamil national question, nor do they possess a consensus or a collective vision on the Tamil issue. What we can observe in the southern political spectrum is division, disunity and mutually divergent, contradictory notions and policies. We are surprised to note that President Kumaratunga is showing concern and interest in resolving the ethnic conflict when political parties aligned to her coalition government are advocating incoherent and irrational policies and articulating brazen forms of racism. We wish to make an open request to all the political parties constituting the governing Freedom Alliance, as well as to the opposition United National Party, to declare publicly their official policy on the fundamentals of the Tamil national question, particularly on the core demands of the Tamil's concerning homeland, nationality and the right to self-determination.

"'It will be meaningful to talk about a permanent settlement if the Sinhala political organisations have a clear, coherent policy, a proper insight and a consensus approach towards the Tamil national question. If not, there is no meaning in engaging in talks about a permanent solution. There is division, discord, confusion, and contradiction within the Sinhala political leadership on the Tamil issue. Having realised the truth that the Sinhala political leadership will not be able to offer a reasonable permanent solution to our people, we submitted an interim solution. We expressed our desire to resume negotiations, based on our proposals for an interim mechanism, to provide relief to our people's urgent existential needs. But the government of Kumaratunga is deliberately impeding the peace efforts by insisting that talks should be about a permanent settlement. Having covered up the serious policy differences and internal contradictions behind the curtain of a loose political alliance, President Kumaratunga is accusing the Tamil Tigers of intransigence. We are confident that the international community will soon be able to see the real face of Chandrika, who is acting with a deceptive mask of peace.

"We cannot continue to be entrapped in a political vacuum without an interim solution or a permanent settlement, without a stable peace and without peace of mind. The Sinhala nation neither assimilates and integrates our people to live in coexistence nor does it allow our people to secede and lead a separate existence. We cannot continue to live in the darkness of political uncertainty, without freedom, without emancipation, without any prospects for the future. There are borderlines to patience and expectations. We have now reached the borderline. At this critical moment we wish to make an urgent appeal to the Sri Lanka government. We urge the government to resume the peace negotiations without conditions, based on our proposal for an Interim Self Governing Authority. If the government of Sri Lanka rejects for an Interim Self Governing Authority. If the government of Sri Lanka rejects our urgent appeal and adopts delaying tactics, perpetuating the suffering of our people, we have no alternative other than to advance the freedom struggle of our nation. We call upon the concerned international governments to understand our predicament and prevail upon the Sri Lanka government to resume peace talks based on our fair and reasonable stand.'

Govt. Responds to LTTE Statement (December 2, 2004 –3.00 GMT)

The government in its response to the LTTE's call for unconditional resumption of peace talks said "insisting unilaterally on a single agenda item is scarcely conducive to good faith negotiations".

On Saturday LTTE leader Velupillai Prabhakaran demanded that the government resume peace negotiations immediately, based on their proposals for an Interim Self Governing Authority.

Appendix

Full text of the government statement:

The government is engaged in a careful study of the statement of the leader of the Liberation Tigers of Tamil Eelam made on November 27.

The absence of direct negotiations since April 2003 is of no benefit to anyone and is unsustainable. Following its election to office in April this year, the UPFA government has, therefore, made serious, sincere and consistent efforts to reopen talks with the LTTE. These efforts are well known to the people of Sri Lanka and to the international community.

A call, couched in threatening language, from the LTTE now for a resumption of negotiations without conditions, while setting conditions itself by insisting unilaterally on a single agenda item is scarcely conducive to good faith negotiations.

The government of Sri Lanka has conveyed publicly, and through the kind facilitation of the Royal Norwegian government, its readiness to discuss the establishment of an interim authority to meet the urgent humanitarian and development needs of the people of the North and East as a priority, while exploring a permanent settlement along the lines of the document signed and accepted by the government and the LTTE in Oslo on December 5, 2002. It also remains firmly committed to the strict maintenance of the Ceasefire Agreement and condemns all violations and actions jeopardising the prevailing ceasefire and which caused fear and thereby tensions among the civil population, leading to the undue rupture of the sensitive balance of ethnic groups presently maintained by the government with the objective of safeguarding the ceasefire and taking the peace process forward.

The government of Sri Lanka is in communication with the Royal Norwegian government on future steps to be taken in the peace process.

APPENDIX – I
Chronology of the 6th Peace Effort Peace Process
Feb 06, 2004

2001	
Dec 05	The UNF government led by Prime Minister Ranil Wickramasinghe *wins* Parliamentary elections on a pledge to open talks with the Liberation Tigers of Tamil Eelam.
Dec 19	LTTE declares a month long unilateral ceasefire beginning midnight on 24 December 2001.
Dec 21	The GOSL *reciprocates;* a bilateral ceasefire in place.
Dec 27	PM officially requests the government of Norway to recommence its facilitator role.
2002	
Jan 01	LTTE leader *writes* to Norwegian PM, requests Norway to continue facilitating between the GOSL and the LTTE.
Jan 02	Government relaxes movement of goods to Wanni area with effect from January 15, 2002.
Jan 08	LTTE suggests India as a venue for talks
Jan 10	A three-member Norwegian peace delegation headed by Vidar Helgessen arrives in Colombo. Norwegian delegation *meets* president. "The ban imposed on the LTTE in Sri Lanka should be lifted immediately to facilitate the commencement of peace negotiations"- TNA tells Norwegian delegation
Jan 12	Norwegian delegation leaves.

Jan 15	PM orders the lifting of economic sanctions on rebel-held areas. The Tigers ease travel restrictions on civilians. The Tigers ease travel restrictions on civilians. Civilian movement to the Vanni allowed on all weekdays; Earlier civilian traffic was permitted only on two days of the week.
Jan 20	Govt, LTTE *extend* ceasefire till February 24, 2002.
Jan 21	LTTE *releases* 10 prisoners as goodwill measure.
Jan 22	"Govt. to consider temporarily lifting the ban on the LTTE" –PM's first *policy* statement to the Parliament.
Feb 01	Civilians protest LTTE extortion, Trincomalee.
Feb 04	Govt. opens Vavuniya-Trincomalee road after a decade.
Feb 05	President *expresses* her deep concern at LTTE's continued child conscription LTTE rejects President's child-recruitment charge.
Feb 06	SLA, LTTE begin de-mining operations at different sites in Omanthai watched by the ICRC.
Feb 12	SLA, LTTE concludes de-mining operations Govt. relaxes travel restrictions to Jaffna.
Feb 19	Govt. reopens Jaffna-Kandy A-9 highway
Feb 22	Ceasefire Agreement (CFA) • Prabhakaran signs CFA copy given by Norwegian Ambassador (February 20, 2002, Vanni) • Shown to the president, Thursday, February 21, evening

	• CFA signed by PM in Vavuniya, Friday, February 22-PM visits Omanthai and meets SL Army Personnel
Feb 24	• SLMM arrives to monitor CFA
	• Status of Mission Agreement (SOMA) – States conditions of SLMM Operations; not made public unlike the MoU.
Feb 27	CBK writes to PM a 9-page letter with her observations on the CFA. • Eleventh hour submission of CFA to the president. • Legality of document? Article 4.1 requires the signature of PM, LTTE leader and not that of the president. • Certain Articles in CFA could impinge on national security • The importance of addressing substantive issues in the talks. Do not make the CFA an end in itself. • CFA should not continue indefinitely without a political solution being reached. • Questions Article 1.2: "offensive naval operations" • Article 1.3: "without engaging in offensive operations against the LTTE", creates impression SLN prohibited from engaging LTTE boats, even if suspected of carrying arms. • SLN should be given clear instructions as to their powers and duties regarding illegal arms shipment

	• LTTE continues to violate assurances given to the UN on child recruitment.
Mar 04	Parliament debates CFA
Mar 11	President, PM discuss CFA
Mar 13	CFA has no legal validity says lawyer H L De Silva, a leading constitutional expert and Sri Lanka's former permanent representative to the UN.
Mar 27	President welcomes announcement of direct peace talks
	Government and LTTE shop for talks venue –India declines
Mar 29	Thailand agrees to play host for peace talks
	Norwegian facilitators meet the president
Apr 04	LTTE charges an entry tax to move beyond Ommanthai.
Apr 10	Prabhakaran holds International Press Conference in the Wanni (First in 12 years he agrees to accept regional autonomy, but says the LTTE will not decommission until a final solution is reached).
Apr 19	Norwegian facilitators call on the president to discuss peace process.
June 25	Tamil-Muslim clashes in the East (Muslims protest against alleged extortion by the LTTE and attacks on them by LTTE supporters).
July 10	Peace talks should begin soon – President.
July 13	LTTE captures two Nordic monitors
July 16	SLMM claims this LTTE act violates CFA
July 19	Peoples' Alliance calls for a revision of the CFA
July 22	UTHR accuses LTTE of child conscription

July 29	Moragoda meets Balasingham in London
Aug 12	Govt. approves sea route for LTTE • A separate sea lane for LTTE vessels sailing off Vanni, to be used twice a week with a SLMM monitor on board, under SLN supervision • Required to inform the govt. 48 hours prior to sea movement • Sea movement permitted only during day time, 6 a.m. – 6 p.m.
Aug 14	Norway announces dates for talks.
Aug 16	President calls for report on Govt.-LTTE sea movement agreement.
Sep 02	President against lifting ban on LTTE
Sep 05	President calls for report on GOSL-LTTE sea movement agreement.
Sep 10	Govt. announces compositions of its delegation for talks.
Sep 13	Stop arms smuggling – President writes to PM.
Sep 14	GOSL Peace team leaves for Thailand Interim Administration – put on the back burner no such demand at 1st round of talks.
Sep 16-18	The first formal peace talks between GOSL-LTTE Rose Garden, Sattahip, Thailand Parties agree on.... Top priority for humanitarian challenges Step by step approach to peace
Sep 25	Seven soldiers of the SLA abducted by the LTTE demanding the release of two cadres in govt. custody.
Sep 27	Abduction issue continues; SLMM says it will not intervene in law of the country.

Appendix – I

Sep 28	GOSL and LTTE swap 18 prisoners in Omanthai
Sep 30	President welcomes prisoner swap
Oct 02	President writes to PM on matters of national security
Oct 04	Moragoda briefs president on Sattahip peace talks
Oct 07	EPDP writes to SLMM 'What the LTTE could not achieve through war it is now achieving through the CFA'
Oct 08	Opposition calls for immediate release of detained soldiers
Oct 10	LTTE releases the 6 soldiers storming of a STF camp in Kanchirankudah, Batticoloa—7 dead. Muslims fear their fate under LTTE control.
Oct 11	Tamil – Muslim clashes in the East again; Vallaichenai
Oct 16	Tamil – Muslim clashes in Akkaraipattu
Oct 18	Release of Muslim civilians in LTTE custody has to be insisted – president writes to defence secretary
Oct 20	Norwegian delegation arrives in Colombo
Oct 29	President says Joint Task Force should be legal.
Oct 31-Nov 03	Colombo High Court sentences LTTE leader Prabhakaran to 200 years imprisonment for 1996 Central bank bombing. **Talks session II**-Rose Garden, Thailand Parties decide to set up sub-committees: SIHRN, SDN, SPM Tigers agree to take up contentious political issues for discussion and enter mainstream politics.

Nov 12	President briefed on second round of talks by Moragoda. President proposes inclusion of LTTE in Commission for Peace.
Nov 15	Norway no longer impartial – Kadirgamar
Nov 18	Westborg meets Kadirgamar
Nov 21	Session III would be political round —GL
Nov 22	President reviews security in the North & East. Ensure law and order in the Delft – president directs defence secretary and IGP.
Nov 25	Norwegian Govt hosts a one-day Peace Support Meeting in Oslo Tigers and the government have their first international outing, going before foreign donors in Oslo and winning up to 85 million dollars in aid to rebuild war-affected areas. President writes to PM urging him to discuss LTTE's intolerance of political opposition at Oslo.
Nov 26	Tactics of terror can never achieve legitimate aspirations —Richard Armitage
Nov 27	Army detects at Omanthai checkpoint a stock of high-powered radio transmitters for Voice of Tigers (VoT) with a permit from the defence secretary.
Dec 02-05	**Talks Session III,** Oslo clashes within SLMC, Hakeem, GOSL negotiator and leader, SLMC, makes hurried return (Dec 3) from Oslo. GOSL-LTTE agrees to explore federal models to find a solution within united Sri Lanka.

	LTTE retains right to self-determination and will resort to secession as "last resort".
Dec 19	JVP writes to president – VoT equipment had arrived October 29, consigned to Norway's Ambassador to Sri Lanka, Jon Westborg – 'Why was the equipment imported in the name of the Ambassador?'
Dec 27	LTTE categorically rejects decommissioning.... (HSZ issue) GOSL acknowledges granting a *Broadcast License* to the LTTE peace secretariat to run an FM radio station and arrange for the recent import of equipment –Licence issued November 11, 2002, in terms of Section 44 of the Sri Lanka Broadcasting Act No. 37 of 1966 – GOSL says request was made on October 18, 2002
Dec 28	High Security Zone issue – president endorses Jaffna SLA Commander Sarath Foneska's proposal, to disarm LTTE cadres before agreeing to the removal of the Jaffna HSZ
Dec 30	President writes to Norwegian PM on VoT issue President writes to PM requesting a report on VoT issue Govt. requests retired Lt. Gen. Satish Nambiar, first UN commander in erstwhile Yugoslavia and retired deputy chief of Indian Army to prepare a report on HSZs. LTTE rejects Nambiar's recommendations

2003

Jan 03	PM replies to the president on VoT issue: "Be cautious to ensure continued Norwegian facilitation"
Jan 06-09	**Talks session IV,** Nakorn Pathom, Thailand
	Tigers and the GOSL in talks in Thailand, agree to appoint the World Bank as custodian of millions of dollars expected in foreign aid.
	Norwegian PM replies president –"The GOSL has already answered your concerns".
Jan 21	Complaints of child recruitment and abductions continue.
Jan 22	President and PM discuss progress in peace.
Jan 23	Retired Maj. Gen. Trygve Tellefsen —new head of SLMM
Jan 27	President directs Army and Police- "Stop LTTE abducting children".
Feb 14	Ceremonial reopening of Jaffna public library opening postponed indefinitely under LTTE threat.
Mar 06	SLMM secure release of soldier and policeman.
Mar 10	Sri Lankan navy sinks a Tiger 'merchant vessel' – arms ship, killing 11 cadres, making it the most serious incident since the truce took effect.
Mar 12	Helgessen meets president and PM.
Mar 18-21	Chinese trawler attacked off eastern coast (Mar 20). LTTE blamed but denies charges.

Appendix – I

Mar 26	LTTE is not the sole interlocutor of the Tamils – Anandasangaree, MP, President, Tamil United Liberation Front.
Mar 29	Norwegian Ambassador, Jon Westborg bids farewell.
Mar 31	Sri Lanka Navy (SLN) vessel attacked, soldiers attacked.
Apr 01	SLN vessel, 'Lanka Muditha', attacked. Peace process will continue – President tells diplomats
Apr 07	President holds bilateral talks with Chief Minister Jayalalitha, of Tamil Nadu, India.
Apr 09	President dissatisfied with final report by SLMM on Chinese trawler issue.
Apr 15	Armitage explains LTTE's exclusion from Washington conference
Apr 21	LTTE unilaterally suspends peace talks, but says it is committed to peace. CFA intact.
Apr 22	President Kumaratunga places security forces on maximum alert as Tigers suspend talks. LTTE pulls out of talks, President says better sense should prevail, hopes talks would recommence
Apr 25	Your reasons unconvincing, get back to talks – US tells LTTE Opposition wants India's intervention.
Apr 28	Opposition concerned over the suspension of talks.
Apr 30	Peace process back on track – GL
May 05	President expresses concern about killing of Intelligence officers. "The Govt. promised us protection" – EPDP writes to President

May 22	S P Thamilselvam, LTTE's political wing leader makes clear LTTE's demand for Interim Administration at press conference in Killinochchi.
Jun 02	PM offers Apex Body to LTTE instead of Interim Administration.
Jun 04	LTTE rejects Apex Body offer.
Jun 05	LTTE boycotts the Tokyo Donor Conference. Continues demand for an Interim Administration. President says no to unconditional Interim Council.
Jun 09	PM offers 'provincial administrative role' to LTTE – speech made in Tokyo.
Jun 10	Tokyo donor conference ends. US $ 4.5 billion in aid pledged by international community.
Jun 14	SLN intercepts two ships that are not carrying any visible registrations. SLN fires, ships sink.
Jun 23	IP Sunil Thabrew who was handling a LTTE informant, killed by the informant himself.
Jun 27	SLMM says "The Navy had a legitimate right" to fire at ships without visible registration.
Jul 01	SLMM requests the LTTE to remove their (Kinniya) camp from the govt. controlled area of Trincomalee.
Jul 24	President appoints a committee to study IA proposals.
Jul 25	"Two versions of IA proposals; substantive discrepancies between them" – Lakshman Kadirgamar

Appendix – I

Jul 28	GOSL spokesman, G L Peiris, claims "No substantive difference between the two IA documents"
Jul 29	SLMM tells PRIU "Ceasefire Agreement undermined" – Kinniya camp issue
Aug 04	President open to discuss IA proposals
Aug 13	Two SLMC supporters killed in Muttur, Trincomalee District.
Aug 14	GOSL spokesman says LTTE to hold 'internal meeting' in Paris from August 21-27, with legal experts, to discuss government's IA proposals.
Sep 11	Special Japanese envoy Yasushi Akashi arrives to chair the post – Tokyo donors' conference. Both parties and the donors invited by the Japanese govt. to attend the meeting.
Sept 12	Follow-up meeting on Tokyo donors' conference held at Hilton Hotel, Colombo. LTTE boycott the meeting. "No aid if peace process is stagnant" – Donors reiterate President writes to PM *'Do not risk national security'* (LTTE threat to the Trincomalee naval base and harbour)
Sept 15	"International community might soon lose interest", warns Akashi. Akashi calls on the president to brief her on the deliberations of the post-Tokyo Donors' Conference. International Community recognised that President Kumaratunga had a key role to play in the peace process to ensure its success, says Akashi

Sept 17	Norwegian Deputy Foreign Minister Vidar Helgesen and Special Advisor Erik Solheim arrive in Colombo
Sept 18	Helgesen, Solheim meet Thamilchelvan Norway hopes talks would recommence mid October *'Let us both pledge to stop parochial political debates on defence issues'* – PM sends a reply to president
Oct 02	USA *redesignates* LTTE as a 'foreign terrorist organisation'
Oct 03	The first batch of LTTE child soldiers *freed* under a UNICEF programme
Oct 04	Reports of more than 20 children abducted by the LTTE in the east.
Oct 06	President *writes* to PM again on LTTE threat to Trincomalee Naval base and harbour. Says his reply (September 17) does not address the important security concerns that she had raised in her letter (September 12)
Oct 07	UNICEF *calls* for the release of the children.
Oct 08	Defence Minister concedes, LTTE military build up around Trincomalee harbour is cause for concern.
Oct 15	**'Third parties who facilitate conflict resolution should avoid mediating or offering guidance'**- Indian Finance Minister Yashwant Sinha *explains* India's reasons for not actively involving itself in Sri Lanka's current peace process.
Oct 21	MoU neglects Muslim concerns *says* Kadirgamar in Parliament.

Appendix – I

Oct 23	President *requests* Norway to remove SLMM Head
Oct 30	SLMM head *recalled* to Oslo for consultation
Oct 31	LTTE *hands over* their much anticipated *proposals* to government through the Norwegian facilitators. LTTE for Interim Self Governing Authority (ISGA)
Nov 04	President *relieves* three ministers of portfolios. The three portfolios are Defence, Interior, and Mass Communications.
Nov 05	Sovereignty not negotiable – SLFP *rejects* Tiger proposals. CFA still stands, *says* President
Nov 12	President *meets* Helgesen and Solheim, says prime minister would continue with peace process
Nov 13	Norwegian delegation *calls on* President. "Peace process in good shape," says Norway
Nov 14	"We will wait" – Norway suspends it's role as facilitator in the Sri Lankan peace process.
Nov 29	Unrest in Trincomalee after three Muslim farmers were brutally murdered in Kinniya.
Dec 01	President *directs* defence authorities to normalise Trinco situation immediately.
2004	
Jan 19	Retired Major General Trond Furuhovde reappointed as Head of SLMM from February 1, 2004 Akashi arrives in Colombo for the second follow-up meeting of Donors' Conference.

APPENDIX – II
Norway Announces Permanent Ceasefire in Sri Lanka
Tamil Net, February 22, 2002

The Norwegian government on Friday declared the commencement from Saturday of a permanent ceasefire between the Sri Lankan government and the Liberation Tigers. In a statement, Jan Petersen, Foreign Minister of Norway, said his government had been asked to make public the agreement signed by LTTE leader Vellupillai Prabhakaran and Sri Lankan prime minister Ranil Wickramasinghe.

The full text of Mr. Petersen's statement follows:

"As from 00:00 hours on 23 February 2002, a ceasefire agreement enters into force between the government of Sri Lanka and the Liberation Tamil Tigers of Eelam (LTTE). The ceasefire document, signed by Sri Lankan prime minister Ranil Wickramasinghe and LTTE leader Vellipulai Prabhakaran, has been deposited with the Norwegian government, and we have been asked to make the agreement public.

"The overall objective of the parties is to find a negotiated solution to the ethnic conflict in Sri Lanka, which has cost 60,000 lives and caused widespread human suffering. The ceasefire will pave the way for further steps towards negotiations.

"Through this formalised ceasefire the parties commit themselves to putting an end to the hostilities. They commit themselves to restoring normalcy for all the inhabitants of Sri Lanka, whether they are Sinhalese, Tamils, Muslims or others. And they commit themselves to accepting an international monitoring mission, led by Norway, which will conduct on-site monitoring.

"Both sides have taken bold steps to conclude the ceasefire, and this agreement is a message that they are prepared to continue taking bold steps to achieve peace. They are embarking on a long road towards a political solution. It will not be easy. It will require determination and courage. The parties will face risks and uncertainties, and they will have to make hard choices. But no hardships are worse than those of conflict and bloodshed. No gains are greater than those of peace and prosperity.

"On the journey to peace and prosperity, the inhabitants of Sri Lanka, and their leaders, will need the solidarity of the international community. It must mobilise political and financial support for peace and reconciliation. Norway will continue to accompany the parties in this demanding process.

"I shall now provide some more detail about the ceasefire agreement.

"First, it outlines the modalities of the ceasefire, including the total cessation of all offensive military operations, the separation of forces, and increased freedom of movement for unarmed troops on both sides.

"Second, measures to restore normalcy for all the inhabitants of Sri Lanka – Sinhalese, Tamils, Muslims and others –putting an end to hostile acts against civilians, allowing the unimpeded flow of non-military goods, opening roads and railway lines, and a gradual easing of fishing restrictions.

"Third, a small international monitoring mission, led by Norway. The mission will conduct international on-site monitoring of the fulfillment of the commitments made by the parties. Let me underline, however, that it is up to the parties to respect the agreement and to impose sanctions on those individuals on either side who act contrary to the agreement."

APPENDIX – III
Text of Sri Lanka Ceasefire Agreement
22 February 2002

Agreement on a ceasefire between the government of the Democratic Socialist Republic of Sri Lanka and the Liberation Tigers of Tamil Eelam

Preamble

The overall objective of the government of the Democratic Socialist Republic of Sri Lanka (hereinafter referred to as the GOSL) and the Liberation Tigers of Tamil Eelam (hereinafter referred to as the LTTE) is to find a negotiated solution to the ongoing ethnic conflict in Sri Lanka.

The GOSL and the LTTE (hereinafter referred to as the parties) recognise the importance of bringing an end to the hostilities and improving the living conditions for all inhabitants affected by the conflict.

Bringing an end to the hostilities is also seen by the parties as a means of establishing a positive atmosphere in which further steps towards negotiations on a lasting solution can be taken.

The parties further recognise that groups that are not directly party to the conflict are also suffering the consequences of it.

This is particularly the case as regards the Muslim population. Therefore, the provisions of this agreement regarding the security of civilians and their property apply to all inhabitants.

With reference to the above, the parties have agreed to enter into a ceasefire, refrain from conduct that could undermine the good intentions or violate the spirit of this agreement and implement confidence-building measures as indicated in the articles below.

Article 1: Modalities of a ceasefire

The parties have agreed to implement a ceasefire between their armed forces as follows:

(1.1) A jointly agreed ceasefire between the GOSL and the LTTE shall enter into force on such date as is notified by the Norwegian Minister of Foreign Affairs in accordance with Article 4.2, hereinafter referred to as D-day.

Appendix – III

Military operations

(1.2) Neither party shall engage in any offensive military operation. This requires the total cessation of all military action and includes, but is not limited to, such acts as:
- a) The firing of direct and indirect weapons, armed raids, ambushes, assassinations, abductions, destruction of civilian or military property, sabotage, suicide missions, and activities by deep penetration units;
- b) Aerial bombardment;
- c) Offensive naval operations.

(1.3) The Sri Lankan armed forces shall continue to perform their legitimate task of safeguarding the sovereignty and territorial integrity of Sri Lanka without engaging in offensive operations against the LTTE.

Separation of forces

(1.4) Where forward defence localities have been established, the GOSL's armed forces and the LTTE's fighting formations shall hold their ground positions, maintaining a zone of separation of a minimum of 600 metres.

However, each party reserves the right of movement within 100 metres of its own defence localities, keeping an absolute minimum distance of 400 metres between them.

Where existing positions are closer than 400 metres, no such right of movement applies and the parties agree to ensure the maximum possible distance between their personnel.

(1.5) In areas where localities have not been clearly established, the status quo as regards the areas controlled by the GOSL and the LTTE, respectively, on 24 December 2001 shall continue to apply pending such demarcation as is provided in article 1.6

(1.6) The parties shall provide information to the Sri Lanka Monitoring Mission (SLMM) regarding defence localities in all areas of contention, cf. Article 3. The monitoring mission shall assist the parties in drawing up demarcation lines at the latest by D-day + 30.

(1.7) The parties shall not move munitions, explosives or military equipment into the area controlled by the other party.

(1.8) Tamil paramilitary groups shall be disarmed by the GOSL by D-day + 30 at the latest. The GOSL shall offer to integrate individuals in these units under the command and disciplinary structure of the GOSL armed forces for service away from the Northern and Eastern Province.

Freedom of movement

(1.9) The parties' forces shall initially stay in the areas under their respective control, as provided in Article 1.4 and Article 1.5

(1.10) Unarmed GOSL troops shall, as of D-day + 60, be permitted unlimited passage between Jaffna and Vavunyia using the Jaffna-Kandy road (A9). The modalities are to be worked out by the parties with the assistance of the SLMM.

(1.11) The parties agree that as of D-day individual combatants shall, on the recommendation of their area commander, be permitted, unarmed and in plain clothes, to visit family and friends residing in areas under the control of the other party. Such visits shall be limited to six days every second month, not including the time of travel by the shortest applicable route. The LTTE shall facilitate the use of the Jaffna-Kandy road for this purpose. The parties reserve the right to deny entry to specified military areas.

(1.12) The parties agree that as of D-day individual combatants shall notwithstanding the two-month restriction, be permitted, unarmed and in plain clothes, to visit immediate family (i.e., spouses, children, grandparents, parents, and siblings) in connection with weddings or funerals. The right to deny entry to specified military areas applies.

(1.13) Fifty unarmed LTTE members shall as of D-day + 30, for the purpose of political work, be permitted freedom of movement in the areas of the North and the East dominated by the GOSL. Additional 100 unarmed LTTE members shall be permitted freedom of movement as of D-day + 60. As of D-day =90, all unarmed LTTE members shall be permitted freedom of movement in the North and the East. The LTTE members shall carry identity papers. The right of the GOSL to deny entry to specified military areas applies.

Article 2: Measures to restore normalcy

The parties shall undertake the following confidence-building measures with the aim of restoring normalcy for all inhabitants of Sri Lanka:

(2.1) The parties shall in accordance with international law abstain from hostile acts against the civilian population, including such acts as torture, intimidation, abduction, extortion and harassment.

(2.2) The parties shall refrain from engaging in activities or propagating ideas that could offend cultural or religious sensitivities. Places of worship (temples, churches, mosques, and other holy sites etc.) currently held by the forces of either of the parties shall be vacated by D-day + 30 and made accessible to the public places of worship which are situated in "high security zones" shall be vacated by all armed personnel and maintained in good order by civilian workers, even when they are not made accessible to the public.

(2.3) Beginning on the date on which this agreement enters into force, school buildings occupied by either party shall be vacated and returned to their intended use. This activity shall be completed by D-day + 160 at the latest.

(2.4) A schedule indicating the return of all other public buildings to their intended use shall be drawn up by the parties and published at the latest by D-day + 30.

(2.5) The parties shall review the security measures and the set-up of checkpoints, particularly in densely populated cities and towns, in order to introduce systems that will prevent harassment of the civilian population. Such systems shall be in place from D-day + 60.

(2.6) The parties agree to ensure the unimpeded flow of non-military goods to and from the LTTE-dominated areas with the exception of certain items as shown in Annex A. Quantities shall be determined by market demand. The GOSL shall regularly review the matter with the aim of gradually removing any remaining restrictions on non-military goods.

(2.7) In order to facilitate the flow of goods and the movement of civilians, the parties agree to establish checkpoints on their line of control at such locations as are specified in Annex B.

(2.8) The parties shall take steps to ensure that the Trincomalee-Habarana road remains open on a 24-hour basis for passenger traffic with effect from D-day + 10.

(2.9) The parties shall facilitate the extension of the rail service on the Batticaloa-line to Welikanda. Repairs and maintenance shall be carried out by the GOSL in order to extend the service up to Batticaloa.

(2.10) The parties shall open the Kandy-Jaffna road (A9) to non-military traffic of goods and passengers. Specific modalities shall be worked out by the parties with the assistance of the Royal Norwegian government by D-Day + 30 at the latest.

(2.11) A gradual easing of the fishing restrictions shall take place starting from D-day. As of D-day + 90, all restrictions on day and night fishing shall be removed, subject to the following exceptions: (i) fishing will not be permitted within an area of 1 nautical mile on either side along the coast and 2 nautical miles seawards from all security forces camps on the coast; (ii) fishing will not be permitted in harbours or approaches to harbours, bays and estuaries along the coast.

(2.12) The parties agree that search operations and arrests under the Prevention of Terrorism Act shall not take place. Arrests shall be conducted under due process of law in accordance with the Criminal Procedure Code.

(2.13) The parties agree to provide family members of detainees access to the detainees within D-Day + 30.

Article 3: The Sri Lanka Monitoring Mission

The parties have agreed to set up an international monitoring mission to enquire into any instance of violation of the terms and conditions of this agreement. Both parties shall fully cooperate to rectify any matter of conflict caused by their respective sides. The mission shall conduct international verification through on-site monitoring of the fulfillment of the commitments entered into in this agreement as follows:

(3.1) The name of the monitoring mission shall be the Sri Lanka Monitoring Mission (hereinafter referred to as the SLMM).

(3.2) Subject to acceptance by the parties, the Royal Norwegian government (hereinafter referred to as the RNG) shall appoint the

Appendix – III

Head of the SLMM (hereinafter referred to as the HoM), who shall be the final authority regarding interpretation of this agreement.

(3.3) The SLMM shall liaise with the parties and report to the RNG.

(3.4) The HoM shall decide the date for the commencement of the SLMM's operations.

(3.5) The SLMM shall be composed of representatives from Nordic countries.

(3.6) The SLMM shall establish a headquarter in such place as the HoM finds appropriate. An office shall be established in Colombo and in Vanni in order to liaise with the GOSL and the LTTE, respectively. The SLMM will maintain a presence in the districts of Jaffna, Mannar, Vavuniya, Trincomalee, Batticaloa, and Amparai.

(3.7) A local monitoring committee shall be established in Jaffna, Mannar, Vavuniya, Trincomalee, Batticaloa, and Amparai. Each committee shall consist of five members, two appointed by the GOSL, two by the LTTE and one international monitor appointed by the HoM. The international monitor shall chair the committee. The GOSL and the LTTE appointees may be selected from among retired judges, public servants, religious leaders or similar leading citizens.

(3.8) The committees shall serve the SLMM in an advisory capacity and discuss issues relating to the implementation of this agreement in their respective districts, with a view to establishing a common understanding of such issues. In particular, they will seek to resolve any dispute concerning the implementation of this agreement at the lowest possible level.

(3.9) The parties shall be responsible for the appropriate protection of and security arrangements for all SLMM members.

(3.10) The parties agree to ensure the freedom of movement of the SLMM members in performing their tasks. The members of the SLMM shall be given immediate access to areas where violations of the agreement are alleged to have taken place. The parties also agree to facilitate the widest possible access to such areas for the local members of the six above-mentioned committees, cf. Article 3.7.

(3.11) It shall be the responsibility of the SLMM to take immediate action on any complaints made by either party to the agreement, and to enquire into and assist the parties in the settlement of any dispute that might arise in connection with such complaints.

(3.12) With the aim of resolving disputes at the lowest possible level, communication shall be established between commanders of the GOSL armed forces and the LTTE area leaders to enable them to resolve problems in the conflict zones.

(3.13) Guidelines for the operations of the SLMM shall be established in a separate document.

Article 4: Entry into force, amendments and termination of the agreement

(4.1) Each party shall notify its consent to be bound by this agreement through a letter to the Norwegian minister of foreign affairs signed by Prime Minister Ranil Wickramasinghe on behalf of the GOSL and by leader Velupillai Prabhakaran on behalf of the LTTE respectively. The agreement shall be initialled by each party and enclosed in the above-mentioned letter.

(4.2) The agreement shall enter into force on such date as is notified by the Norwegian Minister of Foreign Affairs.

(4.3) This agreement may be amended and modified by mutual agreement of both parties. Such amendments shall be notified in writing to the RNG.

(4.4) This agreement shall remain in force until notice of termination is given by either party to the RNG. Such notice shall be given 14 days in advance of the effective date of termination.

APPENDIX – IV
Sri Lanka: Prospects for Peace

Richard L. Armitage, Deputy Secretary of State
Remarks to the Center for Strategic and International Studies
Washington, DC
February 14, 2003

Thank you, Ambassador Schaffer (Director, Center for Strategic and International Studies, South Asia Program). As a diplomat and a scholar, you are a role model. Your actions and your efforts and your care and your devotion to all things in South Asia are well known, and well respected. And I am delighted also to see here the ambassador (Subasinghe, Ambassador of Sri Lanka to the United States). It seems as though it was just last month that you were visiting us to present your credentials. Come to think of it, it was only a month ago. It looks like you're settling in pretty well.

I have to tell you, Tezi (Schaffer), of course I would come here for this occasion. I wouldn't miss it. Twenty years, as far as I'm concerned, between my visits to Sri Lanka, was too long. And I have a feeling it won't be that long again. I suspect I will be out there again in the not too distant future. I am also delighted to be with all of you here today in such a reflective setting. You know, one of the things that is most, sort of, uncomfortable and unpleasant about government service is, there is no time for reflection. You rarely have the luxury of sitting back and actually thinking about something. And I am delighted to have a few minutes here.

The last couple of months — and indeed weeks — have been a busy time of high-stakes diplomacy for our Department of State. Secretary of State (Colin Powell) and I have been to Capitol Hill Six times together in the last two weeks — three testimonies apiece. Of course, we've been talking about such things as Iraq and its biological and chemical weapons and its nuclear intentions; about North Korea's self-inflicted deprivation and desperation, as millions of people are in danger of starving to death from mismanagement and bad luck; and about the high risk of terrorist attacks over this next week. But we've also been talking about the horrible terrorist bombing in downtown

Bogota over the last weekend and the implications for the counter-narcotics efforts in the region, as well as the rockets fired at international forces in Kabul on Monday, which narrowly missed the visiting defence minister of Germany. It certainly did underscore the importance of our reconstruction efforts in that blighted land.

Given these priorities, I think it is important to start today's discussion on Sri Lanka with a baseline question: why should be the United States invest significant attention and resources to Sri Lanka, especially at a time when we have such overwhelming competing interests? Should the United States play a role in this peace process?

Now, I believe the right answer is that the United States should play a role. And there are many credible explanations as to why. There is the pull of opportunity, of ending years of death and years of destruction and bolstering a multiethnic democracy. In the more direct bilateral sense, Sri Lanka is already a solid exporter to the United States and has the potential with peace and the right reforms to become a significant trade partner. And then there is the push of danger. As we have found out far too often, terror and human misery generally will not ebb away on their own or stay neatly within borders if we look at them as someone else's problem.

I have no doubt that the many experts Tezi (Schaffer) has assembled in his audience could provide more answers to my baseline questions. And when taken together, these answers may even add up to a compelling justification. But the problem is that these answers do not really constitute a clear strategic impetus for the United States or for other nations outside of Sri Lanka's immediate neighbourhood, particularly in a time of war and economic uncertainty. It would be tough to make a truly convincing case by sticking to the terms of strict self-interest.

For me, the bottom line in this instance is simple. The United States should be playing a role, in concert with other nations, committing our human and financial resources to settling this conflict because it can be done. And because it's the right thing to do. Because the parties to the conflict appear to be ready to reach a resolution, more so than at any other time in the past twenty years. And because it may well be that it is a resolution that can only be reached with the help of multilateral resources, both moral and material.

Appendix – IV

Indeed, this may be a key moment, when an infusion of such international support can add momentum to the peace process, helping to stop 20 years of abject human suffering and to smooth the ripples of grief and terror that have spread from this tiny island nation through the region and even around the world. This may be the moment when international support can help to spring this country into prominence as a recovering victim of conflict, terrorism, and human rights abuses, but also as a respected participant in the global community. And while I wouldn't want to oversell Sri Lanka as a model —this brew of caste, class, religion and race has its own unique flavour – perhaps this is a nation with lessons to offer the world about how to move from despair to hope, from intractable conflict to workable concord, and indeed, about how the international community can engage and support such conflict resolution.

So, with your permission, I'll share with you a few thoughts about the direction I see Sri Lanka heading in, and the more promising developments as well as the more problematic challenges, and how I believe the United States and the international community can most usefully participate.

Sadly, I have had the chance to see the costs of war up close. Last summer, I travelled to the Jaffna Peninsula. We first flew over the area in a helicopter and saw below us a blasted landscape, pockmarked with thousands of bomb craters and shell craters. For me, that view reminded me strongly of my time in the service in Vietnam. I really don't think I've seen anything quite like it since. And I'm talking both about the physical devastation and the sense of futility that was unmistakable on the ground.

We ventured into one of the cities that had been largely destroyed, where people were nonetheless starting to return, trying to reclaim lives many may have hardly remembered. Today, some 300,000 internally displaced people have returned to the northern and eastern parts of the country, even though these areas lack sanitation, clean water, and other basic amenities. This is, to some extent, a demonstration of confidence in the current ceasefire, but it also confirms something else I saw when I was there. We spoke with a cross-section of Tamil society in the area and the mixture of hope and wariness in their words was an unmistakable reminder that in Jaffna, and across Sri Lanka, a whole generation has grown up knowing little other than war, but is now ready for a change.

It was clear to me at the time that the solution had to start there, in the shattered people and bombed-out villages, in the universal longing for a better life. Because while it is clearly taking a firm decision from the parties to this fight to be partners and to act in the interests of peace, it is also going to take a commitment from all the people of Sri Lanka —Muslims and Buddhists, Christians and Hindus, Sinhalese and Tamils —from all parts of the country, if agreements made around the negotiating table are going to take hold on the ground.

Now, the challenge for the government of Sri Lanka and the LTTE is going to be taking that universal longing and that national commitment and giving people tangible signs of progress and a way to participate in the process. I think they have done a good job to date. First, they have set a powerful foundation. Keeping to the ceasefire for the past year has, as I noted, allowed the public to reach a basic level of confidence. And it is critical that both parties continue to honour and keep this ceasefire. From my point of view, a loss of confidence at this point would be extraordinarily devastating.

December 2002 was also a watershed. The negotiators issued a common statement that called for internal self-determination based on a federal structure within a united Sri Lanka, which created a shared vision for the future of the state, and dealt with many disagreements that destroyed past efforts at a negotiated solution. And in this latest round of talks, which just concluded last week in Berlin, the negotiators turned to concrete issues of humanitarian relief and human rights, including the LTTE's pledge to end child recruitment.

To me, this is all very encouraging. Indeed, two years ago, no one would have believed so much could happen so quickly. But to some extent, the steps taken to date have been the easy ones. And so the negotiations have entered a critical stage, a point at which both sides will have to show the courage to stay the course as they address more difficult issues and make real compromises.

Although the apprehension of an arms-laden trawler during the last round of negotiations and the self immolation by its LTTE crew were most remarkable for failing to derail peace talks, it also called into question the LTTE's commitment to the process. The LTTE is going to have to take a number of difficult steps to demonstrate that it remains committed to a political solution. The Tigers need to honor the restrictions and conditions that the ceasefire —and future negotiations—set on their arms supply. Logically, down the road, this is going to include disarmament issues themselves. Internal self-determination, within the framework of one Sri Lanka, is not going to be consistent with separate armies and navies for different parts of the country. For that matter, the LTTE has often pledged to stop the recruitment of child soldiers, but this time, they will have to prove they can carry through and will carry through on the pledge. The LTTE will also have to respect the rights of Muslims and Sinhalese living in areas under its control. And if the Tigers really want to join Sri Lanka's democratic society on a federal basis, they will also have to accept pluralism within the Tamil community.

Finally, the United States government is encouraged by the vision of the LTTE as a genuine political entity. But for that to happen, we believe the LTTE must publicly and unequivocally renounce terrorism and prove that its days of violence are over. The US will never accept the tactics of terror, regardless of any legitimate Tamil aspirations. But if the LTTE can move beyond the terror tactics of the past and make a convincing case through its conduct and its actual actions that it is committed to a political solution and to peace, the United States will certainly consider removing the LTTE from the list of Foreign Terrorist Organizations, as well as any other terrorism-related designations.

At the same time, the government of Sri Lanka must institute reforms that address the legitimate aspirations of the Tamil people. This means allowing Tamils the simple right to stay in their own homes and to pursue a living, such as fishing in coastal waters, without prejudice or harassment. But it also means protecting the full range of human rights for all the people of Sri Lanka. In particular, the burden will be on the government, military and civilian officials alike to prove that they can accord these rights to residents of the northern and the eastern parts of the nation, including the refugees returning to the area. And that they will hold officials accountable for the conduct.

The government obviously also must tackle key economic reforms. Because ultimately, the people of Sri Lanka, not just Tamils but also the Muslim and Sinhalese communities, particularly in the south, will judge the efficacy of the peace process by how it affects livelihood.

Reaching this vision of prosperity will require a strong and sustained commitment from the government of Sri Lanka. We should all give due credit to President Kumaratunga.

She knew this was the only answer for the country long ago. And her peace plan of 1995 was an important precursor to the progress we see now. Of course today, we owe much of that progress to the government of Prime Minister Ranil Wickramasinghe, who continues to take bold steps in the direction of peace. But it is clear that if Sri Lanka is to continue moving forward, the government must move together as one. No individual, no single political party can carry this burden alone. This must be a concerted effort by the President, the Prime Minister, and the parties.

There are those in Sri Lanka who remain sceptical, and truthfully, many come to their doubts honestly. The President, for one, is understandably cautious. But she also has unusual moral authority when it comes to one of the most difficult challenges facing both the government and the LTTE. As the head of state and inheritor of a powerful political dynasty, she is in a unique position to speak on behalf of everyone who serves or who has served in the government and to ask that those who committed atrocities in the past be forgiven. But she is also a victim of this conflict. She has not only lost loved ones to the violence but will personally bear the scars for the rest of her life. And so her forgiveness of those who have caused her pain is equally important.

In such a close community, everyone of the 65,000 lives lost in the last two decades is a burden of memory the whole society will have to carry. Indeed, perhaps it is too much to ask for forgiveness, but the people of Sri Lanka must somehow find a way to move forward. This may be the most significant challenge. It will require a concept of justice that falls somewhere between retribution and impunity, which will be absolutely necessary if the country is to reconcile with the past and reclaim the future. I believe President Kumaratunga must play a spiritually significant part in this search for truth and for reconciliation.

Appendix – IV

These are tremendous challenges. But these are also largely questions of the political will of the parties involved, something that must come largely from within Sri Lanka. The government of Norway does deserve tremendous credit for catalysing this political will and ushering the parties to the negotiating table. And the Norwegians deserve even more credit for going one step further.

Today, Sri Lanka has pressing humanitarian needs, as well as longer-term reconstruction, rehabilitation, and reintegration needs. Consider, for example, that there are an estimated 700,000 landmines in the country, and that alone is a nearly insurmountable challenge. Yet this is precisely where the government and the LTTE need to show progress and ways for ordinary people to participate. And they have to do this right away if the peace process is to attract the kind of public backing it requires. But the scale and scope of these needs are simply beyond Sri Lanka's means in the near term. And that is one reason international support is so absolutely critical at this time.

In November, Norway hosted a conference to orchestrate this international support, and where the Norwegians led and where they lead, we, the United States, are delighted to follow.

I was pleased to attend on behalf of the United States and to pledge $8 million in support of programmes that meet immediate humanitarian needs, as well as a little over $1 million for de-mining. In June, it is my intention to return for the follow-on meeting of donors, which Japan has graciously agreed to host. And at that time, I believe, with a certain assurance, that I will be able to announce significant further assistance to Sri Lanka for both humanitarian and economic aid.

Of course, such international involvement will come at a cost for Sri Lanka. The price tag for sustaining such interest will be progress – a clear demonstration that all parties to the negotiations have the determination to see this through. As I said at the outset, the fundamental attraction for this outpouring of international interest and certainly for my nation, is that we are not dealing in fantasy but firmly in the art of the possible. By June, both the government, all elements of the government, and the LTTE will need to have made some hard choices and compromises that demonstrate the political will to proceed if they want to meet their ambitions for international support.

Of course, Sri Lanka is hardly the only nation that struggles in the shadow of looming ethnic, racial and religious divides. From Kosovo to Kabul, there are places all over the world that are engaged in a similar fight, many of which have far less going for them in terms of physical infrastructure, in terms of human resources, and in terms of the institutions of democracy. And as Ambassador Schaffer recently wrote, there are other nations, from Northern Ireland to South Africa, that have already dealt with such challenges with some measure of success. From my point of view, and from my government's point of view, it is reasonable to hope that Sri Lanka will not only be able to add to the legacy of optimism of such past success but will also be able to build a model for peace and prosperity in a multifaceted society.

APPENDIX – V
Sinhala nationalists launch de-merger campaign in Trinco
Tamil Net, July 14, 2003

The "Sinhala Sanvidhanaya," a Sinhala nationalist movement on monday launched a signature campaign in Trincomalee to urge the de-merging of the North and East. The first signatory of the memorandum was the president of the organisation, venerable Dehiowitte Piyatissa Thera, sources said.

The signature campaign was launched at the clock tower junction, close to bus stand and general market in the heart of Trincomalee.

A spokesperson of the movement said the temporary merger now in force 1987 under the Indo-Sri Lanka accord should be cancelled and two provincial councils should be established, one for north and the other for east.

The spokesperson added that the signature campaign would be extended to other districts of the eastern province, Batticaloa, and Ampara shortly.

The aim of the movement is to collect one hundred thousand signatures from Sinhala, Tamil and Muslim people and to hand over the memorandum to President Ms Chandrika Kumaratunge, Sri Lanka's Prime Minister Mr Ranil Wickramasinghe and leaders of other political parties, spokesperson said.

APPENDIX – VI
SL President threatens to de-merge northeast province
Tamil Net, August 20, 2003

Sri Lanka's President, Ms Chandrika Kumaratunge, issued a warning through her media spokesman, Mr Harim Periris, on wednesday that she would not hesitate to de-merge the northeast province if the United National Front government failed to quell the violence and restore peace in the east, media sources said.

Mr Peiris, addressing a press conference Wednesday, said that people and religious leaders of the eastern province are making repeated requests to the President to de-merge the province to ensure their rights and safety. "Requests for the de-merger of the northeast province are closely studied by the president and she would take action in this regard at the appropriate time," he said at the press briefing.

"President Kumaratunga is of the view that people have started losing confidence in the Norwegian monitoring mission in the country, as they are not taking prompt steps against the ceasefire violations by the LTTE," said the spokesman for the president.

The northern and eastern provinces were merged according to the Indo-Sri Lanka agreement signed in 1987 by the then Sri Lankan president, J R Jayawardene, and the then Indian prime minister, Mr Rajiv Gandhi, with a condition that a referendum should be held to merge the provinces permanently after one year. However, the temporary merger of the two provinces still continues even after sixteen years and a Governor who has been appointed by the president is now administering the North East Provincial Council established under the 13th Constitutional Amendment.

The NEPC has had no elected administration since it was dissolved by the then President Mr R Premadasa in 1989. The other seven provincial councils in the south are being administered by elected administrations under the 13th constitutional amendment which was intended especially to solve the Tamil national question, political sources said.

APPENDIX – VII
'De-merger of NE a calamity to Sri Lanka' – TNA
Tamil Net, August 28, 2003

"The Tamil National Alliance (TNA) desires to place on record that the de-merger of the northeast province which has existed for the past fifteen years by the president would be a calamity to the whole Sri Lanka, and urges the president to desist from taking this perilous course," TNA said in a press statement issued Thursday in Colombo.

The leaders of Tamil United Liberation Front (TULF), Tamil Eelam Liberation Organisation (TELO), All Ceylon Tamil Congress (ACTC) and Eelam Peoples Revolutionary Liberation Front (EPRLF Suresh wing) have signed the press statement.

The full text of the press release of the TNA follows:-

Statements made by media spokespersons on behalf of the president of Sri Lanka, and the Peoples' Alliance, to the effect that de-merger of the northeast province is under serious consideration by the president have caused most serious concern to the Tamil people, since any such step would strike fatally at the very roots of the current peace process rendering the whole process, meaningless and redundant.

The Tamil National Alliance emphatically state that a Tamil linguistic region in the areas of historical habitation of the Tamil speaking people-the Northeast-constitutes the very foundation of any negotiated solution, and that any attempt to subvert this foundation will inevitably lead to the nullification of all prospects of a negotiated peaceful political solution to the Tamil question.

Such statements emanating from spokesperson on behalf of President Ms Chandrika Kumaratunge, who claimed when she actively entered electoral politics in 1994, that the main objective of her entering politics was to resolve the national question pertaining to the Tamil conflict, reinforces in the minds of the Tamil people the grave doubts they have always held in regard to the sincerity of Sinhala political leadership to evolve a just and acceptable political solution to the Tamil question, and convinces the Tamil people the need to stand together in this hour of peril and fearlessly face this threat.

The Tamil National Alliance reiterates that President Chandrika Kumaratunge made a political commitment to the creation of a region in the Northeast as a unit of power sharing. It was on the basis of such a commitment that the vast majority of the Tamil people at the presidential election in 1994 overwhelmingly supported Chandrika Kumaratunge. Viewed percentage-wise a much larger percentage of the Tamil people than either the Sinhala or Muslim people who voted at the presidential election in 1994 supported Chandrika Kumaratunge. It is indisputable that more than 90% of the Tamils, who voted in the eastern province at the 1994 presidential election, supported Chandrika Kumaratunge.

In 1994, Tamil political leaders for the first and only time in the history of presidential election campaign in Sri Lanka openly campaigned for Chandrika Kumaratunge. This was in view of Chandrika Kumaratunge's political commitment to devolve power to the northeastern region, on the basis of federal principles.

In the above circumstances, the statements made by her spokespersons that the de-merger of the northeastern province which has existed for the past fifteen years, is under her serious consideration, would if implemented, be a gross betrayal of the Tamil people, and an act of political perfidy. Such an act will undoubtedly incur the strongest disapproval of not merely the Tamil people in the northeast but of all Tamils, in all parts of the country, and will irretrievably alienate the President and the Peoples' Alliance from the Tamil people.

The reason attributed for such consideration is that some Muslim people have been killed or have disappeared in some areas in the east. After the signing of the 'Memorandum of Understanding' in February 2002 both Muslims and Tamils have been killed or have disappeared. Though such killings are insignificant compared to what happened prior to the Memorandum of understanding, all killings are unacceptable and must be stopped.

The LTTE is accused of the killings of Muslims. The Tamil National Alliance has raised the question of these killings and its harmful impact on the peace process with the LTTE. The LTTE has denied these killings. No direct evidence is forthcoming against the LTTE. Those who accuse the LTTE allege that if the LTTE is not responsible the LTTE should identify those responsible. It is common knowledge that detection of crime not merely in the northeast, but in all parts of Sri Lanka has reached a sorry state.

Appendix – VII

The LTTE is engaged in talks at various levels with the Muslim people. The leadership of the LTTE and the Sri Lanka Muslim Congress have met. Religious leaders and farmers organisations of the Muslim people are meeting with local LTTE leaders and day-to-day problems are being successfully addressed. Tamil and Muslim peoples very closely interact with each other, and the relationship between the vast majority of the Tamil and Muslim peoples who have lived together in the east or centuries and who enjoy a strong linguistic bond, are quite peaceful and normal. There can be no doubt that with the passage of time and further progress in the talks remaining issues will be discussed and will have to be resolved.

Except for a solitary Muslim parliamentarian who has been estranged from the party to which he belonged when elected, no other member of Parliament representing the Muslim people of the northeast, has sought the de-merger of the northeast. The positions of the Sri Lanka Muslim Congress and the National Unity Alliance, is that there is in existence a merged northeast, and that they expect legitimate Muslim aspirations within the merged northeast as expressed by them, to be adequately addressed. This position has been publicly articulated. This indeed was the clear position of the late Mr M H M Ashraff the leader of the SLMC and the NUA. Democratic Muslim leaders have for over a long period of time discussed these issues with democratic Tamil leaders. This process of discussion has now been extended to the LTTE. There can be no reservation to the Muslim question in the northeast being resolved on a just and equitable basis, so as to ensure the security, the social, economic and cultural well-being of the Muslim people in the northeast to the same inequalities and indignities to which the Tamil people have subjected by the Sri Lankan State.

The well-being of both the Tamil and Muslim peoples demands that these issues be discussed and resolved in a just and equitable manner and with a sense of pragmatism. It is only such a resolution that will bring everlasting peace and amity to the Tamil speaking Tamil and Muslim people who have lived together in the northeast for generations and centuries and who will have to continue to live together. This is primarily their own responsibility and not of anyone else.

Elements opposed to the peace process, who are against the Tamil question being resolved in a just and equitable manner, and who have developed a hatred against the LTTE, are endeavouring to magnify every incident in the east, and drive a wedge between the Tamils and Muslims, and thereby fulfill their own agenda of preventing a just and acceptable resolution of the Tamil question, and the LTTE being brought into the political mainstream. It has also been established that the reports pertaining to some purported incidents in the east have been unfounded and are false.

Some efforts have also been made to project the impression that the Sinhalese in the northeast are in a vulnerable position. Such fears are totally unfounded, as when there is a political resolution of the conflict and in a situation of peace, the Sinhalese people in the northeast, as also the Tamil and Muslim peoples in the rest of the country will have to peacefully co-exist with the majority community wherever they live. Much also has been made of an LTTE camp in Kurankupanchchan in the south of Trincomalee District and the SLMM's ruling that the camp is in government controlled territory and claims that it is within territory under their area, and that they have shown the SLMM evidence of the prior existence of an LTTE camp in this area. The nearest Police post is 8 km away from Soorangal and the nearest army camp is 14 km away at Wan Ela from this LTTE camp. This LTTE camp does not pose a threat to any Police or armed forces installation and is not situated in an area of any strategic importance. The SLMM and others are in continuous contact with the LTTE and there is expectation that this issue is not beyond resolution. It is unfortunate that much is sought to be made on this issue. While this issue definitely needs to be resolved over a period of time it is certainly not an issue on which the success or failure of the peace process in Sri Lanka must depend.

It would be pertinent to point out that the Sri Lanka government forces are not free from breaches of the ceasefire agreement. Some places of worship, school and public buildings are yet in the occupation of the armed forces. Even outside high security zones, displaced Tamil civilians are experiencing difficulties, in resettling and resuming their occupation. New armed forces camps have been set up in government-controlled territory, causing grave inconvenience to returning displaced Tamil civilians.

The matters surely cannot be unknown to President Chandrika Kumaratunge, her advisors, or her spokespersons.

The overall position is that after a protracted conflict lasting around two decades, in the midst of grave suspicion and distrust, efforts are being made to resettle displaced people and restore normalcy in the devastated northeast. This cannot be achieved without the patience understanding and cooperation of all persons in authority. The Tamil National Alliance considers it as singularly unfortunate, that not many persons in high authority have visited the northeast and seen for themselves the immense devastation that has been inflicted to the north particularly in the rural areas and the grave difficulties being experienced by returning displaced Tamil civilians.

It would be a grave mistake to endeavour to misuse the most difficult situation prevalent in the northeast in order to further the political agenda, of individual leaders, or their political parties. The northeast conflict has remained unresolved for several decades in view of the inability of Sinhala political leaders and their parties, to detach this burning issue from their partisan political agendas, and address the same with honesty and objectivity.

The Tamil National Alliance desires to place on record that the de-merger of the northeast province which has existed for the past fifteen years by the president would be a calamity to the whole Sri Lanka, and urges the president to desist from taking this perilous course.

APPENDIX – VIII
LTTE suspends negotiations with Sri Lanka pending implementation of agreements reached
Tamil Net, April 21, 2003

"Dear Prime Minister,
In accordance with the decision of our leadership I am advised to bring to your urgent attention the deep displeasure and dismay felt by our organisation on some critical issues relating to the on-going peace process.

You are well aware that the Ceasefire Agreement that had been in force for more than one year and the six rounds of peace negotiations between the principal parties has been successful, irrespective of the occurrence of some violent incidents that endangered the peace process. The stability of the ceasefire and the progress of the peace talks, you will certainly appreciate, are the positive outcome of the sincere and firm determination of the parties to seek a permanent resolution to the ethnic conflict through peaceful means. The cordial interrelationship, frank and open discussions and the able and wise guidance of the facilitators fostered trust and confidence between the negotiators and helped to advance the talks on substantial levels. The negotiating teams were able to form important sub-committees on the basis of equal and joint partnership. During the early negotiating sessions it was agreed that the government of Sri Lanka and the LTTE should work together and approach the international community in partnership. The Oslo Donor Conference held on 25 November 2002 turned out to be an ideal forum for such joint endeavour.

The LTTE has acted sincerely and in good faith extending its full cooperation to the government of Sri Lanka to seek international assistance to restore normalcy and to rehabilitate the war affected people of the northeast. The LTTE to date has joined hands with the government and participated in the preparation of joint appeals and programmes. In spite of our goodwill and trust, your government has opted to marginalise our organisation in approaching the international community for economic assistance. We refer to the exclusion of the LTTE from the crucial international donor conference to be held in Japan in June. We view the exclusion of the LTTE, the principle partner

Appendix – VIII

to peace and the authentic representatives of the Tamil people from discussions on critical matters affecting the economic and social welfare of the Tamil nation, as a grave breach of good faith. Your government, as legal constraints to invite representatives of a proscribed organisation to their country. In these circumstances an appropriate venue could have been selected to facilitate the LTTE to participate in this important preparatory aid conference. But the failure on the part of your government to do so gives cause for suspicion that this omission was deliberate. The exclusion of the LTTE from this conference has severely eroded the confidence of our people in the peace process.

As you are aware, considerable optimism and hopes were raised among the people when your government, shortly after assuming power, entered into a ceasefire agreement with our organisation, bringing to an end twenty years of savage and bloody conflict. Expectations were further raised when both sides began direct negotiations with Norwegian facilitation. In particular, there was a justifiable expectation that the peace process would address the urgent and immediate existential problems facing the people of the north and east, particularly the million people who are internally displaced by the conflict and are languishing in welfare centers and refugee camps.

As such, the Ceasefire Agreement included crucial conditions of restoring normalcy, which required the vacation, by occupying Sri Lankan troops, of Tamil homes, schools, places of worship and public buildings. Despite the agreed timeframe for this evacuation of troops, which has since passed, there has been no change in the ground situation. We have repeatedly raised the issue of continuing suffering of our people at every round of talks with your government. Your negotiators' repeated assurances that the resettlement of the displaced people would be expedited have proven futile. The negotiations have been successful in so far as significant progress has been made in key areas, such as the agreement to explore federalism on the basis of the right to self-determination of our people. But this progress has not people as a result of your government' refusal to implement the normalisation aspects of the Ceasefire Agreement and subsequent agreements reached at the talks. As a result, considerable disillusionment has set in amongst the Tamil people, and in particular the displaced, who have lost all hope the peace process will alleviate their immense suffering.

Though there is peace due to the silencing of the guns, normalcy has not returned to Tamil areas. Tens of thousands of government troops continue to occupy our towns, cities and residential areas suffocating the freedom of mobility or our people. Such a massive military occupation of Tamil lands, particularly in Jaffna – a densely populated district – during peace times denying the right of our displaced people to return to their homes, is unfair and unjust.

In our view, the conditions of reality prevailing in Tamil areas are qualitatively different from southern Sri Lanka. The Tamils faced the brunt of the brutal war. Twenty years of intense and incessant war has caused irreparable destruction to the infrastructure in the northeast. This colossal destruction augmented by continued displacement of the people and their inability to pursue their livelihoods due to military restrictions and activities have caused untold misery and extreme poverty among the people of the northeast. Continued displacement has also depleted all forms of savings of these people disabling them from regaining their lives on their own. The war-affected people need immediate help to regain their dignity. They need restoration of essential services to re-establish their lives. Reconstruction of infrastructures such as roads, hospitals, schools, and houses are essential for them to return to normal life.

The poverty that is prevailing in southern Sri Lanka is a self-inflicted phenomenon, caused by the disastrous policies of the past governments (both the UNP and the SLFP) in dealing with the Tamil national conflict. In its fanatical drive to prosecute an unjust war against the Tamil people, the Sinhala state wasted all national wealth to a futile cause. The massive borrowings to sustain an absurd policy of 'war for peace' by the former government caused huge international indebtedness. The economic situation of the south has been further worsened by the mismanagement of state funds, bad governance and institutional corruption. Therefore, the conditions prevailing in the south are distinctly different from the northeast where the scale and magnitude of the infra-structural destruction is monumental and the poverty is acute. Ignoring this distinctive reality, your government posits poverty as a common phenomenon across the country and attempts to seek a solution with a common approach. This approach grossly understates the severity of the problems faced by the people in the northeast.

The government's regaining Sri Lanka' document completely lacks any form of identified goals for the northeast. Statistics presented for substantiating the policy totally ignore the northeast and solely concentrate on southern Sri Lanka. However, this has been promoted as the national strategy to the international community to seek aid. It is evident from this that the government lacks any comprehensive strategy for serious development of the northeast. The poverty reduction strategy fails to address the poverty of the northeast as distinct from the rest. In seeking international assistance your government disingenuously speaks of reconstruction being needed in all areas, thereby masking the total destruction of the infrastructure of the northeast which has resulted from the militarist policies of the past three decades.

As we pointed out above, the exclusion of the LTTE from critical aid conference in Washington, the non-implementation of the terms and conditions enunciated in the truce document, the continuous suffering and hardship experienced by hundreds of thousands of internally displaced Tamils, the aggressive Sinhala military occupation of Tamil cities and civilian settlements, the distortion and marginalisation of the extreme conditions of poverty and deprivation of the Tamils of the northeast in the macro-economic policies and strategies of the government have seriously undermined the confidence of the Tamil people and the LTTE leadership in the negotiating process. Under these circumstances the LTTE leadership has decided to suspend its participation in the negotiations for the time being. We will not be attending the donor conference in Japan in June. While we regret that we were compelled to make this painful decision, we wish to reiterate our commitment to seek a negotiated political solution to the ethnic question. We also urge the government of Sri Lanka to restore confidence in the peace process amongst the Tamil people by fully implementing, without further delay, the normalisation aspects of the Ceasefire Agreement and permit the immediate resettlement of the internally displaced people of the northeast. We also request the government to re-evaluate its economic development strategy to reconstruct the Tamil nation destroyed by war."

APPENDIX – IX
The Liberation Tigers of Tamil Eelam (LTTE)

From: *Patterns of Global Terrorism, 2003.* United States Department of State, 17 June 2004.

Other Known Front Organisations
World Tamil Association (WTA)
World Tamil Movement (WTM)
Federation of Associations of Canadian Tamils (FACT)
The Ellalan Force
The Sangillan Force

Description

Founded in 1976, the LTTE is the most powerful Tamil group in Sri Lanka and uses overt and illegal method to raise funds, acquire weapons, and publicise its cause of establishing an independent Tamil state. The LTTE began its armed conflict with the Sri Lankan government in 1983 and has relied on a guerrilla strategy that includes the use of terrorist tactics. The LTTE is currently observing a cease-fire agreement with the Sri Lankan government. First designated in October 1997.

Activities

The Tigers have integrated a battlefield insurgent strategy with a terrorist programme that targets not only key personnel in the countryside but also senior Sri Lankan political and military leaders in Colombo and other urban centers. The Tigers are most notorious for their cadre of suicide bombers, the Black Tigers. Political assassinations and bombings are commonplace.

Strength

Exact strength is unknown, but the LTTE is estimated to have 8,000 to 10,0000 armed combatants in Sri Lanka, with a core of trained fighters of approximately 3,000 to 6,000. The LTTE also has a significant overseas support structure for fundraising, weapons procurement, and propaganda activities.

Location / Area of Operation

The Tigers control most of the northern and eastern coastal areas of Sri Lanka but have conducted operations throughout the island. Headquartered in northern Sri Lanka, LTTE leader Velupillai Prabhakaran has established an extensive network of checkpoints and informants to keep track of any outsiders who enter the group's area of control.

External Aid

The LTTE's overt organisations support Tamil separatism by lobbying foreign governments and the United Nations. The LTTE also uses its international contacts to procure weapons, communications, and any other equipment and supplies it needs. The LTTE exploits large Tamil communities in North America, Europe, and Asia to obtain funds and supplies for its fighters in Sri Lanka.

APPENDIX – X
Press Statement

Richard Boucher, Spokesman
Washington, DC
October 1, 2004

The Peace Process in Sri Lanka

The United State is committed to supporting the Peace Process launched after the 2002 ceasefire between the government of Sri Lanka and the Liberation Tigers of Tamil Elam or LTTE. Only a negotiated settlement according to the agreed terms of the Oslo Declaration can achieve an equitable and long-lasting resolution to the bloody conflict that has divided the nation for too long. The People of Sri Lanka deserve an opportunity to live in peace. Any settlement must preserve the territorial integrity, unity and national sovereignty of Sri Lanka.

Both sides have to take steps to ensure that all provisions of the Ceasefire Agreement are adhered to. We call upon the LTTE to end violence against political opponents and to cease the recruitment of child soldiers.

President Kumaratunga has shown flexibility in her proposals to renew discussions with the LTTE. Further delay in restarting negotiations can only damage the interests of all Sri Lankans who stand to gain from a return to real peace. We urge both parties to return to the negotiating table as soon as possible to bring peace to the island.

APPENDIX – XI
Let us put national interest before our own, for a lasting peace – President
October 4, 2004

The inaugural meeting of the National Advisory Council for Peace and Reconciliation (NACPR) was held today. The event at the 'well of the old Parliament complex' was attended by religious leaders, legislators from several political parties and leaders of civil society.

Full text of President Chandrika Bandaranaike Kumaratunga's address.

"On this important occasion, I would like to thank all of you present here for having accepted my invitation to participate in the National Advisory Council for Peace and Reconciliation (NACPR). We have here with us the Mahanayake Theros, as well as religious leaders from all the religious communities and leaders of important political parties represented in Parliament. We also have present here the leaders and representatives of major non-governmental organisations that have played a role in bringing an end to the armed conflict and building peace in Sri Lanka. I wish to welcome you all and express my gratitude and that of my government for the willingness you have demonstrated to contribute to this great enterprise of collectively seeking solutions as a nation to the most serious challenge posed to our motherland in its post independent history.

The setting up of the NACPR is yet another step along the path of my policy and that of my government for peace.

Our policy for the resolution of the conflict has been made clear and stated often. It has remained consistent and unwavering.

We continue to hold the view that the resolution of the problem lies mainly in negotiations between the government in negotiations between the government and the main protagonist, the LTTE. To this end my governments, for the past ten years; have engaged with the LTTE on four occasions (including the present one) in an attempt to arrive at a negotiated settlement that would be durable and acceptable to the majority of our peoples. In this context we are presently seeking through intense dialogue, to recommence the stalled negotiation process with the LTTE.

Appendix – XI

I wish to state firmly and clearly that the government is committed to do all that is required to persuade the LTTE to return to the negotiating table. But of course, whatever we undertake as a government, will be implemented within the framework of a united Sri Lanka, guaranteeing the sovereignty of the state and the security of the nation and its peoples.

My government also has a stated policy of conducting an open and inclusive process, in its endeavours towards peace. We believe that no lasting peace could be achieved without the involvement of all major players in this country. By this I mean, the people and their elected representatives as well as the religious and civil society leaders and others.

In the course of processes undertaken by my governments for the resolution of the conflict, we have at most times, kept the country informed and obtained their participation in various ways, such as through the "Sudu Nelum" movement, as well as through public briefings by the government. We have now arrived at the conclusion that a more structured forum for a wider and consistent consultation with the people is required.

You are aware of complaints made by leaders of some communities, such as some of the opposition parties, the Muslims and also religious leaders that they have not been consulted sufficiently, during various peace processes undertaken by some governments.

We have taken all these factors into consideration when we formulated the concept of National Advisory Council, to undertake this much-required national consultative process.

We have envisaged the NACPR on the following terms:-

- Firstly, as a national forum for consultation on the peace process between the government and the citizenry, mainly through their elected representatives and also through their religious leaders, as well as leaders of civil society.
- This council will serve as a forum, where the government will keep the country informed of the progress of the negotiations process, as well as measures undertaken for ethnic reconciliation and for reconstruction and development of the North and East.

- It will also serve as a forum for its members to inform the government of their views and concerns, with regard to the peace process and also for them to suggest approaches to move the peace process forward. It will be a forum for everyone of the varied communities that constitute our nation, to have their voices heard on this most crucial issue.
- In addition, interested groups could be invited to express their views and concerns to this council.
- I also hope that this council would serve as a forum for dialogue and advice to the government on measures that need to be adopted for national reconciliation, unity and ethnic harmony.

It is great importance that I reiterate at this point, that the government continues to possess the courage and singularity of purpose in executing its duty and responsibility to resolve. We shall not waver in our commitment to seek solutions for a lasting peace. We remain honestly, totally and forever committed to peace. We are committed to the hilt to a non-violent, negotiated peace; we are committed to end the war and armed conflict.

I must underline that we do not intend to deflect our responsibilities, as a government, which we know has to be total, in resolving the problems faced by the Sri Lankan State, whoever may have caused these problems. Let it be known clearly that the National Advisory Council for peace and reconciliation is not designed and created for such petty and self-interested purposes.

My government shall continue to engage the LTTE, who we recognise as the primary actor, in the process of negotiating an end to the conflict and attaining peace.

My government's dialogue with the LTTE will be a separate and priority process.

But as a democratic, people's government, we are under obligation to keep ourselves properly briefed of the views and concerns of all our peoples. We are aware that many peace efforts have stumbled fee to the non-inclusion of the major players of our body politic in the process.

We believe that any peace process must be open, inclusive and obtain the participation of all the people at various levels. If everyone is not willing to participate, we must endeavour to obtain at least, the inclusion of the majority of our peoples. This is why we believe that a forum or institution such as the NACPR is essential for that part of the peace process which should include the participation of the country.

We see the two processes as moving parallel. The government will engage the LTTE and continue the dialogue with it, through the facilitators, while the government will separately consult with the country through the people's representatives, within the framework of the NACPR.

The first process is not dependent on the second; neither is the second on the first.

We, the government, have clearly stated views on the resolution of the present conflict. My government has repeatedly undertaken numerous programmes for the purpose of implementing these policies. We are not looking for ways to move away from our commitment, nor to shove off our responsibilities on the Advisory Council as a pretext to run away from the challenges of the sacred responsibility which my government undertook to shoulder for better or for worse, when we once again accepted the reigns of government in April this year.

Here I believe that it is important that I reiterate briefly my government's policy on the resolution of the Tamil people's problem.

My governments have attempted since 1994 to adopt a new strategy and radically different attitudes in the resolution of this problem. We studied and attempted to understand the root-causes of the conflict and the particular form it has taken in Sri Lanka, in a scientific and objective manner.

We arrived at the view that our conflict was engendered by the inability of our nation at the moment of decolonisation, 56 years ago, to weld together the separate sets of aspirations of the three main communities living in Sri Lanka, into one collective national vision, in which each community could live freely and in dignity within its own separate identity, in order to comprise one whole harmonious and united whole – a strong, stable and united state.

We recognised that we had to build a new, pluralist, multi-ethnic and multi-cultural state based on the cultural, religious and social identity of the majority Sinhala people who constitute around 75% of our population, as much as the two main smaller communities, the Tamils and the Muslims and the tiny groups of Malays and Burghers, who constitute the rest of the country.

We believe that the solution lies in seeking alternatives to the concept of a monolithic, unitary State – to blend power with principle, to reconcile authority with freedom. We are looking at a form of power sharing with a high level of democratic participation in decision making, law making and governance by the regional authorities or the devolved units.

We do not believe that the dismemberment of the Sri Lankan State, demanded by the LTTE through the employment of terrorist means, would in anyway be a solution to the Tamil people's problems.

We are seeking a compromise that would satisfy the aspirations of all the communities of peoples living within our State – a compromise that would be democratic and pluralistic.

We believe that the State must resolve the contradictions that have arisen between the State and the nationalist consciousness of the Tamil community. We have to find means and procedures to accord expression of this consciousness and to give constitutional, legal and political authority.

I quote here from a recent speech I made in New York at the Asia Society; "We have and we shall – do all that is required of a democratic and responsible government, to ensure that we do not return to armed conflict.

But here I must reiterate – we believe that 'Peace is more than the simple absence of war'. It entails active engagement to identify and rectify the root-causes of conflict".

On the one hand, we have to address the problems of socio-economic of all disadvantaged groups in the South as well as the North and East, marginalisation through an effective programme for poverty alleviation and development. On the other, we have to formulate, in discussion with the adversaries on one hand and the representatives of our polity, new structures and systems to satisfactorily meet the shortcomings and problems faced by the Tamil community, whilst safeguarding the rights and interests of all other communities.

Whilst we believe that peace has to be negotiated, we do not believe in "Peace at any cost". We believe that the sovereignty, the territorial integrity and security of the State must be safeguarded. We believe in a just peace, which means not only the just rights of one community or one group within that community, but the just rights of all Tamil people, as much as all rights of all Tamil people, as much as all other citizens. We believe in a democratic and pluralist polity that rests on the bedrock of the rule of law and the guarantee of human rights in every corner of the country. We believe in a just peace with democracy.

In our search for peace and a lasting resolution of the conflict, we have chosen the path of a negotiated settlement because we believe that even the most unreasonable terrorist group may be persuaded without the use of coercion or arms.

My friends, we believe in life, because we believe in humanity. We believe that even the most ruthless terrorist group must sometime reassume their humanity. We abhor terror and all forms of violence in the pursuit of political aims. We condemn the continuous killings and violence practised against their opponents by the LTTE.

We do not believe that any problem could be resolved through the destruction of life, the protection of which in the last count is the only moral justification for the existence of all human institutions, including the State.

We remain firmly committed to our concept of resolving conflict; based on the assertion that most socio-political conflicts (whether they be expressed in ethnic, religious or other forms) have their origins in some form of injustice and unequal treatment. In the Sri Lankan case, my government was the first to publicly accept that the Tamil people have undergone discriminatory and unjust treatment by consecutive governments, although we do not accept and cannot in anyway condone, the extreme responses of one group claiming to represent the Tamil people. If the government is to turn them away from this extremism, we believe that we must begin with finding solutions to the main causes that generated the conflict.

My government is making every attempt to persuade the LTTE to return to the negotiating table from which it withdrew 18 months ago. The LTTE insists that the government should agree to discuss at first only their ISGA proposals. The government's position has been that we accept the concept of setting up an interim administration in the interim period, whilst a permanent solution is negotiated and implemented. But, we require a commitment from the LTTE that the Interim Administration as well as the final solution would be based on the Oslo Declaration signed by the government of Sri Lanka and the LTTE which declared that the Federal solution should be sought within the framework of a united Sri Lanka. The negotiations with the LTTE as well as the consultation within the NACPR could work out the level and extent of devolution and other details regarding this.

Let it be known clearly and without any doubt that the government will continue to do all that is required of it to make peace a reality. Through the consultations which we will engage in at the NACPR we are making an attempt to include, if not all, at least the majority of our nation in this great national endeavour.

We are all aware that the majority of our peoples expect the political parties to work together on this issue. They wish us to arrive at a consensus in dealing with peace negotiations and in reaching a lasting solution to the problem. I am aware that this view is held by a large majority of people irrespective of their political affiliations, which is also a strongly held view of all religious leaders. The International community has also consistently expressed this view.

The experience of other countries demonstrates that conflicts of this nature have been successfully resolved only when it has been approached as a national issue, which cuts across the limiting boundaries of party politics. The South African case is the best example of this. Also in the UK the main political parties have agreed to a common approach when dealing with the northern Ireland problem.

Since 1994, for ten years, I have made numerous attempts at bringing together the two major political parties, the UNP and the Peoples Alliance (PA). Various proposals for arriving at a consensus and for working together were suggested to the UNP, having overcome many obstacles to obtain the agreement of my party and our partners in government. Everyone of my attempts have been rejected or agreed to and then promises broken. The UNP and the Tamil National

Alliance (TNA) have declined to participate in this initiative whilst, the Sri Lanka Muslim Congress (SLMC) and the Jathika Hela Urumaya (JHU) have requested some clarifications.

The leader of the UNP has informed me that he is of the view that consultation could take place after the government begins talks with the LTTE. The process we begin today is a separate exercise as I have stated earlier, which is designed for all of us here to engage in a free dialogue expressing specific views held by each group represented here, in order that the government be directly and clearly informed of your views. This would serve as an essential and most important input into the planning of the negotiations process and the policies and strategies adopted by the government. We, therefore, need your views not only once talks begin but even before talks can get started.

We are all aware that the LTTE too, has held a similar view for a long time. The LTTE leader Mr Velupillai Prabhakaran has stated on numerous occasions that without the two major political forces of the south, arriving at a consensus on the resolution of the conflict, no effective solution could be implemented to the Tamil people's problem. I quote from his most recent statement in this regard in his speech in 26th November last year.

> "Whenever the party in power attempts to resolve the Tamil issue, the party in opposition opposes it and derails the effort. This mode of conflict continues even when the opposition becomes the ruling party and attempts reconciliation. This Sinhala political drama with its typical historical pattern has been staged regularly for the last fifty years."

> "As a negative consequence of this chess game, in which the Tamils are used as pawns, several peace efforts have failed; several peace negotiations collapsed, several peace agreements torn apart and several peace pacts became defuct. As such, the Tamil conflict continues without resolution. The tragic life of our people continues."

I would, therefore, like to urge the leader of the UNP as well as its members to reconsider their decision and to participate in this great national endeavour we commence today of arriving at a national consensus on the country's one single most important problem.

"Finally, I would like to state in all sincerity that I truly believe that we are today engaged in a bold initiative that could lead to the much desired collective consensus of our nation, hoped for by all our peoples. This should have occurred a long time ago, but even now let us attempt to put national interest before our own and dialogue honestly based on what is realistically possible and arrive at the essential elements to attain a lasting and durable peace.

I have just been informed that the government of USA has issued a statement two days ago endorsing our views with regard to the Oslo Declaration and calling upon the LTTE to end violence against political opponents and to cease the recruitment of child soldiers. The US government has also commended me for the flexibility shown by the government in our efforts to arrive at an agreement with the LTTE to renew discussions.

What I am asking of ourselves may be a tall order. The stars are far away. Yet, I continue to hope and believe in this, our nation's ability and strength to reach for those stars if we work together honestly.

Glossary

CBK	Chandrika Bandaranaike Kumaratunga
CFA	Ceasefire Agreement
EPDP	Eelam People's Democratic Party
GOSL	Government of Sri Lanka
GOVT.	Government
HSZ	High Security Zones
IA	Interim Administration
LTTE	Liberation Tigers of Tamil Eelam
PA	Peoples' Alliance
PM	Prime Minister
SLMM	Sri Lanka Monitoring Mission
SOMA	Status of Mission Agreement
SLA	Sri Lanka Army
SLN	Sri Lanka Navy
SIHRN	Sub-committee on Immediate Humanitarian and Rehabilitation Needs in the North and East
SDN	Sub-committee on De-escalation and Normalisation
SPM	Sub-committee on Political Matters
TNA	Tamil National Alliance
UNF	United National Front
US	United States
UTHR-J	University Teachers for Human Rights, Jaffna
VoT	Voice of Tigers

Index

Adams, Brad, 43-44
Adams Bridge, 110
Afghanistan, 42
Africa
   African-American civil rights movement, 155
   African-American population in Sri lanka, 92
Agampodai Hill, 188
Ahtissari, Martti, 194
Al-Fatah – Revolutiuonary Council, 73
Al-Qaeda, 23, 29
Alahathurai, P, 53
Algeria, 74
Aljazeera. net, 55, 56
All Ceylon Tamil Congress, 60
Alliance of Expatriate Organisations for Peace, 108
Amirthakali, 188
Amman, Pottu ('Beria' of LTTE), 40
Amnesty International (AI), 62, 63, 207, 208
Ampara, 40, 48, 64, 79, 204
Appapillai Amrithalingam, 181
Annan, Kofi, 214
Anti-LTTE Tamil Broadcasting Corporation, London-based, 64
Armitage, Richard L, 88

Asia, 21, 74
   East, 70
   South, 21, 75, 108, 190
   Southeast, 75
   West, 78
Asian Development Bank, 22, 208
Athulathmudali, Lalith, 79
Australia, 70, 71, 188, 214

Baddewela, Mahinda, 156
Balachanddran, P K, 110, 111
Balakumar, 76
Balasingham, Anton, 40, 101, 167, 168, 215-16
Bandaranaike, Sirimavo, 141, 159, 173, 175, 176, 179, 182, 183
Bandaranaike-Chelvanayakam Pact (29 July 1957), 182
Bandaranaike, Solomon West Ridgeway Dias (Bandaranaike, SWR), 174, 176, 178, 183
Bandaranaikes, 159, 176
Bangladesh, 147
Basque Liberation Movement ETA, 73
Batticaloa, 11, 21, 40, 41, 44, 47, 52, 53, 54, 55, 64, 76, 188, 204
   Batticaloa-Ampara region, 39, 48
Bhanu, 63

Bindunuwewa Rehabilitation Centre, Bandarawela, Tamil youths done to death at, 139-41
Bismark, Otto von, 127
Black, J Cofer, 22-26, 28, 88, 89
Brattskar, Hans, 48
Buddha, Lord, 149
Buddhism, 174, 175, 180 (*see also* Sinhalese)
Buddhists, 3, 5, 26, 30, 33, 79, 149, 173, 174, 175, 180, 182, 192, 197, 199, 203
Bundunuwewa incidents, 150
Burghers, 28, 87
Burma, 42, 74
Burundi, 42
Bush administration, 88

CMI, 194
Cambodia, 74
Cameron, David, 124
Canada, 71
Cass, Frank, 155
Ceasefire Agreement (CFA) between Sri Lankan State and LTTE, 2, 5, 8, 9, 15, 20, 52, 71, 85-88, 167, 190, 202, 203, 204, 215, 216
Centre for Alternative Policy, 55
Colombo, 121, 124
Ceylon Petroleum Corporation (CPC), 111, 112
Ceylon Workers' Congress, 172
Chamberlain, Houston, 177
Charles Anthony brigade, 63
Chavakachcheri AGA division, 81
Chechen rebels, 29
Chelvanayakam, SJV, 126, 177, 180, 181
Chennai (earlier Madras) Port, 133

Chilaw, 146
Children
 child abductions, 42-45
 child labour, 45
 child soldiers, 44, 45
 UN Children's Fund, 43, 208
 UNICEF, 43, 44, 45
China, 209, 214
 fishermen of, 108
Christians, 175, 207
Citizens
 Citizens Movement for Good Governance (CIMOGG) Colombo, 144-47, 150
 Citizenship Act of December 1948, 176-77
 Citizenship laws, 181
 Civil Society Forum, Colombo-based, 121-22
Claridge, David, 74
Coastline, 131
Cold War, scenario
 Anglo-American block in emerging, 174
Colombia, 42
Colombo's Youth Council Centre, 32
Commonwealth, 147, 174
 Commonwealth Heads of government, Cyprus meeting of, 82
Congo, Democratic Republic of, 42, 74
Cyprus, 82
 meeting of Commonwealth Heads of government at, 82

de Silva, Colvin R, 180
de Silva, H L, 125, 126, 129
de Silva, K M, 74, 173, 174, 175, 176

Devananda, Douglas, 6, 29, 50, 54, 55, 57, 58-59, 61, 213
Dhanapala, Jayantha, 3, 6, 7, 48, 60, 103, 120, 192, 212
Dhileepan, Amirthalingamhunger strike near Kandaswamy temple at Nallur, 76-77
Dixit, JN, 79, 105, 108

EROS Bala (Balanandarajah Iyer), 11
ETA, 93
Easwaran, 54
Edirisinha, Rohan, 125
Eelam (Tamil homeland), 217
Eelam People's Democratic Party(EPDP), 6, 10, 11, 29, 52, 57, 58-59, 65, 66, 73, 90, 126, 164
Eelam People's Revolutionary Liberation Front (EPRLF), 52, 53, 54, 65, 66, 84, 121
EPRLF-led NEPG (Northeast Provincial Government), 84-85
Eelam Revolutionary Organisation of Students, 76
Elections, 119, 179, 183
Parliamentary Elections Amendment Act of 1949, 176-77
Elilan, S, 137
Ethnic issue (problem), 127, 129
Ethnic communities, 136
Ethnic Tamils, 84
Ethnic war, 2, 3
Presidential Truth Commission on Ethnic Violence (1981-84), 137
Europe, 71, 175, 181, 195, 217
European Union (EU), 10, 11, 12, 22, 26, 114, 147, 214

Fanaticism, 71
Federal Party, 126, 180, 181
Federalism (federal system), 125, 127, 143, 151, 154, 161, 183, 184, 210
concept of, 121, 124
Forum of Federation (Canada based international network on federalism), 124
Fernando, Chandra, 212
Foreign Correspondent's Club, 3, 58, 59

Galle, 110
Galle Face Green, 133, 180, 181
Gandhi, Mohandas Karamchand (Mahatma Gandhi), 77, 92-93, 100, 111
non-violence of, 92-93
satyagrahis, advice to, 93
Gandhi, Rajiv, 13, 79
assassination of, 100, 104, 132, 215
Geneva, 62, 63
Germany, 73, 127
Godage, Kalyananda, 113-14
Goonawardene, Leslie, 180
Goonetilleke, Bernard A B, 215
Gross, Feliks, 91
Gulf of Mannar, 110
Gunaratna, Rohan, 79
Guerrillas, 156
degenerate guerrillas, 73

Hakeen, Rauff, 105, 106, 197
Hambantota, 110
Handagama, Ashoka, 152
Harrold, Peter, 208
Helgesen, Vidar, 1, 8-10, 18, 63, 197, 201, 215, 216

Index

Helsinki, 194
Herath, Vijitha, 30-31, 32
High Security Zones (HSZs), 6, 203
Hindus, 136
Hilter, Adolph, 177
Horgan, John, 74, 75, 155
Howen, Nicholas, 63
Human rights, 44, 80, 141
   Human Rights Commission of Sri Lanka, 139, 141
   Human Rights Watch (HRW), 43, 44, 52, 53, 54, 62, 63
   National Human Rights Commission (NHRC), 207

IRA, 195
India, 147, 181, 214
India-USSR Peace, Friendship and Cooperation Treaty of 1971, 113
Indian Intervention (1987), 78-79
Indian Oil Corporation, 109
Indian Peace Keeping Force (IPKF), 76, 77, 133, 134
Indian Tamil question (1949), 177
Indo-Sri Lanka Agreement of 1987 (Indo-Sri Lanka Accord), 13, 15, 103, 108, 127
Indo-Sri Lanka defence agreement, 115-16
Indo-Sri Lankan relations, 13, 15, 100-29, 133-35
   comprehensive treaty of peace, friendship and cooperation, proposals for, 113-14
   policy of strict neutrality, 104
   Tamil Nadu fishermen's intrusion in Sri Lankan water, 116-17
Indian Ocean island, 1, 3
Indonesia, 21, 74, 192-95
   Aceh, 193-95

Acehnese deaths due to tsunami, 195
Free Aceh Movement (GAM), 193, 194
Krueng Raya, 195
rebels, 193
tsunami devastation in, 192-95
Information
   high-technology information system, 109
Interim Self Governing Authority (ISGA), 3, 4, 5, 6, 7, 10, 13,19, 25, 26, 27, 30, 31, 32, 33, 42, 58, 86, 89, 90, 91, 105, 114, 115, 117, 118, 119, 121, 122, 123, 124, 125, 127, 131, 132, 143, 145, 155, 169, 170, 171, 172, 184, 198, 201
Internally displaced persons (IDPs), 5, 6
International Commission of Jurists (ICS), 62, 63
Interpol, 217
Iran, 29
Iraq, 29
Irish Republican Army, 73
Island newspaper, 54
Israel, 31
   Israeli-Palestinian conflict, 108
   Iyer, Balanadarajah (*see* EROS Bala)

Jaffna Peninsula, 41, 51, 52, 54, 62, 75, 76, 77, 79, 80, 81, 123, 160, 182, 183, 187, 204, 214, 218
"Offensive in Jaffna leaves many homeless", 81
Janatha Hela Urumayu (JHU), 3, 30, 106

Janatha Vimukthi Paramuna (JVP), 3, 19, 30, 31, 32, 33, 34, 95, 106, 107, 145, 149, 171, 172, 184, 186, 190, 191, 192, 195, 198, 199, 200, 203, 209
  rebellions, 145
  uprisings, 149
Japan, 22, 147, 214
Jakarta, 193, 194
Jayatilleka, Dayan, 126, 127, 129
Jayewardene, Junius Richard, 13, 15, 78, 79, 83, 139, 141, 169, 182
Jennings, Ivor, 173
Jeyanathan Regiment (brigade), 11, 63, 64
Jeyarani, Thiagaraja (Sathya Leeda), 54-55
Jongman, A J, 72

Kadirgamar, Lakshman, 104-05, 107, 162, 189, 190, 212, 213, 214, 215, 216
  assassination of, 212, 213, 215, 216
Kallady, 188
Kandy, 182-196
Kandyan aristocracy, 159
Kankasenthurai, 181, 204
Kannapattai, 53
Kantha, K D Lal, 31
Karadiyanaru, 63
Karuna, V Muralitharan (Karuna Amman)
  defection of 1, 2, 3, 6, 11, 12, 21, 38-66, 83, 158, 200, 208, 218
  Karuna group, 155-56
  LTTE – Karuna tussle, 48
Katcheri, 80

Katkovalam, 188
Kausalyan, 48
Kenya, 74
Ketheeswaran, Loganathan, 121
Killings, 52, 78, 79, 162
Killinochchi, 47, 49, 86, 104, 167, 187, 201, 204
Kittu, 133
Koizumi, Junichiro, 214
Kollupitiya, 54
Kosovo Liberation Army, 73
Kotelawala, John, 159, 174, 178, 179
Kudathanai, 189
Kulatunge, B, 156
Kumara, Sarath, 138
Kumaratunga, Chandrika, 3, 9, 12, 16-18, 20, 27, 28, 30, 34, 48, 58, 59, 83, 84, 87, 90, 95, 103, 107, 122, 123, 128, 131, 135-36, 137, 138, 141, 159, 160, 161, 162, 163, 164, 166, 167, 168, 169-70, 171, 172, 178, 184, 190, 191, 197, 198-99, 200, 203, 206, 208, 212, 214, 216, 218
Kurdistan Workers' Party, 73

LTTE (Liberation Tigers of Tamil Eelam) 1, 2, 3, 4, 6, 7, 8, 9, 10, 11, 12, 13, 17, 18, 19, 20, 21, 22, 23, 24, 25, 26, 27, 28, 29, 30, 31, 32, 33, 34, 38, 39, 40, 41, 42, 43, 44, 45, 46, 47, 48, 49, 50, 51, 52, 53, 54, 55, 56, 57, 58, 59, 60, 61, 62, 63, 64, 65, 66, 71, 72, 73, 74, 75, 76, 77, 78, 79, 80, 81, 82, 83, 84, 85, 86, 87, 88, 89, 90, 91, 94, 101, 102, 103, 104, 105, 106, 107, 114, 115, 116, 117, 118,

119, 120, 121, 122, 123, 124, 125, 126, 127, 128, 129, 131, 132, 133, 134, 137, 139, 140, 141, 142, 143, 145, 146, 147, 150, 152, 153, 155, 156, 158, 160, 161, 162, 163, 164, 165, 166, 167, 168, 169, 170, 171, 172, 173, 184, 185, 186, 187, 188, 189, 190, 191, 192, 196, 197, 198, 200, 201, 202, 203, 204, 206, 207, 208, 210, 212, 213, 214, 215, 216, 217, 218
F M radio, 107
LTTE-Karuna tussle, 48
special forces of, 11
split in military machine of, 1
voice of Tiger, 107
LSSP, 179-80, 183
Lanka Indian Oil Company (LIOC), 109, 111, 112
Lanka Sama Samaj Party, 177
Leach, James A, 70-71
Liberation movements, 70-95 (*passim*)
distinguished from pure terrorism, 72-73
Liberation Tigers, newspaper, 18
Liberia, 42
Long Range Reconnaissance Patrols (LRRPs) Sri Lankan's army's, 22, 46

MILF, 195
Madras (renamed Chennai) Port, 133
Malays, 28, 87
Mandur, 53
Manikawasagar, K, 80
Manikkalingam, Ram, 157
Marine and off-shore resources, 118, 131

Marxists
JVP (Marxist organisation)
Marxist allies, 186
Marxist left, 176
Marxists, 175, 176
Mendis, G C, 148-49
Mile Post (Kuchchaveli Road), 188
Millennium Account facility, 22
Moulana, 59
Mount Lavinia, 53
Mullaitivu, 39, 78, 187, 204, 217
Muslims, 21, 28, 31, 87, 90, 91, 106, 114, 125, 136, 150, 152, 160, 188, 191, 196- 97, 202, 203, 207, 218
Eastern Muslim Council, 197
Sri Lanka Muslim Congress (SLMC), 105, 196-97
Muttur, 126

NEPG (Northeast Provincial Government), 84-85
NGOs, 199, 200
Nagaventhurai
battle at, 80
Nallur, 54, 77
Kandaswamy Temple, 77
Narayan Swamy, M R, 84
Narcotics smuggling, 71
Natalagawa, Marty, 194
National Advisory Council for Peace and Reconciliation, 27, 128, 169
National Bhikku Front, 203
National Police Commission, 207
National Water Supply and Drainage Board, 109
Nationalism, 157, 173, 175, 183
Natwar Singh, K, 105
Navalady, 188
Navy (naval force), 115-17, 188

Nesiah, Devanesan, 119
New Zealand, 188
Niththy, 11
Norway
  Norwegian mediation in Sri Lanka Peace process, 1, 9, 14, 15, 17, 25, 48, 54, 63, 102-03, 106-08, 145, 147, 167, 190, 197, 201-02, 216

Oddusuddan, 40
Omadiyamadu, 11
Omanthai, 40
Operation Liberation (1987), 79
Operation Yal Devi, offensive code-named, 81
Oslo Declaration (2-5 December 2002), 121, 126, 164, 216

PKK, 73
Pacific, 70
Pakistan, 147
Palihakkara, H M G S, 215
Palk Strait, 110
Palestine
  Democratic Front for the Liberation of Palestine, 73
  Palestine Liberation Organisation, 72-73
  Popular Front for the Liberation of Palestine, 73
Pallai assistant government agent (AGA), 81
Panchchankerni, 64
Paramathan, Mylvaganam, 53
Pararajahsingham, Joseph, 45, 57, 59, 122
Patten, Chris, 12
Peace negotiations (talks) (process), 1-2, 3, 4, 7, 8, 13, 14, 17, 18, 19, 20, 49, 63, 65, 85, 88, 92, 105, 106, 126, 163, 167, 190, 191, 197, 201-02, 214, 215, 216
  Alliance of Expatriate Organisations for Peace, 108
  Norwegian mediation in (*see also* Norway)
Peiris, G L, 101, 165, 171, 172
Peiris, Harim, 56, 162, 163, 164
People's Alliance (PA), 15, 17, 91, 161, 166, 170
  United National Front-People's Alliance, 91
People's Liberation Organisation of Tamil Eelam (PLOTE), 52
  PLOTE Mohan (Kandiah Yogarasa), 45, 46, 53
People's Liberation Organisation of Tamil Nadu, 45
People's movement, 70-95 (*passim*)
Perera, Amantha, 65
Perera, N M, 177
Petersen, Jan, 214
Philippines, 21, 195
Point Pedro, 188, 189
Pol Pot's Khmer Rouge of 1970s, 75
Polannaruwa-Batticaloa, 11
Ponnambalam, Gajen, 60-61
Pooneryn, battle at, 80
Porativu local council, 53
Prabhakaran, Velupillai, 3, 12, 39, 41, 46-47, 49, 52, 56, 58, 60, 82, 102, 104, 108, 165, 167, 216, 217
  annual 'Heroes Day' radio address (26 November 2001), 70-72
Prakash, Arun, 115-17
Premadasa, Ranasinghe, 76, 83, 133, 215
Puthukudiyiruppu, 39

Index

Racialism, 177
Radicalism, 181
Rae, Bob, 124, 126-27
Ragupathy, Kadiragamanathan, 53, 54
Rajapakse, Mahinda, 128
Rajasingham, KT, 107
Ramesh, 48, 63
Ramiah Rajendran (Rajan), 53
Reggie (Sivasundari, Vinayagamoorthi), 63, 64, 65
Rice, Condoleezza, 214
Richardson, Louise, 75-76
Riots
   anti-Tamil, 163, 180, 182
   Riot Act, 27
Rocca, Christina B, 190
Rupasinghe, Kumar, 26-27, 121-22
Russia, 103

Sahara, Western, 74
Samaraweera, Mangala, 4, 9, 108, 109-10
Sampanthan, R, 24, 25, 89
Sandagiri, Daya, 115, 117
Saravanamuttu, Paikiasothy, 55, 84
Sathya Leela (Thiagaraja Jeyarani), 54-55
Scandinavian countries, 71
Schmid, A P, 72
Sea Tigers, 116, 118, 132, 133, 189
Secessionism, 126, 127
Senadhirajah, 48
Senanayake, D S, 159, 173, 174, 176, 177, 183
Senanayake, Dudley, 174
Senanayakes, 159
Seneviratne, Sudharshan, 148-49
Separatism, 71
   groups, 74-75
   movements, 74

Sethusamundram navigational channel dredging project (Sethusamudran Ship Canal project), 109-10, 111, 117
Sharvananda, S, 137
Silva, Tilvin, 192
Sinha, Yashwant, 104
Sinhala language, 178-80, 181
Sinhala Only Act, 179
Sinhala Only Bill, 180
Sinhalese, 4, 6, 13, 14, 17, 26, 28, 30, 33, 79, 83, 85, 86, 90, 91, 108, 114, 117, 118, 119, 120, 121, 122, 123, 125, 126, 127, 128, 129, 131, 136, 138, 141, 142, 143, 145, 146, 147, 148, 149, 150, 151, 152, 155, 156, 157, 159, 160, 161, 166, 168, 169, 173, 174, 175, 177, 179, 180, 181, 182, 183, 186, 191, 192, 197, 198, 199, 203
   cinema of (film makers), 152
Sinhalese-Buddhist chauvinism, 33, 34, 173, 174, 180, 181-82, 183, 198, 206
Sinhalese-Buddhist communalism, 181
Sinhalese-Tamil conflict, 148
Sinhalese-Tamil relations, 156
Sivakumar, Mylvaganam, 53-54
Social scientists groups, 151
Solheim, Eric, 103
Somalia, 42
South Africa, 74
Spain, 195
Special Task Force, 52
Splinter, Peter, 63
Sri Lanka Development Forum, 196
Sri Lanka Directorate of Military Intelligence, 53

Sri Lanka Freedom Party (SLFP), 4, 33, 34, 83, 118, 119, 120, 138, 142, 159, 160, 161, 166, 167, 173, 176, 178, 179, 184, 199
Sri Lanka Inter Netball Association, 156
Sri Lanka Monitoring Mission (SLMM), 2, 8, 43, 50, 51, 57, 108, 167, 216
SLMM Trond Furuhovde, 8
Sri Lankan Muslim Congress (SLMC), 91, 105, 106
Sunday Leader, 65
Subathiran, Thambirajah (Robert), 54
Suntheralingam, C, 126
Sutarto, Endriartono, 194
Switzerland, 71, 145
Syria, 29

TELO (Varathan), 52
TNAMP, 143
Taleban, 29
Tamil Congress, 177
Tamil Eelam (Tamil homeland), 33, 76, 191
Tamil Eelam Liberation Organisation, 52
Tamil Eelam People's Liberation, 47
Tamil guerrilles, 131
Tamil language, 181
Tamil militant or terrorist groups, 28-29
Tamil National Alliance (TNA), 24, 29, 45, 47, 57-58, 60, 83, 88-89, 102, 122, 198, 217
Tamilnet website, 156
Tamil rebels, 2, 3, 4, 80, 81
Tamil Rehabilitation Organisation (TRO), 200
Tamil United Liberation Front (TULF), 84, 146
Tamils (Tamil communities) (Sri Lankan Tamils), 16, 17, 24, 28, 29, 30, 31, 50, 57, 58, 59, 71, 74, 75, 78, 82, 83, 84, 86, 87, 88, 89, 90, 91, 92, 114, 119, 120, 121, 123, 125, 126, 128, 129, 133, 136, 138, 139, 142, 146, 147, 148, 149, 150, 151, 152, 156, 157, 158, 160, 165, 175, 176, 177, 179, 180, 181, 182, 183, 186, 187, 188, 191, 192, 197, 217
  migrants living in Germany, 73
  Sinhalese-Tamil relations, 148, 156
Taraki, 26
Taylor, Max, 74, 75, 155
Terrorism 29, 59, 70, 71, 72, 145, 155
  counter-terrorism, 22
  definition(s) of, 72, 75-76
  foreign terrorist groups, 26
  foreign terrorist organisations, 88, 190
  future of, 74, 75
  global war on, 21, 72
  liberation movements distinguished from, 72-73
  legal definition, 72
  Prevention of Terrorism Act, 140
  social science definition, 72, 74
Tamil militants or terrorist group, 28-29
  terrorist acts, 73
  terrorist-liberation groups, 72-73
  terrorist movements, 74
  terrorist organisation, 72
  terrorist violence and political,

Index

distinction between, 75
terrorists, 104, 129, 195
terrorists and freedom fighters, distinction between, 71
'Terrorists as Transnational Actors"75
to fight terrorism, 23
U S global alliance against, 71
Thailand, 108, 164
Thalayasingam, Lakshman, 213
Thamilchelvan, SP, 4, 5, 10, 11, 47, 49, 51, 62, 65, 66, 86, 124, 187, 201, 212, 214
satire, 122
Thapa, Tej, 44
Thoppigala, 46
Tiger Organisation Security Intelligence Service (TOSIS), 39, 40
Tigerism, 157
Tirukkovil, 181
Tokyo Declaration, 172
Trincomalee, 52, 116, 181, 183, 188, 203-04
Trincomalee harbour, 117
Trincomalee Bay, 51
Tsunami, 186-209 (*passim*)
affected areas, 187
devastation on 26 December 2004 and after, 187, 195
Post-Tsunami Operation Management Structure (P-TOMS) (Tsunami Relief Council), 186, 192, 197, 198, 200, 201, 202, 203, 204, 205, 206, 209
relief distribution, 189-190
Tsunami Relief Council, 192
Tsunami-wrecked parts of Sri Lanka, 186

UK (United Kingdom) (Britain), 70, 71, 91, 133, 174, 195, 214
UN (United Nations), 94, 141, 194, 195, 214
Convention on Law of Sea, 110
Security Council, 42-43
UN Children's Fund, 43, 208
UNICEF, 43, 44, 45
UNF (United National Front), 14-15, 33-34, 59, 142, 168, 170
UNP (United National Party), 13, 27, 32, 59, 83, 138, 139, 142, 159, 160, 161, 163, 166, 167, 169-70, 171, 172, 176, 177, 178, 179, 182, 184, 185, 195, 198, 206
UPFA (United People's Freedom Alliance), 15-16, 32, 91, 95, 118, 123, 171, 172, 187,200
US (America) (Americans), 22, 23, 25, 26, 27, 31, 61, 70, 71, 73, 88, 91, 92, 103, 114, 128, 147, 164, 168, 190, 214, 215, 216
American population in Sri Lanka, 92
USSR, 127
India-USSR Peace Friendship and Cooperation Treaty of 1971, 113
Uganda, Northern, 42
Unceasing Waves, 40
Union of Regions, 30
Uyangoda, Jayadeva, 13, 14, 15, 17, 120, 123, 142, 143, 155, 169

Vadamaratchchi, 77, 79, 189
Vaddukoddai Resolution of 1976, 126, 146
Vaharai, 44
Vajpayee, Atal Behari, 104

Vakarai, 11
Varathan faction, 53
Varnakulasingam, Somasunderam, 73
Vavuniya, 42, 156, 167
Vembadi Girls College, 7, 54
Vicky, 11
Veitnam, 74
Vigneswaram, K, 126
Voice of Tiger, 107

Wadduwa, 124
Walawe, 146
Wanni,, 39, 41, 57, 64, 156
Weerakoon, Bradman, 159
Weerawanse, Wimal, 32-33, 199

Westborg, Jon, 107-08
Wickremanayake, Ratnasiri, 108-09
Wickremasinghe, Ranil, 14, 15, 32, 34, 52, 59, 91, 101, 103, 107, 118, 122, 123, 128, 137, 142, 159, 160, 161-62, 165, 166, 167, 168, 169, 170-71, 172, 184, 185, 198
  googly of, 171
Wijeratne, Ranjan, 134
Wilkinson, Paul, 92-94, 155
World Bank, 208
World War second, 91
Yugoslavia, 127

Zimbabwe, 74